ELECTRONICS AND INSTRUMENTATION
FOR THE CLINICAL LABORATORY

ELECTRONICS AND INSTRUMENTATION FOR THE CLINICAL LABORATORY

Arthur A. Eggert, Ph.D.

Associate Professor of Pathology and Laboratory Medicine
University of Wisconsin Hospital
Madison, Wisconsin

A WILEY MEDICAL PUBLICATION
JOHN WILEY & SONS
New York · Chichester · Brisbane · Toronto · Singapore

Cover and interior design: Wanda Lubelska
Production Supervisor: Audrey Pavey

Chapter 11 was prepared based on material provided by Bausch & Lomb Instruments and Systems Division, which also provided technical assistance in the preparation of Section 13-1. Some figures in Chapter 11 and Section 13-1 were redrawn with permission of Bausch & Lomb.

Library of Congress Cataloging in Publication Data:

Eggert, Arthur A.
  Electronics and instrumentation for the clinical laboratory.

  Bibliography: p. 421
  Includes index.
  1. Medical laboratories—Equipment and supplies.
2. Medical electronics. I. Title. [DNLM: 1. Computers.
2. Diagnosis, Laboratory—Instrumentation. 3. Electronics. QY 26 E29e]
  RB36.2.E35 1983   616.07′5′028   83-10524
  ISBN 0-471-86275-4

Printed in the United States of America

10 9 8 7 6 5 4 3 2 1

PREFACE

In the third quarter of the twentieth century the automation of analytical methods has caused the clinical laboratory to mushroom from a small support group to a major component of medical care. In the last quarter of the century the advance of computer hardware and informational technique promises to make automated instrumentation ever more complex.

The growing trend toward automation has radically changed the jobs performed by medical technologists, chemists, and microbiologists who work in the clinical laboratory. While these workers must still understand the chemistry and biology behind the methods they employ, they must also understand how the instruments they use operate. Without such knowledge they cannot detect instrumental errors or maintain the instruments properly.

There are four areas of knowledge, exclusive of chemistry and biology, needed to understand modern instrumentation: the physical principles of measurement, sample handling, electronics, and data processing. Each of these areas will be explored in this text.

The first area to be covered is electronics. The basic circuit elements that are commonly encountered are discussed at a level intended to give the reader an adequate background for understanding their actual operation. These chapters also set the background for electrochemical measurements, electronic detectors, and data processing.

Data processing is next presented in terms of computing hardware and data structures. These topics are then integrated into the discussion of actual instruments throughout the remainder of the text. A separate chapter considers the problems in making instruments intelligent.

The physical principles upon which instrumental measurements are based are the primary topics of the second part of the book. After discussing the theory and implementation of a specific principle, the text covers relevant methods for handling the samples to take advantage of that principle. The use of light and electricity are explored first. Later chapters deal with the principles involved in nuclear methods, chromatographic separation, and mass spectrometry.

I have tried to discuss instruments in as generic a manner as possible. To emphasize some points, however, it has been necessary to look at specific commercial products. This allows the reader to see how all the principles work together to give an operating instrument. In no way do I intend to endorse any of the commercial products mentioned, although I wish to thank their vendors for supplying key figures illustrating their operation.

To facilitate the understanding of the material covered, each chapter has review questions and many chapters have worked examples as well as problems for the reader to solve. Answers to selected problems are given in the appendix. Also in the appendix are some mathematical aids, a symbol table, and a glossary.

In writing this book I am attempting to raise the understanding of the bench-level clinical laboratory worker beyond the "black box" or "gee whiz" stage. This book is not intended as either an operator's manual or an engineering text. Its function is rather to give an adequate theoretical background in automated analysis that will permit the medical technologist, clinical chemist, and microbiologist to readily master the operation and control of any new laboratory instrument.

A.A.E.

v

ACKNOWLEDGMENTS

I wish to express my deep appreciation to my colleagues for their critical review of the materials herein presented.

Joan E. Eggert, M.T. (ASCP) Whole book

Joan E. Emmerich, M.T. (ASCP) Whole book

George S. Cembrowski, M.D., Ph.D. Numerous sections

Thomas J. Blankenheim, A.S. Electronics and computers

Isabel J. Barnes, Ph.D. Electronics, computers, and optics

Susanne J. Ames, M.S., M.T. (ASCP) Laboratory instruments

Carl C. Garber, Ph.D. Laboratory instruments

James O. Westgard, Ph.D. Emission, absorption and chemical analyzers

David D. Koch, Ph.D. Electronics and liquid chromatography

William C. Zarnstorff, Ph.D. Computers

James W. Taylor, Ph.D. Chromatography and mass spectrometry

E. Clifford Toren, Ph.D. Electrochemistry

Richard A. Proctor, M.D. Microbiology

Robert S. Helman, M.D. Nuclear methods

Leonard M. Uhr, Ph.D. Pattern recognition

Caroline M. Stieghorst, M.T. (ASCP) Cell counters

Glennda L. Brandt, M.T. (ASCP) Microbiology

I also wish to thank my illustrator, *Lucy Ebisch.*

A.A.E.

CONTENTS

ELECTRONICS AND INSTRUMENTATION
FOR THE CLINICAL LABORATORY

CHAPTER 1
CURRENT AND RESISTANCE

Perhaps the easiest way to envision electric current is by comparison with water current. As water responds to gravitational force, so electrons respond to electromotive force. We shall therefore begin with aqueous models and gradually abandon them as the nature of electric current becomes more familiar.

Section 1-1
OHM'S LAW

If one has a beaker of water and tips it so the water can flow over the edge, the water will fall to the floor. This is a direct result of gravity, but it is illustrative of a more basic principle. The water in the beaker has more potential energy than water on the floor. Water will therefore "seek its own level," that is, attempt to move to a position of minimum potential energy. Any substance will, given the chance, move to a state of lower potential energy. This is a result of the principle expressed in the second law of thermodynamics. In the case of water, the potential energy exists relative to the force of gravity. This is the key to the concept of potential energy; it can have a value other than zero only if there is a force being exerted to pull it toward a lower level, that is, a more stable state. Without such a force, there is no reason for an item to seek a lower energy level, and its potential energy is zero. When a substance is acted on by a force and moves to a lower level of potential, it acquires kinetic energy equal to the potential energy it loses. In the case of the water, the kinetic energy is the energy with which it strikes the floor and is dissipated by the splash. When the water comes to rest on the floor, its potential energy has

been lost owing to its reduction in height above the floor, and the kinetic energy gained by the fall has been dissipated by the collision with the floor. The potential energy left to the water is zero, at least relative to the floor.

Let us formalize the water example as in Figure 1-1. The water in the reservoir is at zero potential energy. The pump raises the water to a height at which its potential energy (E) is equal to the height reached (h) times the force of gravity (g) times the amount of water (a) that falls.

$$E = hga \qquad (1\text{-}1)$$

The water then falls through the height h to reach the reservoir, losing all the potential energy E. This is converted into kinetic energy, which is dissipated by the splash when the reservoir is reached. This process leaves the water in the same condition as when it started in the reservoir. The complete operation can be called a "circuit," and the flow of water can be called a "current."

A completely analogous situation exists in the second part of Figure 1-1. This is a diagram of an electrical circuit, that is, a closed path through which an electric current can flow. In order to make the current flow, it is necessary that we have something that can generate electrical potential, just as the pump generated gravitational potential. For now, we will generate such potential, called the electromotive force, using a battery.

A battery is represented by a series of long and short lines. The number of pairs of these lines is usually arbitrary, but can be used to represent the relative potential-generating ability of the battery, more pairs of lines meaning more potential. The end of the battery with the long line is called positive, and the end with the short line is called nega-

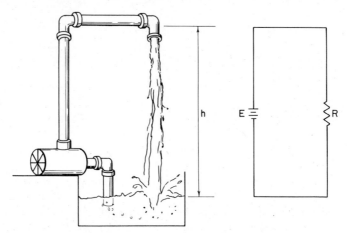

Figure 1-1   On the left the water is pumped to a height h from which it falls back to the level of the reservoir. On the right the charge is pumped up to a voltage E, which is lost by traversing a resistance R.

tive. Units of electricity at the negative end of the battery are said to be of relative potential zero. Those at the positive end of the battery are said to be of relative electrical potential E, and E is called the voltage of the battery. The voltage is measured in units called volts. The unit of electricity moved by the battery is called a coulomb (q), which is equal to the charge of 6.24×10^{18} electrons. In terms of the more basic units of physics, 1 volt is equal to 1 joule (a unit of energy) divided by 1 coulomb.

$$1 \text{ volt} = \frac{1 \text{ joule}}{1 \text{ coulomb}} \quad \textbf{(1-2)}$$

The battery, also called the voltage supply, therefore raises coulombs of electricity from the potential of zero to the potential of E. The coulomb units, however, will try to return to zero potential by traversing the rest of the circuit. To do so, they must pass through the components that make up the circuit. Most of these components are wire, which usually has negligible resistance to the flow of coulombs of charge. Other elements of the circuit offer more resistance to the flow of the charge and are called resistors. The effectiveness of a resistor at retarding the flow of charge is measured in ohms, a unit named after George Ohm, a nineteenth century German physicist who discovered the rela-

tionship between voltage and resistance. This discovery, called Ohm's law, stated that the amount of current (I) that a voltage supply of E volts could force through a resistance of R ohms is voltage (E) divided by resistance (R). The current is measured in amperes.

$$\text{Current} = \frac{\text{voltage}}{\text{resistance}} \quad \textbf{(Ohm's law)}$$

or

$$I = \frac{E}{R} \quad \textbf{(1-3)}$$

Ohm's law is usually written in the form of Eq. 1-4.

$$E = IR \quad \textbf{(1-4)}$$

A current is the amount of something flowing past a point during a certain length of time. The units of electric current were defined so that 1 ampere is equal to 1 coulomb flowing past a point each second.

$$\text{Current} = \frac{\text{charge flow}}{\text{time}}$$

or

$$I = \frac{q}{t} \quad \textbf{(1-5)}$$

$$1 \text{ ampere} = \frac{1 \text{ coulomb}}{1 \text{ second}} \quad \textbf{(1-6)}$$

Table 1-1 Metric Prefixes

Name	Factor
giga	10^9
mega	10^6
kilo	10^3
milli	10^{-3}
micro	10^{-6}
nano	10^{-9}
pico	10^{-12}

The ohm is then defined so that 1 ampere will equal 1 volt divided by 1 ohm.

$$1 \text{ ampere} = \frac{1 \text{ volt}}{1 \text{ ohm}} \qquad \textbf{(1-7)}$$

An ampere is frequently called an "amp" and abbreviated A. The respective abbreviations for coulomb and ohm are C and Ω (the Greek letter *omega*). All electrical units are metric and therefore prefixable as other metric values. Table 1-1 gives the common metric prefixes.

In Figure 1-1 the resistor is indicated by a zigzag line, while the wire, which we will usually assume is of negligible resistance, is indicated by a straight line. Most resistors are drawn with three or four zigzags, but occasionally resistors are drawn with more zigzags to indicate that they are of higher resistance or are very precisely made. The length of wire is immaterial in the drawing. There is no relationship between the length or shape of the wire in electrical drawings and the same wire in the real circuit. Drawings are made to be easy to understand and are not intended to be a snapshot of the real hardware. Wires in a drawing may be thought of as rubber bands that can be stretched as necessary to see most easily how the circuit works. Figure 1-2 presents three totally different drawings of the same circuit.

Current, as mentioned, is the flow of charge. This flow can be accomplished in two ways. The first is for positively charged ions to move in the direction of the current, from positive to negative. The second is for negative ions or electrons to travel from negative to positive, that is, opposite the current flow (Fig. 1-3). The effect of this latter situation is exactly the same as the former because nature is symmetrical. Negative charge flowing backward is equivalent to positive charge flowing forward. In most electrical circuits, the flow of charge is carried by electrons moving opposite to the indicated flow of current. The convention that current flows from positive to negative is always used, however, regardless of the actual mechanism of charge transfer.

A unit of charge in a circuit has zero voltage when it reaches the negative end of the battery after traversing the circuit. But where does the energy go that was generated by the battery to raise the charge units to a potential E? Since there is no "splash" as in the case of water, the energy must be lost while passing through the resistance R. This is, in fact, the case, and the amount of energy dissipated per unit of time, usually in the form of heat, is

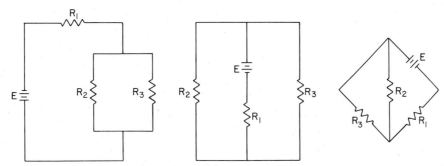

Figure 1-2 Three drawings of the same circuit to demonstrate how diagrams can be rearranged for clarity.

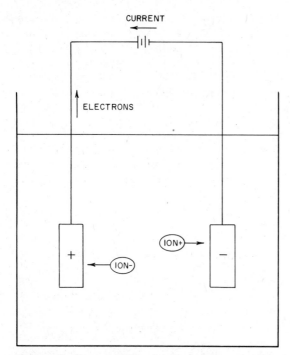

Figure 1-3   Current in the wire is carried by negative electrons moving in the backward direction. Current in the solution is carried by ions moving toward the oppositely charged electrode.

the product of the amount of current flowing and the potential lost across the resistance.

$$P = EI \qquad (1\text{-}8)$$

This new quantity power (P) has units of energy per time and is measured in watts (W). A watt is 1 volt times 1 ampere. If Ohm's law is substituted into this expression, we find that

$$P = I^2R \qquad (1\text{-}9)$$

EXAMPLE 1-1

A battery of 20 volts sends 0.4 amps through a resistor R. What is the resistance of R?

Solution:

$$E = IR$$

Therefore

$$R = \frac{E}{I}$$

$$R = \frac{20 \text{ volts}}{0.4 \text{ amps}} = 50 \text{ ohms} \qquad \blacksquare$$

EXAMPLE 1-2

How much power did the resistor in Example 1-1 dissipate?

Solution:

$$P = EI$$

$$P = 20 \text{ V} \times 0.4 \text{ A} = 8 \text{ watts} \qquad \blacksquare$$

Section **1-2**
SERIES CIRCUITS

Figure 1-4 shows another example of a water system. In this example, the water is pumped to the same height and gains the same potential energy hga as the water in Figure 1-1. However, instead of falling in one step to the reservoir and losing its potential energy, it first falls to an intermediate platform and then falls off the end of that platform into the reservoir. We note that the amount of water that can flow through the system is the same as in the previous case and that the total height that the water falls is equal to the sum of the two heights of the two component falls ($h_1 + h_2$). We can rewrite the energy equation as

$$E = (h_1 + h_2)ga \qquad (1\text{-}10)$$

Note that this equation can be rewritten by the rules of algebra (distributiveness) as

$$E = h_1 ga + h_2 ga \qquad (1\text{-}11)$$

In this latter form, it is easy to see that the potential energy lost in the first fall was $h_1 ga$, leaving the water with a potential energy of only $h_2 ga$ at the beginning of the second fall.

Figure 1-4 also contains an electrical circuit, which is similar to that of the water system. The resistor R has been replaced by two resistors (R_1

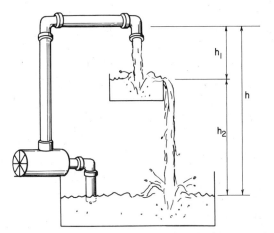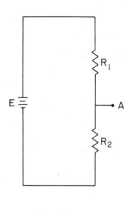

Figure 1-4 On the left water is pumped to a height *h* from which it falls in two cascades back to the reservoir. On the right charge is raised to a voltage *E*, which is dissipated by traversing two resistors in series.

and R_2) whose total resistance is equal to the previous R (i.e., $R = R_1 + R_2$). Consequently, we can substitute this expression into Ohm's law to get

$$E = IR = I(R_1 + R_2) = IR_1 + IR_2 \quad \textbf{(1-12)}$$

From this example we can learn three valuable principles. The first is that the resistance R in Ohm's law is the total resistance and can be composed of a number of individual resistances. Second, when the resistances are in series, that is, when the current must pass through each one of them in turn, then the total resistance is the sum of the individual resistances. Mathematically, this is written

$$R = \Sigma R_i = R_1 + R_2 + R_3 + \cdots \quad \textbf{(1-13)}$$

The summation sign Σ (sigma) provides a convenient shorthand method to indicate that the number of items summed is arbitrarily large. The number of resistors in series can vary from two to infinity. Ohm's law is sometimes written $E = I\Sigma R$ when applied to a series circuit.

EXAMPLE 1-3

The current through a circuit is 2.03 A and the voltage is 124 V. If the circuit has two resistors in se-

ries, what is the resistance of the second, if the resistance of the first is 43.6 Ω?

Solution:

$$E = I(R_1 + R_2)$$

$$R_2 = \frac{E}{I} - R_1$$

$$= \frac{124}{2.03} - 43.6$$

$$= 17.5 \ \Omega \qquad \blacksquare$$

For the third principle involved, it is necessary to go back to the example. The height of the first falls is totally independent of the height of the second falls. In other words, the first falls would behave the same way whether the second falls were there or not. The amount of potential energy lost going over the first will always be $h_1 ga$. If we call this term E_1 and refer to $h_2 ga$ as E_2, then

$$E = hga = (h_1 + h_2)ga = h_1 ga + h_2 ga = E_1 + E_2$$
$$\textbf{(1-14)}$$

The amount of potential energy lost totally is the sum of the component energy losses.

Electrical potential behaves exactly the same way. Just as potential energy is lost over the first falls and is not available to be lost over the second, so voltage (i.e., electrical potential) is lost over the first resistor and not available to the second. If we say that the voltage E_1 is equal to IR_1 and voltage E_2 is equal to IR_2, then

$$E = IR = I(R_1 + R_2) = IR_1 + IR_2 = E_1 + E_2 \tag{1-15}$$

Since the voltage at the negative end of the battery is 0 in Figure 1-4, then the voltage at point A (between R_1 and R_2) must be E_2, that is, the total voltage E minus E_1, the voltage lost over the first resistor. The amount of voltage lost over a resistor is always just the product of the current through that resistor times the resistance of the resistor. This reduction in voltage is called the "voltage drop" or "IR drop" across the resistor, since $E = IR$.

EXAMPLE 1-4

If resistor R_1 in Figure 1-4 is twice the size of R_2, and if the battery voltage is 60 volts, what is the voltage at point A?

Solution:

$$E = I(R_1 + R_2)$$

$$I = \frac{E}{R_1 + R_2}$$

$$E_2 = IR_2 = \left(\frac{E}{R_1 + R_2}\right)R_2$$

Since $R_1 = 2R_2$,

$$E_2 = \frac{ER_2}{2R_2 + R_2} = \frac{ER_2}{3R_2} = \frac{E}{3}$$

$$E_2 = \frac{60}{3} = 20 \text{ volts} \qquad \blacksquare$$

This drop of voltage over each resistor in series is called "voltage division" because the voltage is divided among the resistors, each taking its share before passing the remainder on to the next resistor.

This principle of voltage division is the basis for many measuring circuits. When the resistance of one of the resistors in a series is altered, a redivision of the voltage occurs; this can be measured by various methods discussed later. One of the most common uses of this principle is a voltage divider. Figure 1-5 shows its operation. Figure 1-5A shows a circuit with five resistors of 1,000 ohms each. The 100 volts of the power supply is divided evenly over the five equal resistors, as can be readily calculated. The voltage across each resistor is 20 volts. One can therefore get voltages between 0 and 100 volts in steps of 20 volts by attaching leads to the appropriate places in the circuit. Although this is convenient if one needs voltages in these step increments, Figure 1-5B shows an even better arrangement. Here the 5,000 ohms are in one long resistor that can be accessed along its entire length by a movable contact. At whatever point the contact touches the resistor, the voltage is divided between that which has been lost up to that point and that which will be lost before reaching the end of the resistor. If the contact is at the end attached to the positive terminal of the battery, 0 volts have been lost and the voltage is 100 compared with the negative terminal of the battery. If the contact is at the end of the resistor attached to the negative terminal of the battery, 100 volts have been lost, and the voltage is 0 volts compared with the negative terminal of the battery. If the contact is placed anywhere between the ends, the voltage between that position and the negative terminal of the battery is somewhere between 0 and 100 volts. This device is called a potentiometer and is built so that the resistance of the resistor varies linearly with its length. One can determine the voltage division of the potentiometer by measuring the distance between the contact and the negative end of the potentiometer. Similarly, if one knows the voltage division, one can determine how far the contact arm has been moved. This is an important device in producing an electrical signal proportional to a mechanical movement.

EXAMPLE 1-5

A potentiometer is 12.00 cm long. The voltage over the potentiometer is 8.72 V and the voltage measured at the contact was 6.21 V. How far from the positive terminal is the contact located?

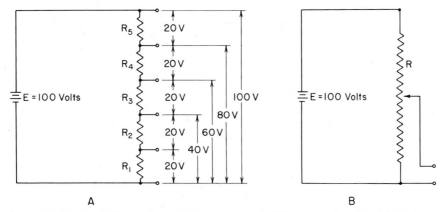

Figure 1-5 On the left is a voltage divider composed of five resistors, each of 1000 ohms. On the right is a potentiometer, a device that allows a variable voltage division to be made by a movable contact arm. It too has 5000 ohms of total resistance.

Solution:

$$E = IR$$

$$E_1 = IR_1$$

Therefore

$$\frac{IR_1}{IR} = \frac{E_1}{E} \Rightarrow R_1 = \frac{E_1}{E} R$$

R in this example is proportional to centimeters, so we can use that unit:

$$R_1 = \frac{6.21}{8.72} \times 12.00 = 8.55 \text{ cm from negative end}$$

Distance from positive end $= 12.00 - 8.55$

$$= 3.45 \text{ cm} \qquad \blacksquare$$

The final item of significance regarding resistance in series is the dissipation of power. Each resistor dissipates power independently of all the rest. For a particular circuit, $P = EI = I^2R$ (Eq. 1-9). By substituting for R its components, we get

$$P = I^2 \Sigma R_i = I^2(R_1 + R_2 + R_3 + \cdots) \quad \textbf{(1-16)}$$

$$P = I^2R_1 + I^2R_2 + I^2R_3 + \cdots$$

$$P = P_1 + P_2 + P_3 + \cdots \qquad \textbf{(1-17)}$$

By splitting R into components, we do not get more power dissipated. However, increasing R for a

given voltage has an interesting effect. Let us use a special form of resistor, a light bulb, with a resistance of 100 ohms. If we place this alone in a circuit with a 100-volt battery, we have the following situation:

$$I = \frac{E}{R} = \frac{100 \text{ V}}{100 \ \Omega} = 1.00 \text{ A} \qquad \textbf{(1-18)}$$

$$P = I^2R = (1\text{A})^2 \times 100 \ \Omega = 100 \text{ W} \quad \textbf{(1-19)}$$

This power is dissipated in the form of heat and light. If we now place a second light bulb in series with the first, we double the resistance (100 + 100 = 200 ohms). The circuit equation then gives us

$$I = \frac{E}{R} = \frac{100 \text{ V}}{200 \ \Omega} = 0.50 \text{ A} \qquad \textbf{(1-20)}$$

$$P = I^2R = (0.50 \text{ A})^2 \times 200 \ \Omega = 50 \text{ W} \quad \textbf{(1-21)}$$

The amount of power that can be dissipated in the latter case is only half as much as before. Moreover, since each bulb is only giving off half that amount, each bulb is radiating only 25 watts, one-quarter of the value in the previous case. Why is this so? Increasing the resistance decreases the current. Since the power dissipated is proportional to the square of the current, it decreases as well, even though the resistance term is rising. Putting light bulbs in series is a poor way to get more light.

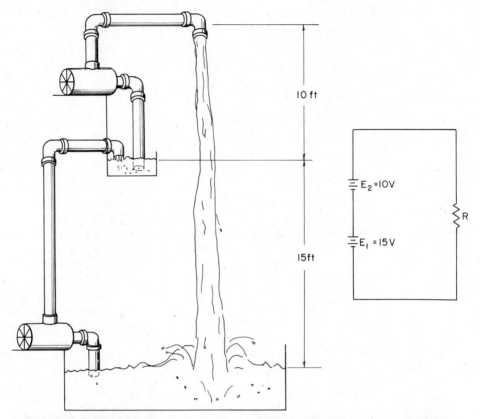

Figure 1-6 On the left water is pumped to a height of 25 feet by two pumps, the first raising it 15 feet and the second 10 feet. The water then falls back to the reservoir. On the right the charge is raised to a voltage of 25 volts by two batteries in series, which have voltages of 15 and 10 volts, respectively. The charge returns to zero potential through resistor R.

As shown in Figure 1-6, it is also possible to put batteries in series. When batteries are in series their voltages add. It is very much like two successive water pumps. If the first pump raises the water 15 feet and the second 10 feet, the water is then 25 feet high and has the corresponding potential energy. In the same way, if the first battery raises the voltage 15 volts and the second battery raises the voltage 10 volts, the total voltage over the two batteries in series is 25 volts.

Simply put, in a series circuit,

$$E = \Sigma E_i \qquad \text{(1-22)}$$

EXAMPLE 1-6

Calculate the voltage at the point between each circuit element in Figure 1-7.

Solution: The first step in the solution is to write Ohm's law in the proper form for this circuit:

$$\Sigma E_i = I \Sigma R_i$$

$$\Sigma E_i = E_1 + E_2 = 20 + 12 = 32 \text{ V}$$

$$\Sigma R_i = R_1 + R_2 + R_3 = 100 + 250 + 290 = 640 \text{ } \Omega$$

$$I = \frac{\Sigma E}{\Sigma R} = \frac{32 \text{ V}}{640 \text{ } \Omega} = 0.050 \text{ A}$$

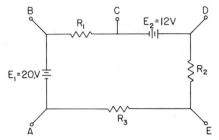

Figure 1-7 Two batteries and three resistors form a series circuit. The electrical potential of any point around the circuit can be calculated compared to an arbitrary ground point. ($R_1 = 100$ Ω, $R_2 = 250$ Ω, $R_3 = 290$ Ω.)

It is now necessary to define a point as 0 voltage (or ground). Let us pick point A.

$$E_A = 0$$

Since voltage increases over batteries placed in the forward direction,

$$E_B = E_A + E_1 = 0 + 20 = 20 \text{ V}$$

But voltage drops over resistors,

$$E_C = E_B - IR_1 = 20 - 0.05 \times 100 = 15 \text{ V}$$

$$E_D = E_C + E_2 = 15 + 12 = 27 \text{ V}$$

$$E_E = E_D - IR_2 = 27 - 0.05 \times 250 = 14.5 \text{ V}$$

$$E_A = E_E - IR_3 = 14.5 - 0.05 \times 290 = 0 \text{ V},$$

as assumed. ■

To solve resistor and battery problems, it is usually necessary to find the unknown quantity in Ohm's law before one can proceed. Note that if a battery is in a series circuit backward to the current flow, it lowers the voltage just as does a resistor.

Section **1-3**
PARALLEL CIRCUITS

Figure 1-8 shows a new wrinkle to the pump diagram. Instead of one discharge opening at height h, there are two, and water will fall from both of them. The total amount of water to fall is still a, but now a has two components, a_1, the amount of water going through the left pipe and a_2, the amount of water going through the right pipe. Substituting this into the potential energy equation, we get

$$E = hga = hg(a_1 + a_2) = hga_1 + hga_2 \quad \textbf{(1-23)}$$

The amount of potential energy is again independent in each branch.

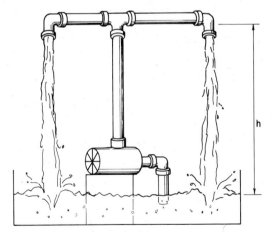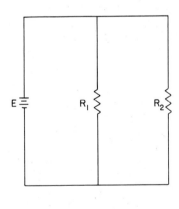

Figure 1-8 On the left water is pumped to a height h from which it falls from two openings to the reservoir. The total water going up the pipe is equal to the sum of what falls from the two orifices. On the right the current pumped by the battery can flow through either resistor, but not both, to the negative end of the battery.

The corresponding electrical circuit appears in the second part of Figure 1-8. The total current I through the battery must equal the sum of the current through resistor 1, called I_1, and the current through resistor 2, called I_2. Substituting into Ohm's law gives us

$$E = IR = (I_1 + I_2)R = I_1R + I_2R \quad \textbf{(1-24)}$$

Oops! All this math is fine, except what is R? It cannot be either R_1 or R_2 because all the current does not flow through R_1 or R_2; in fact, there is no common resistor. Faced with this problem, we must go back to the basic law governing a resistor in a circuit, that is, that the potential drop over a resistor is equal to the current through the resistor times its resistance. The voltage across both resistors in Figure 1-8 is just E, the battery voltage, while resistances are R_1 and R_2, respectively. Therefore, we can define I_1 and I_2 in terms of resistance and voltage.

$$I_1 = \frac{E}{R_1} \quad \textbf{(1-25)}$$

$$I_2 = \frac{E}{R_2} \quad \textbf{(1-26)}$$

If we substitute Eqs. 1-25 and 1-26 into Eq. 1-24, we get

$$E = (I_1 + I_2)R = \left(\frac{E}{R_1} + \frac{E}{R_2}\right)R$$

$$E = \left(\frac{1}{R_1} + \frac{1}{R_2}\right)ER$$

$$\frac{1}{R} = \frac{1}{R_1} + \frac{1}{R_2} \quad \textbf{(1-27)}$$

$$R = \frac{R_1 R_2}{R_1 + R_2} \quad \textbf{(1-28)}$$

The total resistance R, called the equivalent resistance, is a combination of the two resistances in the circuit. Because the resistors lie next to each other in a simple drawing, this type of circuit, in which any element of the current can go through only one of several branches, is called a "parallel" circuit. The equivalent resistance for a parallel circuit is given by

$$\frac{1}{R} = \sum \frac{1}{R_i} = \frac{1}{R_1} + \frac{1}{R_2} + \frac{1}{R_3} + \cdots \quad \textbf{(1-29)}$$

Note that this expression cannot be rewritten in either of the following two forms:

$$\frac{1}{R} = \sum \frac{1}{R_i} \neq \frac{1}{R_1 + R_2 + R_3 + \cdots}$$

$$R \neq \frac{\Pi R_i}{\Sigma R_i}$$

where $\Pi R_i = R_1 \cdot R_2 \cdot R_3 \cdots$.

A few items about parallel circuits are worth noting. First, the current through any resistor is totally independent of the presence or value of any other resistor. Varying the resistance of other resistors in the parallel arrangement does not affect the amount of current flowing through a fixed-value resistor, nor does it change the voltage across any of the resistors. Current division is not analogous to voltage division. Second, the equivalent resistance is always less than any of the component resistances, that is, $R < R_1, R < R_2, R < R_3$. That this should be true becomes obvious after a little reflection. If we have a circuit with only one resistor, the voltage E and resistance R will cause a current I in accordance with Ohm's law. Now, if a second resistor is placed in parallel with the first, the same amount of current will flow through the first resistor as before and an additional amount of current will flow through this second resistor as well. Since all current has to come from the power supply, the amount of current drawn from the power supply must increase to meet the new demand. The voltage of the power supply is fixed; the only way this can happen and keep Ohm's law true is for the equivalent resistance to decrease (E = constant = IR, if $I \uparrow$, R must $\downarrow$). Therefore, the equivalent resistance is less than whatever resistor is chosen as the initial resistor. Since this is an arbitrary choice, the equivalent resistance is less than that of any of the parallel resistors. As an example, let $R_2 = R_1$ in Figure 1-8. Then

$$\frac{1}{R} = \frac{1}{R_1} + \frac{1}{R_2} = \frac{1}{R_1} + \frac{1}{R_1} = \frac{2}{R_1} \quad \textbf{(1-30)}$$

$$R = \frac{R_1}{2}$$

For n equal resistors in parallel of value R, the equivalent resistance is R/n.

EXAMPLE 1-7

A circuit has three resistors of 300., 540., and 680. ohms, respectively, in parallel attached to a 12.0 V battery. What is the total current drawn?

Solution: This problem can be solved in two ways. The first way is to do a summation of the currents:

$$I = I_1 + I_2 + I_3$$

$$I = \frac{E}{R_1} + \frac{E}{R_2} + \frac{E}{R_3}$$

$$I = \frac{12.0 \text{ V}}{300 \ \Omega} + \frac{12.0 \text{ V}}{540 \ \Omega} + \frac{12.0 \text{ V}}{680 \ \Omega}$$

$$I = 0.0400 \text{ A} + 0.0222 \text{ A} + 0.0176 \text{ A}$$

$$I = 0.080 \text{ A}$$

The second way is to find the equivalent resistance:

$$\frac{1}{R} = \frac{1}{R_1} + \frac{1}{R_2} + \frac{1}{R_3}$$

$$R = \frac{R_1 R_2 R_3}{R_2 R_3 + R_1 R_3 + R_1 R_2}$$

$$R = \frac{300 \times 540 \times 680}{540 \times 680 + 300 \times 680 + 300 \times 540}$$

$$R = \frac{110160000}{367200 + 204000 + 162000} = 150. \ \Omega$$

$$I = \frac{E}{R} = \frac{12.0}{150} = 0.080 \text{ A}$$

The power dissipation of a parallel circuit is equal to the sum of the power dissipations by each resistor.

$$P = \Sigma(E \cdot I_i) \qquad (1\text{-}31)$$

Since

$$I_i = \frac{E}{R_i}$$

$$P = \sum \frac{E^2}{R_i} = E^2 \sum \frac{1}{R_i} \qquad (1\text{-}32)$$

Since *E* is constant,

$$P = \frac{E^2}{R_1} + \frac{E^2}{R_2} + \frac{E^2}{R_3} + \cdots \qquad (1\text{-}33)$$

If we use our example of 100-ohm light bulbs with a 100-volt power supply again,

$$P = \frac{(100 \text{ V})^2}{100 \ \Omega} = 100 \text{ W} \qquad \text{for one bulb} \qquad (1\text{-}34)$$

$$P = \frac{(100 \text{ V})^2}{100 \ \Omega} + \frac{(100 \text{ V})^2}{100 \ \Omega} = 200 \text{ W}$$
$$\text{for two bulbs} \quad (1\text{-}35)$$

and so forth. This is clearly the way to wire light bulbs in order to get more light. ∎

Although it is possible to put any two batteries in series (because their voltages add), batteries placed in parallel must have identical voltages. Parallel resistors have the same voltage drop over them because they are wired between the same points. The same is true for batteries. If batteries of different voltages are placed in parallel, one battery will try to drive the other backward with an uncertain outcome for the final combined voltage.

Section **1-4**
SIMPLE NETWORKS

A simple network is composed of a voltage supply and a group of resistors, which are, in fact, merely grouped series and parallel combinations. We will examine both an elementary and a complicated example of a simple network in this section.

To solve a network it is necessary to apply a method called successive reduction. By this method the circuit is reduced in steps to a circuit with a single resistor and battery. The following rules constitute the method of successive reduction for a resistor network.

1. Redraw the figure to emphasize the part being reduced.
2. Replace all parallel resistors with an equivalent resistor.
3. Combine all series resistors into an equivalent resistor.

4. Repeat steps 1 through 3 until only one resistor remains.

5. Apply Ohm's law to find the current.

EXAMPLE 1-8

Calculate the total current flowing through the battery in Figure 1-9A.

Solution: It is not necessary to redraw the figure, since it is adequate, so we start by replacing resistors R_2 and R_3 with an equivalent resistor R_A.

$$R_A = \frac{R_2 R_3}{(R_2 + R_3)} = \frac{89 \times 111}{89 + 111}$$

$$R_A = 49.4\ \Omega$$

We have now "reduced" the circuit to Figure 1-9B, which should be drawn. Next, we combine the series resistors to form a new resistor R_B.

$$R_B = R_1 + R_A = 137 + 49.4$$

$$R_B = 186.4\ \Omega$$

We now have Figure 1-9C. Here we can apply Ohm's law to get the current:

$$I = \frac{E}{R_B} = \frac{38}{186.4}$$

$$I = 0.20\ A$$

Thus we have the total current from the battery shown in Figure 1-9A. ∎

EXAMPLE 1-9

Find the current through all branches of Figure 1-10A.

Solution: Although the circuit is complicated, a brief examination will show that it is a combination of series and parallel elements, which can therefore be resolved by the reduction methods previously discussed. To solve this problem, we must divide it into two phases: (1) find the total current I_t from the battery, and (2) divide this current appropriately among the various pathways that the current can traverse. Let us begin accomplishing step 1 by systematically applying the rules discussed above. Initially we can perform two reductions. In the first we combine resistors R_2 and R_3 to form a new resistor R_8.

$$R_8 = R_2 + R_3$$

$$R_8 = 100 + 680 = 780\ \Omega$$

For the second reduction, we replace resistors R_5 and R_6 with an equivalent resistor R_9:

$$R_9 = \frac{R_5 R_6}{R_5 + R_6} = \frac{560 \times 490}{560 + 490}$$

$$R_9 = 261\ \Omega$$

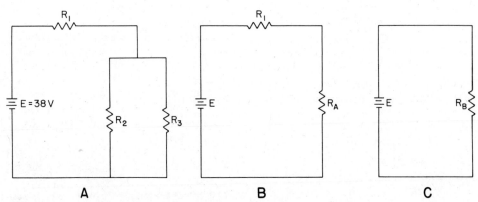

A **B** **C**

Figure 1-9 The circuit in part A is reduced to B by replacing two parallel resistors with an equivalent resistor. The circuit is further reduced to C by replacing two series resistors with an equivalent resistor. ($R_1 = 137\ \Omega$, $R_2 = 89\ \Omega$, $R_3 = 111\ \Omega$.)

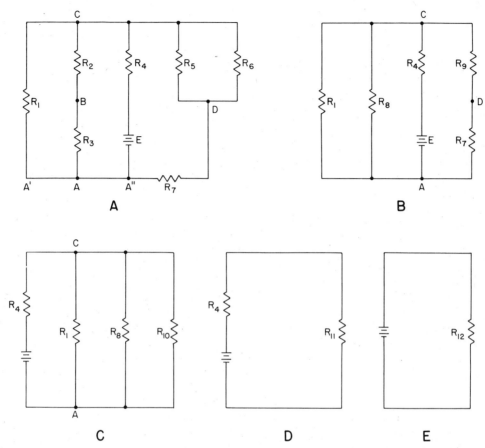

Figure 1-10 The item-by-item reduction of a complicated network to a basic Ohm's law circuit. ($E = 27.0$ V, $R_1 = 370$ Ω, $R_2 = 100$ Ω, $R_3 = 680$ Ω, $R_4 = 68$ Ω, $R_5 = 560$ Ω, $R_6 = 490$ Ω, $R_7 = 220$ Ω.)

After completing these replacements, it is time to redraw the figure before confusion sets in. As we do this it is important to note that junction A′ is at the same voltage as the junctions A and A″. In fact, these points are electrically equivalent and can collectively be denoted as A. The same is true for C or for any other similar situation. When a figure is redrawn, it is important to carry along these junction designations, for which alphabet letters are used, to facilitate seeing what has been done to the circuit. The resistors should also be labeled again to prevent confusion. Note that Figure 1-10B shows the circuit after the above reduction.

Figure 1-10B can be reduced by both a series and a parallel reduction, similar to what was done in Figure 1-10A. Nevertheless, it is advantageous to delay the parallel reduction of R_1 and R_8 until after the next redrawing of the circuit. While the advantage may not seem obvious now, it will become easy to spot with some practice. The series reduction of R_9 and R_7 to form R_{10} is, however, essential.

$$R_{10} = R_9 + R_7$$

$$R_{10} = 261 + 220 = 481 \text{ Ω}$$

The circuit is then redrawn to produce Figure 1-10C. Note that a major change has taken place. The battery has been moved to one side of the diagram, and most of the remaining resistors are now in parallel. This rearrangement can be performed because all the elements are attached to point A on one side and to point C on the other and because the order in which things are drawn in such a case is unimportant. Since these resistors are in parallel, it is possible to replace all of them at once rather than in pairs, as would have had to be done if we had done a parallel reduction from Figure 1-10B. Equivalent resistor R_{11} can be used to replace R_1, R_8, and R_{10}:

$$\frac{1}{R_{11}} = \frac{1}{R_1} + \frac{1}{R_8} + \frac{1}{R_{10}}$$

$$\frac{1}{R_{11}} = \frac{1}{370} + \frac{1}{780} + \frac{1}{481}$$

$$\frac{1}{R_{11}} = 0.00270 + 0.00128 + 0.00208 = 0.00606$$

$$R_{11} = 165 \ \Omega$$

At this point the circuit has been reduced as shown in Figure 1-10D. A simple series combination of R_4 and R_{11} gives us Figure 1-10E.

$$R_{12} = R_4 + R_{11}$$

$$R_{12} = 68 + 165 = 233 \ \Omega$$

From this diagram the total current can be quickly calculated:

$$I_t = \frac{E}{R} = \frac{27.0}{233}$$

$$I_t = 0.116 \ A$$

Part 1 of the problem is solved, but it is now necessary to work backward to find all the currents through the individual resistors. Since all parts of Figure 1-10 are true and equivalent, we can use any of them as necessary to determine these current values, which we seek.

From Figure 1-10D

$$I_4^* = I_t = 0.116 \ A$$

* Final current.

From Figure 1-10C

$$E_A = 0$$

$$E_C = E + E_A - I_4 R_4$$

$$E_C = 27.0 + 0 - 0.116 \times 68$$

$$E_C = 19.1 \ V$$

$$I_1 = \frac{E_C - E_A}{R_1} = \frac{19.1 - 0}{370}$$

$$I_1^* = 0.052 \ A$$

$$I_8 = \frac{E_C - E_A}{R_8} = \frac{19.1 - 0}{780}$$

$$I_8 = 0.0245 \ A$$

$$I_{10} = \frac{E_C - E_A}{R_{10}} = \frac{19.1 - 0}{481}$$

$$I_{10} = 0.0397 \ A$$

From Figure 1-10B

$$I_7^* = I_9 = I_{10}$$

$$= 0.040 \ A \ \text{(rounded for significant fig.)}$$

$$E_D - E_A = I_7 R_7$$

$$E_D = I_7 R_7 + E_A = 0.0397 \times 220 + 0$$

$$E_D = 8.73 \ V$$

From Figure 1-10A

$$I_2^* = I_3^* = I_8 = 0.024 \ A$$

$$I_5 = \frac{E_C - E_D}{R_5} = \frac{19.1 - 8.73}{560}$$

$$I_5^* = 0.018 \ A$$

$$I_6 = \frac{E_C - E_D}{R_6} = \frac{19.1 - 8.73}{490}$$

$$I_6^* = 0.021 \ A$$

■

Section 1-5
KIRCHHOFF'S LAWS

If the same methods used above were applied to the circuit in Figure 1-11, they would fail to resolve the

* Final current.

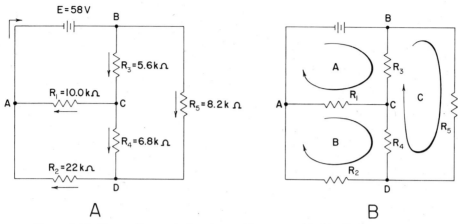

Figure 1-11 The assignment of nodes and loops to a Kirchhoff's laws problem.

circuit. This is because this circuit is not a simple combination of elements in series and parallel. There are so-called crossresistors, such as R_4, which prevent a redrawing of the circuit into a form in which the previous rules will work. In such cases it is necessary to resort to the rules developed by Robert Kirchhoff, a German physicist of the nineteenth century.

Kirchhoff's First Law

The sum of the currents flowing into a junction point must equal the sum of the currents flowing out. Therefore, the algebraic sum of the current around a junction is 0, that is,

$$\Sigma I_i = 0 \qquad \textbf{(1-36)}$$

Kirchhoff's Second Law

The algebraic sum of all voltage sources around a closed loop is equal to the algebraic sum of all IR drops in the loop:

$$\Sigma E - \Sigma IR = 0 \qquad \textbf{(1-37)}$$

Note the following points: (1) a closed loop is any path through a circuit that can be drawn with no wires that cross, but are not connected; (2) the voltage increases over batteries that are negative to

positive in the direction of current flow and falls over batteries of reverse polarity; and (3) voltage *drops* over resistors in a loop that are encountered in the direction of current flow but *increases* over resistors encountered going opposite to current flow.

Because both Kirchhoff's laws are true for any circuit, either or both may be applied in analyzing a circuit. Numerous ways of using these laws have been devised to make circuit analysis easier. All these methods of analysis are mathematically identical, but some make certain circuits easier to solve because they isolate the quantity of interest from the rest. Two of the most common methods of analysis are nodal analysis and loop analysis, which come from the direct application of the first and second laws, respectively. In nodal analysis there are N-1 independent equations if there are N nodes, because the Nth nodal equation is the sum of the previous N-1 equations and is therefore not independent. Nodal analysis is most easily applied to circuits in which the current in some of the branches is known, such as when constant current supplies are present. Since in our simplified approach to electronics we have been dealing only with constant voltage supplies, we will restrict our attention to loop analysis. Loop analysis is best shown by an example.

EXAMPLE 1-10

Find the current in each branch of Figure 1-11.

Solution: There are clearly three loops in Figure 1-11, labeled A, B, and C. If we postulate that a current flows around each of the loops, we have current I_A, I_B, and I_C. The direction of these currents is taken to be clockwise around the loops. The real current through any circuit element is then the sum of the loop currents flowing through it, since current can neither be gained nor lost. Using this approach, one can then write equations for the voltage around the three loops on the basis of Kirchhoff's second law, Eq. 1-37. These are:

Loop A

$$E - (I_A - I_C)R_3 - (I_A - I_B)R_1 = 0 \qquad (1)$$

Loop B

$$-(I_B - I_A)R_1 - (I_B - I_C)R_4 - I_B R_2 = 0 \quad (2)$$

Loop C

$$-I_C R_5 - (I_C - I_B)R_4 - (I_C - I_A)R_3 = 0 \quad (3)$$

Note that because the power supply was crossed negative to positive, its voltage has a plus sign. If more than one current flows through a resistor, the currents must be algebraically summed before the final current is multiplied by the resistance.

The next step is to write the equations in terms of the unknowns by regrouping.

Loop A

$$-(R_1 + R_3)I_A + R_1 I_B + R_3 I_C = -E \qquad (4)$$

Loop B

$$R_1 I_A - (R_1 + R_2 + R_4)I_B + R_4 I_C = 0 \qquad (5)$$

Loop C

$$R_3 I_A + R_4 I_B - (R_3 + R_4 + R_5)I_C = 0 \qquad (6)$$

If we now substitute for the known resistances and voltages, we have three equations in three unknowns. These can be solved by various methods of substitution, elimination, or matrices. The method of elimination is shown below.

From (4)

$$-15.6\, I_A + 10.0\, I_B + 5.6\, I_C = -5.8 \times 10^{-2} \quad (7)$$

From (5)

$$10.0\, I_A - 38.8\, I_B + 6.8\, I_C = 0 \qquad (8)$$

From (6)

$$5.6\, I_A + 6.8\, I_B - 20.6\, I_C = 0 \qquad (9)$$

Note that all equations were divided through by 10^3.

Eliminate I_C (from 7 and 8):

$$-23.83\, I_A + 41.95\, I_B = -5.8 \cdot 10^{-2} \quad (10)$$

Eliminate I_C (from 8 and 9):

$$35.89\, I_A - 110.74\, I_B = 0 \qquad (11)$$

Eliminate I_B (from 10 and 11):

$$-27.02\, I_A = -1.53 \cdot 10^{-1} \qquad (12)$$

$$I_T{}^* = I_A = 5.7 \text{ mA} \qquad (13)$$

Having calculated one value, it is now possible to back-substitute into the various equations in order to get the rest of the values.

From Eq. (11):

$$I_2{}^* = I_B = \frac{35.89 \times 5.7 \cdot 10^{-3}}{100.74} = 1.8 \text{ mA} \quad (14)$$

From Eq. (9):

$$I_5{}^* = I_C = \frac{5.6 \times 5.7 \cdot 10^{-3} + 6.8 \times 1.8 \cdot 10^{-3}}{20.6}$$
$$= 2.1 \text{ mA} \qquad (15)$$

$$I_3{}^* = I_A - I_C = (5.7 - 2.1)10^{-3} = 3.6 \text{ mA} \qquad (16)$$

$$I_1{}^* = I_A - I_B = (5.7 - 1.8)10^{-3} = 3.9 \text{ mA} \qquad (17)$$

$$I_4{}^* = I_B - I_C = (1.8 - 2.1)10^{-3} = -0.3 \text{ mA} \qquad (18)$$

∎

The above method is a bit complicated, but it will work on any network. If, however, the network can be drawn in two dimensions without any unconnected wires crossing, the network is called a mesh. In a mesh one can simplify the set of Eqs.

---

* Final current values.

(4)–(6) of Example 1-10. Let us multiply them by −1 and rewrite them as below.

$$E = (R_1 + R_3)I_A - R_1 I_B - R_3 I_C \qquad (19)$$

$$0 = -R_1 I_A + (R_1 + R_2 + R_4)I_B - R_4 I_C \qquad (20)$$

$$0 = -R_3 I_A - R_4 I_B + (R_3 + R_4 + R_5)I_C \qquad (21)$$

Note that the coefficients of these equations are symmetrical around a line from the I_A term in the upper left to the I_C term in the lower right (main diagonal). These equations can be written by inspection of the circuit if the following rules are observed:

1. The voltage is written on the left side with a plus sign if the power supply is traversed negative to positive and with a minus sign if traversed positive to negative. Voltage supplies in series are added. If no supplies are present, a zero is written.
2. The terms on the main diagonal are positive, and the coefficients are the sum of the resistors around the loop.
3. The off-diagonal terms are negative. They are the product of the resistor value times the current of the other loop in which the resistor is included. As a result, these values must be symmetrical around the main diagonal. If two loops do not have a resistor in common, the corresponding off-diagonal term will be zero.

Using the above rules, it is possible to set up the equations for any mesh quickly. These can then be solved as shown in the solution by Example 1-10.

Section 1-6
DELTA–WYE TRANSFORMATION

While Kirchhoff's laws can be used to solve any circuit problem, sometimes one can do a circuit transformation that will permit an easier solution by successive reduction. One of the most common transformations is that by delta–wye. Figure 1-12 shows how one moves from a delta configuration of resistors to a wye configuration, or vice versa. Figure 1-12B does not represent a legitimate equivalent circuit, but merely shows how the two superimpose on each other.

To go from the delta to the wye, a point O must be added. To go from wye to delta, this point must be lost. Almost all simplifying transformations are from delta to wye. The equations below permit calculation of the corresponding resistor values for one type of circuit when the values for all the resistors in the other type of circuit are known.

From delta to wye

$$R_A = \frac{R_{AB} R_{AC}}{R_{AB} + R_{AC} + R_{BC}} \qquad \textbf{(1-38)}$$

$$R_B = \frac{R_{AB} R_{BC}}{R_{AB} + R_{AC} + R_{BC}} \qquad \textbf{(1-39)}$$

$$R_C = \frac{R_{AC} R_{BC}}{R_{AB} + R_{AC} + R_{BC}} \qquad \textbf{(1-40)}$$

In general

$$R_x = \frac{\text{product of two adjacent resistors}}{\text{sum of all three resistors}} \qquad \textbf{(1-41)}$$

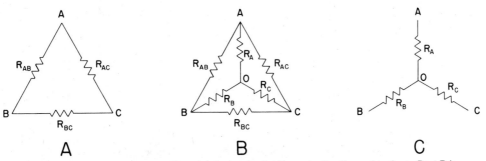

Figure 1-12 The transformability of delta to wye is shown by the three drawings. Part B is not a legitimate equivalent to parts A and C, but merely a superposition.

From wye to delta

$$R_{AB} = R_A + R_B + \frac{R_A R_B}{R_C} \qquad \textbf{(1-42)}$$

$$R_{AC} = R_A + R_C + \frac{R_A R_C}{R_B} \qquad \textbf{(1-43)}$$

$$R_{BC} = R_B + R_C + \frac{R_B R_C}{R_A} \qquad \textbf{(1-44)}$$

In general

$$R_{xy} = \text{resistor } x + \text{resistor } y$$

$$+ \frac{\text{product of resistors } x \text{ and } y}{\text{remaining resistor}} \qquad \textbf{(1-45)}$$

While no proof for the validity of these equations is given here, you can check the consistency of the equations by substituting one set into the other.

EXAMPLE 1-11

Find the total current in Figure 1-13.

Solution: Figure 1-13A shows the same circuit as Figure 1-11 only it has been redrawn to emphasize the location of the delta's present. (This circuit is a type of Wheatstone bridge, which will be discussed later.) To demonstrate the usefulness of this approach, we will apply the delta–wye transformation

to the top delta of this new diagram. Figure 1-13B shows the wye in place of the delta in the circuit.

$$R_6 = \frac{R_3 R_5}{R_3 + R_5 + R_4}$$

$$R_6 = \frac{5.6 \cdot 10^3 \times 8.2 \cdot 10^3}{5.6 \cdot 10^3 + 8.2 \cdot 10^3 + 6.8 \cdot 10^3} = 2.23 \text{ k}\Omega$$

$$R_7 = \frac{R_3 R_4}{R_3 + R_5 + R_4}$$

$$R_7 = \frac{5.6 \cdot 10^3 \times 6.8 \cdot 10^3}{20.6 \cdot 10^3} = 1.85 \text{ k}\Omega$$

$$R_8 = \frac{R_4 R_5}{R_3 + R_5 + R_4}$$

$$R_8 = \frac{6.8 \cdot 10^3 \times 8.2 \cdot 10^3}{20.6 \cdot 10^3} = 2.71 \text{ k}\Omega$$

The solution from this point can be obtained by the use of series and parallel formulae. A brief mathematical summary without explanation is given below.

$$R_9 = R_7 + R_1$$

$$R_9 = 1.85 \cdot 10^3 + 10 \cdot 10^3 = 11.85 \text{ k}\Omega$$

$$R_{10} = R_8 + R_2$$

$$R_{10} = 2.71 \cdot 10^3 + 22 \cdot 10^3 = 24.71 \text{ k}\Omega$$

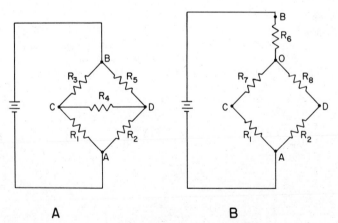

A   B

Figure 1-13   The use of a delta to wye transformation to reduce a bridge circuit to a simple network. This is the same circuit as Figure 1-11.

$$R_{11} = \frac{R_9 R_{10}}{R_9 + R_{10}}$$

$$R_{11} = \frac{11.85 \cdot 10^3 \times 24.71 \cdot 10^3}{11.85 \cdot 10^3 + 24.71 \cdot 10^3} = 8.01 \text{ k}\Omega$$

$$R_{12} = R_6 + R_{11}$$

$$R_{12} = 2.23 \cdot 10^3 + 8.01 \cdot 10^3 = 10.24 \text{ k}\Omega$$

$$I_t = \frac{E}{R_{12}} = \frac{58}{10.24 \cdot 10^3}$$

$$I_t = 5.7 \cdot 10^{-3} \text{ A}$$

This is effectively the same answer, with allowance for rounding, that we got before. It is now possible through back substitution to obtain all the currents and voltages in the circuit. ■

The delta–wye transformation probably does not reduce the total length of the solution of most problems, but it certainly permits a closer connection between the mathematics and the problem. It is easier to find a mistake or realize that the solution is making nonsense. Consequently these transformations are frequently used on complicated problems.

Section 1-7
SUPERPOSITION

The last method to be discussed here as a means of analyzing a complex circuit is superposition. This method is only applicable when two or more power supplies are present in a circuit. A typical example is given in Figure 1-14. We could use Kirchhoff's laws to solve this problem by creating two loop equations. Superposition, however, enables us to avoid these multiple equations and to solve the problem as the sum of two simple circuits. To apply superposition to a problem with N power supplies, one draws N figures that have the resistors and wires in the same place as the initial figure, but that have only one power supply each. The remaining power supplies are replaced with wires. One solves each of these single-power problems separately and then algebraically adds the individual solutions together to get the final solution.

EXAMPLE 1-12

Find the current in all branches of the circuit in Figure 1-14A.

Solution: The first step is to draw two new circuits (number of power supplies equals 2) each with only one battery, as done in Figure 1-14B. Next, as in any current problem, we pick the most probable current direction in each new circuit separately. These need not be the same between the various diagrams for any branch. Next we proceed to find all the currents in the various diagrams separately.

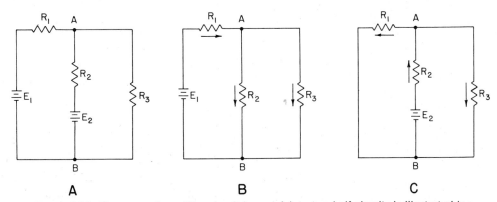

Figure 1-14 The separation of the circuit in part A into two half circuits is illustrated in part B. The technique is called superposition and requires all corresponding values to be re-added to give a final solution. (E_1 = 30 V, E_2 = 40 V, R_1 = 220 Ω, R_2 = 330 Ω, R_3 = 560 Ω.)

In the first diagram,

$$R'_p = \frac{R_2 R_3}{R_2 + R_3}$$

$$R'_p = \frac{330 \times 560}{330 + 560} = 208 \ \Omega$$

$$R'_t = R_1 + R'_p$$

$$R'_t = 220 + 208 = 428 \ \Omega$$

$$I'_1 = \frac{E_1}{R'_t} = \frac{30}{428}$$

$$I'_1 = 0.070 \ A$$

$$E'_A = E_1 - I'_1 R_1$$

$$E'_A = 30 - 0.070 \times 220 = 14.6 \ V$$

$$I'_2 = \frac{E'_A - E'_B}{R_2}$$

$$I'_2 = \frac{14.6 - 0}{330} = 0.044 \ A$$

$$I'_3 = \frac{E'_A - E'_B}{R_3}$$

$$I'_3 = \frac{14.6 - 0}{560} = 0.026 \ A$$

In the second diagram,

$$R''_p = \frac{R_1 R_3}{R_1 + R_3}$$

$$R''_p = \frac{220 \times 560}{220 + 560} = 158 \ \Omega$$

$$R''_t = R_2 + R''_p$$

$$R''_t = 330 + 158 = 488 \ \Omega$$

$$I''_2 = \frac{E_2}{R''_t} = \frac{40}{488}$$

$$I''_2 = 0.082 \ A$$

$$E''_A = E_2 - I''_2 R_2$$

$$E''_A = 40 - 0.082 \times 330 = 12.9 \ V$$

$$I''_1 = \frac{E''_A - E''_B}{R_1}$$

$$I''_1 = \frac{12.9 - 0}{220} = 0.059 \ A$$

$$I''_3 = \frac{E''_A - E''_B}{R_3}$$

$$I''_3 = \frac{12.9 - 0}{560} = 0.023 \ A$$

This completes all the preliminary calculations. The final currents are obtained by the algebraic sum of the individual currents. Note well that this means the direction of the current must be taken into account. Currents in the same direction through a wire add; currents in the opposite directions subtract.

$$I_1 = I'_1 - I''_1$$

$$I_1 = 0.070 - 0.059 = 0.011 \ A$$

$$I_2 = I'_2 - I''_2$$

$$I_2 = 0.044 - 0.082 = -0.038 \ A$$

$$I_3 = I'_3 + I''_3$$

$$I_3 = 0.026 + 0.023 = 0.049 \ A$$

(all signs relative to Figure 1-14B)   ■

This brings us to the end of the discussion of current flow in resistance circuits. The material presented here is by no means exhaustive, but it should give you a feel for how current distributes itself among the resistors in a circuit. This knowledge will serve as necessary background when you study the more complicated elements of the circuits that make up real instruments in the clinical laboratory.

REVIEW QUESTIONS

1. Define potential energy.
2. How are potential energy and kinetic energy related?
3. Define circuit.

4. Define current. What physically is "electrical current"?

5. What is Ohm's law?

6. Define electromotive force.

7. Define ampere.

8. Define volt.

9. Define ohm.

10. Define coulomb.

11. Give the metric prefixes and their meanings.

12. Define watt.

13. Define distributiveness.

14. Define series. How is Ohm's law written for series resistors?

15. Define voltage drop. Why is it also called *IR* drop?

16. Define voltage division.

17. What is a potentiometer?

18. Why is a potentiometer more useful than a group of equal resistors in series?

19. How does the position of a contact arm of a potentiometer vary compared with the voltage?

20. Why does putting more resistors in series with the same power supply decrease the total power dissipated?

21. How is Ohm's law written for series batteries?

22. Why does one pick the negative end of a battery to be zero volts?

23. Define parallel. How is Ohm's law written for parallel resistors?

24. Define equivalent resistance.

25. Why is the equivalent resistance less than any of the component resistances in a parallel circuit?

26. Derive the formula for three parallel resistors in the same form as Eq. 1-28.

27. Write the power dissipated in terms of the total current for a parallel circuit.

28. Why is Ohm's law stated $E_A - E_B = IR$ over resistors?

29. What is the purpose of redrawing figures?

30. Which figure in a series of network reductions is most valid?

31. What is a simple resistor network?

32. What is Kirchhoff's first law?

33. What is Kirchhoff's second law?

34. How many independent equations from Kirchhoff's laws are there for a network with N nodes? With M loops?

35. What is the general formula for the delta to wye transformation?

36. What is the general formula for the wye to delta transformation?

37. What is the criterion for applying superposition?

38. Why is the algebraic sum used to combine the currents when using superposition?

39. What are the essential considerations in assigning directions to current flow?

40. How does one realize if current flow was chosen incorrectly?

PROBLEMS

1. A resistor of 47 kΩ is attached across a battery of 4.5 V. How much current will flow? What amount of power is dissipated?

2. If a kilowatt-hour is 1 kW being dissipated for 1 hr, how many joules are equal to 1 kW-hr?

3. If a battery of 20. V is attached to a resistor of $1.0 \cdot 10^4$ Ω, what is the current through the resistor?

4. By how much would one have to reduce the voltage in Problem 1-1 to reduce the power dissipated by one-half?

5. A circuit has two resistors in series with a battery. The voltage is 9.3 V and the current is 0.074 A. If one resistor is 41 Ω, what is the value of the other resistor?

6. In Figure 1-15A, the voltage is 42 V; R_1, R_2, and R_3 are, respectively, 27 Ω, 330 Ω, and 560 Ω. What is the current?

7. What is the resistance of R_2 in Figure 1-15A if the voltage is 4.0 V, the current is 0.100 A, R_1 is 5.0 Ω, and R_3 is 10.0 Ω?

8. What would the current be if the resistance of R_2 in Problem 1-7 were doubled?

9. Give the voltage drop across each component in Problem 1-7.

10. The voltage in Figure 1-15A is 89 V and the current is 21.3 mA. If resistor R_2 is 1.14 kΩ and resistor R_3 is 1.92 kΩ, what is the value of R_1?

11. What would the current be if the resistance of R_3 in Problem 1-10 were increased by 50%?

12. Give the voltage drop across each component in Problem 1-10.

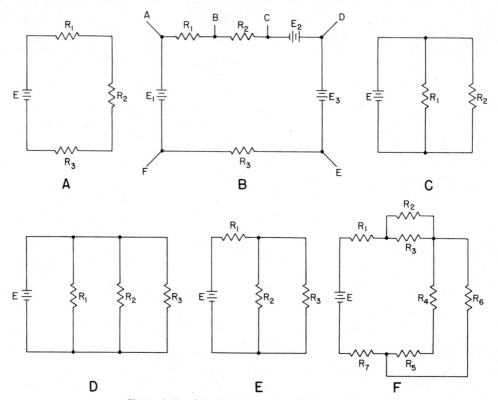

Figure 1-15 Circuits for Problems 6 through 29.

13. Two resistors are in series with a battery producing 31.6 V. If R_1 is 72% as large as R_2, what is the voltage drop across each resistor?

14. Calculate the voltage needed in Figure 1-15A to dissipate $3.0 \cdot 10^2$ W of power if R_1, R_2, and R_3 are 20 Ω, 37 Ω, and 18 Ω, respectively.

15. A potentiometer is 8.00 cm long and has a voltage of 14.9 V applied across it. What is the voltage measured with respect to the negative end of the battery at 6.81 cm from the negative terminal?

16. Redo the calculations asked for in Example 1-6 assuming that point C of Figure 1-7 is 0 volts.

17. Assuming that point F Figure 1-15B is ground ($E = 0$), give the voltages at points A through E. In this circuit $E_1 = 20.0$ V, $E_2 = 10.0$ V, and $E_3 = 5.0$ V. The values of R_1, R_2, and R_3 are 0.150 kΩ, 0.050 kΩ, and 0.300 kΩ, respectively.

18. Assuming that E_2 is replaced in the circuit backward, redo Problem 1-17.

19. Assuming that E_2 is replaced by a resistor of 0.250 kΩ, redo Problem 1-17.

20. In Figure 1-15C, if $E = 50.0$ V, $I = 0.83$ A, and $R_1 = 1.00 \cdot 10^2$ Ω, what is the value of R_2?

21. What is the current in Figure 1-15C if the voltage is 7.7 V, $R_1 = 28$ kΩ, and $R_2 = 2.2$ kΩ?

22. What is the current in Figure 1-15D if the voltage is 14.5 V, $R_1 = 56$ kΩ, $R_2 = 48$ kΩ, and $R_3 = 39$ kΩ?

23. What percentage of the current flows through each resistor in Figure 1-15D if R_1, R_2, and R_3 are 21 Ω, 26 Ω, and 41 Ω, respectively?

24. What is the current through each branch of Figure 1-15E if the voltage is 1.84 V, $R_1 = 4.7 \cdot 10^4$ Ω, $R_2 = 9.1 \cdot 10^4$ Ω, and $R_3 = 1.36 \cdot 10^5$ Ω?

25. The voltage in Figure 1-15E is 20. V, the current is 0.40 A, and R_2 is 60. Ω. If $R_1 = R_3$, what is the value of R_1?

26. The voltage in Figure 1-15E is 32.2 V, the current is 54.5 mA, and R_3 is 587 Ω. If $R_2 = 79\%$ of R_1, what are R_1 and R_2?

27. If the resistors in Figure 1-15E are light bulbs of resistance 100. Ω and E supplies 100. V, how much power is dissipated?

28. If the power supply in Figure 1-15E produces 73 V and the resistors R_1, R_2, and R_3 are 119 kΩ, 82 kΩ, and 67 kΩ, respectively, how much current flows through R_2?

29. Using successive reduction, calculate the current in all branches of Figure 1-15F. (*Note:* Use I_i to indicate current through R_i.) In this network, $E = 100.0$ V, $R_1 = 10.0$ kΩ, $R_2 = 20.0$ kΩ, $R_3 = 30.0$ kΩ, $R_4 = 40.0$ kΩ, $R_5 = 50.$ kΩ, $R_6 = 60.$ kΩ, and $R_7 = 70.$ kΩ.

30. Using successive reduction, calculate the current in all branches of Figure 16A. In this network $E = 9.8$ V, $R_1 = 17.2$ Ω, $R_2 = 25.1$ Ω, $R_3 = 38.3$ Ω, $R_4 = 44.6$ Ω, $R_5 = 58$ Ω, $R_6 = 66$ Ω, and $R_7 = 81$ Ω.

31. Using successive reduction, calculate the current in all branches of Figure 1-16B. Give the voltage between each of the components. In this diagram, $E_1 = 21.6$ V and $E_2 = 9.7$ V. R_1 through R_6 are, respectively, 740 Ω, 1.33 kΩ, 680 Ω, 2.02 kΩ, 202 Ω, and 88 Ω.

32. Interchange resistors R_1 and R_3 in Figure 1-11A and solve the problem again.

33. Using Kirchhoff's laws and successive reduction, calculate the current in all branches of Figure 1-16C. In Figure 1-16C, $E = 50.$ V, $R_1 = 100.$ Ω, $R_2 = 80.$ Ω, $R_3 = 60.$ Ω, $R_4 = 50.$ Ω, $R_5 = 40.0$ Ω, and $R_6 = 20.0$ Ω.

34. Assume that R_4 is attached at B instead of A in Figure 1-16C. Find the current through all the resistors, using the values in Problem 1-33.

35. For the following resistors in a delta configuration, calculate the corresponding values of resistors in a wye configuration.

    A. $R_{AB} = 218$ Ω B. $R_{AB} = 6.7$ kΩ
        $R_{AC} = 251$ Ω $R_{AC} = 12.8$ kΩ
        $R_{BC} = 309$ Ω $R_{BC} = 9.1$ kΩ
    C. $R_{AB} = 36$ kΩ
        $R_{AC} = 3.6$ kΩ
        $R_{BC} = 360$ Ω

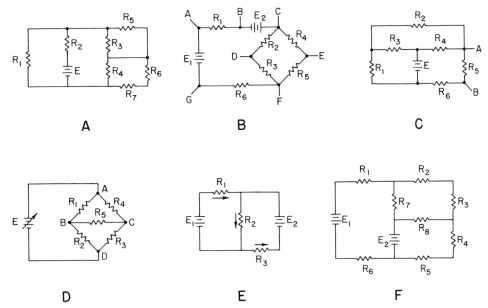

Figure 1-16 Circuits for Problems 30 through 42.

36. For the following resistors in wye configuration, calculate the corresponding values of resistors in a delta configuration.

    A. $R_A = 22.0$ kΩ   B. $R_A = 14.0$ Ω
    $R_B = 57$ kΩ $R_B = 23.0$ Ω
    $R_C = 64$ kΩ $R_C = 31.0$ Ω
    C. $R_A = 770$ Ω
    $R_B = 930$ Ω
    $R_C = 1.02$ kΩ

37. Calculate the voltage so that 0.100 A flows through R_5 in Figure 1-16D. In this circuit, $R_1 = 70.$ Ω, $R_2 = 60.$ Ω, $R_3 = 30.0$ Ω, $R_4 = 40.0$ Ω, and $R_5 = 50.$ Ω.

38. Calculate the voltage so that 0.100 A flows through R_4 in Figure 1-16D, using the values given in Problem 1-37.

39. In Figure 1-16E, $E_1 = 22.7$ V, $I_1 = 12.7$ mA, $I_2 = 50.8$ mA, $I_3 = 38.1$ mA, $R_1 = 470$ Ω, $R_2 = 330$ Ω, and $R_3 = 560$ Ω. What is the value of E_2?

40. Assume that voltage E_1 and resistors are the same as given in Problem 1-39 for Figure 1-16E. If $E_2 = 29.6$ V, what are I_1, I_2, and I_3?

41. Assume that the polarity of battery E_2 is reversed in Problem 1-40. What are the current values?

42. Figure 1-16F gives a challenging network. By any means that you care to try, calculate the current through each branch of the circuit. Each of the power supplies and resistors in this network has the value of its subscript times 100 and is known to a precision of 1 part in 200.

CHAPTER 2
MEASUREMENT OF ELECTRICITY

If voltage, current, and resistance have a definite value in a circuit, it ought to be possible to measure them. To make such measurements will require that we use principles of nature not yet discussed. These involve the interaction between electricity and magnetism, a phenomenon discussed in some detail later in this book. The place we must start is current meters.

Section 2-1
CURRENT METERS

One observable effect of the interaction between electricity and magnetism is that if a wire runs through a magnetic field perpendicular to it, and if a current flows through that wire, then a physical force will occur on the wire that will attempt to push it perpendicular to both the field and the current. Figure 2-1 illustrates the previous statement, showing in which direction that wire will be pushed. The amount of force applied to the wire will be proportional to both the strength of the magnetic field and the amount of current passing through the wire. By holding the field strength constant, which can be done by using a permanent magnet, the force becomes directly proportional to the current. While this is theoretically possible, it has not been practical to build a device that applies this principle so directly.

The way in which the principle is actually applied is illustrated in Figure 2-2. In Figure 2-2A, a wire loop is placed in the magnetic field. As the current flows through the wire, it flows upward through one side of the loop, but downward through the second side. Thus one side is pushed away from the viewer and the other side toward the viewer. If the center

of the loop of wire is fixed, the effect of the current flowing through the magnetic field in the loop will be to turn the loop until each side of the loop is equidistant from the magnetic poles. The tendency to turn the loop, called the torque, is again proportional to both the magnetic field strength and the current passing through the loop. Since the torque of a single loop is very small for modest-size currents, the torque is increased by wrapping a large number of loops (dozens to hundreds) in the same plane as the first loop. This multiplies the torque of a single loop by the number of loops, thereby making the effective torque relatively large. As shown in Figure 2-2B, the object around which these wire loops are wrapped is a soft iron cylinder that improves the quality of the magnetic field.

Two additional elements are necessary to make reliable measuring devices. The first is a pair of coil springs that can be unrolled only by applying an increasingly larger amount of torque (Fig. 2-2C). If these are used to hold the wire-wrapped metal core in place, the core will turn only until the torque resulting from the current passing through the magnetic field is balanced by the force exerted by the springs as they try to regain their unextended position. To determine how far the coil moves, a needle is attached to the axis of the core and a scale is placed below the needle. This scale is calibrated in units of current that are going through the coil. A drawing of such a device is shown in Figure 2-3. It is called a moving-coil galvanometer or a D'Arsonval meter, after Jacques Arsène d'Arsonval, the French physicist who devised it.

Note that the meter described and pictured is of the simplest type. Numerous enhancements have been added over the years to improve the reliability of the meter, such as jeweled pivots, needle stops, multiple scales, and shunts. Some of these will be

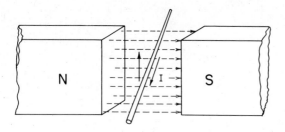

Figure 2-1 When current flows through a wire perpendicular to a magnetic field, the wire is pushed in a direction perpendicular to both the direction of the magnetic field and the current flow.

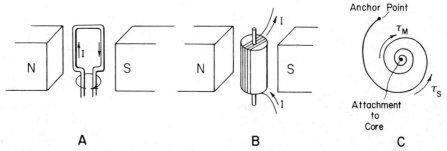

A   B   C

Figure 2-2 The wire loop in part A turns in the magnetic field because the forces on the opposite sides are in opposite directions. The core in part B tends to rotate with a force proportional to the number of turns of wire, the amount of current, and the strength of the field. The spring in part C unwinds as the core turns, exerting a force proportional to the distance it has been turned.

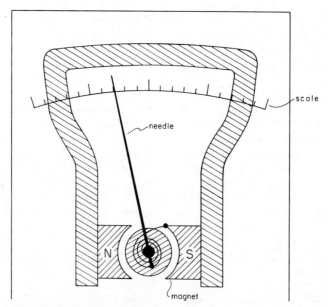

Figure 2-3 A simple D'Arsonval meter is used to measure the flow of current.

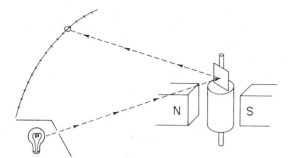

Figure 2-4 A light shines on a mirror and is reflected onto a scale.

discussed later. This type of meter is used extensively in electronics today.

A less commonly used current measuring device based on this same principle is the reflecting galvanometer. This device has the core suspended by filaments, and a mirror is mounted on top of the core. As the core attempts to rotate, the filaments are twisted. Their resistance to this twisting becomes proportionally stronger as they are twisted further, until they counteract the torque of the current. The final position is therefore proportional to the current applied. A light is shone on the mirror from a fixed position. As the mirror turns, this light is reflected at a greater angle. The distance the image of the light appears from its rest (no current) position is a measurement of the value of the current (Fig. 2-4).

Early reflecting galvanometers for sensitive work were huge, filling an entire room and using marks on the wall to indicate current values. Experimenters would follow the position of the light beam and mark its location versus time to follow an experiment. The extensive use of mirrors and lenses has reduced the size of the laboratory galvanometer to about the size of a bread box. Because of the advent of the oscilloscope and operational amplifier, the galvanometer has lost its previous usefulness in chemical laboratory investigations.

Section 2-2
THE AMMETER

The common D'Arsonval meter is very sensitive, deflecting to full scale (maximum reading at 100 to

200 μA; that is, 1.0–2.0 · 10^{-4} amps). The meter is also a weak resistor, owing to the inherent resistance of the wire and the energy absorbed in traversing the magnetic field. This resistance is usually less than 100 ohms. To use such a meter successfully it is necessary to keep in mind its inherent full scale and resistance properties.

To measure current we must have the current flow through the meter. A D'Arsonval meter used as an ammeter (to measure amps) must therefore be in the current stream; that is, it must be in series, as shown in Figure 2-5A. The current flowing through the circuit must go through the meter, thereby giving its value to the meter position. The meter can be used for any value of current up to its full-scale readings, although current less than a few percent of full scale will be difficult to see because there is very little needle movement.

Unfortunately, most currents in common electronic equipment are far above 100 μA, and our meter appears to be doomed for general work. The usefulness of the meter can be extended, however, by the use of a shunt around the meter. Figure 2-5B shows a shunt in position. Because the shunt is in parallel with the meter, some of the current flows through the shunt, avoiding the meter. The percentage of the total current that flows through the shunt instead of through the meter is a function only of the value of the meter and shunt resistances and is independent of the amount of current flowing. Consequently, if one picks the right value of shunt resistance, one can move most of the current around the meter, thereby protecting it from burning up. An example will illustrate the point.

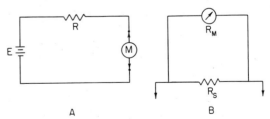

Figure 2-5 The position of a current meter in part A is in series with the circuit being measured. A shunt in part B is placed in parallel with a current meter to allow most of the current to be diverted around the meter. (The arrows indicate the leads for attachment to a circuit.)

EXAMPLE 2-1

The meter in Figure 2-5B has a full-scale deflection at 131 μA and a resistance of 87 Ω. What is the value of the shunt resistor needed to make an instrument that has a full-scale deflection of 0.0100 amps?

Solution: Note that at full scale only $1.31 \cdot 10^4$ A can flow through the meter, and the resistance of the meter is 87 Ω. Therefore, at full scale the voltage over the meter must be *IR* or $1.31 \cdot 10^{-4} \times 87 = 1.14 \cdot 10^{-2}$ V. Because the shunt resistor R_s is in parallel, the voltage over it must be the same. All the current that does not flow through the meter must flow through the shunt; therefore, $0.0100 - 1.31 \cdot 10^{-4} = 9.87 \cdot 10^{-3}$ A must flow through the shunt. If we know the voltage over the shunt and the current through it, Ohm's law gives us its resistance:

$$R_s = \frac{E}{I} = \frac{1.14 \cdot 10^{-2}}{9.87 \cdot 10^{-3}} = 1.16 \; \Omega \quad \blacksquare$$

One problem with the manufacture of the shunt resistors is worth noting. Resistors of small resistance, much less than 1 ohm, are extremely hard to build accurately, since their resistance is so close to that of wire. Consequently, when a meter must be built to handle relatively large currents, it may be necessary to artificially increase the resistance of the meter and therefore the size of the needed shunt resistor by placing a resistor in series immediately before the meter (e.g., if the added resistor increases the effective meter resistance tenfold, the shunt resistor can also increase tenfold with no change in current division).

The use of a shunt greatly extends the usefulness of the moving coil meter. Moreover, there is no reason to limit oneself to only one combination of resistors. Figure 2-6 shows a number of resistors so positioned that only one of them at a time can be used to augment the meter resistance. Each of these resistors is so calibrated compared with the shunt that it will take a known percentage of the current when added in series to the meter resistance. It is therefore possible to have a series of parallel scales on the meter face. The selection knob at A allows the desired current division to be

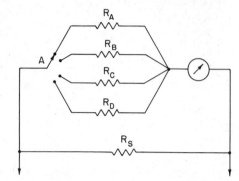

Figure 2-6 A group of shunts can be used to allow one meter to make measurements in several different current ranges.

chosen and the value of current to be read on the corresponding scale.

Although the shunt greatly extends the useful range of the meter, it does not protect the meter from careless use. It is still possible to damage or destroy the meter by connecting it to a current supply that is too large for the selected scale. Before inserting a meter, one should estimate the amount of current present. To minimize the chances of damage, a meter should always be set on its least sensitive (largest) range, and initial contact should be momentary to determine whether even this scale of the meter is exceeded. If so, the meter cannot be used directly in making the measurement. If not, the meter should be placed into the circuit, the power applied, and the approximate value noted. If the value is smaller than the maximum of the next scale, the selection knob should be moved to the next most sensitive scale and the observation repeated. When it is no longer possible to move to a more sensitive scale and still keep the needle on scale, the best possible value has been obtained and should be noted.

The ammeter, as mentioned, must be placed in series in the circuit in order to be useful. Since it is in itself a resistor, the ammeter adds to the total resistance in the circuit. Because the voltage in the circuit remains constant, the current must drop. Therefore, the introduction of an instrument to measure current causes a change in the current being measured. The amount of the error is called the relative error (*E%*) and is given by the expression

$$E\% = \frac{I - I_\text{m}}{I} \times 100\% \qquad (2\text{-}1)$$

I is the current with the meter absent, and I_m with the meter present. Since it is impossible to obtain I (if the meter is present one gets I_m, and if it is absent one gets no reading at all), it is necessary to rearrange this expression by substituting for I and I_m. Let E be the total voltage, R the total resistance without the meter, and R_m the resistance of the meter. (Note that all these quantities can be measured independently.) Then,

$$I = \frac{E}{R} \qquad (2\text{-}2)$$

$$I_\text{m} = \frac{E}{R + R_\text{m}} \qquad (2\text{-}3)$$

Substituting in Eq. (2-1),

$$E\% = \frac{E/R - E/(R + R_\text{m})}{E/R} \times 100\%$$

$$E\% = \frac{1/R - 1/(R + R_\text{m})}{1/R} \times 100\% \qquad (2\text{-}4)$$

Multiplying by R,

$$E\% = \left(1 - \frac{R}{R + R_\text{m}}\right) \times 100\%$$

$$E\% = \frac{R_\text{m}}{R + R_\text{m}} \times 100\% \qquad (2\text{-}5)$$

EXAMPLE 2-2

A meter with 53 Ω resistance reduced the current in a circuit to 83% of its previous value. What was the resistance of the circuit?

Solution:

$$E\% = 100 - 83 = 17\%$$

$$E\% = \frac{R_\text{m}}{R + R_\text{m}} \times 100\%$$

$$17\% = \frac{53}{R + 53} \times 100\%$$

$$0.17R + 9.0 = 53$$

$$R = 260 \ \Omega \qquad \blacksquare$$

Section 2-3
THE VOLTAGE METER

Meters respond to current and not to voltage. This is because the deflection of the meter is proportional to the movement of a wire in a magnetic field, which is proportional to the product of the current and the field strength. Very fortunately, the voltage is equal to the current times the resistance, in accordance with Ohm's law. Therefore, if the resistance is a constant for a certain meter, the voltage is proportional to the current, which is proportional to the deflection of the meter. If the meter is calibrated in units of voltage, it can be used to measure that quantity, provided it is properly inserted in the circuit.

Let us first examine the construction of a voltmeter. Over any simple meter there is a voltage drop when the meter is placed in a circuit. This occurs because the meter has a small internal resistance. Since a meter cannot tolerate a very large current, the maximum voltage drop that a simple meter can have over it is also small, on the order of a few hundredths or thousandths of a volt, as calculated in the previous section (e.g., $E = IR$, if $I = 10^{-4}$ A and $R = 50$ Ω, then $E = 5 \cdot 10^{-3}$ V). To measure larger voltages, therefore, it is necessary to increase the resistance of the meter. This is accomplished, as shown in Figure 2-7A, by placing a larger resistor in series with the simple meter. The resistance of the voltmeter is then the total of that of the meter and the supplemental resistor. By making this resistance high enough, it is possible to measure voltage of thousands of volts with a meter that deflects full scale to 10^{-4} A.

The voltmeter, as we have constructed it, will measure the potential difference between the two ends of the meter. To use this meter, we must attach it at two points of different potential in a circuit. Instead of placing the meter in series, as with the ammeter, the voltmeter is attached "across" an element in the circuit, that is, in parallel with part of the circuit, as shown in Figure 2-7B. Note that the circuit element measured across need not be a battery. Any element over which there is a potential difference may be measured across, and the potential difference across the device will be the value read on the meter. If no potential difference exists, the reading is zero.

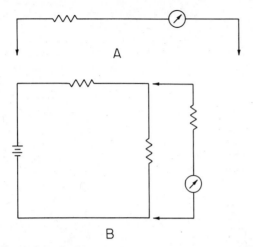

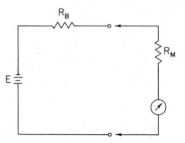

Figure 2-9   When a voltmeter is used to measure the voltage of a battery, the internal resistance of the battery and the meter form a voltage divider so that only the portion of the voltage lost over the voltmeter is measured by it.

Figure 2-7   A resistance in series with a meter is used to reduce the flow of current through the meter in part A. To measure the voltage across an element in a circuit, the voltmeter must be placed in parallel with the element as shown in part B.

The voltmeter, like the ammeter, can have several scales on the same meter face. This is accomplished as demonstrated in Figure 2-8 with a switch-selectable resistor nest. As with the ammeter, the highest available scale should be used initially, and only momentary contact should be made. In case of the wrong polarity or a too insensitive scale, the appropriate adjustments should be made to get the most accurate reading possible.

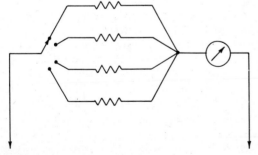

Figure 2-8   A group of attenuating resistors can be used to allow one meter to make measurements in several different voltage ranges.

When a voltmeter is used to measure the voltage of a battery, the circuit shown in Figure 2-9 is formed. Note that the battery has an internal resistance R_B as well as a voltage. The reading of the meter E_m is only the part of the voltage dropped over the meter and not the total voltage of the battery because part of the voltage of the battery is lost in the IR_B drop over the battery. Only when no current is being drawn from a battery can the voltage of the battery be measured accurately. At all other times, the voltage of the battery will be decreased by the IR_B drop. If I is large, this can be substantial. The relative error in a voltage measurement by a meter that draws a finite amount of current is given by

$$E\% = \frac{E - E_m}{E} \times 100\% \qquad \textbf{(2-6)}$$

The total voltage is composed of the voltage over the battery resistance and that over the meter

$$E = E_B + E_m$$

Substituting this value gives

$$E\% = \frac{E_B + E_m - E_m}{E_B + E_m} = \frac{E_B}{E_B + E_m} \times 100\% \qquad \textbf{(2-7)}$$

Since $E_B = IR_B$ and $E_m = IR_m$, we have

$$E\% = \frac{IR_B}{IR_B + IR_m} = \frac{R_B}{R_B + R_m} \times 100\% \qquad \textbf{(2-8)}$$

This final equation shows that the smaller the resistance of the battery and the larger the resistance of the meter, the more accurate the measurement of the voltage and, incidentally, the better the performance of the battery as a power source.

Not only does a voltmeter affect the voltage of a battery, it also affects the voltage drop over any component across which it is attached. For example, the voltage drop over resistor R_1 in Figure 2-10 is 10 volts without a meter being present. This is because it is one of three equal resistors in series with a 30-volt battery. If a meter is attached across R_1, a parallel circuit is formed. In a parallel circuit, as shown in Chapter 1, the equivalent resistance is less than that of either component. Consequently, the $R_1 \| R_m$ combination has a lower resistance than R_2 and R_3. Since the same amount of current flows through each element in the series, the voltage drop must be lower as well. The voltage drops over R_2 and R_3 are each greater than 10 volts, and the drop over R_1 is less than 10 volts. Consequently, the introduction of the meter affects the entire circuit. This effect can be minimized by using a voltmeter with a high internal resistance compared with the resistance over which the measurement is being made. If R_m is greater than $10^2 \cdot R_1$, the $R_1 \| R_m$ combination effectively equals R_1 to the ability that most simple meters can measure.

EXAMPLE 2-3

The resistance of the meter in Figure 2-10 is $98 \cdot 10^3$ Ω. What is the relative error that the presence of the meter introduces into the circuit?

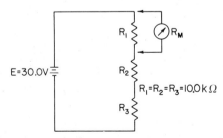

Figure 2-10 A voltage division occurs when resistance is in series. Placing a meter across one resistor will reduce its value, perhaps significantly, and cause a redistribution of voltages over all resistors.

Solution:

$$R_T = R_1 + R_2 + R_3 = 30.0 \text{ k}\Omega$$

$$I = \frac{E}{R} = \frac{30.0}{30.0 \cdot 10^3} = 1.00 \cdot 10^{-3} \text{ A}$$

$$E_{R_1} = IR_1 = 1.00 \cdot 10^{-3} \times 10.0 \cdot 10^3 \text{ A}$$

$$E_{R_1} = 10.0 \text{ volts}$$

$$R_1 \| R_m = \frac{R_1 R_m}{R_1 + R_m}$$

$$= \frac{10 \cdot 10^3 \times 98 \cdot 10^3}{10 \cdot 10^3 + 98 \cdot 10^3}$$

$$R_1 \| R_m = 9.07 \cdot 10^3 \ \Omega$$

$$R_T = R_1 \| R_m + R_2 + R_3$$

$$= (9.07 + 10 + 10) \cdot 10^3$$

$$= 29.1 \cdot 10^3$$

$$I = \frac{E}{R_T} = \frac{30.0}{29.1 \cdot 10^3}$$

$$= 1.03 \cdot 10^{-3} \text{ A}$$

$$E_m = I \times R_1 \| R_m = 1.03 \cdot 10^{-3} \times 9.07 \cdot 10^3$$

$$= 9.35 \text{ V}$$

$$E\% = \frac{E_{R_1} - E_m}{E} \times 100\%$$

$$E\% = \frac{10.0 - 9.35}{10.0} = 6.5\%$$
∎

Section 2-4
THE RESISTANCE METER

We have measured current in a circuit because the meter deflection was proportional to a constant magnetic field times the current. We have been able to measure the voltage by using Ohm's law and holding the resistance constant to permit the voltage to vary directly with the current. If we try to measure the resistance with our simple current meter, we must again use Ohm's law, only this time holding the voltage constant. With the voltage constant, the current will vary inversely with the resistance ($I = E/R$) so that greater resistance will mean less, not more current. This inverse relationship is bound to increase the complication of measuring resistance.

Figure 2-11 shows the circuit for a simple resistance meter, called an ohmmeter. It consists of a constant voltage supply E, a meter with a maximum scale current I_{max}, and a variable resistance R_v. Note that for the sake of simplicity, the resistance of the voltage supply R_B and the meter R_m is incorporated into R_v, since all the resistances are in series. When not in use, no current flows through the meter. When the meter is in use, an unknown resistance R_u is placed between A and B, the probes of the meter. Since the resistances are in series, the expression for the current is

$$I = \frac{E_B}{R_v + R_u} \qquad (2\text{-}9)$$

To use this meter, it is necessary to calibrate it. When R_u is 0, that is, when the probes of the meter are touched to each other (shorted), a certain amount of current flows. Consequently, we can set the meter to the full scale mark by changing R_v until $I = I_{max}$.

$$I = I_{max} = \frac{E_B}{R_v} \qquad (2\text{-}10)$$

On the other hand, any nonzero value of R_u reduces the value of I. If $R_u = \infty$, that is, if the probes are unattached and no closed circuit exists, the current is 0. This is the second point of our calibration. The undeflected position means infinite resistance and the full deflected position means zero resistance for R_u.

If we examine several other points on the meter, we come to an alarming conclusion. If $R_u = R_v$, then $I = \frac{1}{2}I_{max}$.

$$I = \frac{E_B}{R_v + R_u} \qquad (2\text{-}11)$$

If $R_u = R_v$

$$I = \frac{E_B}{R_v + R_v} \qquad (2\text{-}12)$$

$$I = \frac{1}{2}\frac{E_B}{R_v}$$

$$I = \frac{1}{2}I_{max}$$

since

$$I_{max} = \frac{E_B}{R_v}$$

If $R_u = 2R_v$, then $I = \frac{1}{3}I_{max}$, and so forth. This means that the midpoint on the scale between ∞ and 0 is R_v. Moreover, one-half the distance between ∞ and R_v is $3R_v$. In short, the scale is not linear. Resistances less than R_v are spread out on the right side of the typical meter, while all the resistances from R_v to ∞ fall on the left side of the meter. Figure 2-12 shows the typical face of an ohmmeter. Unlike the measurements of the voltmeter and ammeter, the reading of the ohmmeter shows no relative er-

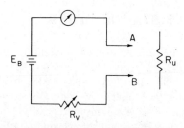

Figure 2-11   The ohmmeter consists of a circuit which can be calibrated to a known current when the probes are shorted and which will give a percentage of that current when an external resistor is inserted between the probes.

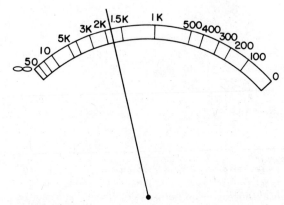

Figure 2-12   The ohmmeter is nonlinear in resistance.

ror, because the component being measured is isolated from any other circuit effects.

In order to use an ohmmeter with resistors of different sizes and still obtain precise readings of the resistance, it is necessary to have multiple scales, so when possible, readings can be made on the right half of the scale. Since R_v, the value of the resistance of the meter, is the center of the scale, one must increase or decrease the resistance of the meter to scale the unknown resistance. This is not as straightforward as it sounds, however, because the meter must still read full scale after the resistance is altered; several schemes are available to do this, one of which is shown in Figure 2-13. The selection switch is connected so as to change both sets of resistors simultaneously. Therefore, when R_{1A} is selected, so is R_{1B}, and so on. The resistors are matched so that as the value of the A resistance is reduced to decrease the resistance of the meter, the B resistance is also reduced, so less of the available current flows through the meter. A small variable resistance is still needed in series with the meter to compensate for the slight imbalance in the resistor networks as one moves from scale to scale. Each scale should be calibrated separately as it is used in order to get accurate readings.

EXAMPLE 2-4

When a 470 Ω resistor is tested with an ohmmeter, the meter deflects to 82% full scale. What is the internal resistance of the ohmmeter?

Solution:

With resistor

$$I = \frac{E_B}{R_v + R_u}$$

Without resistor

$$I_{max} = \frac{E_B}{R_v}$$

Substituting for E_B

$$I = \frac{R_v I_{max}}{R_v + R_u}$$

$$R_v + R_u = \frac{R_v I_{max}}{I}$$

$$\left(1 - \frac{I_{max}}{I}\right) R_v = -R_u$$

$$R_v = \frac{R_u}{(I_{max}/I) - 1}$$

$$R_v = \frac{470}{(1/0.82) - 1}$$

$$= 2,140 \ \Omega \qquad \blacksquare$$

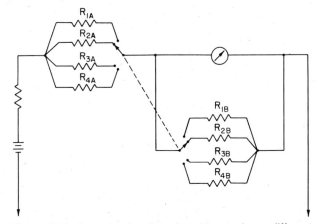

Figure 2-13 In order for the ohmmeter to have different ranges and still read full scale when shorted, a connected double set of resistors is needed to control the total current flowing and the percent of the current going through the meter.

Section 2-5
THEORY OF MEASUREMENT

To make a measurement, one must engage in a process called "mapping." The quantities that we wish to measure in the laboratory—the physical properties, such as conductivity, color, density, or turbidity—are useful only if they vary in magnitude for different samples of the same type. The concentration of sodium, for example, varies between specimens, and this is meaningful. In order to compare these magnitudes of quantities, we must attach numbers to them. The physical properties are in what one can call the physical domain, whereas the numbers are in the numeric domain. Mapping is the method of defining numbers to represent the magnitude of physical properties. The physical domain is mapped into the numeric domain to give us numbers that represent real quantities.

To get from the physical domain to the numeric domain, it is frequently, but not always, convenient to go through the electronic domain whose properties (attributes) include voltage, current, and resistance. To get from one domain to another, it is necessary to use a conversion device called a transducer. The transducer converts a physical attribute (e.g., color) into an electronic quantity (e.g., voltage) or an electronic quantity (e.g., voltage) into a numeric value (e.g., 43). Various transducers from the physical to the electronic domain will be discussed later in this book. Transducers from the electronic to the numeric domain are the meters that we introduced in the first part of this chapter. The quality of a measurement is totally dependent on the accuracy of the transducer, that is, how closely the transducer renders the value of the equivalent quantity in the new domain to the value of the quantity in the old domain. In complex measurements, domain boundaries may be mapped across numerous times to get a numeric result, and each transducer in the process is important. On the other hand, a weight transducer, such as a scale, goes directly from a physical quantity weight to the corresponding number that represents that weight.

The purpose of performing a measurement is to measure the quantity of interest both accurately and precisely. Precision can be gained by having an appropriate scale on the meter that gives good significance within the range of the answer, that is, in the middle or upper part of the scale, where relative error is small. Accuracy depends on the principle used in the measurement and on how badly the circuit is disturbed by the presence of the measuring device. As we have seen, resistance can be accurately measured by a current meter, albeit nonlinearly, but voltage and current cannot be. Moreover, the precision of each of these measurements is affected by the inability to get more than two significant figures from the average meter face.

To circumvent these difficulties in making accurate measurements, a new technique must be used. It is called "null balance." When using the current meter as a direct measuring tool, it may (1) be nonlinear, (2) have decreased sensitivity caused by resistor networks, or (3) affect the circuit being investigated. To avoid these inaccuracies, the null balance approach uses the current meter only to check whether the desired quantity being measured is electronically balanced against a similar quantity generated by the measuring device. The current meter in this approach will be measuring those small current differences that it is best designed to handle. We will begin our study of this principle with an examination of a Wheatstone bridge.

The Wheatstone bridge, as pictured in Figure 2-14, is composed of 4 resistors and a meter. Two of the resistors are fixed in value and are chosen for the particular measurement at hand. The third resistor is a variable resistor whose value is linearly proportional to the position of some contact arm. Such variable resistors are known in electronics as

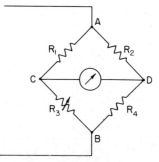

Figure 2-14 A Wheatstone bridge is a null balance device that can be used to measure resistance very accurately.

potentiometers or "pots" because they can be used to divide the "potential" over the resistor into two parts in certain usages. The fourth resistor is the unknown resistor that we wish to measure. The meter is very sensitive to current flow and can deflect in either direction.

To understand how a Wheatstone bridge works, one must derive the equation governing it. Let us begin by assuming that the meter portion of the circuit does not exist. By Ohm's law,

$$I_3 = \frac{E_A - E_B}{R_1 + R_3} \qquad (2\text{-}13)$$

$$I_4 = \frac{E_A - E_B}{R_2 + R_4} \qquad (2\text{-}14)$$

$$E_C = E_B + I_3 R_3 \qquad (2\text{-}15)$$

$$E_C = E_B + \left(\frac{E_A - E_B}{R_1 + R_3}\right) R_3 \qquad (2\text{-}16)$$

$$E_D = E_B + I_4 R_4 \qquad (2\text{-}17)$$

$$E_D = E_B + \left(\frac{E_A - E_B}{R_2 + R_4}\right) R_4 \qquad (2\text{-}18)$$

At balance

$$E_C = E_D \quad \text{(i.e., the meter reads zero)} \quad (2\text{-}19)$$

Therefore,

$$E_B + \left(\frac{E_A - E_B}{R_1 + R_3}\right) R_3 = E_B + \left(\frac{E_A - E_B}{R_2 + R_4}\right) R_4 \qquad (2\text{-}20)$$

$$\frac{(E_A - E_B)R_3}{R_1 + R_3} = \frac{(E_A - E_B)R_4}{R_2 + R_4}$$

$$\frac{R_3}{R_1 + R_3} = \frac{R_4}{R_2 + R_4} \qquad (2\text{-}21)$$

$$R_3 R_2 + R_3 R_4 = R_1 R_4 + R_3 R_4 \qquad (2\text{-}22)$$

$$R_3 R_2 = R_1 R_4 \qquad (2\text{-}23)$$

$$\frac{R_4}{R_3} = \frac{R_2}{R_1}$$

$$R_4 = \frac{R_2 R_3}{R_1} \qquad (2\text{-}24)$$

This equation governs the operation of the Wheatstone bridge when in balance. When out of balance,

the calculation becomes much more complex, as seen in Chapter 1.

EXAMPLE 2-5

When an unknown resistor is placed as R_4 in the Wheatstone bridge, the value of R_3 at balance is 431.3 Ω. If resistors R_1 and R_2 are reversed, the value of R_3 needed to balance the bridge is 108.8 Ω. What is the value of R_4?

Solution: Write the equations for the two cases

$$R_3' = \frac{R_4 R_1}{R_2} = 431.3$$

$$R_3'' = \frac{R_4 R_2}{R_1} = 108.8$$

Solve each for R_1/R_2 and set them equal:

$$\frac{R_1}{R_2} = \frac{431.3}{R_4} = \frac{R_4}{108.8}$$

$$R_4^2 = 431.3 \times 108.8$$

$$R_4 = 216.6 \ \Omega \qquad \blacksquare$$

What can be applied to resistors can also be applied to a voltage source isolated from a circuit. The standard device for doing this is a laboratory potentiometer, as shown in Figure 2-15. Let us first examine the top loop of the circuit. A battery capable of generating a relatively constant current of 10 mA at a constant voltage over a number of minutes is necessary. The voltage may vary over the period of several days, but must not vary significantly during the experimental period. An accurately known resistor, 101.8 Ω in this example, is needed as well as a uniform slidewire resistor (or potentiometer) that has 10.00 Ω resistance at full length. The final variable resistor need not be calibrated, but must be able to be adjusted very accurately. To use the laboratory potentiometer in measuring a voltage source, this upper circuit must be adjusted by use of the variable resistor to allow 10.00 mA to flow. When this is accomplished, the voltage drop across the 101.8 Ω precision resistor will be 1.018 V.

To determine when this voltage drop is reached, the lower left-hand circuit is used. This loop con-

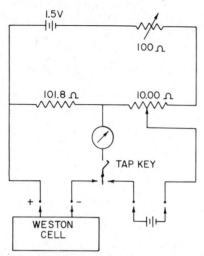

Figure 2-15 A laboratory potentiometer is a device that has a main circuit whose current flow can be very accurately calibrated against a reference. Unknown voltages can then be measured by balancing them against a percentage of a known voltage drop over a variable resistor. The voltage of a Weston cell is 1.018 V.

tains a tap key for making momentary contact, a meter or a galvanometer for noting the direction of the current deflection, a selection switch, and a standard Weston cell. The Weston cell is diagrammed in Figure 2-16. It is represented by the following cell expression:

$$Cd(Hg)\|CdSO_4 \cdot 8/3\ H_2O_{sat}, Hg_2SO_{4sat}\|Hg$$

At 25°C, the saturated cell has a voltage of 1.018 V, which it holds accurately if no current demands are made and if the temperature is held constant. The chemical equation supplying the voltage is

$$Cd + Hg_2SO_4 \rightleftharpoons CdSO_4 + 2Hg$$

In the potentiometer circuit, when the voltage drop across the precision resistor is 1.018 V, it is exactly equal to the voltage drop over the Weston cell, which is in the circuit backward. When this condition is reached, the voltage on each side of the meter is the same when the tap key is pushed, and therefore no deflection occurs. Consequently, it is possible to set the current precisely in the upper

circuit without polarizing, and therefore destroying, a precision voltage reference source.

If the current in the upper circuit is precisely 10.00 mA, then the voltage over the slidewire is exactly 100.0 mV. Because the slidewire is precisely calibrated with regard to the contact position, it is possible to set the contact arm accurately for any voltage between 0 and 100 mV. If we have an unknown voltage source within this range, it can be inserted between the contacts in the lower right-hand circuit and the selector switch thrown to that loop. The slidewire is then positioned so that the voltage drop over the slidewire up to the contact arm is exactly equivalent to the voltage of the battery. When this happens, as before, the meter sees no net current and is undeflected when the tap key is pushed. One can then read the voltage from the position of the slidewire. This device can be accurate to a few tenths of a percent. A regular voltmeter is accurate to within a few percent.

The principle employed here is null balance. Because no current is drawn from the unknown volt-

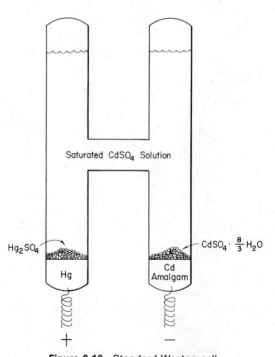

Figure 2-16 Standard Weston cell.

age source during the measurement, the resistance of the voltage source is irrelevant. By use of larger batteries and different resistors it is possible to extend this technique to other voltage ranges. Because null balance involves the negating of current flow, it cannot be applied directly to current measurement.

The major limitation of the laboratory potentiometer is that it is too slow to use in monitoring many ongoing reactions. To follow a chemical reaction, the readings have to be taken every few seconds in many cases, and preferably continuously. The solution to this problem is to automate the laboratory potentiometer. To accomplish this, the calibration scheme must be simplified, the slidewire contact must be connected to a motor that runs in either direction, depending on the current polarity, and the meter must be replaced with an amplifier as illustrated in the block diagram of Figure 2-17. There is no tap key in the circuit. When the voltage of the source is larger than that of the reference, the

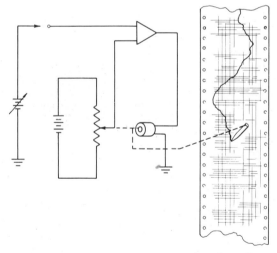

Figure 2-17 In a servo-driven recorder, the voltage difference between an unknown source and the reference source is amplified and used to drive the reference source in the direction needed to reduce the voltage difference to zero. A pen on a moving chart is so attached that its position reflects the voltage of the reference source, and therefore also the unknown source. (The triangle indicates an amplifier.)

motor runs to increase the reference voltage. When the voltage is less, the motor runs in the opposite direction to decrease the reference voltage. The position of the reference voltage contact indicates the value of the unknown voltage. To present these data to the experimenter, the same mechanical system that drives the position of the reference voltage drives a pen on a recorder as well. A time axis is added to the recorder by driving the chart paper past its pen at a constant speed (Fig. 2-17).

The device that results from this modification is a strip chart recorder. It is frequently called a servo recorder or a servomechanical recorder because it is self-correcting and uses mechanical means to accomplish the correction. The quality of the recorder is highly dependent on the quality of the amplifier and the mechanical linkage. The amplifier must amplify the difference between the two signals and produce a large output voltage in the appropriate direction, depending on which signal is greater. It is very important that the output rapidly flip from one state to the other when the amplifier inputs pass through equality. If this does not happen, the pen will drive in the wrong direction for too long, and the recorder will overshoot the correct position. The original amplifiers were chopper stabilized, which meant that they cut back and forth between the two signals rapidly to get reproducibility by comparing values with zero. Today adequately stable difference amplifiers exist to handle this task, as will be discussed in Chapter 6.

The second problem of the servo recorders is in the mechanical linkage. It is necessary to eliminate all play in the linkage. Such play can cause the motor to move slightly without corresponding changes in the reference voltage or pen position. This type of occurrence reduces the sensitivity of the instrument. Linkage inertia can also be a problem. It may take time for the movement of the motor to be translated into action throughout the recorder. This can cause overshooting and inexact pen positioning for a fast reaction. Such problems must be tested for before a recorder can be used for a particular experiment.

Most servo recorders have a series of scales to permit the experimenter to keep the pen on the chart paper. These can be implemented either electronically or mechanically. The servo recorder is designed to measure voltage, but it can be used with current sources as well, if the appropriate input circuits are used. The electronic principles will be considered in our discussion of operational amplifiers.

Section 2-6
OSCILLOSCOPE

While the servo-driven recorder is one of the most important inventions for scientific investigation and laboratory analysis, it also has the limitations mentioned above. In particular, it responds too slowly to signals that occur within fractions of a second. This means that many phenomena cannot be measured by these recorders. To measure these more rapid phenomena, the oscilloscope was developed, the active portions of which are sketched in Figure 2-18. The prime advantage of the oscilloscope is that it is a totally electronic device; there are no moving parts as in a meter or recorder pen. Consequently, the motion of the signal is several orders of magnitude (powers of 10) faster than the partially mechanical measuring devices. Because oscilloscopes are frequently used as parts of analytical equipment, a thorough examination of this instrument is well warranted.

The device sketched in Figure 2-18 is properly called a cathode ray tube (CRT); it is the heart of both the oscilloscope and the television. At the left end is a negatively charged metal plate, which is heated so that electrons boil off the surface. This is called the electron gun or cathode because it is the source of the electrons that make the CRT work.

Electrons emitted from the cathode can fall back to the cathode or they can leave the area. The design of the tube enables electrons to leave in only one direction. In this direction there is a porous grid, which is slightly negative with respect to the cathode. The more negative this grid is, the fewer electrons can leave through it.

The electrons do leave through it, however, because there is a charged ring that is 500–600 volts more positive than the cathode. The charge difference causes the electrons to accelerate toward this ring (called an anode). Because the ring is hollow, the place of greatest attraction is the center. The electrons tend to rush toward this spot and thereby focus into a beam or ray. This gives the tube its name, "cathode ray," because a ray comes from the cathode. The momentum of the electrons carries them through the first ring anode and then into the field of a second ring anode whose voltage is 10–15 times more positive than the first. This causes the beam to accelerate rapidly through the middle of the anode and into the space between the deflection plates.

The deflection plates are used to position the beam as it emerges into the right end of the tube. The plates are basically flat surfaces whose trailing edges curve away from the beam so that it does not collide with them as it bends. There are two sets of two plates each. The first set of plates is horizontal and is called the vertical deflection plates. A difference in voltage between these two plates will cause the beam to bend in the direction of the more positive plate. Since this deflection is toward one of the plates, it is perpendicular to the plane of the plates; therefore, the horizontal plates really do cause verti-

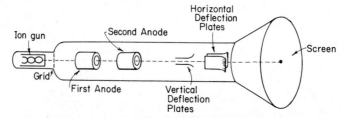

Figure 2-18 A cathode ray tube directs a beam of electrons onto a phosphorized screen. The position of the beam is determined by the value of signals placed on the vertical and horizontal deflection plates.

cal deflection. The second set of plates is vertical, being perpendicular to the first, and is called the horizontal deflection plates. The beam is again bent toward the more positive plate. As a result, the path of the emergent beam is bent at an angle in both the horizontal and vertical direction to that of the incident beam.

The beam proceeds until it encounters a fluorescent screen at the far right end of the tube. The electrons activate the phosphors they strike, causing them to emit light, which is visible against an otherwise dark screen. If the screen is ruled, the position of the dot caused by the electron beam striking the screen can be measured to within 1 or 2%. If several electron guns are focused on the screen and a correct choice is made of differently colored phosphors, one has a color television.

The various parts of the CRT must be accurately controlled to get good results. Several control knobs work with the parts already discussed. The grid voltage is manipulated by the intensity control. By making the grid voltage more negative, the number of electrons that can get through the grid is decreased, as is the number of phosphors activated on the screen. The converse is also true. The focusing control adjusts the voltage on the first anode relative to the second. This changes the point at which the beam reaches its focus. By appropriate adjustment, this focus can be moved to the surface of the screen, giving a sharp image.

The signal measured by the oscilloscope is applied to the horizontal and vertical plates. The circuit to accomplish this is extremely complex, but the principle is illustrated by the circuit in Figure 2-19. The lower plate has half the voltage of the power supply across it. The voltage on the upper plate can be varied from zero to the total voltage of the power supply. By changing the position of the contact point, we can vary the potential on the upper plate from highly positive to highly negative relative to the lower plate. Therefore, the electron beam will be deflected up or down accordingly. The actual input circuit behaves in much the same way. Ground is offset by a voltage generated internally and is applied to one plate. The signal is amplified, offset by the same amount, and applied to the other plate.

Two controls on the front of the scope are associ-

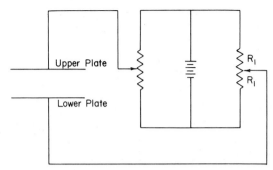

Figure 2-19 In an oscilloscope, one plate is offset from zero and the other is offset either more or less depending on the input signal. In this diagram the voltage on the lower plate is fixed while the voltage on the upper plate can be made greater or less than the lower.

ated with the input circuit. The first is the offset. The offset voltage applied to the signal plates can be varied slightly by the user so that the point at which the signal is at ground need not be in the center of the screen, but can be moved up or down, depending on whether the phenomenon one wishes to observe is mostly above or below ground. A switch to short the signal to ground for such "zero positioning" is usually provided so that it is not necessary to touch the probe to ground to make this adjustment. The second control changes the amplification factor applied to the signal before it is offset. This is similar to the scaling function on a volt-ohm meter.

Oscilloscopes generally have two input channels. Frequently the oscilloscope permits one signal to be applied to the vertical deflection plates and the other signal to the horizontal deflection plates. A dot is formed at the coordinate determined by these two inputs. If either or both signals vary rapidly, this dot will move quickly across the screen and will be hard to follow. If the pattern is regular, however, the eye will see what appears to be a line along the path that the rapidly moving dot is tracing over again and again. For this reason these lines are called traces.

Most measurements made with the oscilloscope are not done with one input against the other, the so-called x–y plot. Instead, for most measurements, one or both inputs are graphed against time. To accomplish this, the input signal is applied to the vertical deflection plates, and a time signal is applied to the horizontal deflection plates. This time signal is generated as shown in Figure 2-20A. When the voltage is zero, the deflection occurs to the left side of the screen (viewed from the front). As the voltage rises, the deflection moves toward the right-hand edge until it crosses it. At this instant in time, the voltage is suddenly reduced to zero, causing the beam to return rapidly to the left side of the screen. A voltage signal that increases or decreases at a uniform rate is called a ramp. Because this ramp is restarted periodically, it looks jagged and is called a "sawtoothed" ramp. The generation of such a ramp is relatively simple and will be discussed in Chapter 6. To prevent the returning-to-zero portion of the time signal from showing on the screen, the intensity of the beam is diminished momentarily while the beam passes over the screen from right to left. This process is called blanking.

The movement from left to right across the screen permits changes in the voltage signal input with time to be seen as irregularities in the otherwise smooth line. By having the time sweep continually restarted, it is possible to follow an event over a period of time. Unfortunately, most events of interest are so fast that only if they repeat themselves at regular intervals will they reinforce the image on the screen often enough to be seen. If the time signal source, called the time base generator, reinitializes the sweep as soon as it reaches the edge of the screen, the signal phenomena will appear randomly on the screen and will not reinforce each other unless, by chance, the frequency of the restart is exactly a multiple of the frequency of the phenomena.

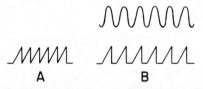

A   B

Figure 2-20 In part A the sweep is free running, restarting as soon as it has reached the maximum position. In part B the sweep is triggered (started) only when a specific voltage level on the rising wave is reached.

Such an occurrence is called synchronization. Continuous sweeping is called a free running trigger because the signal is "fired" as soon as the ramp is discharged. Synchronization can be obtained by careful varying of the output frequency of the time base generator, but this is difficult to achieve.

To handle many repetitive signals, it is desirable to hold the frequency of the time base generator to a known value, so that accurate measurements of the frequency of the signal can be made. Figure 2-20B shows that this is accomplished by not reinitializing the sweep as soon as possible, but by waiting until some predetermined point on the input signal is seen. Such a point can be picked by a triggering control that permits the user to select an appropriate voltage magnitude and direction (rising or falling) at which the trace should be started. Because each new trace begins at the same position on the input wave, the signals reinforce and can be seen as a solid line on the screen. In addition to picking the frequency of the time base generator (speed at which the ramp rises) and the triggering point, the user can position the start of trace with respect to the left side of the screen.

When two input channels exist, it is possible to display both at once on the screen. This permits the comparison of two signals. When doing so, it is frequently desirable to offset the zero voltage position of the two traces so that they do not fall directly on top of each other. To show the two signals simultaneously, they are either displayed in rapid succession, one trace and then the other (called alternate mode), or the input signals are applied alternately to the plates in such a rapid fashion that the two lines are actually drawn at the same time, alternating points. The last method is called "chopped mode" and is most commonly used at low frequencies. Alternate mode is used at high frequencies so the frequency of the chopper will not distort the traces.

The oscilloscope is not a null balance device. It differs from a voltmeter only in that its input resistance is so high (1 or 10 MΩ) that the effects on ordinary circuits are insignificant. But because all measurements are made in comparison with ground, in order to get a true measurement of the signal voltage across a circuit element, it is necessary to attach one probe to each side and apply the difference between them to the vertical deflection plates.

The above discussion of the oscilloscope is much simplified and generalized. The use of several grids and anodes is common. Magnetic as well as electronic deflection is used in some instances. Such refinements are not necessary to understand the working of the oscilloscope, but can be found in advanced texts for the interested reader.

The making of measurements involves various trade-offs. The most accurate technique, null balance, is limited by the speed of the equipment. Measuring current is limited by the ability to cut into the circuit, a difficult task if it is a printed circuit. An oscilloscope is good, but costs 20 times as much as a volt-ohmmeter (VOM) and can only measure voltage. The selection of the appropriate means of measurement depends on what is to be measured and how accurately it must be measured. A careful application of the rules of electronics that have been covered can serve as a useful guide.

REVIEW QUESTIONS

1. On what physical principle is the D'Arsonval meter based?
2. What is the deflection of a wire in a magnetic field proportional to?
3. Why does a loop in a magnetic field turn when current is applied?
4. What is torque?
5. Why are multiple loops of wire used to wrap a core?
6. How does the D'Arsonval meter work?
7. How does a reflecting galvanometer work?
8. What principle is used to reduce the sensitivity of the D'Arsonval meter?
9. Give two reasons why the scheme described in the text to reduce the current meter sensitivity is used instead of simply reducing the number of wire loops on the meter core.
10. Why are multiple shunts used in the ammeter?
11. Suggest an ammeter design that would have multiple scales but that would only add about 1 ohm of resistance to the circuit being measured, regardless of the scale used.
12. Why is low resistance desirable in an ammeter?
13. How can a D'Arsonval meter be used to measure voltage?
14. Why is a voltmeter placed in parallel instead of in series?
15. How does the use of attenuating resistors in a voltmeter differ from the use of shunts in an ammeter?
16. Graph the effect of increased current flow on the measurable voltage of a battery.
17. Why does the resistance of a voltmeter affect the reading it produces?
18. Why is an ohmmeter nonlinear in resistance?
19. How is an ohmmeter calibrated? What is its relative error?
20. What is the center position on an ohmmeter?
21. Why is scaling on an ohmmeter so complicated?
22. What is a domain?
23. What is a transducer?
24. Define null balance.
25. What is the advantage of null balance over direct techniques?
26. Draw the Wheatstone bridge circuit.
27. Why is a Wheatstone bridge better at measuring resistance than an ohmmeter?
28. How does a laboratory potentiometer work?
29. What is the reaction in a Weston cell?
30. Diagram a laboratory potentiometer and label its parts.
31. Sketch a Weston cell and label its parts.
32. What is the voltage of a standard Weston cell?
33. What is the function of a tap key?
34. Diagram a servo recorder and label its parts.
35. How does a servo recorder work?
36. What are potential problems with a servo recorder?
37. Diagram a CRT and label its parts.
38. How does a CRT work?
39. How is the electron beam focused?
40. How are signals applied to the CRT?
41. What is the purpose of the grid, anodes, and deflection plates in a CRT?
42. How is offset accomplished? What is it?
43. Why does a trace appear on the screen?
44. What is the x–y plot?
45. What is a sawtoothed wave?
46. How is a time axis put on the screen?

47. What is triggering?
48. What is blanking?
49. What is the difference between alternate mode and chopped mode?
50. Why is an oscilloscope more like a VOM than a laboratory potentiometer?
51. Why does one use an oscilloscope in place of a VOM or a laboratory potentiometer?

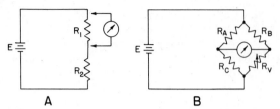

Figure 2-21 Circuits for Problems 8 and 13.

PROBLEMS

1. A meter, like the one in Figure 2-5A, has a full-scale deflection for a current of 189 μA. Its internal resistance is 114 Ω. What is the value of the shunt resistor needed to make an instrument that has a full-scale deflection of 0.0150 A?

2. An ammeter has a full-scale deflection of 12.0 mA. Its shunt resistance is 1.27 Ω and its current meter deflects full scale at 108 μA. What is the resistance of the current meter?

3. An ammeter with an internal resistance of 39 Ω reduces the current in a circuit by 5.2%. What was the resistance of the circuit initially?

4. A circuit with a resistance of 984 Ω and a voltage of 2.95 V has a current measuring 2.83 mA on an ammeter. What is the resistance of the meter?

5. If the relative error is 8% when a voltmeter with an internal resistance of $2.0 \cdot 10^4$ Ω is used to measure a battery, what is the internal resistance of the battery?

6. When a voltmeter with an internal resistance of 33.6 kΩ was used to measure the voltage of a battery, the relative error was only 64.0% as great as when a voltmeter with 20.0 kΩ of internal resistance was used. What is the internal resistance of the battery?

7. In Figure 2-10, assume that the resistance of the meter is 67 kΩ and the value of the resistors is 10kΩ times their subscripts. What is the relative error in voltage measurement if the voltage is 30.0 V?

8. Estimate the internal resistance of the voltmeter in Figure 2-21A if the relative error in the voltage over R_1 is to be less than 1%; E is 65.3 V, R_1 is 2.87 kΩ, and R_2 is 9.61 kΩ.

9. If an ohmmeter has an internal resistance of 1,560 Ω, what percentage of full scale will the meter deflect to when measuring a 2,200 Ω resistor?

10. If the needle on an ohmmeter deflects 60% of full scale for resistor R_1, what will be the deflection for a resistor R_2 that has twice the resistance of R_1?

11. In Figure 2-14, assume R_1 is 735.7 Ω and R_2 is 843.8 Ω. What is the value of resistor R_3 if resistor R_4 is 644.3 Ω?

12. In a Wheatstone bridge in which resistor R_1 is 1.276 times R_2 and resistor R_4 is 0.916 times R_3, what is the value of R_1 in terms of R_2 at balance?

13. In the Wheatstone bridge shown in Figure 2-21B, resistors R_A, R_B, and R_C are unknown at balance. R_V is 48 Ω. If R_A, R_B, and R_C are interchanged to all possible positions, at balance, R_V is either the original 48.0 Ω, 3.0 Ω, or 8.33 Ω. What are the values of R_A, R_B, and R_C, respectively?

CHAPTER 3
PHYSICAL BASIS
OF ELECTRONIC PRINCIPLES

In the first two chapters we have looked at the flow of electrical current in terms of quantities that we called voltage and resistance. We have discussed various devices used to assign numeric values to these quantities. The quantities, as well as the other electrical concepts we shall soon encounter, have their basis in the physical properties of atoms and molecules. By examining these, we can better understand why materials exhibit the electrical properties they do.

Section 3-1
CURRENT AND RESISTANCE

In nature, the number of positive and negative charges is equal. If one chooses the appropriately sized box, one will always find the number of positive charges (protons) equal to the number of negative charges (electrons). The smallest box is the atom. A neutral atom has the same number of protons and electrons. Most atoms can form molecules, and these too are electrically neutral, that is, they have the same number of positive and negative charges in their natural state.

Both atoms and molecules can become ionized. In order for this to happen, they must lose or gain electrons and, in the process, become positively or negatively charged. At this point the box called an "atom" or a "molecule" is no longer big enough to be electrically neutral, so a larger box must be defined. This may be an ion pair, a molecular cluster, or a beaker. It may even be cubic miles of sky, as when a thunderstorm occurs. Nevertheless, a box of finite size always exists which encloses an electrically neutral collection of particles.

An electric field is created when positive and negative charges are separated inside an appropriate box. In chemistry, such a box can be a beaker or flask holding an ionic solution (Fig. 3-1). If electrodes are placed into the solution and an external power source is applied to the electrodes to create a potential difference between them, an electric field is created. There will be a force of attraction F between the electrically charged species that will be directly proportional to the product of their charges q and inversely proportional to the square of the distance d between the charges:

$$F \propto \frac{q_1 q_2}{d^2} \tag{3-1}$$

Since electrodes cannot move toward each other, the ions in the solution will move. Therefore, a physical displacement of positive and negative charge in the solution will occur. This movement of charge is, of course, nothing but the flow of electrical current. In this case, both the positive ions and the negative ions carry the current. The amount of current that can be carried will be directly proportional to the concentration of the ions present, a fact that will be used as a measurement method later, and inversely proportional to the size and mass of the ions. This ability to carry current when a voltage is applied is called conductivity and is given the symbol σ (sigma). In order for the conductivity to go up, the resistance to current flow must decrease. Therefore, resistance times conductivity is equal to a nonzero constant. By choosing

43

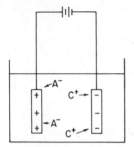

Figure 3-1 A beaker is a box that contains electrical neutrality. Current is carried internally by the movement of ions toward fixed electrodes.

the appropriate unit size, this constant can be made to be 1:

$$R\sigma = 1 \quad \text{or} \quad R = \frac{1}{\sigma} \qquad (3\text{-}2)$$

This means that it is possible to relate the electrical quantity of resistance to more elementary physical properties as mass, size, charge, temperature, and concentration.

When one looks at a solid, the carriers of charge, that is, current, cannot be ions. Even when ions exist, such as in solid NaCl, they are locked into a crystal structure that does not permit them to move freely. The only charged particle capable of moving in a solid is the free electron.

Electrons exist in solids in atomic or molecular orbitals. Within the shells of every atom, there are a number of locations for electrons to occupy. When all the positions are full in a shell, there is no room for any additional electrons to enter. These configurations are so stable that it is hard to remove an electron. This means there are few "holes" for electrons to fall into and few electrons moving around. As a consequence, electrons do not move, and current does not flow through materials with full shells.

In most atoms the outer shells are not full. These shells can react with the shells of other atoms to form molecules, ionic species, or coordinate clusters. The outer shell is called the valence shell, and atoms customarily have valences that reflect the number of electrons that must be lost or gained to leave the atom with a full shell. When atoms are

together in a nonionic solid, the valence electrons interact, regardless of whether an actual compound is formed. These interactions involve the hybridizing (rearranging) of the atomic orbitals into molecular orbitals. This arrangement is called the "valence band" because the valence electrons have occupied an energy level (band) that is the minimum possible for the electrons involved. As long as the electrons remain in the valence band, as little will happen as in the case of atoms with full electron shells.

In addition to orbitals in the valence band, molecules also have orbitals of higher energy levels that are normally not filled. These levels result from the unfilled levels that existed in each atom that joined the molecule. When electrons are given more energy, they will be excited to these higher levels. Electrons in these higher levels are capable of drifting away from the molecule because they no longer contribute to its bonding. These orbitals constitute what is called the "conduction band." Electrons in these orbitals can flow from one molecule or atomic coordinated cluster to another relatively unimpeded by the atoms in the solid.

Electrons are "allowed" to be in the valence band or the conduction band, but not in any level between these bands, by the exclusion rules of quantum mechanics. The energy required for the transition from the valence band to the conduction band differs, depending on the substance. For example, for conductive metals, it is effectively zero (Fig. 3-2); for semiconductive elements, it is small; and for insulators, the transition energy is large. The ability of a substance to conduct current is thus

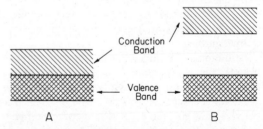

Figure 3-2 For metals the conduction and valence bands are adjacent. For insulators and semiconductors, there is an energy gap caused by the rules of quantum mechanics.

dependent on the amount of energy necessary to promote electrons from the valence band to the conduction band.

When an electron leaves its position in the valence band and is promoted to the conduction band, it leaves a hole behind it. In a conductive metal in which attraction for the valence electrons is weak, this loss is inconsequential because an electron from elsewhere is bound to fall into the position rapidly. In such a conductive metal, therefore, electrons flow freely between bands and positions randomly until an electric field is applied. Such a field causes the free electrons to move toward the positive end of the field. Since these are continually replaced with electrons from the negative end of the field, current flows through the wire from the positive to the negative end of the field. The resistance of the metal to this flow of current will vary depending on certain properties of the metal. The first is the energy difference between the valence and conduction levels for particular electrons. Although this difference is small for metals, any given electron requires some energy to move from one band to the other, thereby drifting away and causing a charge deficiency. Since all atoms of an element have the same electron structure, the energy differences can be tabulated for the various species. The second major factor affecting the resistance is the availability of pathways through the metal. The packing structure of the metal is of major importance, since it determines the molecular orbitals available for the migrating electrons, some of which conduct much better than others. Such packing schemes of the atoms can be cubic, face centered, body centered, and so forth. The particular structure that exists will be the one most energetically favorable. The molecular orbitals then act as paths for the migrating electrons. Anything that disturbs these pathways increases the resistance to electron flow. Two such disturbances are impurities and heat. The impurities cause imperfections in the packing structure, interrupting the smooth flow of electrons. Heat causes increased vibration of the atoms and distorts the pathways, making them a less effective means of carrying electrons. In contrast, when metals are cooled to near absolute zero, they become superconductive because the pathways are nearly ideal. Figure 3-3 shows the resis-

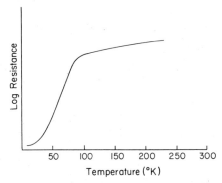

Figure 3-3 The resistance of a metal is very low near absolute zero, but increases as a function of temperature to the fifth power until near 100° Kelvin, after which it is almost linear with temperature to near the melting point of the metal.

tance of a typical metal as a function of temperature.

If one looks at insulators, one finds that they are composed of materials that have a large energy gap between the valence and conduction bands. Electrons are not able to take advantage of any conductive paths that may exist because they cannot escape their host atoms. Covalently bonded compounds of different atoms featuring mostly single bonds are particularly good insulators because they have no way of delocalizing electrical charge (e.g., nylon, wood). Note that structure can make a big difference, since carbon as graphite is conductive while carbon as a diamond is not.

Between the metal conductors and insulators in conductivity are the semiconductors. Semiconductors fall primarily in the middle of the fourth column of the periodic table. These elements, like carbon, have half-filled valence shells. Each atom in a crystal is bonded to four neighboring atoms (Fig. 3-4), and therefore reasonable pathways exist for electrons to traverse the matrix. The problem, just as it was for insulators, is that few electrons escape from their positions in the valence band to enter the conduction band. For each electron that does leave, a hole is left behind. The silicon or germanium atom, for these are the elements in the appropriate part of the periodic table, immediately attracts an electron from a neighboring atom, and

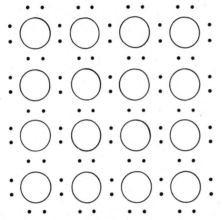

Figure 3-4 The atoms of column IV in the periodic table can form crystals in which they are bonded to their four nearest neighbors.

the hole moves over. Since the hole causes a negatively charged electron to move in one direction, it appears to be a positive charge moving the other direction. Moreover, since the electron that falls into the hole is in the valence band rather than in the conduction band, it moves independently of the initially promoted electron and behaves as an additional charge carrier. Each electron that is moved from the valence band to the conduction band therefore generates two charge carriers, the negative electron and the positive hole. Unfortunately, at room temperature, there are only on the order of 10^{13} electrons per mole in the conduction band, which means $2 \cdot 10^{13}$ total carriers. This is an ineffective number for good conductivity, and such elements have thousands of ohms of resistance per centimeter.

While semiconductors are poor conductors, they are also poor insulators, because current does flow. The small number of free electrons and holes that naturally exist are called intrinsic carriers. The number of holes is equal to the number of electrons. The product of the number of holes and electrons is like an equilibrium constant:

$$N_h \times N_e = K \qquad \textbf{(3-3)}$$

However, this constant is temperature dependent, being roughly 10^{26} at room temperature. As the temperature rises, the constant does too, causing the number of holes and electrons to rise. The greater the number of available carriers, the more current is carried, and the lower the resistance becomes. Note that this process is exactly the opposite of that which occurs when a metal conductor is heated. Although the pathways are distorted in the heating of a semiconductor, this decrease is easily overwhelmed by the increase in the conductors available. Even so, this increase in carriers is inadequate to permit a large quantity of current to flow.

To make semiconductors more conductive, it is necessary to dope them. Doping is a method of artificially increasing the number of holes or electrons. This is accomplished by adding impurities to the silicon or germanium crystal. While impurities adversely affect the conductivity of metal conductors, a small amount of the right impurity can greatly enhance the conductivity of a semiconductor.

To add an extra electron to a silicon matrix, one replaces the silicon atom with an arsenic or antimony atom. These atoms are from the fifth column of the periodic table and have five electrons. When placed in the silicon matrix, the arsenic atom must surrender one of its electrons to the conduction band, since there is no place in the valence band for it. This creates a positive electrical charge embedded in the matrix, because there is no orbital hole for the electron to occupy. The doped semiconductor is electrically neutral. It is a positive matrix containing an equal number of free negative charges. Because the electrons are free to roam and the positive charges are not, the semiconductor behaves as a ready source of electrons. This overall negative atmosphere causes semiconductors so doped to be called n-type semiconductors. Doping levels are usually one atom in 10^8 of host atoms. This increases the number of electrons to 10^{15} per mole, equal to Avogadro's number ($\sim 10^{23}$) times the extent of doping ($\sim 10^{-8}$). Since the number of electrons times the number of holes is fixed for a specific temperature (Eq. 3-3) and is not significantly affected by the minute amounts of impurities, only 10^{11} holes per mole remain ($10^{15} \cdot 10^{11} = 10^{26}$). The total number of carriers is $10^{15} + 10^{11}$, which is approximately 10^{15} carriers per mole, or 50 times that of the undoped semiconductor. Obviously, the resistance experiences a 50-fold reduction.

It is also possible to make positively doped or p-type semiconductors. In this case it is necessary to add more holes to the matrix. This can be accomplished by using atoms such as gallium or indium, which come from the third column of the periodic table. These elements have one less electron than is found in silicon. When placed in the matrix, all the molecular orbitals form, but one is empty because none of the atoms has an electron to fill it. While the area is electrically neutral, the positional hole will nevertheless draw in an electron from a neighboring silicon atom, and the hole will begin to migrate just as if it were formed by the promotion of an electron. Consequently, while the p-type semiconductor is electrically neutral just as the n-type, it has a tendency to absorb electrons to fill the holes. The p-type semiconductors are doped to the same extent as the n-type and therefore possess the exactly opposite number of holes and electrons.

As has been shown, electrical resistance can be directly related to the physical properties of atoms, molecules, and ions. One can make resistance work to one's advantage by appropriate manipulation of the physical properties on which it is based. For example, a light bulb is composed of a wire of moderate resistance which is heated by the flow of electricity to the point of incandescence. As the metal gets hotter, the resistance fortunately increases to reduce the flow of current. If the resistance were to decrease with temperature, more and more current would flow until something would burn up. The potentiometer is another example of controlled resistance. By making a special wire very uniform in diameter, the voltage division can be made a function of the position on the wire. The construction of carbon resistors for control circuits in radio and television, as well as in laboratory instruments, is possible because carbon granules that conduct can be mixed with an insulator that does not conduct. By varying the amount of carbon and insulator present and how tightly these are mated, one can produce a wide range of resistance values in resistors that are almost the same physical size, making design work considerably simpler. The concept of resistance is not magic—it is merely the inverse of

conductivity, which is the degree to which the physical properties of a substance will allow it to move charge.

Section **3-2**
BATTERIES

To move charge, one needs a potential difference. To understand the nature of such a potential difference, it is necessary to return to solution chemistry. When powdered zinc metal is placed into a suitably buffered copper sulfate solution, the zinc will begin to dissolve into solution and the copper will begin appearing on the zinc particles. This occurs because having copper metal in a solution of zinc sulfate gives a lower potential energy than having zinc metal in a copper sulfate solution. The reaction is

$$Zn + Cu^{2+} \rightleftharpoons Zn^{2+} + Cu \qquad \textbf{(3-4)}$$

The difference in potential energy will appear as kinetic energy in the form of a heated solution. While this energy may warm the room, it is lost, as far as electrical applications are concerned. We can, however, recover this energy if we construct an apparatus as shown in Figure 3-5. Here a zinc plate is placed in a dilute zinc sulfate solution, and a copper plate is placed in a concentrated copper sul-

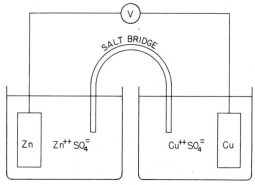

Figure 3-5 By separating two half-reactions, it is possible to obtain electrical energy rather than heat energy as one half-reaction drives the other one backward. This is the basis of the battery.

fate solution. The two solutions are connected by a salt bridge that allows a displacement of ions to occur. The copper and zinc plates are attached to the leads of a voltmeter. The following chemical reactions occur:

$$Zn \rightleftharpoons Zn^{2+} + 2e^- \qquad -0.763 \text{ V} \quad \textbf{(3-5)}$$

$$2e^- + Cu^{2+} \rightleftharpoons Cu \qquad -0.337 \text{ V} \quad \textbf{(3-6)}$$

Since the solutions cannot readily diffuse into each other, these reactions must occur at the respective metal surfaces. The electrons freed at the zinc electrode will therefore follow the path of most favorable flow and move through the meter to the copper plate. Here the extra electrons will be seized by copper ions, which then plate onto the copper strip. This reaction would quickly stop as the solutions would become charged from the net transfer of negative charge if it were not for the salt bridge. This bridge allows negative ions to flow into the bridge from the copper solution and out of the bridge into the zinc solution. As a result, the two beakers are kept electrically neutral, and the reaction continues to occur. The meter measures the difference in potential between the two electrodes, in this case the sum of the two equations given because one has already been inverted. The negative sign implies that energy is being given off, which should be obvious since electrons are being moved from one place to another. This entire system is identical in every way to the first simple reaction except that we have separated the two half-reactions such that one can use the energy from them as they occur.

The apparatus we have created here is a battery. It is called the zinc–copper battery. All batteries rely on the same basic principle—separation of two chemical half-reactions. These reactions occur at separate plates called electrodes, and the voltage they produce is the difference in the energy given up by one reaction going forward and driving the other reaction backward. Several batteries used in laboratory instruments are discussed below.

A common battery is the zinc–carbon battery, which is used in many applications. It is referred to as a dry cell because it does not involve a solution. Instead of a solution, an electrolyte paste containing manganese dioxide connects the two electrodes. One electrode is the zinc case, which en-

closes the cell and is gradually dissolved. The other electrode is a carbon rod. The carbon rod is inert, but its surface allows the transfer of an electron to the manganese dioxide. The half-reactions are given in Eqs. 3-7 and 3-8. The cell works because the electrons lost by the zinc go through an external circuit and back to the carbon rod.

$$Zn \rightarrow Zn^{2+} + 2e^- \qquad \textbf{(3-7)}$$

$$2e^- + 2H^+ + 2MnO_2 \rightarrow Mn_2O_3 + H_2O \quad \textbf{(3-8)}$$

Here they reduce MnO_2 in the paste. The paste, which also contains acid, water, manganese oxide, and salts of zinc, acts as the salt bridge between the two electrodes. The potential of a carbon–zinc battery is about 1.5 V.

The same general half-reactions are used in the alkaline battery, except that Eq. 3-9 replaces 3-8. The anode is again zinc, but the cathode is made from manganese dioxide. The electrolyte is hydrated potassium hydroxide.

$$2e^- + H_2O + 2MnO_2 \rightarrow Mn_2O_3 + 2OH^- \quad \textbf{(3-9)}$$

The alkaline battery has a much longer life than the carbon–zinc battery and can produce more current without damage. Since the same basic reactions are involved in the two batteries, the voltage is effectively the same, which makes the batteries interchangeable.

The nickel–cadmium battery adds another dimension to the dry cell because it is rechargeable. Rechargeable batteries are called secondary cells in contrast to nonrechargeable batteries, called primary cells. The anode is a cadmium–cadmium oxide electrode and the cathode is a mixture of nickel oxides. The half-reactions are given in Eqs. 3-10 and 3-11. The battery is recharged with rectified alternating current from a wall outlet (see Chapter 7).

$$Cd \rightleftharpoons Cd^{2+} + 2e^- \qquad \textbf{(3-10)}$$

$$e^- + Ni^{2+} \rightleftharpoons Ni^+ \qquad \textbf{(3-11)}$$

Although it only puts out 1.3 V, the nickel–cadmium battery is extremely durable, holding the same potential under heavy use. Being rechargeable, it has an indefinite life. However, the nickel–cadmium battery is very expensive, costing 20 or more times the price of a carbon–zinc battery.

The mercury cell is frequently used as a voltage reference in instruments. This is because it has a very constant potential during discharge. Its anode is a zinc amalgam, and its cathode is mercuric oxide. The half-reaction of the battery is given in Eqs. 3-12 and 3-13. The battery has a long shelf life and low internal resistance, but its current capacity will decrease with temperature and heavy use. Like all primary cells, it is not rechargeable.

$$Zn + H_2O \rightarrow ZnO + 2H^+ + 2e^- \quad \textbf{(3-12)}$$

$$2e^- + 2H^+ + HgO \rightarrow Hg + H_2O \quad \textbf{(3-13)}$$

The reactions in any of these batteries cannot be indefinitely sustained. While all reactions are written as proceeding in one direction, in fact, there is always a reverse reaction. As the materials on the left side of the equations are depleted and those on the right side of the equations build up, the reverse reaction becomes significant, reducing the potential of the battery. Finally equilibrium is reached, and no potential difference remains between the two electrodes. The battery is dead. The voltage sources for all circuits previously discussed have been batteries. Although individual chemical batteries have relatively low voltage, they can be used in series to generate very large voltages. The resistance we have seen in batteries is a result of internal ionic movement, which compensates for the external movement of electrons through the circuit. Later in this chapter we will introduce another type of voltage source.

Section 3-3
CAPACITANCE

Anyone who has witnessed a thunderstorm realizes how much energy is dissipated when lightning (current) moves between two oppositely charged electrified objects. What one is witnessing is the discharge of the world's largest capacitor. A capacitor is composed of three parts: two objects that can hold charge and a third between that prevents the charge from flowing from one of the charge-containing objects to the other. In the case of a thunderstorm, either the clouds and the earth or two clouds are the chargeable objects, and the air is the separator.

It is not practical to bring a thunderstorm into a laboratory or kitchen, yet capacitance is still a very useful natural phenomenon. In order to build capacitors of reasonable size, we must make some substitutions into nature's model. For the chargeable devices we will use metal plates or metal foil (Fig. 3-6). Because metals have conduction bands near their valence bands, it is relatively easy to remove a large number of electrons from one of the plates. Similarly, since the conduction band is merely a lot of unused molecular orbitals, it is relatively easy to dump a large number of electrons onto the other plate. In most capacitors, the plates are identical, and either may be made positive or negative. Each capacitor has a number that indicates the amount of charge that can be stored by that capacitor at a given voltage. This number is called the capacitance and is given by the equation

$$C = \frac{q}{E} \quad \textbf{(3-14)}$$

Capacitance is measured in farads, named after Michael Faraday. One farad is equal to 1 coulomb per volt.

The value of the capacitance will be affected by several factors. The first is the size of the capacitor plates. The more area there is, the farther the electrons or holes can spread out from each other, and the easier it is to pack in more charge. The capacitance is therefore directly proportional to the area of the plates A. The distance between the plates is also important. As the plates move closer together, the positive field around the positively charged plate attracts the electrons of the negatively charged plate, and vice versa. The result is a stabilizing effect that makes it easier to hold a larger

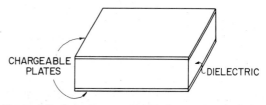

Figure 3-6 A common capacitor is composed of two chargeable plates with a nonconducting substance called a dielectric between them.

amount of charge. The capacitance is therefore inversely proportional to the distance between the two plates d. The third quantity needed to calculate the capacitance is the factor ε_0, the permittivity of free space. Its value is a constant equal to $8.85 \cdot 10^{-12}$ farads per meter and is effectively a coefficient that acts as a conversion factor between two sets of units.

The last factor affecting the capacitance is the material lying between the two plates. This material is called a dielectric and must be a very good insulator. Since the dielectric is in contact with both sides of a potential difference, it is, in effect, the wire of a circuit. The current will try to flow through it. Only by having very poor pathways for electrons and a very large energy difference between the valence and conductive bands can a dielectric prevent the current from flowing. The resistivity of a dielectric to its electrical breakdown is called the dielectric constant K, a unitless number defined as 1.0000 for vacuum. The constants of all other materials are calculated as ratios of their effectiveness to that of vacuum. These values vary from a little over 1 for gases to about 3 for organic polylmers to 5 or more for mica. Therefore, the final equation for capacitance is as follows:

$$C = \frac{K\varepsilon_0 A}{d} \qquad \textbf{(3-15)}$$

Two other comments should be made about the nature of capacitors. While the dielectric will attempt to prevent the spontaneous discharge of electrons from the negative to the positive plate, it is possible that, as in the case of a lightning bolt, the electrons will simply jump as a unit through the dielectric without resorting to typical pathways. This occurs if the voltage across the dielectric gets too high. Discharge through the dielectric will usually fuse the dielectric and thereby destroy the capacitor.

Second, not all capacitors are bipolar, meaning that they can have either plate charged negatively. Some capacitors are electrolytic. These capacitors have a metal anode (positive end) coated with a thin oxide film that serves as the dielectric between the anode and the solution, which is the cathode (negative end). Because the distance between the two charged objects is so small, the capacitance is very

large. At neutrality, or when charged in the forward direction, the capacitor works properly. If charged in the reverse direction, the oxide film dissolves and the dielectric disappears. We will discuss the use of capacitors in electrical circuits in Chapter 4.

Section **3-4**
INDUCTANCE

In order to explain the wavelengths of light generated when electrons within atoms of certain elements are excited, it was necessary to postulate an electronic spin. This spin creates a magnetic field that interacts with that of the nucleus to give the results observed. Other constraints, however, limit the spin to two possible orientations, up or down, either in line with the nuclear spin or opposite to it. When substances have a large number of atoms with all their electron spins in one shell aligned in the same direction, these substances are said to be magnetized. Because of various constraints involving the necessary electron shell levels, only iron, and to a lesser extent those elements adjacent to it in the periodic table, has the ability to become significantly magnetized.

Magnetism, as seen in a bar magnet, for example, is the result of polarizing electronic spins. The electron, however, also creates a magnetic field wherever it moves. Figure 3-7 shows that a field is set up in the plane perpendicular to a current-carrying wire. A small free-floating magnet placed at various locations around the wire will show that a magnetic field is present by its deflection, which will change

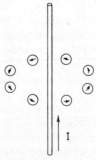

Figure 3-7 Electrons moving through a wire cause a circular magnetic field around it.

depending on where the magnet is placed. This is circular magnetism, since there is no discernible north or south from whence the field radiates. The direction of the field is determined by the right-hand rule; that is, if the thumb of the right hand points in the direction of the current, the fingers of the right hand point from the direction of magnetic north and to magnetic south around the wire. The strength of the field is proportional only to the current.

When two wires carrying current in the same direction lie close to each other, there is an attraction between them, because where the fields overlap, they are of the opposite magnetic polarity (Fig. 3-8). When the currents are in the opposite direction, however, the wires repel each other because the overlapping fields are in the same direction. The force generated is proportional to the length of the wire times the product of the currents divided by the distance between the wires.

All these attributes of nature become important when we wrap the wire around to form a loop (Fig. 3-9). It can now be seen that the circular magnetism all around the wire is directed in the same way from north to south. This means that the circular lines of magnetism place north on one side of the loop and south on the other. Since the loop is symmetrical,

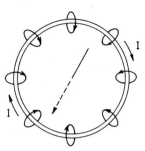

Figure 3-9 When a wire forms a loop, all the individual lines of magnetism are made parallel in the same direction. This causes a north pole to exist on one side of the loop and a south pole on the other side.

the axis of it must therefore be the line perpendicular to the plane of the loop and through its center. The direction of north can be found by wrapping fingers of the right hand around the loop in the direction of current flow and taking the direction of the thumb as north. The strength of this field is proportional to the current divided by the radius of the loop.

When current is flowing at a constant rate, the voltage across the coil of wire is very low, equal only to the resistance of the wire. If the current attempts to change, however, the voltage will suddenly increase. The change of current induces a change in voltage over the coil. This process occurs because the magnetic field is dependent on the amount of current flowing and must increase or decrease in order to accommodate the new current level. Energy to maintain the magnetic field is either gained or lost. Since energy can be expressed in terms of current times voltage, a certain amount of voltage must exist across the coil while the change takes place. Because a change in current induces a voltage in a coil, a coil is frequently called an inductor; the process is called induction.

The key feature of an inductor is that the voltage that exists across it is not a steady function of either the voltage applied or the amount of current flowing through it. The voltage across an inductor is instead proportional to the change in the amount of current flowing (dI) with respect to time (dt).

$$E = -L \frac{dI}{dt} \qquad \textbf{(3-16)}$$

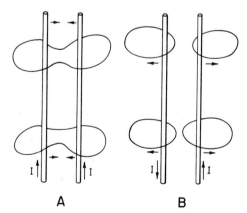

A   B

Figure 3-8 When the currents in two parallel wires are in the same direction, the overlapping magnetic fields reinforce and cause the wires to be attracted toward each other. When the currents are in the opposite direction, the magnetic fields cancel each other, and the wires repel each other.

The proportionality constant L is the inductance of the coil. The unit of inductance is the henry (H), named after Joseph Henry, a nineteenth-century American physicist. Practical inductors range in size from a few microhenrys to hundreds of henrys. The minus sign exists because the potential generated is in the opposite direction to the attempted change in current level. Because inductors tend to resist changes in the flow of current, they are sometimes called "chokes," for they "choke" the large amount of current that tries to flow when a switch is first closed. The way in which this occurs in actual circuits will be discussed in Chapter 4.

A magnet or inductor can be made more efficient if the hole in the coil is filled with a substance that is easily magnetized, such as a soft iron core. This substance causes the lines of force to become more concentrated and more energy to be stored. The inductance can be varied by moving the metal core further into or out from the center of the coil.

Moving electrons through a wire loop produces a magnetic field. In Chapter 2 we saw how a simple current meter operated by generating a field that aligned itself with a permanent magnet. If, on the other hand, we move the wire through the field of a permanent magnet, we witness the formation of a current. As the wire moves across the lines of force, the rotation of the electrons in the wire is disturbed. Like a spinning top, the electrons try to maintain their angular momentum by moving perpendicular to the force applied. If the wire is moved through a magnetic field perpendicular to it, the electrons will be forced toward one end of the wire, as shown in Figure 3-10. If these electrons can escape from the end at which they are accumulating and can move to the other end of the wire, a circuit is formed that will carry current as long as the wire continues to move perpendicular to the magnetic field.

The distance that a wire can travel is very short before physical constraints such as the length of the wire and the magnetic field size come into play. Consequently, a circular arrangement, such as that shown in Figure 3-11, has been devised. In this case, the current flow is zero as the wire is at point A, moving parallel to the field. It increases rapidly as point B is approached and then falls back to zero

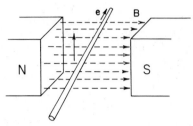

Figure 3-10 As a wire is moved perpendicular to a magnetic field, many of the electrons are forced to one end of the wire due to the force applied on their magnetic fields by the larger magnetic field of the permanent magnet.

as point C is reached. As the loop continues to point D, the current reverses direction as the wire is now moving in the opposite direction in the field. At point A the current is back to zero. Slip rings allow the current to be transmitted without breaking the wire.

When many loops of wire are moved through such a field, the voltage is proportional to the number of loops (N), as well as the strength of the field ($\mathbf{B}$) and the velocity (v) with which the wire is moving:

$$E = kN\mathbf{B}v \qquad (3\text{-}17)$$

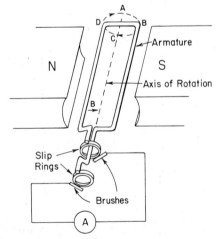

Figure 3-11 When an armature is rotated in a magnetic field, the electrons are forced around a closed exterior loop.

The voltage then from this type of generator is a sine wave versus time, centered about zero voltage. The current is of the same shape when the output is applied across a constant resistance. All power used for transmission is generated this way (by atomic reactors, dams, and so forth) and is called alternating current (ac), as opposed to direct current (dc), which is unidirectional. The properties of ac are defined more fully in the next four chapters in which the reaction of various components to it is studied.

The properties of the submicroscopic atom and the electron can readily be used to explain all the effects observed in electronics on the macroscopic scale. This chapter provides a brief discussion of the fundamental aspects of electronic behavior. We now turn to the implementation of these properties in working electronic devices.

REVIEW QUESTIONS

1. What does electrical neutrality mean?
2. Define conductivity.
3. What is the relationship between conductivity and resistance?
4. To what is the force of attraction between two charged bodies proportional?
5. What is an electrical hole?
6. What is the valence band?
7. What is the conduction band?
8. What are the charge carriers in a wire?
9. What are the charge carriers in a solution?
10. What is the relationship between the valence band and the conduction band in metals? In insulators? In semiconductors?
11. What is a semiconductor?
12. From which part of the periodic table do semiconductors come? List several.
13. List the things that affect the conductivity of a metal.
14. Describe the conductivity of a metal as a function of temperature.
15. Why does a hole move in the opposite direction from an electron?
16. How many holes exist in a mole of undoped semiconductor?

17. What is the relationship between holes and electrons in a piece of semiconductor?
18. What effect does temperature have on a semiconductor?
19. How does one dope a semiconductor?
20. What kind of material does one use to make p-type semiconductor? List several examples.
21. What kind of material does one use to make n-type semiconductor? List several examples.
22. Explain how n-type material works.
23. Explain how p-type material works.
24. To what level is a semiconductor doped?
25. Why can resistors of various values be made the same size?
26. How does a zinc–copper battery work?
27. What is the function of the salt bridge?
28. What is a dry cell?
29. What is a primary cell? A secondary cell?
30. What are the half reactions in a zinc–carbon cell? In an alkaline battery? In a nickel–cadmium battery? In a mercury battery?
31. Why do batteries become discharged?
32. What causes the internal resistance of a battery?
33. List the components of a capacitor.
34. Define capacitance.
35. What is an electrolytic capacitor, and how is it different from a regular capacitor?
36. What is the dielectric constant? How is its numeric value assigned?
37. What are the units of capacitance? What more standard units is this equivalent to?
38. Why can the plates of a capacitor hold either a positive or negative charge?
39. What is capacitance proportional to?
40. What is inductance?
41. What causes magnetism?
42. What is circular magnetism?
43. Why do parallel wires carrying current in the same direction attract each other?
44. Why does a loop carrying current have a north and a south pole?
45. What is the purpose of the soft iron core in an electromagnet?
46. How is voltage over a coil related to the current through it?

47. What happens when a wire moves through a magnetic field parallel to the lines of force? Perpendicular to them?

48. Why does a generator produce alternating current?

49. What is alternating current?

50. To what is the voltage of a generator proportional?

51. How is the twisting of the wire in a generator prevented?

52. Why is more than one wire loop used in a generator?

CHAPTER 4
CAPACITORS AND INDUCTORS

The principles of capacitance and inductance are essential to modern electronic circuits. They are used to construct power supplies, smooth signals, tune radio equipment, and create large voltages and currents. Capacitors and inductors are used extensively in laboratory equipment, either as individual components or as part of integrated microcircuits.

Section 4-1
CAPACITORS

The general properties of capacitance were discussed in Chapter 3. The fundamental use of a capacitor in a circuit is to try to hold the voltage across itself constant by acquiring and relinquishing charge. In other words, the capacitor fights the change in voltage by changing the current in the circuit. Capacitors can be placed in circuits with direct current and effectively constant voltage or with alternating current where the voltage may change in either direction, either regularly or irregularly.

When a capacitor is placed in the simplest possible circuit (see Fig. 4-1), the voltage across the capacitor almost instantly becomes the same as that across the battery. Without the capacitor present, the voltage between points A and B would be E_B, the voltage of the battery. Since one plate of the capacitor is attached to point A and the other to B, these plates will also have a potential difference of E_B, because, as with an open switch, no current can flow between them. The charging of the capacitor is almost instantaneous because there is little resistance in the circuit. The charge necessary to cause a voltage E to exist is $q = CE$, the equation in the previous chapter. We can substitute Ohm's law

into this expression to get:

$$q = CE = C(IR) \qquad \textbf{(4-1)}$$

If we now substitute the definition of current $(I = q/t)$, we than have

$$It = CIR$$

or

$$t = RC \qquad \textbf{(4-2)}$$

If R is small, t is small, and the current needs to flow for only a very short time to charge the capacitor. (Common capacitors have values on the order of 10^{-6} farads or less.)

While this looks very straightforward, it is, in fact, much more complex. Ohm's law was intentionally misapplied in the previous mathematical derivation. To see how a capacitor really works in a circuit, let us examine Figure 4-2A. A resistor is positioned to retard the flow of current and slow down the charging of the capacitor as the capacitor increases its voltage to match that of the battery. The capacitor will indeed reach the battery voltage; it will just take longer. When the switch is closed, the circuit becomes a voltage divider. The battery voltage is divided between the voltage over the resistor and the voltage over the capacitor.

$$E_B = E_R + E_C \qquad \textbf{(4-3)}$$

We have an equation for each of these two voltages, so we can substitute to get

$$E_B = IR + \frac{q}{C} \qquad \textbf{(4-4)}$$

It is important to note that this voltage division is not constant. When the switch is first closed, the capacitor is completely discharged ($E_C = 0$). This

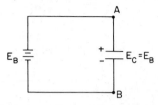

Figure 4-1 A capacitor placed across a battery quickly acquires the voltage of the battery.

means from Eq. 4-3, $E_B = E_R$ and current is given by

$$I = \frac{E_R}{R} = \frac{E_B}{R} \qquad \text{(4-5)}$$

As the current continues to flow, the charge begins to build up on the capacitor, since it cannot go through. E_C is no longer zero, and the current is given by

$$I = \frac{E_R}{R} = \frac{(E_B - E_C)}{R} \qquad \text{(4-6)}$$

Since E_C is positive, the current has decreased and will continue to drop until $E_C = E_B$. At that time, the resistor is effectively between two voltage sources of equal potential, but opposite polarity, so no current flows.

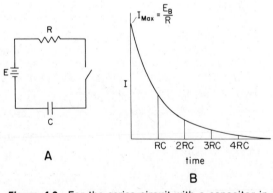

A

B

Figure 4-2 For the series circuit with a capacitor in part A, the voltage of the battery is divided between the two, based on how much current is flowing. In part B the decrease of the current in the circuit is a result of the increasing charge on the capacitor.

To determine how much current is flowing at each instant, one must use Eq. 4-7. It can be derived by use of calculus and is graphically displayed in Figure 4-2B.

$$I = \frac{E_B}{R} e^{-t/RC} \qquad \text{(4-7)}$$

Note that it is a continuously decreasing function, as one would expect. This type of process is called exponential decay and obeys first-order kinetic principles. The current approaches zero asymptotically, that is, zero is the lowest value that can exist, but in theory, it is never equaled. In reality, after five time constants, it is approached so closely that the difference is insignificant for all practical purposes. The last statement introduces the concept of the time constant. This is a quantity which appears in numerous natural phenomena and is defined as the length of time required for a quantity to fall to $1/e$ of its original value, where e is the natural number 2.71828. . . . In this case, the time constant (τ) is equal to RC, since substituting RC for t in Eq. 4-7 gives the exponential the power of -1, which is the same as 1 over the exponential base (in this case, $1/e$). The interested reader can find the derivation of Eq. 4-7 in electronics texts.

Once the current is known, it is possible to determine the voltage division at any time after the switch is closed. Since E_R is given by Eq. 4-5, it is possible to define E_R in terms of R, C, and t by substituting into Eq. 4-7.

$$E_R = IR = \left(\frac{E_B}{R} e^{-t/RC}\right) \times R$$

$$E_R = E_B e^{-t/RC} \qquad \text{(4-8)}$$

The voltage over the capacitor can be determined from Eq. 4-6.

$$IR = E_B - E_C$$

$$E_C = E_B - IR$$

$$= E_B - \frac{E_B}{R} e^{-t/RC} \times R$$

$$E_C = E_B(1 - e^{-t/RC}) \qquad \text{(4-9)}$$

The graphs for these two equations are shown in Figure 4-3. Note that the sum of E_R and E_C is always equal to E_B (Eq. 4-3).

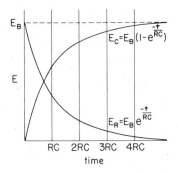

Figure 4-3 The voltage over the resistor decreases as the voltage over the capacitor increases to keep the sum constant.

EXAMPLE 4-1

How long will it take for E_R to equal E_C in Figure 4-2A if R is 2.3 kΩ and the capacitance is 12.3 μF?

Solution:

$$E_R = E_C$$

Substituting from Eqs. 4-8 and 4-9:

$$E_B\, e^{-t/RC} = E_B(1 - e^{-t/RC})$$

$$2\, e^{-t/RC} = 1$$

$$\frac{-t}{RC} = \ln \tfrac{1}{2} = -\ln 2$$

(ln = log to the base of e)

$$t = RC \ln 2$$

$$= 2.3 \cdot 10^3 \times 12.3 \cdot 10^{-6} \times 0.693$$

$$t = 0.020 \text{ seconds} \qquad \blacksquare$$

Figure 4-4 shows another type of resistor-capacitor circuit. This circuit is noteworthy in that it has no power supply. Nevertheless, it is a functional circuit if the capacitor is charged when the switch is closed. Under such conditions, one plate of the capacitor serves as the source of charge and forces current through the resistor to the other plate of the capacitor, thereby discharging itself. The capacitor is behaving as a battery, although it is a very weak one. As the charge moves off the plates to form the current, the voltage drops rapidly.

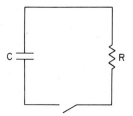

Figure 4-4 A circuit in which the capacitor discharges exponentially through the resistor.

This is more easily understood from the equations. When the switch is closed, the whole voltage drop between the ends of the capacitor is seen over the resistor. Therefore, the voltages over the resistor and capacitor are equal. Initially,

$$E_R^\circ = E_C^\circ \qquad \textbf{(4-10)}$$

As the capacitor discharges, the voltage undergoes exponential decay, as given in Eq. 4-11.

$$E_R = E_C = E_C^\circ\, e^{-t/RC} \qquad \textbf{(4-11)}$$

Unlike the previous case, the voltages over R and C remain identical at all times and can be represented by the E_R curve in Figure 4-3.

Thus far we have dealt with the total circuit capacitance as represented by one capacitor. We have seen with resistors that it is possible to have more than one element contribute to the total resistance in a circuit. The same situation exists with capacitance. Let us therefore look at how capacitors combine their individual values to form the total capacitance in a circuit. Figure 4-5 shows three capacitors in series. The total voltage drop over all the capacitors must equal the charge that

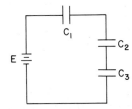

Figure 4-5 Capacitors in series behave like resistors in parallel.

flowed from the battery divided by the circuit capacitance:

$$E = \frac{q}{C} \qquad (4\text{-}12)$$

On the other hand, this voltage must also equal the sum of the voltage drops over the individual capacitors because a series circuit causes voltage division.

$$E = E_1 + E_2 + E_3 \qquad (4\text{-}13)$$

Each of these voltages is determined by the corresponding capacitor's charge and capacitance.

$$E = \frac{q_1}{C_1} + \frac{q_2}{C_2} + \frac{q_3}{C_3} = \frac{q}{C} \qquad (4\text{-}14)$$

The same amount of positive charge that left the battery must be deposited on the left plate of the first capacitor. Consequently, the same amount of positive charge must leave the right plate of the first capacitor and migrate to the upper plate of the second. This must then continue in like fashion until that same amount of positive charge finally makes it to the negative end of the battery, thereby completing the circuit. The result is that all the charges must be the same:

$$q_1 = q_2 = q_3 = q \qquad (4\text{-}15)$$

Therefore

$$\frac{q}{C_1} + \frac{q}{C_2} + \frac{q}{C_3} = \frac{q}{C} \qquad (4\text{-}16)$$

and

$$\frac{1}{C} = \frac{1}{C_1} + \frac{1}{C_2} + \frac{1}{C_3} \qquad (4\text{-}17)$$

These equations show that capacitors in series act like resistors in parallel. This makes sense when we realize that capacitors in series each have a lower voltage drop across them than would an individual capacitor and therefore can hold less charge at the same capacitance. By adding capacitors in series, one decreases the voltage over each of them and therefore the charge they can hold, which has the same effect as decreasing the capacitance.

Figure 4-6 shows capacitors in parallel. The voltage across each of the capacitors is the same. Since

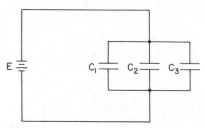

Figure 4-6   Capacitors in parallel behave like resistors in series.

each capacitor will therefore function independently of the others, the total charge held will be the sum of the individual charges on the capacitors.

$$q = q_1 + q_2 + q_3 \qquad (4\text{-}18)$$

Substituting the basic capacitor equation for the individual charges, we get

$$q = E_1 C_1 + E_2 C_2 + E_3 C_3 \qquad (4\text{-}19)$$

But we already observed that all the voltages are the same; therefore,

$$q = E(C_1 + C_2 + C_3) \qquad (4\text{-}20)$$

By definition, the equivalent capacitance must be $C = q/E$; consequently,

$$EC = E(C_1 + C_2 + C_3) \qquad (4\text{-}21)$$

and

$$C = C_1 + C_2 + C_3 \qquad (4\text{-}22)$$

Extra capacitors at the same voltage serve as extra repositories of charge, which means more total capacitance.

EXAMPLE 4-2

What is the effective capacitance in Figure 4-7?

Solution: Capacitors C_1 and C_2 are in parallel. We can replace them with capacitor C_A.

$$C_A = C_1 + C_2 = 5.8 \ \mu\text{F} + 19.1 \ \mu\text{F}$$
$$= 24.9 \ \mu\text{F}$$

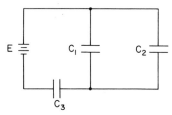

Figure 4-7 Capacitor networks can be made similar to resistor networks. In this case, $C_1 = 5.8~\mu F$, $C_2 = 19.1~\mu F$, and $C_3 = 8.7~\mu F$.

Capacitors C_A and C_3 are in series:

$$\frac{1}{C_T} = \frac{1}{C_A} + \frac{1}{C_3} = \frac{1}{24.9} + \frac{1}{8.7}$$

$$C_T = 6.4~\mu F \qquad\blacksquare$$

The above equations apply to a capacitor network, but are far from a complete set. Further mathematical development, however, is not necessary for subsequent work. Let us now consider what happens when capacitors are placed in sinusoidal ac circuits.

Figure 4-8A shows the simplest example of an ac generator attached to a capacitor. To understand what happens, one must follow current and voltage through one complete cycle of the sine wave. As the generator begins to raise the voltage, current will flow onto the upper plate of the capacitator, because the voltage of the generator is higher. This will continue until the voltage of the generator reaches a peak. After this, the voltage of the gener-

ator will begin to decrease, and the current will flow from the upper plate of the capacitor toward the generator, which is now at a lower voltage, and on through to the lower plate of the capacitor. As the voltage drops toward zero, the current will continue to flow backward through the generator from the more positive side of the capacitor. The voltage of the generator will continue to drop past zero until it reaches a negative maximum. During this entire process the current will flow backward. When the generator turns and begins getting less negative, the current will reverse and start flowing in the forward direction because the reverse voltage of the capacitor is greater than the reverse voltage of the generator. Figure 4-8B shows the relative position of the current to the voltage in a pure capacitive sinusoidal circuit. Since the current reaches a position on the sine wave curve a quarter cycle before the voltage, the current is said to lead the voltage by 90°. This difference is called the phase angle (ϕ). It is measured from the current toward the voltage. Therefore, the phase angle for a pure capacitive circuit is −90°.

All components placed into an ac circuit can be thought to have a phase angle. For a resistor, the phase angle is zero because the value of the current through the resistor corresponds exactly to the value of the voltage, being tied together by Ohm's law. If both a resistor and a capacitor are present in series (Fig. 4-9A), it is not possible for each to operate at its usual phase angle, and a compromise phase angle must be worked out.

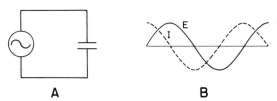

A   **B**

Figure 4-8 When a capacitor is placed in series with an ac voltage supply, the current will flow in both directions during one cycle, depending on whether the power supply or the capacitor momentarily has the greater voltage. In such a pure capacitive circuit, the current leads the voltage by 90°.

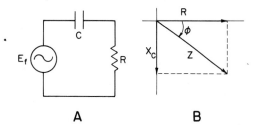

A   **B**

Figure 4-9 The presence of resistance and capacitance must both be taken into consideration to determine the phase angle and the impedance. The vector representing them is the sum of the two vectors representing the resistance and capacitive reactance in a series circuit.

To determine the magnitude of this compromise, a new quantity has to be defined that will relate capacitance to effective resistance. This quantity is called capacitive reactance and is symbolized as X_C. It is given by the equation

$$X_C = \frac{1}{2\pi f C} \tag{4-23}$$

The frequency of the sine wave (f) is given in cycles per second (now called Hertz). Since 2π has the effective units of "per cycle" and capacitance is given in farads, the physical equivalent of seconds per ohm, the units cancel to give a result in ohms. The dependence on frequency is as significant as the dependence on capacitance. At high frequency the reactance is small and has little effect on the circuit. This means that the capacitor "passes" the high frequency signal while weeding out the low frequency signal. The same effect is caused by the size of the capacitor. Small capacitors cause a much greater distortion of an ac circuit than a large capacitor.

The total retarding effect on current flow is called the impedance and is given the symbol Z. The capacitive reactance and the resistance act as vectors due to the phase angle. The direction of these is shown in Figure 4-9B. Impedance is the vector along the diagonal of the box formed by the reactance and resistance. The magnitude of the impedance is calculated as is the hypotenuse of a right triangle,

$$Z = \sqrt{X_C^2 + R^2} \tag{4-24}$$

The angle between the resistance and the impedance is the phase angle. As one can see, this is zero for a pure resistance and $-90°$ for a pure capacitance. The tangent of this angle is the opposite side over the adjacent side and the sign is negative because X_C is a positive quantity pointed in a negative direction:

$$\tan \phi = \frac{-X_C}{R} \tag{4-25}$$

EXAMPLE 4-3

The frequency of the signal source in Figure 4-9A is 60. Hz. If the resistance is $1.00 \cdot 10^4 \ \Omega$ and the capacitance 340. nF, what is the impedance and phase angle?

Solution:

$$X_C = \frac{1}{2\pi f C}$$

$$= \frac{1}{2 \times \pi \times 60 \times 340 \cdot 10^{-9}}$$

$$= 7,800 \ \Omega$$

$$Z = \sqrt{X_C^2 + R^2}$$

$$= \sqrt{(7,800)^2 + (10,000)^2}$$

$$= 1.27 \cdot 10^4 \ \Omega$$

$$\tan \phi = \frac{-X_C}{R} = \frac{-7,800}{10,000}$$

$$\phi = - \arctan 0.78$$

$$\phi \doteq -38° \qquad \blacksquare$$

The work required to charge a capacitor is given by Eq. 4-26:

$$W = \frac{qE}{2} \tag{4-26}$$

Note that there is no direct dependence on either the time or the capacitance in the equation. There is no dependence on the time because it takes as much work to charge a capacitor regardless of the time taken, and there is no dependence on the capacitance because the presence of charge and voltage implies a relationship between them, namely the capacitance.

In laboratory instruments, capacitors are used extensively for noise elimination and the accumulation of the analog signal response. Wires running in parallel for a long distance (such as to a computer interface) develop a capacitance between them, and this capacitance must be "matched" by capacitors in the instrument to prevent distortion of the information being transmitted. High-frequency noise generated by electronic discharges in various instruments or by turning on equipment are picked up by circuits containing long wires (the wires act as antennas). Using capacitors in parallel with analytical circuitry can provide a path of low impedance to the high-frequency noise not available to the much slower analytically significant signals, thereby reducing noise. A voltage proportional to a rate of a reaction or to the sum of counts can be accumulated on a capacitor to prevent noise from having any effect on the signal at the instant of measurement.

Section **4-2**
INDUCTORS

Inductors, like capacitors, react to prevent changes in the operation of a circuit. While the capacitor fights voltage change by releasing or absorbing current, the inductor fights the change in current by the expansion or collapse of its magnetic field. The similarity becomes even stronger if we realize that the charge built up on a capacitor is an electrical field. A capacitor, then, captures current on its plates to form an electrical field. An inductor uses the current flowing through it to create a magnetic field.

When an inductor is placed in the simple circuit shown in Figure 4-10, and the switch is closed, the current begins to flow through the inductor. As the current begins to circle the coil, a magnetic field begins to expand. As it does, the magnetic lines of force move across the wires of the coil, generating a voltage which is in the opposite direction to the voltage shoving the current. This backward voltage or "back emf" (*electromotive force*) retards the flow of current through the inductor. As the field grows, the lines of force expand out from the coil

and less retarding effect is experienced by the current. Eventually, the current assumes a value determined solely by the resistance in the circuit. At this point, the magnetic field is stationary, and no energy is entering or leaving it.

A magnetic field is indeed a field that contains energy. Just as it requires energy to separate the charges over a capacitor, in the same way it requires energy to build the magnetic field. That energy (W) is given by Eq. 4-27 and is a function of both the current (I) and the inductance (L). Note that a $\frac{1}{2}$ again appears, since the field starts at zero and builds to full, thus giving the average as $\frac{1}{2}$. This energy is absorbed from the electrical circuit during the time that the back emf is retarding the flow of current:

$$W = \tfrac{1}{2}LI^2 \qquad (4\text{-}27)$$

The difference is energy between what the battery puts in and the circuit loses in resistance is what builds the field. Once built, the field is inert to the circuit since the electrons do not cut cross the lines of force of the field, but rather circle between them.

In Figure 4-11A, we have the next basic inductor circuit. The maximum current that can flow is determined by the resistor. If the inductor is having no effect on the current flow, the current is given by Ohm's law, $I = E_B/R$. This then serves as the upper

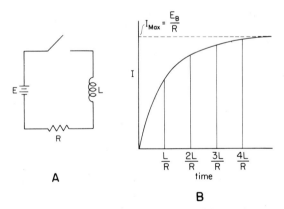

A

B

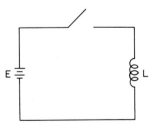

Figure 4-10 The magnetic field over an inductor builds up from the flow of current through it, reaching a steady value when the current becomes constant.

Figure 4-11 The current in a circuit with a series resistance and inductance rises until it is at the quotient of the battery voltage and the resistance. The voltage over the resistor rises because the voltage over the inductor decays exponentially.

limit that the current will reach. During the initial moments after the switch is closed, however, the inductor will fight the current flow, and its back emf must be subtracted from the battery voltage to determine the effective voltage across the resistor and therefore the current. The magnitude of the back emf is limited by the battery voltage. An applied voltage cannot generate a back emf greater than itself, otherwise, logically, the current would start to flow backward toward the positive end of the battery. Consequently, the initial back emf equals the battery voltage, and the effective initial current is zero, as no potential difference exists across the resistance. This condition is only momentary because the back emf can only be maintained by current flowing through the coil. In order to fight the flow of current by means of back emf, the coil must have current flowing. This is clearly a losing proposition for the inductor. As the magnetic field expands, the amount of current necessary to generate a specific back voltage grows, and the amount of current racing through the coil also grows. A limit is reached when the resistor will allow no further current to enter the inductor, and the back emf, dependent on the *change* in the amount of current flowing, becomes zero.

The voltage division is given by Eq. 4-28, where E_L is the back emf.

$$E_B = E_R + E_L \qquad \textbf{(4-28)}$$

This equation can be expanded by substituting Ohm's law and the inductor equation (3-10).

$$E_B = IR + L\frac{dI}{dt} \qquad \textbf{(4-29)}$$

If this equation is integrated, the current at any moment is given by:

$$I = \frac{E_B}{R} \times (1 - e^{-Rt/L}) \qquad \textbf{(4-30)}$$

The equation for the current is plotted in Figure 4-11B. To find the equation for the voltage over the resistor, it is only necessary to multiply Eq. 4-20 by R.

$$E_R = IR = E_B(1 - e^{-Rt/L}) \qquad \textbf{(4-31)}$$

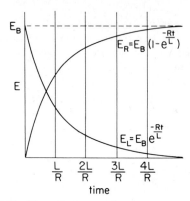

Figure 4-12 The voltage over the resistor increases as the voltage over the inductor decreases to keep the sum constant.

To find voltage over the inductor, one must substitute Eq. 4-31 into Eq. 4-28.

$$E_B = E_B(1 - e^{-Rt/L}) + E_L$$

or

$$E_L = E_B e^{-Rt/L} \qquad \textbf{(4-32)}$$

These two equations are plotted in Figure 4-12. Note the similarity to Figure 4-3. The voltage curve over the resistor and over the second device are just the opposite for the capacitor as for the inductor. Note that there is again a time constant. This constant is given by the ratio of inductance to resistance and again has the units of seconds.

$$\tau = \frac{L}{R} \qquad \textbf{(4-33)}$$

EXAMPLE 4-4

How long will it take for the current to reach 4.2 mA in Figure 4-11A if the voltage is 15.2 V, the resistance is 3.0 kΩ, and the inductance is 8.2 H?

Solution: Start with Eq. 4-30.

$$I = \frac{E_B}{R} \times (1 - e^{-Rt/L})$$

Solve for t:

$$e^{-Rt/L} = 1 - \frac{IR}{E_B}$$

$$\frac{-Rt}{L} = \ln\left(1 - \frac{IR}{E_B}\right)$$

$$t = \frac{-L}{R} \times \ln\left(1 - \frac{IR}{E_B}\right)$$

Then substitute as necessary:

$$= \frac{-8.2}{3.0 \cdot 10^3} \ln\left(1 - \frac{4.2 \cdot 10^{-3} \times 3.0 \cdot 10^3}{15.2}\right)$$

$$= -2.73 \cdot 10^{-3} \times \ln 0.171$$

$$= (-2.7 \cdot 10^{-3})(-1.766)$$

$$t = 4.8 \cdot 10^{-3} \text{ sec} \qquad \blacksquare$$

As with resistors and capacitors, it is possible to place inductors in series and in parallel with each other. Because the inductance term appears in the numerator of the voltage definition equation, as it does for resistors, instead of in the denominator, as it does for capacitors, inductances combine with inductances by the same equations that resistances combine with resistances.

$$L_S = \Sigma L_i = L_1 + L_2 + L_3 + \cdots$$
$$\text{(series)} \quad \textbf{(4-34)}$$

$$\frac{1}{L_P} = \Sigma \frac{1}{L_i} = \frac{1}{L_1} + \frac{1}{L_2} + \frac{1}{L_3} + \cdots$$
$$\text{(parallel)} \quad \textbf{(4-35)}$$

Naturally, one cannot combine resistances with inductances by these equations because they have different units and properties.

Figure 4-13A shows the simplest ac circuit containing an inductor. As with capacitors, it is necessary to work through a complete voltage cycle to see what happens to the current in the circuit. When the voltage first begins to rise in the positive direction, the current also will rise until the voltage maximum is reached. In the process the field will expand. As the maximum in voltage is passed, the field begins to collapse, shoving current through in the forward direction more enthusiastically than

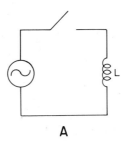

A

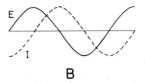

B

Figure 4-13 When an inductor is placed in series with an ac voltage supply, the current will flow in both directions during one cycle, depending on which end of the coil has developed the north magnetic pole. In such a pure inductive circuit, the voltage leads the current by 90°.

ever. As the voltage passes zero, the current continues flowing in the positive direction until the voltage reaches a maximum in the reverse direction. As the voltage now begins to get less negative, the coil, having a reversed magnetic field, begins to shove current through in the reverse direction. This continues with greater enthusiasm until the voltage again reaches zero. It then gradually subsides as the voltage again approaches a maximum in the positive direction. If we skip what happens during the first quarter-cycle of our explanation (the one-time charging cycle), we see that we have a situation in which the current follows the voltage by a quarter-cycle (Fig. 4-13B). This occurs because the coil attempts to keep the current flow constant. When the current flow tries to change, the field will expand or collapse to try to prevent it from doing so.

The description of the phenomenon of induction explains the difference in phase between current and voltage. If we follow the convention of measuring from the current to the voltage, the phase angle is +90°. It is also necessary, as in the case of capacitance, to define a quantity which represents the retarding effect of inductance on a circuit. This quantity is called inductive reactance and is given by

$$X_L = 2\pi f L \qquad (4\text{-}36)$$

The frequency of the sine wave is given by f. Since the 2π term has the unit of "per cycle" and the frequency is in units of cycles per second, henries (H) can be expressed in terms of standard units as ohm seconds. The dependence on frequency is significant as in the case of capacitive reactance. For inductors, increases in frequency cause increases in the reactance. This makes sense since the inductor resists the change in the amount of current flowing. A higher frequency means an effort is being made to change the amount of current flowing more often, which causes the coil to become more stubborn and to resist more strongly.

The impedance for a resistor–inductor circuit is calculated in the same fashion as for a resistor–capacitor circuit.

$$Z = \sqrt{X_L^2 + R^2} \qquad (4\text{-}37)$$

The phase angle is calculated in the same manner, except that no negative sign is present because the phase angle is in the positive direction.

$$\tan \phi = \frac{X_L}{R} \qquad (4\text{-}38)$$

EXAMPLE 4-5

If the impedance of the circuit in Figure 4-14 is 8.3 kΩ, the inductance 30.1 H, and the frequency 23.5 Hz, what is the resistance?

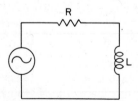

Figure 4-14 The presence of resistance and inductance must both be taken into consideration to determine the phase angle and the impedance.

Solution:

$$X_L = 2\pi f L$$
$$= 2\pi \times 23.5 \times 30.1$$
$$= 4.44 \cdot 10^3 \ \Omega$$
$$Z = \sqrt{X_L^2 + R^2}$$
$$R = \sqrt{Z^2 - X_L^2}$$
$$= (\sqrt{(8.3)^2 - (4.44)^2}) \cdot 10^3$$
$$= 7.0 \cdot 10^3 \ \Omega \qquad \blacksquare$$

The most common use of inductors in the laboratory is as current filters. Because of their resistance to the change in the amount of current flowing, they are used in circuits where a constant current supply is necessary. Coulometric titrations and power supplies are such constant current devices. The use of inductors is much less frequent than is that of capacitors.

Section 4-3
COMPLEX CIRCUITS

The combination of inductance, capacitance, and resistance gives us the ability to build even more complex circuits. If one uses a battery as a voltage source in Figure 4-15A, then solving the differential equation for the interaction between the variable

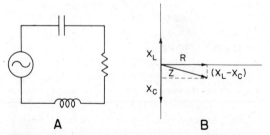

A   B

Figure 4-15 When inductance and capacitance are placed in series in the same circuit, their reactances are 180° out of phase and partially cancel each other. Resistance, inductive reactance, and capacitive reactance can be combined, using vectors, to give a total impedance and phase angle.

components becomes complex because voltages are changing over all three devices. If, however, one uses an ac source, one observes an interesting occurrence. Since the capacitive reactance leads the voltage by 90° and the inductive reactance follows the voltage by 90°, the capacitive and inductive reactances are 180° out of phase and are mutually destructive. Therefore, the effective reactance in the circuit is the difference between the inductive and capacitive reactance.

The reactances for the inductive and capacitive components are calculated in the same way as when each is present separately. The impedance, however, shows the result of the canceling effect.

$$Z = \sqrt{(X_L - X_C)^2 + R^2} \qquad \textbf{(4-39)}$$

Similarly, the phase angle is also affected by the opposition of the inductance and capacitance (see Fig. 4-15B).

$$\tan \phi = \frac{X_L - X_C}{R} \qquad \textbf{(4-40)}$$

The most interesting feature of such circuits occurs when $X_L = X_C$. At this point, regardless of their size, the inductance and capacitance do nothing to impede the flow of current. If all resistance is removed from such a circuit, there is no impedance at all to current flow! Figure 4-16 shows such a circuit. If the capacitor is initially charged to a given voltage, an incredible phenomenon will occur. The capacitor will try to discharge spontaneously through the piece of wire that is the inductor coil. As the charge tries to leave the capacitor, the coil will build up its magnetic field to oppose it. When the capacitor reaches zero voltage, the magnetic field will have reached its peak. With no current to sustain it, it will begin to collapse and con-

tinue to shove current in the direction in which it was originally flowing (recall that a coil fights the *change* in current flow). As the field collapses, the capacitor begins to charge in the reverse direction. When the field finally reaches zero, the capacitor is equally charged as when it started, but is of the opposite polarity. Since the situation is equivalent to the initial situation, the process is repeated to recharge the capacitor in the forward direction. Because of the difference in phase angle, there is no happy medium or rest state. The fields of the capacitor and the inductor are fully developed out of phase, and the collapsing phase of one is the building phase of the other. The frequency of this oscillation can be determined by setting $X_L = X_C$ and solving for f.

$$X_L = 2\pi f L$$

$$X_C = \frac{1}{2\pi f C}$$

If

$$X_L = X_C \qquad \textbf{(4-41)}$$

$$2 f L = \frac{1}{2\pi f C}$$

$$f = \frac{1}{2\pi \sqrt{LC}} \qquad \textbf{(4-42)}$$

EXAMPLE 4-6

What inductance is needed to make the frequency of the circuit in Figure 4-16 equal 6.4 kHz if the capacitance is 5.2 μF?

Solution:

$$f = \frac{1}{2\pi \sqrt{LC}}$$

$$LC = \frac{1}{(2\pi f)^2}$$

$$L = \frac{1}{(2\pi f)^2 C}$$

$$= \frac{1}{(2\pi \times 6.4 \cdot 10^3)^2 \cdot 5.2 \cdot 10^{-6}}$$

$$= 1.19 \cdot 10^{-4} \text{ H} \qquad \blacksquare$$

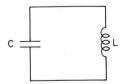

Figure 4-16 A circuit with only capacitance and inductance will be sensitive to the frequency at which resonance occurs.

There are, of course, no perfect inductive–capacitive circuits. There is always a slight amount of resistance in the circuit that will gradually disperse the energy of the circuit through heat. On the other hand, anything of the same frequency will tend to give the circuit a "kick," that is, will tend to strengthen the oscillation of the circuit. This type of circuit then can be used to tune a radio or television to the appropriate station. Each station has a frequency of broadcasting radiation that can be matched by changing the relative value of inductance to capacitance in a tuning circuit in a radio receiver. When the frequencies are the same, the receiver picks up the energy from the radiation and amplifies it; it can produce sound and even a picture. A common way to do such "tuning" is to use a capacitor that has two sets of interleafed plates and that uses air for a dielectric. One set of plates can be rotated away from the other by turning a dial. Such movement of the plates increases the frequency that will stimulate a particular circuit.

In the laboratory, such pick-up of radiated energy can be an annoyance. The inadvertent twisting of circuit wires creates inductance, and parallel wires create capacitance. When other equipment in the vicinity emits radiated signals caused by energy dissipation, they can be picked up by a sensitive analytical instrument to give a noisy signal. The greatest noise source is the 60-cycle radiation given off by the line voltage that is ubiquitous in the laboratory.

In Chapter 7, we will look at some positive uses of inductor–capacitor circuits in the laboratory.

REVIEW QUESTIONS

1. How does a capacitor fight the change of voltage in a circuit?
2. What does a capacitor in series with a battery act like?
3. What is the equation used to define capacitance?
4. What is a time constant? How is it defined for capacitors? For inductors?
5. What happens to the voltage over a capacitor in series with a resistor and a battery? Over the resistor? What happens to the current?
6. What is exponential decay?
7. What is e?
8. What is ln?
9. Why do capacitors in series combine like resistors in parallel?
10. Why is the charge on all capacitors in series, regardless of size, the same?
11. Why does the capacitance of capacitors in parallel add?
12. What is the relationship between the current and the voltage in a pure capacitive ac circuit? Why?
13. What is reactance? Give the formulas for capacitive and inductive reactance.
14. What is a phase angle? Give the general formula.
15. How does capacitive reactance differ from inductive reactance?
16. What is a hertz?
17. What is impedance? Give the general formula.
18. What is the relationship between resistance, capacitance, and impedance?
19. How much work does it take to charge a capacitor to a specific voltage?
20. What are some uses for capacitors?
21. What problems does capacitance cause in the laboratory?
22. How does an inductor fight the change in current in a circuit?
23. How is the charging of a capacitor and inductor similar?
24. How is the energy stored when a specified current goes through an inductor?
25. What is the relationship between current and voltage in a pure inductive ac circuit? Why?
26. What happens to the voltage over an inductor in series with a resistor and a battery? Over the resistor? What happens to the current?
27. To what is the voltage over an inductor proportional?
28. Why do inductors in series combine like resistors in series?
29. What is the effect of having capacitance and inductance in series?
30. List some uses of inductors.
31. What is resonance?
32. What inhibits resonance?
33. What increases resonance?

34. Of what use is resonance?

35. What problems does resonance cause in the laboratory?

PROBLEMS

1. The voltage of the battery in Figure 4-2A is 8.87 V. What is the voltage over the resistor 1.042 sec after the switch is closed if the resistor has a value of 43.0 kΩ and the capacitor, initially discharged, has a value of 30.2 μF?

2. If the voltage of the battery is 16.8 V in Figure 4-2A and the resistor is 94 kΩ, what must the size of the capacitor be to permit the voltage over the capacitor to reach 12.1 V at 0.271 sec after the switch is closed?

3. If the resistance in Figure 4-4 is 23.2 kΩ and the capacitance is 68.2 μF, how long will it take for the voltage over the capacitor to drop from 6.00 V to 2.00 V when the switch is closed?

4. If the three capacitors shown in Figure 4-5 are 91, 68, and 94 μF, respectively, what is the total capacitance in the circuit?

5. If the voltage of the battery in Problem 4-4 is raised by 13.0%, what must be the new value of C_2 for the amount of work done in charging the capacitor network to remain the same if C and C_3 remain unchanged?

6. The energy required to charge all the capacitors in Figure 4-6 is 0.0100 joule (watt second) if the battery is 20.0 V. If C_1 is doubled in capacitance, the energy required is $12.4 \cdot 10^{-3}$ J, and if instead C_2 is tripled, $1.64 \cdot 10^{-2}$ J is required. What are the values of C_1, C_2, and C_3?

7. What is the total capacitance of the circuit in Figure 4-7 if C_1 is 77 μF, C_2 is 41 μF, and C_3 is 131 μF?

8. If the battery provides 58 V, what is the voltage over each of the capacitors in Problem 4-7?

9. If C_3 is 20 μF and C_1 is 24 μF in Figure 4-7, what value of C_2 is needed to give a total capacitance of 12 μF?

10. What is the total capacitance in the circuit shown in Figure 4-17A?

11. What is the time constant for the circuit shown in Figure 4-17A? What is the voltage over the resistor after three time constants?

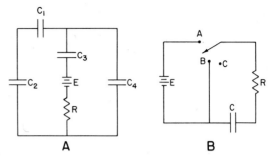

Figure 4-17 Circuits for Problems 10 through 13. In Part A, C_1 = 20.0 μF, C_2 = 10.0 μF, C_3 = 30.0 μF, C_4 = 40.0 μF, R = 10.0 kΩ, and E = 5.00 V.

12. Assume that the power supply in Figure 4-17A is a 76-Hz source rather than a battery. What is the reactance of the total circuit and each individual capacitor?

13. In Figure 4-17B, the capacitor is initially discharged. The switch is closed to point A for $1.00 \cdot 10^{-2}$ sec, then moved to point B for the same length of time and then moved to point C. When the switch reaches point C, the capacitor is measured and found to have 20.0% of the voltage of the battery E. If the resistor is 2.80 kΩ, what is the value of the capacitor?

14. The frequency of the signal source in Figure 4-9A is 21.5 Hz. If the capacitance is 2.77 μF and the resistance is 3,190 Ω, what is the impedance and the phase angle?

15. If the capacitance in Figure 4-9A is 64.2 μF and the resistance is 47 kΩ, what is the frequency necessary to produce a phase angle of $-14.6°$?

16. The voltage of the battery in Figure 4-11A is 21.68 V. What is the voltage over the resistor 0.843 sec after the switch is closed if the resistor has a value of 28.7 Ω and the inductor has a value of 59.0 H?

17. In Problem 4-16, how long does it take for the voltage over the inductor to fall from 12.0 V to 3.0 V?

18. How much energy is required to fully charge the inductors in Problem 4-16?

19. Assume that the capacitors in Figure 4-6 are replaced with inductors. If the total inductance is 114 H, L_1 is 382 H, and L_2 is 413 H, what is L_3?

20. The frequency of the power supply of Figure 4-14 is 60.0 Hz and its voltage is 213 V. If the inductance is 5.70 H and the impedance 6.90 kΩ, what is the phase angle?

21. What effect would changing the frequency from 45.0 to 90.0 Hz have on the impedance and phase angle in Figure 4-15A if the resistance is 21.8 kΩ, the capacitance is 348 nF, and the inductance is 104 H?

22. In Figure 4-15A, the resistance in ohms is numerically 100 times the inductance in henrys and 10^{10} times the capacitance in farads. If the frequency is 42.2 Hz, what is the resistance when the phase angle is 45.0°?

23. What capacitance is needed to make the circuit in Figure 4-16 oscillate at 12.6 kHz if the inductance is 0.097 H?

24. Calculate the impedance and phase angle for the circuit in Figure 4-18A if $R_1 = 1000.$ Ω, $R_2 = 400.$ Ω, $C_1 = 4.00\,\mu\text{F}$, $C_2 = 7.00\,\mu\text{F}$, $L = 5.00$ H, and $f = 60.0$ Hz.

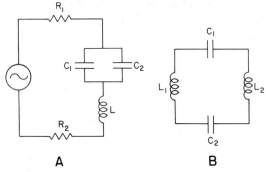

Figure 4-18 Circuits for Problems 24 through 26.

25. What is the resonance frequency of the circuit in Figure 4-18B if $C_1 = 20.0\,\mu\text{F}$, $C_2 = 30.0\,\mu\text{F}$, $L_1 = 1.54$ H, and $L_2 = 2.7$ H?

26. Changing only C_2, double the frequency in Problem 4-25.

CHAPTER 5
TUBES AND TRANSISTORS

The circuit components discussed thus far are called "linear" elements. This is because some entity associated with the component responds linearly to an applied voltage. In the case of a resistor, this entity is current flow. For a capacitor it is charge build-up. For an inductor it is the magnetic field. In each case a constant relates voltage to this other entity, and it is this constant that we use to characterize the circuit element. The value we assign to a resistor, for example, is just the constant R from Ohm's law. There are, however, circuit elements that do not respond linearly to voltage. These are called "nonlinear elements," and they are essential for amplification and rectification. Before investigating these elements, it will be necessary to review some basic physics.

Section 5-1
THERMAL ELECTRONS

The process we call "heating" is actually the physical act of increasing the velocity of atoms in a substance. This can be seen if we combine the two equations for energy that were encountered in general physics.

$$E = kT \qquad (5\text{-}1)$$

$$E = \tfrac{1}{2}mv^2 \qquad (5\text{-}2)$$

Equation 5-1 says that energy is proportional to absolute temperature T and Eq. 5-2 says that energy is proportional to the velocity squared. Combining and rearranging gives us Eq. 5-3.

$$v = \sqrt{2kT/m} \qquad (5\text{-}3)$$

In any quantity of matter, however, all the atoms will not be traveling at the same speed, even though the whole quantity of material appears to be at the same temperature. While the most probable velocity will be that given in Eq. 5-3, a distribution of velocities will exist as shown in Figure 5-1. This is called a Maxwell distribution. Note that it is not symmetrical because an atom cannot move more slowly than zero velocity, but nothing prevents it from having a very high velocity. As the temperature rises, the curve shifts to the right and, as the temperature decreases, it shifts to the left.

Moreover, atoms are not immutable spheres. The outer shells that collide are composed of electrons, and the mechanism of collision is repulsion between the outer electron shells. In the process, bonds are stretched in a solid, and energy is imparted to individual electrons. This causes ionization and exchange of electrons. If an individual electron acquires enough energy, it may be able to escape from the atom holding it and drift off into space. A dashed line in Figure 5-1 represents the velocity at which an atom has enough energy to lose an electron. As the temperature rises, a larger percentage of the electrons become dislodged as the curve shifts to the right, while the dashed line on the graph stays at the same velocity. This process is called "boiling off" electrons because it resembles a boiling liquid.

When electrons leave a solid and meander off into space, they leave a positively charged material behind. Consequently, some of the electrons will be attracted back again. The positive material will also try to reclaim electrons from any other nearby source, particularly the atmosphere. The effect of this is to cause a chemical reaction at the surface of the heated material which, after a period of time,

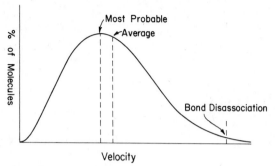

Figure 5-1 Maxwell distribution of velocities of molecules with a given average energy. Since $E = \frac{1}{2}mv^2$, this curve is also similar in shape to the energy distribution.

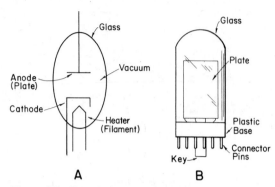

Figure 5-2 Part A shows a schematic diagram of a vacuum tube diode. Part B is a pictorial sketch of a vacuum tube. The plate surrounds the cathode and the filament (heater).

corrodes the surface and perhaps destroys the material. Therefore, it is necessary to prevent this by removing the atmosphere from the area around a substance off which one wishes to boil electrons.

If one does want to boil electrons off a material, the best material to use would be a conductor, that is, a metal, since metals have electrons that can easily be removed. One could further increase the number of electrons boiled off by placing a negative charge on the metal. This would cause electrons that leave to be less likely to return. One could then collect these electrons by putting a positive metal plate somewhere in the near vicinity to attract them.

Section 5-2
VACUUM TUBE DIODE

If one did what was suggested in the last paragraph, one would have what is called a "vacuum tube diode." A schematic diagram and sketch of such a tube are given in Figure 5-2. The tube consists of an evacuated glass envelope containing three electrical elements. The first is the heater that is made of a metal with a high resistance-to-current flow, so that a lot of heat is generated. This heater has two leads that are not necessarily attached to the other electronics in the tube, but rather to a special power supply. The presence of the heater circuit is critical to the operation of the vacuum tube diode, but it is

not usually included in circuit diagrams to improve clarity.

The last two electrical elements in the tube are attached to the circuit of interest, sometimes called the analytical or plate circuit. These elements are the anode and the cathode, the two "odes" that give rise to the name "diode." The cathode is a piece of metal positioned around the heater so that electrons can be boiled off the cathode. (Occasionally, the heater and cathode are combined.) It has a negative charge when conducting. The anode or plate is the positive electrode at an appropriate distance from the cathode.

If one gradually increases the potential difference between the cathode and the anode of a vacuum tube diode, beginning at zero, nothing happens initially. The electrons in the metal cathode are bound too tightly for any significant number to escape. As a result, no current flows through the tube. As the cathode becomes more negative, electrons jump the gap to the plate and current flows through the tube. Note that the current flows from the plate to the cathode, opposite the direction of the electron movement, because current always flows from positive to negative. As the voltage continues to increase, the current rises at a faster and faster rate, until finally the tube becomes saturated as the cathode cannot produce enough electrons to carry more current. This relationship between current and voltage is graphically represented in Figure 5-3 and

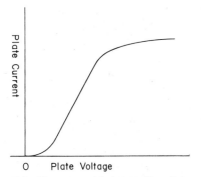

Figure 5-3 The current between the plate and cathode of a vacuum tube diode is a nonlinear function of the voltage applied to the plate relative to the cathode.

must be determined experimentally for each diode. It is clearly nonlinear, that is, not a straight line.

The effect of reversing the polarity of the electrodes should be considered as well. If the plate is gradually made more negative than the cathode, the tube sits there inertly. The now positive cathode already has an electron deficiency and will not tolerate the loss of additional electrons. The plate has a surplus of electrons, but being unheated, cannot force the electrons off. The result is no current flow. The fact that current will flow in one direction through a diode, and not the other, gives rise to the

main use of diodes: rectification. This phenomenon is discussed later in this chapter.

When one places a vacuum tube diode into a dc circuit such as in Figure 5-4, one can write an equation for what will happen. The voltage of the battery (E) is divided between the resistor (E_R) and the diode (E_T). Since the voltage across the resistor must obey Ohm's law, we obtain Eq. 5-5, which is the basis of all diode and transistor operation:

$$E = E_R + E_T \qquad (5\text{-}4)$$

$$E = IR + E_T \qquad (5\text{-}5)$$

The mystery quantity in the equation is E_T, the voltage over the tube. It is clearly affected by the current if E and R are fixed, but on the other hand E_T determines the current. This gives us a chicken-and-egg dilemma. To solve it, we need two pieces of information. The first is the graph relating the current through the diode to the voltage across it. This is called a characteristic curve because it is characteristic of what happens when the tube is in a circuit. This is what Figure 5-3 represents. We can obtain the second piece of information by analyzing Eq. 5-5. The form of this equation is simply $y = ax + b$, which is a straight line. For a particular set of E (substituted for b) and R (substituted for a), one can compute where this line would lie by determining any two value pairs that satisfy the equation,

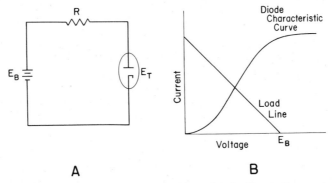

Figure 5-4 When a diode is placed in a circuit with a battery and a resistor, the voltage of the battery is divided between the other two elements. Part B shows the graph of the current versus the voltage for both the resistor and the diode. The intersection of the two lines is where the circuit operates.

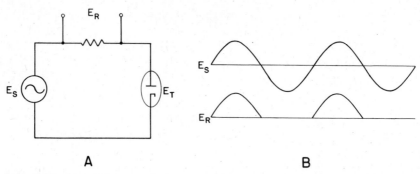

Figure 5-5 Part A shows a diode and a resistor in series with an ac source. The voltage over the resistor rises on the positive part of the cycle but is zero on the negative portion, as is shown in Part B.

since two points determine a straight line. The easiest two points to determine are when E_T is zero and when I is zero.

$$\text{If} \quad E_T = 0 \quad \text{then} \quad I = \frac{E}{R} \quad \textbf{(5-6)}$$

$$\text{If} \quad I = 0 \quad \text{then} \quad E_T = E \quad \textbf{(5-7)}$$

If we plot these two points on the same graph as the characteristic curve of the diode and connect them with a straight line, we have the interesting phenomenon of two curves, both of which must be true, on the same coordinate system. From your experience in doing graphic solutions to algebra problems, you will recall that the only point on the graph that satisfies both Eq. 5-5 and the operating characteristics of the tube is where the lines intersect. From the graph, it is therefore possible to obtain the values of I and E_T that will exist in the circuit for the particular diode indicated and the values of E and R specified.

The line representing Eq. 5-5 is called the "load line." (Fig. 5-4B) It comes from the fact that resistor R limits the current in the circuit and therefore "loads" the circuit. Resistor R is called the load resistor. The graphic use of load lines and characteristic curves is as essential to nonlinear elements as is algebra to linear elements.

While the use of a diode with direct current is not particularly valuable, its use with alternating current is much more important. Suppose we place an ac source into the circuit (Fig. 5-5) and measure the current in the circuit in terms of the voltage across

a resistor (to which it is linearly proportional by Ohm's law). As the voltage on the plate becomes more positive, current begins to flow through the circuit, making the voltage over the resistor rise. As the source voltage reaches a maximum and declines, so does the voltage over the resistor. When the voltage reaches zero, no current flows and $E_R = 0$. As the voltage of the plate continues to get more negative with respect to the cathode, E_R continues to be zero. Finally, the source voltage will complete the negative portion of the loop and will begin to rise again. E_R then will rise as well. The net result is that only positive voltage appears over the resistor, and current only flows one way through the resistor. The current is therefore "righted" or "rectified" by the vacuum tube diode.

The effect of rectification is to change ac to dc. Granted, it is not what we normally consider dc, but it does only flow in one direction. It is called "pulsed dc" because the current comes only in pulses, separated by intervals of no current. The diode is very important, however, because many devices cannot run on ac; therefore, the ac must be converted to dc before it can be used. Most laboratory instruments require dc in at least some internal circuits.

Section 5-3
VACUUM TUBE TRIODE

Nonlinear element technology would be limited if it only consisted of rectifying alternating current. The

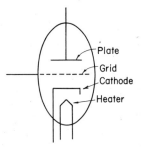

Figure 5-6 A triode is a tube with a grid between the plate and cathode to regulate current flow.

vacuum tube becomes much more versatile if one installs another electrode, called a grid. The tube now has three "odes" and is called a triode. The grid is a wire mesh placed between the cathode and the anode, as indicated in Figure 5-6.

The purpose of the grid is to control the flow of electrons from the cathode to the plate. This is accomplished by making the grid slightly more negative than the cathode. Because the grid is near the cathode and in a direct line with the plate, its negative field discourages the migration of electrons from the cathode. The electrons are, in effect, repelled back to the less negative cathode. The grid must be negative with respect to the cathode or current will flow from the cathode to the grid and destroy the delicate grid.

Figure 5-7A shows a triode in a typical circuit. As one views this diagram, it immediately becomes clear that there is another circuit in addition to the heater circuit (not shown) and the cathode-plate

circuit (hereafter called the plate circuit). This circuit is the one between the grid and the cathode that is used to make the grid slightly negative compared with the cathode. The grid is said to be "negatively biased" compared with the cathode. Since no current flows from the cathode to the more negative grid (it is cold like the plate), the function of the voltage source E_g is solely to bias the grid, that is, give it a more negative potential than the cathode. There is no equation relating grid current to grid voltage, since I_g is effectively zero.

In the plate circuit, however, current does flow. Moreover, the equation for this circuit is Eq. 5-5, since the outside circuit cannot distinguish whether the tube is a diode or a triode. It follows then that there should be a characteristic curve for the triode as for the diode. In reality, there is a whole series of curves, one for each value of E_g, as shown in Figure 5-7B. For any particular value of E_g, the triode behaves like a diode. Changing the value of E_g causes the triode to behave like a different diode. The family of characteristic curves in Figure 5-7B is obtained by choosing representative values of E_g. It must be remembered that there are an infinite number of curves corresponding to the infinite number of E_g's possible. The triode is then a variable diode.

Unlike the diode, the triode finds its primary use in dc rather than ac circuits, as diagrammed in Figure 5-8. Here the grid bias is determined not by a preset battery, but by the varying voltage signal of some other circuit. We must therefore investigate what happens when E_g varies. We can start by observing that no matter what happens to E_g, Eq. 5-5

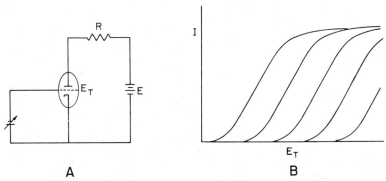

A   B

Figure 5-7 The triode, shown in a typical circuit in Part A, has a whole family of characteristic curves depending on the bias voltage E_g applied to the grid.

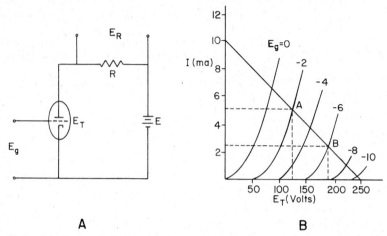

A   B

Figure 5-8   In a typical triode circuit the signal applied to the grid affects the voltage across the load resistor. The values of E_T and I are determined from the load line in Part B.

must still be true. As a consequence, it is possible to calculate a load line and place it on the graph of the characteristic curves, as shown in Figure 5-8B. The operating conditions of the circuit will be the point where the characteristic curve determined by E_g intersects this load line, which is determined by the power supply E and load resistor R. As E_g goes from -2.0 to -6.0 volts, for example, the operating point of the circuit moves from point A to B.

EXAMPLE 5-1

What is the change in E_R as E_g goes from -2.0 V to -6.0 V if $E = 250$ V and $R = 25$ kΩ for the circuit given in Figure 5-8A?

Solution:

If $E_T = 0$ then $I = \dfrac{250 \text{ V}}{2.5 \cdot 10^4 \ \Omega} = 10.$ mA

If $I = 0$ $E_T = E = 250$ V

This line is drawn in Figure 5-8B. Changing E_g from -2.0 to -6.0 volts causes the operation of the circuit to move from point A to point B.

At point A

$I' = 5.1$ mA

Therefore

$E'_R = IR = 5.1 \cdot 10^{-3}$ A $\times$ 25 $\cdot$ 10^3 Ω

$E'_R = 128$ V

At point B

$I'' = 2.6$ mA

Therefore

$E''_R = IR = 2.6 \cdot 10^{-3}$ A $\times$ 25 $\cdot$ 10^3 Ω

$E''_R = 65$ V

$\Delta E_R = E''_R - E'_R = 65$ V $-$ 128 V

$\Delta E_R = -63$ V   ∎

In this example, a change of four volts in E_g produced a 63-volt change in E_R. What has happened is that the signal E_g has been amplified. The amplification factor is given by the quotient of the change in output divided by the change in input.

$$A = \frac{\Delta E_{\text{out}}}{\Delta E_{\text{in}}} \tag{5-8}$$

EXAMPLE 5-2

What is the amplification factor in Example 5-1?

Solution:

$$A = \frac{\Delta E_R}{\Delta E_g} = \frac{-63}{-6-(-2)} = 16$$

(rounded for significant figures)   ■

One of the key uses of a triode is as an amplifier. A small voltage signal fed on to the grid can produce a much larger voltage change over a load resistor. In many applications, the output of one triode amplifier is fed into another to increase a small signal to a measurable one. The amplification is linear only as long as the characteristic curves are parallel to each other for the voltage values that are input. Once outside this area on the graph, amplification may still occur, but a change in E_g will no longer produce a proportional change in E_R. In short, A is no longer constant. To be useful, amplifiers must be built so that A is constant in operation. Even so, changes in temperature and aging can cause A to drift over a period of time. In a real vacuum tube amplifier, R would have to be variable so that the output voltage could be adjusted to be the proper value for an accurately known input. Feedback techniques explained in Chapter 6 are also used to provide stabilization.

There is another important use of a triode. For Figure 5-9, the load resistor is relatively small. Consequently, if $E_g = 0$, the load line intersects the characteristic curve in the region where the plate

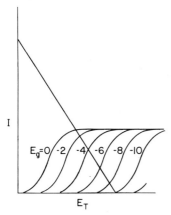

Figure 5-9 The triode can be used as a switch by varying E_g between saturation and shutdown voltages.

current has saturated. On the other hand, if $E_g = -12$ V, the intersection occurs at the x axis, and no current flows. By changing the voltage applied to the grid from 0 to −12 volts, the plate current is effectively turned off. When the grid voltage is returned to ground, the plate current is turned back on. The result is an electrically controlled switch, which is the second major way in which triodes are used.

The diode and triode are by no means the only types of vacuum tubes available. More electrodes can be added and the geometry changed to give numerous effects. The three basic uses of nonlinear elements have, however, been introduced and are rectification, amplification, and logic (switch) control. Vacuum tubes are no longer widely used because the same operations can be accomplished by use of solid state devices that require less power, are more stable, and have a longer lifetime. Nevertheless, vacuum tubes more clearly demonstrate the principles mentioned, and consequently they were discussed first.

Section 5-4
SEMICONDUCTOR DIODE

As was mentioned in Chapter 3, chemical elements exist that are semiconductors (column IV of the periodic table), neither allowing charge to pass as easily as a metal conductor nor completely blocking it as an insulator. These semiconductors can be made more conductive by the addition of very small amounts of impurity from the third and fifth columns of the periodic tables. These doped materials are then called p-type semiconductors if an excess of positional holes exists and n-type if an excess of roving electrons exists. If placed in a circuit with a battery, semiconductors function as resistors slowing the discharge of the battery.

A more electrically useful situation occurs if we attach a piece of p-type semiconductor to a piece of n-type semiconductor. Any time two different conductors are placed in contact, a "junction potential" develops between them. This is because the affinity each has for electrons is not the same. Some electrons will migrate from one conductor to the other to achieve the most stable thermody-

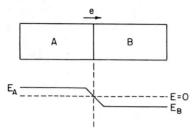

Figure 5-10 The electrical junction potential at the interface between two materials is shown as a function of distance from the boundary.

namic state, that is, the lowest overall potential energy. When this happens, as is shown in Figure 5-10, one of the conductors becomes slightly positive and the other slightly negative compared with their unattached state. When p-type and n-type materials are placed next to each other, they are a perfect match. One has excess free electrons and the other excess places for electrons to reside. As a result, electrons migrate across the interface from the n region to the p region. Figure 5-11 shows what happens. As soon as the electrons begin to move across the interface, the n-type material, which previously had an equal amount of positive and negative charges, becomes depleted of electrons in the region near the interface and takes on a slightly positive charge. On the other hand, the p-type material, also originally electrically neutral, begins to accumulate electrons in the region next to the interface and becomes slightly negatively charged.

One might reasonably wonder why all the free electrons do not wander over the interface from the n-type material to the p-type material and fall into positional holes. The reason is that two competing

processes are at work. One process is causing free electrons to fall into the positional holes, which is an energetically more favorable situation. To accomplish this, however, one must separate the electrons from the fixed positive charges in the n-type material and physically transport them to the p region. This process involves the separation of charges and requires a goodly amount of energy. The electrical stability of the filled orbital fights the electrical instability of charge separation. Somehow, these forces must be resolved.

As in all natural processes, the final situation is reached when the forces balance each other. This is called equilibrium. For a p–n semiconductor junction, this equilibrium occurs when a small region of positive charge develops along the n-type side of the interface and a similar region of negative charge develops along the p-type side of the interface. Because excess free electrons and holes no longer exist in this area, it is called the "depletion layer." This layer electrically blocks the passage of more electrons from the n region to the p region. On the other hand, since the n region is positively charged (albeit slightly) and the p region is negatively changed and there is a conductor between them, current should flow. Current does not flow because the voltage difference is offset by the positional stability of the electrons in the previously vacant orbitals. Nevertheless, if the situation could be stabilized by some outside force which would replenish the electrons, current would indeed flow. This current is called the intrinsic current because it is an intrinsic property of how the semiconductor junction is designed and independent of any external potential. The intrinsic current is very small, frequently less than 1 μA.

In Figure 5-12 the p–n device has been placed

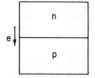
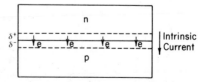

Figure 5-11 Electrons migrate from n-type to p-type semiconductors, leaving a slight positive charge on the n-type and creating a small negative charge on the p-type.

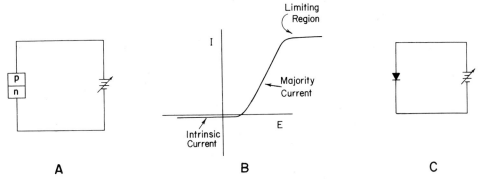

Figure 5-12   A p–n junction device acts in the same manner as a vacuum tube diode when put in series with a power supply. Part C is the standard representation of Part A, while Part B shows the characteristic curve.

into a circuit. As shall be seen shortly, this device is just a semiconductor version of the diode. Initially, the electrons in the n region remain at home due to a negatively charged layer on the p side of the interface and the attraction of the excess positive charges in the n material. As the voltage begins to rise over the diode in Figure 5-12, more electrons enter the n region, thereby making it less appealing for an electron to remain there. At the same time the negative layer in the p material is being depleted by the attraction of the positive end of the power supply. At a few tenths of a volt (much less than for a vacuum tube diode), the electrons begin breaking through the depletion layer and current begins to flow through the diode. It should be noted that this current flows in the direction opposite that of the intrinsic current, which, in effect, has to be overcome. This current is called the "majority current" because it flows in the direction that a majority of the current carriers, holes and electrons, want to go, that is, electrons out of the n-type material. The current flow is plotted as a function of voltage in Figure 5-12B. The circuit in Figure 5-12A is redrawn in Figure 5-12C, using the electrical symbol for the diode. Note that there is a maximum amount of current that can be carried by the diode in this forward direction, and the relationship between current and voltage is nonlinear, as in the case of the vacuum diode.

Let us suppose that the diode in Figure 5-12 had

been put in backward. As the potential of the battery is increased, electrons are poured into the p-type material and extracted from the n-type material. The electrons left in the n-type material begin to retreat from the interface with its growing negative charge on the other side. Similarly, electrons in the p-type material preferentially move into the holes near the n-type material which is nearer the growing positive charge. The result is that the depletion layer grows thicker. Moreover, since the charge for the intrinsic current is being replenished from the outside, we actually see a small flow of current in the reverse direction, unlike in the vacuum tube diode, where it cannot flow backward. This procedure of putting the diode in backward is called "reverse biasing." A p–n junction where the n region is made more positive than the p region is said to be reversed biased. When the p region is more positive than the n region, the junction is called forward biased. Reverse biasing a diode virtually eliminates the flow of current, except for a very small amount of intrinsic current. In most cases this amount of current is insignificant.

If one continues to increase the reverse bias voltage, the n region of the diode is gradually totally depleted of electrons, while the p region has all its holes filled. In effect, the depletion layer is now the whole diode. Any additional electrons forced into the p region by the power supply cannot find stable orbitals and are repelled out of the very negative p

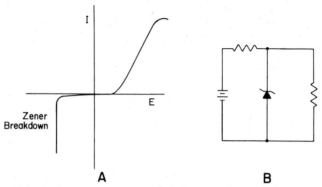

Figure 5-13   When an adequately high voltage is applied in the reverse direction to a semiconductor diode, it will experience a Zener breakdown. Those diodes that can sustain such a breakdown without damage are called Zener diodes and are symbolized as shown in Part B of this figure.

region into the highly positive n region, from which they are rapidly sucked out by the even more positive power supply. In fact, each electron literally flies through the diode backward, with all factors encouraging its rapid transit. The result is called the Zener breakdown. The diode can do nothing to prevent the flow of any amount of current the power supply cares to send through. This breakdown, as shown in Figure 5-13, happens at a specific voltage, depending on the design of the diode. When it occurs, the ordinary diode rapidly heats up and is destroyed.

Diodes have been developed that can withstand this Zener breakdown, appropriately called Zener diodes. When the back biasing of a Zener diode reaches the breakdown point, it begins to conduct all the current the power supply can send through it. The power supply cannot be raised to a higher voltage because it cannot generate enough current to produce an *IR* drop over the Zener diode equal to a higher voltage. In effect, any voltage greater than the Zener voltage is shorted out. A Zener diode can therefore be used to fix the maximum voltage of a power source if it is put in parallel with a load across the supply. We will explore this use more when power supplies are discussed in Chapter 7. Naturally, to be useful the Zener diode must be installed in the circuit backward. The electrical

symbol for the Zener diode is shown in a sample circuit in Figure 5-13.

Section 5-5
BIPOLAR JUNCTION TRANSISTOR

One can increase the complexity of the diode by adding another layer of semiconductor material to it. In particular, Figure 5-14A shows an extra layer of n-type material that has been added to form a sandwich, and the new device, called a transistor,

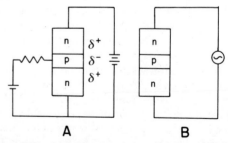

Figure 5-14   A bipolar junction transistor is in a typical circuit in Part A. A small layer of p-type material is sandwiched between two n regions in this type of BJT. In Part B no current will flow in either direction because one p–n junction is always back-biased.

has been placed in a typical circuit. The transistor is interesting because it has two p–n interfaces in the opposite directions, almost like two diodes with the p-type semiconductor ends attached together. It should be immediately apparent that current cannot flow in either direction through the device since one or the other of the p–n junctions must always be reverse biased (Fig. 5-14B). Let us examine what is happening in terms of electrons and holes. The n-type semiconductor attached to the positive end of the battery has become an electron-depleted positive region. The n-type material attached to the negative end of the battery, which already had an abundance of electrons, is now literally saturated with them. Between these two layers is a narrow piece of p-type material. This material has acquired a slight negative charge and is bordered by slightly positively charged layers in each piece of the n-type material. This region acts as a fence preventing the passage of electrons. Although one can break this fence by applying enough voltage to force the Zener effect to occur on the reverse biased junction, this would destroy the transistor and would therefore be counterproductive.

The key to the operation of the transistor is the p-region. If one attaches a second power supply between the p-type material and the negative end of the first battery (Fig. 5-14A), one can force current into the p-type material. As the voltage on the auxiliary battery rises, the excess electrons in the p-type material are removed. When this happens, the fence between the two n-type pieces disappears and electrons, which initially enter the p-type material from the bottom n region simply to replenish the lost charge, are attracted into the more positive n-type material on the top. As a consequence, current flows through the transistor. The transistor described above is called a bipolar junction transistor (BJT) and is very similar to the vacuum tube triode. The names of the electrodes even correspond to the older technology. The end of the BJT attached to the negative end of the battery, which corresponds to the cathode, is called the emitter, since it "emits" electrons through the device. The other attachment to the power supply is the collector, collecting the emitted electrons. The circuit corresponding to the plate circuit is called the collector

circuit. The control element that replaces the grid is called the base. The BJT obeys Eq. 5-5, just as the triode does. The characteristic curves for a typical BJT are shown in Figure 5-15. Note that as the current at the base increases, the current at the collector increases as well. This is just the opposite of what happens in a triode (Fig. 5-8). A limit is reached beyond which increases in the collector voltage will no longer produce more collector current for a given base current. Work through the diagram to be sure you understand the effect of changing the base current.

The BJT runs at relatively low voltages and currents. For comparison, the voltage in the collector circuit of a BJT is only a small percentages of that in the plate circuit of a triode. Like the triode, the base must be very fragile to make the transistor work, and a large amount of base-emitter current cannot be tolerated. Only a slight amount is necessary to make the transistor work. It is necessary to protect the base with a large resistor to prevent substantial current from flowing and destroying the transistor.

It should be noted that while the transistor in Figure 5-14 appears to be symmetrical between the collector and the emitter, it is a rare transistor in which they are actually interchangeable. Transistors are made in many sizes, current capacities, and sensitivities. To get the characteristics one wants requires various physical distortions of the three components. The transistor discussed above is

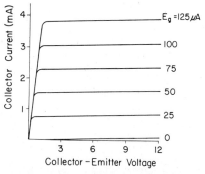

Figure 5-15 The characteristic curves of a BJT show that more base current implies more collector current.

called an n–p–n transistor because of the arrangement of the semiconductor components. Its electrical symbol is shown in Figure 5-16.

Also shown in Figure 5-16 is the p–n–p transistor. Unlike a vacuum tube, in which only one configuration is possible because electrons cannot jump from the cold anode to the hot cathode, it is possible to build a "backward" transistor. Everything in the circuit is reversed. While the current still flows from the collector to the emitter, the operation of the transistor is best explained in terms of the flow of holes rather than electrons. Whereas in reality it is always electrons that move, it is much clearer to see what is happening if one just interchanges the polarity of all the terms in the n–p–n explanation.

The uses of the BJT parallel those of the triode that it has replaced. Amplification can be obtained from appropriately designed transistors in a very similar manner to that obtained from triodes, although the magnitude of the voltage will be considerably less. The use of the common transistor as a switch is so widespread in laboratory instrumentation that a few examples of circuits are worth considering.

The first two circuits are shown in Figure 5-17. In Figure 5-17A, the transistor switch is in series with a resistive load of some sort. When the voltage applied to the base (E_B) is low (effectively zero), the

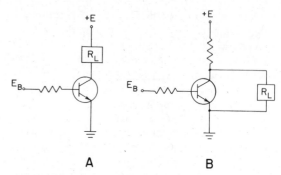

Figure 5-17   Two typical transistor circuits show how loads can be switched on and off.

transistor will not conduct. If the transistor does not conduct current, it acts like an open switch, and no current will flow through the load resistance. If E_B is high enough, the transistor will conduct readily. The effect is like a closed switch with the collector shorted to the emitter. This means the collector is virtually at ground and current will flow through the load.

In Figure 5-17B, the BJT is in parallel with the load. If the base of the transistor is held low, then the current cannot flow through it but must flow through the parallel load. Thus the load is "on" when the transistor is "off." If a positive voltage is applied to the base, the emitter attached to one side of the load is effectively shorted to the collector attached to the other side of the load. The current takes advantage of this easy route to ground and bypasses the load, turning it off. The on–off polarity of the load is therefore opposite to that of the transistor switch. Note the presence of a resistor in series with the transistor. This is necessary to prevent excessive current from passing through the transistor and destroying it by overheating. The resistor, of course, must be before the collector-load branch in order to make the switch effective. Note that this is not necessary in Figure 5-17A because the load itself is between the positive power supply and the transistor.

Figure 5-18 shows a more complicated transistor switch. Here two BJTs are used to control a resistive load. When point A is grounded, transistor T_1 will be turned off. This will cause point B, which is

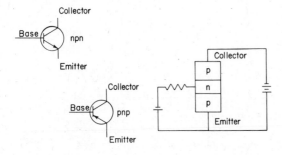

Figure 5-16   Part A shows the electrical symbols for n–p–n and p–n–p transistors. Part B shows a diagram of a p–n–p transistor circuit.

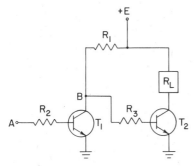

Figure 5-18 A two-transistor circuit is used to control a load.

now electrically attached only to the power supply, to be at nearly the power supply voltage (there is very little current to produce a significant IR drop across R_1). This means that the base of transistor T_2 will be high and current will flow through T_2. As a consequence, the load is on when point A is low. If a voltage is applied to point A, the base of T_1, T_1 will conduct and point B becomes attached to ground. Now significant current will flow through R_1. Since the resistance of R_1 is much greater than that of T_1, most of the voltage is lost over R_1, and point B is very close to ground potential. With point B low, the base of T_2 is low and T_2 will shut off. As a result, no current flows through the load when point A is high. Note that R_1 protects T_1 and the load protects T_2 from too much current flowing through them when they are turned on. R_2 and R_3 protect the bases of the transistors. Because of the design of the circuit, R_3 may not be necessary if R_1 is large enough.

It is reasonable to ask why two transistors are used when a similar action could be obtained by use of only one transistor in parallel with the load. There are several possible reasons. First, transistors come in many power ratings. It is sometimes necessary to control a high current circuit with a weak input signal which would be unable to saturate the base of the larger power transistor. The first transistor acts as an input signal amplifier to drive the second. On the other hand, it is possible to get the whole voltage of the power supply over the load by this arrangement, which is not possible

if a simple transistor is put in parallel with the load (Fig. 5-17B).

Figure 5-19 shows a three-transistor circuit in which one transistor is p–n–p. When the voltage is high at point A, T_1 will conduct. This will cause point B to be shorted to $+E$ (a positive power supply) and to rise to that voltage value. Current will flow from point B to the ground. When point A is of high potential, T_2 will also turn on. This will short the base and emitter of T_3 together and will prevent current from flowing through T_3 because point C will have effectively the same voltage as point B. If point A is low (ground), then T_1 will stop conducting, and point B will be electrically disconnected from $+E$. At the same time T_2 will also stop conducting because its base is also low. Points B and C will then not be connected electrically. The only electrical attachment now to point C is $-E$ (a negative voltage supply), which will cause the voltage at point C to drop. Since T_3 is a p–n–p transistor, this will turn it on, which will short point B to $-E$. This will cause current to flow through R_4 from the more positive ground to the more negative point B. This is the opposite of how the current flowed through R_4 when point A was high. Circuits that can have

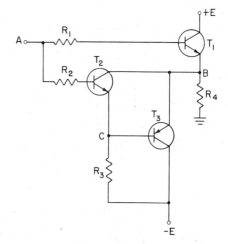

Figure 5-19 This three-transistor circuit allows current to flow in either direction through resistor R_4. ($+E$ indicates a positive voltage supply and $-E$ a negative voltage supply.)

current flow either into or out of them, depending on the input, are essential to the functioning of operational amplifiers, as we shall see in Chapter 6.

Section 5-6
FIELD-EFFECT TRANSISTORS

The bipolar junction transistor is only one of a number of transistors and transistorlike devices. Another popular type of transistor is the field-effect transistor (FET), diagrammed in Figure 5-20.

The body of this transistor is composed of one type of semiconductor. Pieces of the other type of semiconductor are implanted on either side of this slab. For simplicity, we will discuss in detail only one of the two possible transistors, the one where the slab is n-type material and the side pieces are p-type. When in operation, current flows through the body of the n-type semiconductor from one end to the other. This passage is called the "channel." The end where the electrons enter the FET corresponds to the cathode and is called the "source." The end where they leave acts as the anode and is called the "drain." The two p-type regions, attached by a wire, function as the control element and are collectively called the gate. This type of FET is called n-channel-p-gate.

Figure 5-21A shows an n-channel-p-gate FET in a circuit. Because there is contact along the interface, the p-type material has become slightly negative and the n-type material slightly positive, as we have seen before. This means the p–n junction is back biased. If E_g is 0 with respect to the source, the current flows through the channel of the FET as if it were a very small resistor. If, on the other hand, we attach a battery between the source and the gate so that E_g becomes more negative (Fig.

5-21A), the holes in the p-type material become filled with electrons. This makes the p-type material more negative and causes the electrons in the neighboring n-type material to be driven away from the negative p region. A positive field is created in the neighborhood of the gate through which electrons cannot travel freely. The size of the channel is effectively squeezed (Fig. 5-21B), making the passage through the channel more difficult, so that less current can flow for a given voltage. The FET acts as a variable resistor, much as the triode. If the gate is made negative enough, the field completely cuts the channel, and the source-drain current ceases. The field-effect transistor works because the field of the gate affects the flow of the current, hence the name.

As with the BJT, the possibility exists for a transistor with the opposite polarity. The p-channel-n-gate FET works analogously to the FET discussed above, except all the electrical connections and polarities are reversed. The symbols for both types of transistors are given in Figure 5-22, as is the basic circuit for the p-channel-n-gate FET. The FET works similarly to the triode in that the voltage which is applied to the control element (gate) is for the purpose of charging that element and not to establish a current as with the BJT. The FET has a very high input impedance at the gate which makes it a good input stage in a measuring circuit.

The characteristic curves for a FET are shown in Figure 5-23. At any particular gate voltage E_g, the drain current rises linearly with the drain voltage for the first few volts and then reaches saturation. After this, moderate increases in drain voltage will have no effect on the drain current until dielectric breakdown occurs (similar in effect to a Zener breakdown). Different E_g's give different saturation currents. Each FET will have its own family of characteristic curves. By placing a FET into a circuit such as that in Figure 5-24A, one gets an amplifier similar to the triode amplifier. The equation for the drain circuit is again simply

$$E = IR + E_T \tag{5-5}$$

If this equation for the load line is graphed with the characteristic curves, one gets Figure 5-24B. The transistor will operate at the point of intersection between the load line and the characteristic curve

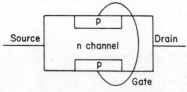

Figure 5-20   A diagram of the n-channel-p-gate field effect transistor (FET).

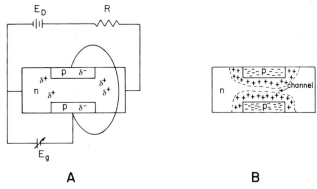

A   B

Figure 5-21 Part A shows a FET in a circuit with the appropriate voltage polarities. Part B shows the constriction of the channel as the gate becomes more negative.

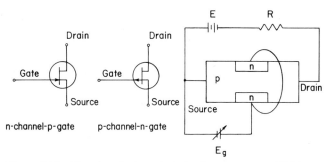

Figure 5-22 The electrical symbols for the two types of FETs are shown in this figure as is the manner in which a p-channel-n-gate FET is placed in a circuit.

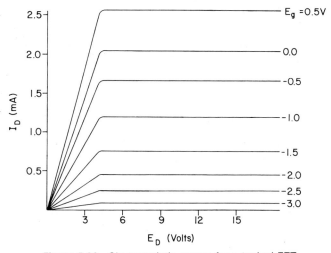

Figure 5-23 Characteristic curves for a typical FET.

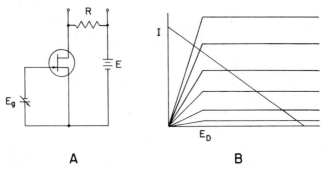

A   **B**

Figure 5-24 Part A shows a typical FET amplifier circuit, and Part B shows the load line superimposed on the characteristic curves.

determined by the gate voltage, just as in the case of the triode. By varying the gate voltage, the current can be changed from one value to another. Since the voltage over resistor R is dependent on the current, this voltage will also change as happened for the triode. The amplification then is just the ratio of the changes in the voltage over R divided by the voltage on the gate. The amplification factor is given by

$$A = \frac{\Delta E_{\text{out}}}{\Delta E_{\text{in}}} = \frac{\Delta E_R}{\Delta E_g} \qquad \textbf{(5-8)}$$

Numerous circuits are possible using FETs, two of which are shown in Figure 5-25. In Figure 5-25A we have a follower, in this case a source follower.

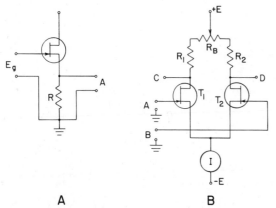

A   **B**

Figure 5-25 A source follower and a differential amplifier are diagrammed.

As the voltage at the gate decreases (becomes more negative), the gate closes down the flow of current through the transistor. Since the voltage at point A is equal to IR, this voltage also decreases (approaches zero). On the other hand, if E_g increases (approaches zero), then current flow increases, and E_A approaches $+E$, the voltage of the power supply. The name "source follower" comes from the fact that the source voltage "follows" the direction of voltage change at the gate. Because of the ground between them, the output circuit is isolated from the input circuit, and the polarity with respect to ground is switched (ground being high to ground being low). Such circuits are frequently used to convert negative to positive voltage levels and to electrically isolate a signal source from a measuring device. They can also be made using BJTs.

Figure 2-25B shows a FET differential amplifier, similar to what would be found in the input stage of an operational amplifier as discussed in the next chapter. The circuit has a constant current device, an element which draws a constant current by varying its own resistance. This device forces the sum of the currents in the two branches of the circuit to be constant. R_B is adjusted so that the same amount of current flows through each branch when $E_A = E_B$ (i.e., the circuit is balanced). If the voltage at A becomes more negative, less current is allowed to flow through T_1. This causes a smaller IR drop over R_1, and the voltage at C becomes more positive. Because the total current must be the same, the constant current source must increase the voltage over both branches of the circuit. Since the resistances of R_2 and T_2 have not changed, the current through this branch will increase with the higher voltage. This causes a larger *IR* drop across R_2 and causes point D to fall in voltage. Therefore, a more negative voltage at A produces a more positive voltage at C and a less positive voltage at D. The identical effect can be accomplished by making the voltage at B *less* negative. A less negative voltage at B causes T_2 to increase the amount of current that flows. This causes a larger *IR* drop over R_2 and point D to be less positive. Since more current is coming through the second branch, the constant current source must decrease the voltage over both branches of the circuit to keep the total current the same. This lower voltage causes a current reduction in the first branch of the circuit. When this happens, the *IR* drop over R_1 is less and point C becomes more positive.

The fact that the two inputs have the opposite effect on certain points in the circuit gives rise to the name "differential amplifier." The circuit allows the subtraction of two voltage levels, a frequently needed ability in measurement devices. The amplifier will only work in that range in which the drain current is directly proportional to the gate potential and the drain voltage. This is the left portion of the graph in Figure 5-23. This limited working range can be expanded through additional circuitry.

Section 5-7
OTHER SOLID-STATE DEVICES

Several other solid-state devices are of particular interest to the laboratory professional. The first of these is the light-emitting diode (LED). The LED is constructed in the same manner as a basic diode except that the material from which it is made is capable of light emission. An ordinary diode, which is made of silicon or germanium, dissipates the energy that evolves from electron-hole recombination in the form of heat. However, when diodes are made from combinations of gallium, arsenic and phosphorous (GaAs, GaP, GaAsP), the energy is radiated as light. This light is usually of a restricted wavelength band somewhere in the upper half of the visible or near infrared region (550–900 nm).

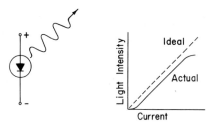

Figure 5-26 A light emitting diode (LED) symbol and its emission curve.

The symbol of the LED is given in Fig. 5-26 along with a graph of the response curve. As can be seen, the light intensity is not directly proportional to the current through the diode. There is an initial period of low response before a linear relationship develops. Moreover, there is eventually current saturation beyond which no additional light is generated. Consequently, the operating range of the LED must be restricted appropriately if the light is to be used as a measure of the current flow.

The counterpart of the light-emitting diode is the photosensitive diode or photodiode. Unlike the LED, the photodiode is reversed biased. As a result, appreciable current is not expected to flow through the photodiode. The photodiode is designed, however, so that the depletion layer can be reached by electromagnetic radiation (light). Light of a certain wavelength will cause the production of an electron–hole pair by providing the energy to excite the electron. The number of conductors produced by this means exceeds that produced by random motion and is proportional to the amount of exciting radiation. As a consequence, the depletion

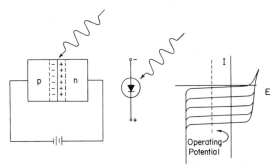

Figure 5-27 A diagram of a photodiode in a circuit, its symbol, and its characteristic curves when operating.

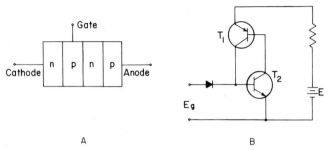

Figure 5-28 The basic layout of a silicon controlled rectifier and how it works, as simulated by two transistors.

layer becomes leaky and permits some current to flow. The amount of current is proportional to the number of conductors, which is proportional to the intensity of the light. Therefore, the current response is proportional to the light stimulus. What happens next is depicted graphically in Figure 5-27. The increase in light intensity (flux) causes the intrinsic current to appear to increase. To operate the photodiode successfully one must pick a voltage somewhere between zero and the Zener breakdown. The photodiode is very quick in response, but only generates currents in the microampere range. An LED–photodiode pair can be used to isolate one circuit from another. Such a couple is called an optical isolator. It prevents high frequency electrical noise from being propagated through the circuit and eliminates grounding problems.

The final device we shall examine in this chapter is the silicon controlled rectifier (SCR). The SCR is one of a class of devices called "thyristors" and has four semiconductor layers, as shown in Figure 5-28A. An SCR will allow current to follow in only one direction, from the anode to the cathode. To understand how it works, it is necessary to make a two-transistor equivalent drawing (Figure 5-28B). Note that this is for pedagogical purposes only and cannot be used in place of an SCR in a circuit. If the voltage at the gate (E_g) is zero or negative, then T_2, an n–p–n transistor, will not conduct. In this case, the base of T_1, a p–n–p transistor, will have no current drawn from it, and it too will not conduct. If E_g is raised to some positive value, T_2 will be turned on. This will cause current to be drawn from the base of T_1, and it will also conduct. This will cause

current to flow through T_1 into the base of T_2, which will keep it conducting once E_g falls to zero or below. Once the SCR is activated by a positive pulse at the gate, it will stay on. Note that a diode is placed in the gate circuit to prevent current draining from the SCR into the circuit driving the gate.

One may well ask: What good is a circuit that goes on and stays on once it is pulsed? For a dc circuit, this would be pointless. If the power supply were ac instead, or a signal source that fluctuated around zero, the main circuit would switch off any time E fell to zero and would not switch back on again until pulsed. The SCR is indeed a rectifier, but a controllable one, that will allow one to select when one wants to start receiving the positive signal.

The use of nonlinear elements is essential to the operation of modern laboratory equipment. Scientific progress has allowed us to advance from bulky tubes to incredibly small solid-state components. This makes practical the use of sophisticated detection and calculation circuitry in even the most mundane laboratory instrument. Knowing the basic principles of such electronics is essential to understanding how instruments work. In Chapter 6 we will continue the exploration of nonlinear technology in terms of signal amplification.

REVIEW QUESTIONS

1. What is the difference between a linear element and a nonlinear one?
2. What is the effect of temperature on the kinetic energy of a molecule?

3. What is the effect of temperature on molecular velocity?

4. What is a Maxwell distribution?

5. How are electrons "boiled off"?

6. Why are vacuum tubes evacuated?

7. Why is a metal used as the cathode of a vacuum tube?

8. What is a diode?

9. What is the function of the heater in a vacuum tube?

10. Why does current only flow one way through a vacuum tube diode?

11. What is a load line?

12. What is a characteristic curve?

13. What is rectification? Why is a rectifier used?

14. What is "pulsed" dc?

15. What is the purpose of the grid?

16. Where is the grid located?

17. How does the grid operate?

18. Why is the grid negatively biased?

19. Why does a whole family of characteristic curves exist for triodes?

20. Why is a triode used in a dc rather than an ac circuit?

21. What is amplification? How is it accomplished with a triode?

22. What does a negative sign in an amplification result mean?

23. What is the easiest way to draw a load line on a graph?

24. What are the major uses of a triode?

25. What is the major use of a diode?

26. Define junction potential.

27. What happens at the interface between n-type and p-type semiconductors?

28. What are the charges at the p–n junction at equilibrium?

29. What are the opposing forces that control the equilibrium at a p–n junction?

30. What is the depletion layer?

31. What is intrinsic current?

32. What is the majority current?

33. How does a vacuum tube diode differ from a semiconductor diode?

34. What is the effect on the depletion layer of reverse biasing a diode?

35. What is Zener breakdown?

36. How does a Zener diode differ from a regular diode?

37. How does a Zener diode work?

38. What is a transistor?

39. What is a BJT?

40. What are the functions of the base, emitter, and collector?

41. Why can current not flow through a BJT if the base is disconnected?

42. Compare the voltage levels for a BJT with those of a vacuum tube.

43. What is the difference between a p–n–p and n–p–n transistor?

44. List several uses of a BJT.

45. Why is a resistor necessary in Figure 5-17B? Why is the resistor before the branch instead of after it?

46. Why might the circuit in Figure 5-18 be used instead of the one in Figure 5-17B?

47. Explain how the circuit in Figure 5-19 works.

48. What is a FET?

49. What are the functions of the source, channel, drain, and gate?

50. What are the two types of FETs? Sketch them in a simple circuit and label the parts.

51. In what way is the control of the BJT different from that of the FET and vacuum tube?

52. What is a source follower? How does it work?

53. What is a differential amplifier?

54. What is an LED? How does it work?

55. What is a photodiode? How does it work?

56. How does an SCR work? In what type of circuits is it used?

57. What is an optical isolator and why is it used?

PROBLEMS

What will happen in the circuit indicated in Figure 5-29 for various combinations of inputs (A low, B low; A high, B low; and so on)?

1. Figure 5-29A

2. Figure 5-29B

3. Figure 5-29C

4. Figure 5-29D

For Problems 5–8, you may use a 5-volt power supply (plus and minus voltages available), n–p–n and p–n–p transistors, resistors, and diodes to build the circuits described. Protect the inputs as necessary.

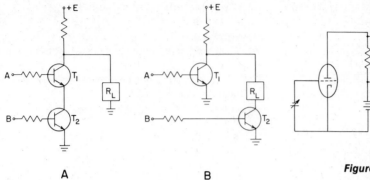

A   B

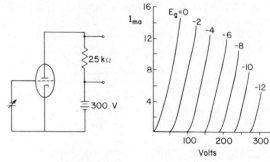

Figure 5-30 A triode amplifier.

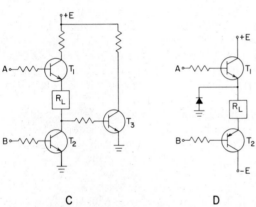

C   D

Figure 5-29 BJT circuits for Problems 1 to 4.

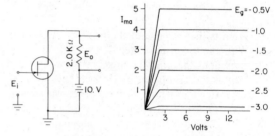

Figure 5-31 A FET amplifier.

5. The circuit has one input and two outputs. If the input is low (0), the output 1 is high (+) and the output 2 is low (0). If the input is high, the opposite is true.

6. The circuit drives a load R_L and has three inputs. If at least two of the inputs are high (+), the load is activated; otherwise, it is off.

7. The circuit has one input and one output. When the input is initially low, the output is low. As soon as the input becomes high, the output goes high and stays high no matter what the input does.

8. Using only five transistors, design a four-input circuit that drives R_L only if the first and fourth inputs are high (+) and the second and third inputs are low (0).

9. For the circuit in Figure 5-30, what is the voltage change over the resistor if the grid voltage goes from -2.0 to -5.0?

10. Resolve Problem 5-9, assuming that the resistor is only 20. kΩ.

11. In Figure 5-31, what is ΔE_R if E_i goes from -1.0 V to -2.0 V? What is the voltage gain?

12. Resolve Problem 5-11 assuming that the battery is 12 V and the resistance is 3.0 kΩ. What is the voltage gain over the transistor?

CHAPTER 6
OPERATIONAL AMPLIFIERS

Chapters 1–5 have made reference to amplification. The concept of amplification is simple to understand–something is made larger. Nature, however, is very stingy and will not arbitrarily allow us to increase electrical quantities. All electrical quantities, so you will recall from Chapter 1, are related to the storage or flow of energy. Amplifying an electrical quantity requires that more energy be expended. Energy is conserved in nature; if more energy is needed at one place, then the extra energy must be lost at some other place.

Section 6-1
OPERATIONAL AMPLIFIERS

Various electronic amplifiers have been built in the past, some examples of which were seen in Chapter 5. The major amplifier currently used in laboratory equipment is the operational amplifier. Figure 6-1 shows the symbolic representation of an operational amplifier. This amplifier has two circuits attached to it that have totally separate identities. One circuit is the circuit of interest, the one that has the analytical signal. The other is a power circuit that provides the energy to amplify the analytical signal. The power circuit generally has three leads: one to a positive voltage supply (frequently +15 V), one to a negative voltage supply (frequently −15 V), and one to ground. (Some integrated circuit amplifiers do not require a ground or treat the negative supply voltage as ground.) To obtain good quality output, these supply voltages must be relatively stable. This power circuit always exists for an operational amplifier, even though it is seldom mentioned. For simplicity throughout the remainder of the book, we will not include it in our figures or

descriptions, but it is important that it is always present.

The analytical circuit also has three attachments to the amplifier. These are called the inverting input (−), the noninverting input (+), and the output (o). A voltage level applied to the noninverting input will be amplified by the gain of the amplifier (A), usually between 10^3 and 10^8 times, and will appear at the output. A voltage level applied to the inverting input will be amplified by the negative gain of the amplifier and will appear at the output. The output voltage in terms of the input voltages and gain is

$$E_o = A(E_+ - E_-) \qquad \textbf{(6-1)}$$

The output voltage is limited by the power supply voltage; it cannot be higher than the positive supply voltage or lower than the negative supply voltage. If the power supply voltages are +15 V and −15 V and the gain is 10^5, then from Eq. 6-1, we get the working range of the amplifier:

$$-1.5 \cdot 10^{-4} \text{ V} < E_+ - E_- < 1.5 \cdot 10^{-4} \text{ V}$$

The working range for the input difference, then, is very small. In fact, it is usually so small that in most circuits we say that

$$E_+ \approx E_- \qquad \textbf{(6-2)}$$

This approximate equality is used to solve many operational amplifier problems. When the amplifier inputs exceed this range, the amplifier output goes to "limit"; that is, it goes to the power supply level, either positive or negative, and stays there until the input difference falls back within the working range. Amplifiers at limit are of no use in analytical measurement, but they can be used to drive servo systems. The constant voltage output of an ampli-

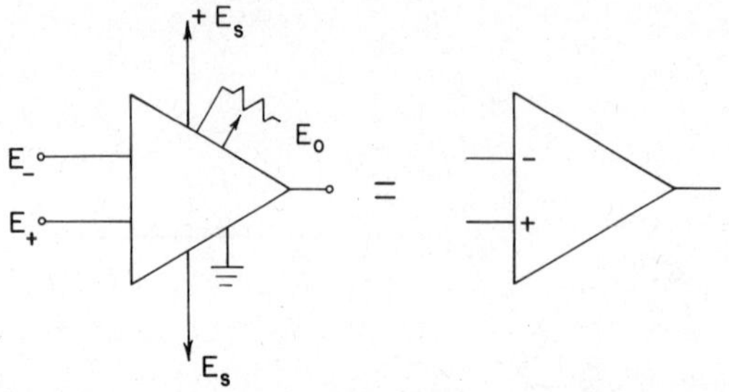

Figure 6-1 An operational amplifier is represented by a triangle. It contains an analytical circuit with attachments E_+, E_-, and E_o; a power circuit consisting of attachments $+E_s$, $-E_s$, and ground; and a calibrating circuit consisting of two potentiometer leads.

fier can drive the feedback circuit motor until compensation is reached. At that point, the voltage rapidly falls off, and the motor stops until some further change in the input voltage occurs (Section 2-5).

The nature of the analytical connections of an operational amplifier is important to understand. The inverting and noninverting inputs are gates of field effect transistors. As a consequence, their input impedance (resistance to current flow) is very high, on the order of 10^8–10^{10} ohms. Current, therefore, will not flow into or out of the inputs of an operational amplifier. On the other hand, current will flow both into and out of the output of the operational amplifier. The output impedance is very low, a few ohms at most, because the output is formed by the emitter of one transistor and the collector of another, which are attached to the positive and negative power supplies, respectively. The excess current is therefore taken from or given to the power supply circuit.

Another small circuit is indicated in Figure 6-1. This is called the balance circuit and consists of an external variable resistor used to balance the gain of the inverting and noninverting circuits within the amplifier. Because of manufacturing inaccuracies and aging, these gain circuits are never quite identical and must be balanced to allow Eq. 6-1 to be true and the amplifier to work properly. For simplicity, this circuit too is omitted in subsequent drawings and discussions. In fact, many integrated circuit amplifiers are stable enough not to require this circuit external to the amplifier.

Section 6-2
COMMON MODE REJECTION RATIO

If one grounds the inverting input and applies $1.0 \cdot 10^{-4}$ V to the noninverting input of an operational amplifier with a gain of 10^4, the output will be 1.0 V. If one applies 10.00000 V to the inverting input and 10.00010 V to the noninverting input, one still has a difference of $1.0 \cdot 10^{-4}$ V in the input and should still get 1.0 V as the output. In the latter case, however, this is not likely to happen. The reason is that there is 10.00000 V of common mode voltage, that is, voltage common to both inputs. The ability of the input circuits to balance each other perfectly under such conditions is called common mode rejection. The more effectively this common mode is ignored, the better the amplifier will do at producing a result proportional to the difference of its inputs. The common mode rejection ratio is the ratio of the common mode value to the signal input that would cause the same effect:

$$\text{CMRR} =$$

$$\frac{\text{change in output per unit change in input}}{\text{change in output per unit change in common mode}}$$

$$(6\text{-}3)$$

If the CMRR of the amplifier above were 10^5 (no units), then having a 10 V common mode would be equivalent to an input difference of $\pm 1.0 \cdot 10^{-4}$ V. In the above example, such a voltage is of the same magnitude as the analog signal. The output, being a combination of the analytical contribution and the common mode contribution, will fall somewhere between 0 (1 − 1) and 2 (1 + 1) V. Because the difference in the input values is always small, it is desirable to keep down the input voltages to minimize common mode problems. The CMRR for common operational amplifiers is about 10^5.

Section 6-3
VOLTAGE FOLLOWERS

Although an operational amplifier may be good at increasing the magnitude of a signal, it is not very good at doing so reproducibly. The gain of the amplifier is affected by temperature and aging. It will

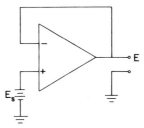

Figure 6-2 A voltage follower has the output fed back into the inverting input to nullify the unstable amplifier gain.

drift significantly over even a short period of time. To use an amplifier successfully requires designing circuits that compensate for the drift in the gain. The first application that we shall examine is that of a voltage follower. In Figure 6-2, we have an amplifier that has been wired into an unusual circuit. To understand what happens in the circuit it will be necessary to work through the mathematics of the circuit. We start with Eq. 6-1 and note that we must find the values for E_+ and E_- in order to solve for E_o. E_+ is simply the voltage of the battery source, E_s, but E_- is attached to E_o, so it must be the same voltage. We substitute and solve

$$E_o = A(E_+ - E_-)$$

$$E_+ = E_s \tag{6-4}$$

$$E_- = E_o \tag{6-5}$$

Therefore

$$E_o = A(E_s - E_o) \tag{6-6}$$

$$E_o + AE_o = AE_s$$

$$E_o = \frac{E_s A}{A + 1} \tag{6-7}$$

Now, if A is larger, 10^3 or greater, $A/(A + 1)$ is less than one-tenth of 1% different from 1. Since electrical circuits are less stable than that, we can assume that for all practical laboratory purposes the ratio is 1 and the output voltage equals the source voltage.

$$E_o = E_s \tag{6-8}$$

The importance of this equation is monumental. The gain of the amplifier, with all its inherent insta-

bility, has been removed from the final operating equation. The gain is free to drift as long as it is great enough to make true our assumption that $A/(A + 1) = 1$ at the level of precision we seek. If a device that puts out the same voltage it takes in seems a bit mundane, it must be realized that the input effectively draws no current and therefore does not affect the circuit it is attached to, while the output has the ability to generate enough current to run any meter (or other circuit) without having any effect on the voltage. The voltage follower then is the perfect isolation device to place between a sensitive voltage source and circuits that draw significant current.

A circuit like the one in Figure 6-2 is called a "feedback" circuit. The output voltage is "fed back" into the input. The function of this arrangement is to stabilize the circuit. As the voltage at the noninverting input begins to rise, the output begins to rise much more rapidly. Since this output is attached to the inverting input of the same amplifier, the increasing signal there has the effect of trying to cause the output to swing sharply negative. If this were to happen, however, this negative output would enter the inverting input and drive the output positive again. The final result of the forces that are trying to move the output more positive and more negative is to compromise on an output effectively equal to the signal at the noninverting input. The voltage at the noninverting input is E_s, and the voltage at the inverting input is very slightly less than E_s. This gives a net difference of a small positive input that is then amplified into the voltage of the output; since it is connected to the inverting input, it is also slightly less than E_s. This is apparent from an examination of Eq. 6-7. If the amplifier gain varies, the output will try to change, but this will affect the inverting input which will immediately bring the output voltage to its previous level.

Section 6-4
VOLTAGE FOLLOWERS WITH GAIN

Figure 6-3 shows a circuit with some similarities to that in Figure 6-2, but with two resistors added, one in the feedback part of the circuit and one between the inverting input and ground. To determine how

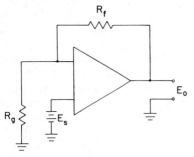

Figure 6-3 The voltage follower with gain uses the feedback principle to obtain a stable circuit gain based on the relationship between the ground and feedback resistors.

the circuit works, we will substitute into Eq. 6-1 as before:

$$E_o = A(E_+ - E_-)$$

From Figure 6-3

$$E_+ = E_s \qquad \text{(6-9)}$$

Note that the resistors R_f (feedback) and R_g (ground) form a voltage divider between the output voltage and ground. The voltage at the inverting input is just the voltage dropped over R_g.

$$E_- = IR_g \qquad \text{(6-10)}$$

$$I = \frac{E_o - 0}{\Sigma R}$$

$$= \frac{E_o}{R_f + R_g} \qquad \text{(6-11)}$$

$$E_- = E_o \frac{R_g}{R_f + R_g} \qquad \text{(6-12)}$$

Substituting into Eq. 6-1

$$E_o = A\left(E_s - E_o \frac{R_g}{R_f + R_g}\right) \qquad \text{(6-13)}$$

$$E_o \frac{1 + AR_g}{R_f + R_g} = AE_s$$

$$E_o = E_s A \left(\frac{R_f + R_g}{R_f + R_g + AR_g}\right) \qquad \text{(6-14)}$$

This is a messy equation, but we can greatly simplify it if we make two assumptions. The first is the

same as before, namely that the gain is large compared with 1. The second is that the ratio R_f/R_g is much less than the gain. If both of these are true, then AR_g is much greater than $R_f + R_g$, and these latter terms can be dropped from the denominator. If

$$AR_g \gg R_f + R_g \qquad \text{(6-15)}$$

then

$$E_o = E_s A \left(\frac{R_f + R_g}{AR_g}\right)$$

or

$$E_o = E_s \left(\frac{R_f + R_g}{R_g}\right) \qquad \text{(6-16)}$$

The output voltage has been amplified by the factor $(R_f + R_g)/R_g$, a number always greater than 1. This amplification occurs because only a part of the output voltage is fed back to the inverting input. Since the same voltage value is needed at the inverting input to stabilize the amplifier as in the voltage follower, the output voltage must be greater so that a fraction of it can equal that value. The $(R_f + R_g)/R_g$ factor is called the gain of the circuit. Note well that this is neither the same as, nor bears a relationship to, the gain of the amplifier, except that it must be significantly less for Eqs. 6-15 and 6-16 to hold. This circuit gain, unlike the amplifier gain, is stable, since it contains no A term.

EXAMPLE 6-1

The feedback resistor in Figure 6-3 is 2,400 Ω. If the signal is 1.9 V and the output 5.2 V, what is the value of the ground resistor?

Solution:

$$E_o = E_s \frac{R_f + R_g}{R_g}$$

$$E_o R_g - E_s R_g = E_s R_f$$

$$R_g = \frac{E_s R_f}{E_o - E_s}$$

$$= \frac{1.9 \times 2.4 \cdot 10^3}{5.2 - 1.9}$$

$$= 1.4 \text{ k}\Omega \qquad \blacksquare$$

In a simple follower there is no current flow around the amplifier. The only current in the circuit flows to or from the output. In the follower with gain, there can be a significant flow of current around the amplifier. Although current does not enter the inverting input, current does flow between it and ground and between it and the output. Since no current can flow into or out of the input, the current through R_f and R_g must be of the same magnitude and direction. In addition, current will flow between the output and whatever circuit is attached to the amplifier. These currents are separate and distinct, and there is no relationship between them. The former is determined solely by the circuit elements around and before the amplifier, and the latter, by the elements after the amplifier. The amplifier output generates or absorbs the extra current necessary to make everything balance. The energy to do this comes from the external power circuit.

Section 6-5
INVERTORS

While followers with and without gain have numerous uses, even more circuits are based on the invertor concept. Figure 6-4 shows a simple invertor circuit that we will analyze with the methods used on previous amplifiers. We start with the amplifier equation:

$$E_o = A(E_+ - E_-) \qquad (6\text{-}1)$$

We note immediately that we can simplify this equation because the noninverting input is grounded.

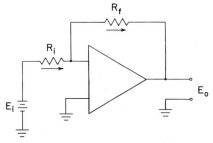

Figure 6-4 The invertor uses the feedback concepts, but attaches the signal source to the inverting input to make the gain easier to calculate and also invert the output.

$$E_+ = 0 \qquad (6\text{-}17)$$

Therefore

$$E_o = -AE_- \qquad (6\text{-}18)$$

We observe that the circuit attached to the inverting input is a voltage divider. We need first to calculate the current through the circuit, so that we can find the voltage E_-.

$$I = \frac{E_i - E_o}{R_i + R_f} \qquad (6\text{-}19)$$

$$E_- = E_i - IR_i \qquad (6\text{-}20)$$

$$E_- = E_i - \frac{(E_i - E_o)\, R_i}{R_i + R_f}$$

Putting everything over the same denominator

$$E_- = \frac{E_i R_i + E_i R_f}{R_i + R_f} - \frac{E_i R_i - E_o R_i}{R_i + R_f}$$

$$E_- = \frac{E_i R_f + E_o R_i}{R_i + R_f} \qquad (6\text{-}21)$$

If we now substitute for E_- in Eq. 6-18, we get

$$E_o = \frac{-A(E_i R_f + E_o R_i)}{R_i + R_f} \qquad (6\text{-}22)$$

$$E_o(R_i + R_f) = -AE_i R_f - AE_o R_i$$

$$E_o(R_i + R_f + AR_i) = -AE_i R_f$$

$$E_o = \frac{-AR_f E_i}{R_i + R_f + AR_i}$$

$$E_o = \frac{-A}{1 + R_f/R_i + A} \times \frac{R_f}{R_i} \times E_i \qquad (6\text{-}23)$$

If the amplification is large compared with both 1 and R_f/R_i, then these latter two items can be dropped from the denominator of the first term of Eq. 6-23 to give us

$$E_o = \frac{-A}{A} \times \frac{R_f}{R_i} \times E_i$$

or

$$E_o = -\frac{R_f}{R_i} \times E_i \qquad (6\text{-}24)$$

Several points should be noted about this equation. First, the sign of the output voltage is the

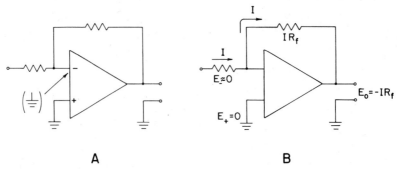

Figure 6-5 When the noninverting input is grounded, the inverting input assumes a value near zero volts, called "virtual ground." All current flowing into the virtual ground must flow out through the feedback part of the circuit.

opposite of the sign of the input voltage, giving rise to the name "invertor." Second, the amplification factor of the circuit is R_f/R_i. Unlike the follower with gain, the gain can be greater or less than 1, permitting output voltages that are larger or smaller in magnitude than the input voltages.

To find the current that flows around the amplifier, we substitute the output voltage equation (6-24) into the current equation (6-19):

$$I = \frac{E_i - E_o}{R_i + R_f}$$

$$= \frac{E_i - (R_f/R_i)E_i}{R_i + R_f} \qquad \textbf{(6-25)}$$

$$= \frac{E_i(R_f + R_i)/R_i}{R_i + R_f}$$

$$I = \frac{E_i}{R_i} \qquad \textbf{(6-26)}$$

The current flows down from the battery toward the inverting input. If we substitute this current into Eq. 6-20, the equation for E_-, we get

$$E_- = E_i - \frac{E_i}{R_i} R_i$$

$$E_- = 0 \qquad \textbf{(6-27)}$$

Wait just one minute! That's not possible! If $E_- = 0$ (Eq. 6-27) and $E_+ = 0$ (Eq. 6-17), then by Eq. 6-1, $E_o = 0$, and nothing happens; everything is grounded! All of this is almost true—almost. It would be true if Eq. 6-25 were rigorously true math-

ematically, but it is not. To get that equation, we assumed $A \gg 1$ and $A \gg R_f/R_i$ and ignored these terms. While these terms are too small to measure, they do, in fact, exist. Therefore, E_o is not quite equal to $-E_iR_f/R_i$, I is not quite equal to E_i/R_i, and E_- is not quite equal to 0.

As we saw with the voltage follower, the inverting input voltage E_- must be very close to the noninverting input voltage E_+ for the circuit to work. The same thing is true for the inventor; only here, since $E_+ = 0$, E_- is very close to zero. This condition in an invertor is called "virtual ground" because the inverting input is virtually at ground (Fig. 6-5A). Naturally, really grounding this point will cause the amplifier to stop working in a useful manner. Working with both inputs near ground eliminates common mode difficulties.

From Eq. 6-26 it should be clear that the current flowing into an invertor is independent of anything in the circuit after the virtual ground. This point electrically isolates the inputs from the outputs even though they are physically connected through the feedback resistor. The current through the feedback resistor is determined by the current flowing into or out of the virtual ground from the input circuit, since none can enter the amplifier. One can therefore think of the output voltage as being the voltage needed to maintain an IR drop from the zero voltage that exists at the virtual ground in order that all the input current will be able to flow through the feedback resistor (Fig. 6-5B).

After analysis of several circuits, the methodology to analyze amplified circuits should be becoming apparent. To determine the equation for the amplifier, one starts with Eq. 6-1 and replaces E_+ and E_- with suitable definitions in terms of the input or output voltages (or ground). One then solves the equation for E_o, makes the necessary restrictive assumptions to allow the gain of the amplifier to be eliminated, and writes the final equation. To really use the circuit one must be sure that the assumptions are justified by the choice of components.

EXAMPLE 6-2

Figure 6-6 shows a two-amplifier circuit with the resistor values as shown. Calculate the output voltage of the second amplifier.

Solution: To solve the problem, it is necessary to divide it into two parts and solve each separately. The appropriate division point is point A, since this point can be regarded as the output of the first amplifier and the input of the second.
For the first amplifier

$$E_A = E_i \frac{R_f + R_g}{R_g}$$

$$= 1.00 \frac{10.0 + 5.0}{5.0}$$

$$= 3.0 \text{ V}$$

For the second amplifier

$$E_o = -E_A \frac{R_f'}{R_i'}$$

$$= -3.0 \times \frac{20}{15}$$

$$= -4.0 \text{ V} \qquad \blacksquare$$

Section 6-6
ADDERS

By Kirchhoff's first law, all the current that enters a point on a circuit must leave it. The algebraic sum of current at any point must be zero. At the virtual ground of an inverting amplifier circuit, this law must hold true. Since none of the current can enter or leave the inverting input, all the extra current that comes in through the input resistor must leave through the feedback resistor. Let us assume that we attach a second battery and resistor to the virtual ground point (Fig. 6-7). Because of the way an operational amplifier works, the attachment point remains at virtual ground. The amount of current entering is now the sum of the currents from the two sources, and all this current must exit through the only available avenue, the feedback resistor.

$$I_f = I_1 + I_2 \qquad \textbf{(6-28)}$$

There is nothing magic about two sources of current. It is possible to attach an arbitrary number of input circuits to the point of virtual ground.

This situation leads to tremendous possibilities. If we generalize Eq. 6-28, we get

$$I_f = \Sigma I_i \qquad \textbf{(6-29)}$$

This equation tells us that at the virtual ground all input currents are added together before passing through the feedback resistor. The virtual ground point therefore acts as a "summing point" for current. This phenomenon allows the invertor to be used to add currents and to produce a voltage proportional to them. The current through a feedback resistor can be expressed in terms of Ohm's law.

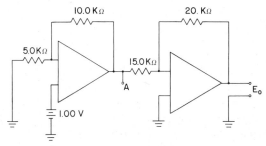

Figure 6-6 This two-amplifier circuit consists of a voltage follower with gain and an invertor with gain.

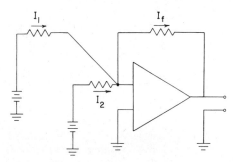

Figure 6-7 The virtual ground becomes a summing point when several current sources are attached.

$$I_f = \frac{E_- - E_o}{R_f} \qquad (6\text{-}30)$$

Since $E_- \approx 0$

$$E_o = -I_f R_f \qquad (6\text{-}31)$$

$$E_o = -R_f \Sigma I_i \qquad (6\text{-}32)$$

It must be noted here that the output voltage is proportional to the sum of the input currents, *not* the input voltages.

The input current need not even be generated by a battery–resistor combination; any current source will do. Moreover, the currents need not be in the same direction (Fig. 6-8). Current can flow in from one source and out through another without harm. The feedback circuit will make up the difference either way. By inverting one source before the summing point, one can perform subtraction between two signals. It should further be observed that there is effectively electrical isolation between the inputs as well as between the inputs and output. This is true because the virtual ground acts as a separation point just like a real ground would. The amplifier fights to keep this point fixed; as long as its operating conditions are not exceeded, it will hold this point so close to zero that isolation is assured.

EXAMPLE 6-3

In Figure 6-8, the resistors have the following values: $R_1 = 10.0 \text{ k}\Omega$, $R_2 = 6.8 \text{ k}\Omega$, $R_3 = 4.9 \text{ k}\Omega$, and $R_f = 5.6 \text{ k}\Omega$. The output voltage is -4.1 V, while input E_1 is 1.21 V and $E_2 = -2.93$ V. What is E_3?

Solution:

$$E_o = R_f \Sigma I_i$$

$$E_o = -R_f \left(\frac{E_1}{R_1} - \frac{E_2}{R_2} + \frac{E_3}{R_3} \right)$$

Solving for E_3

$$E_3 = -R_3 \left(\frac{E_o}{R_f} + \frac{E_1}{R_1} - \frac{E_2}{R_2} \right)$$

$$= -4.9 \cdot 10^3$$

$$\times \left(\frac{-4.1}{5.6 \cdot 10^3} + \frac{1.21}{10.0 \cdot 10^3} - \frac{2.93}{6.8 \cdot 10^3} \right)$$

$$E_3 = 5.1 \text{ V} \qquad \blacksquare$$

To make effective use of invertors as adders of voltages, it is necessary to use other than random resistors in the design. The first step is to make all the input resistors be the same value. Using Figure 6-8 as an example, we get

$$E_o = -R_f \left(\frac{E_1}{R_1} + \frac{E_2}{R_2} + \frac{E_3}{R_3} \right) \qquad (6\text{-}33)$$

If

$$R_1 = R_2 = R_3 = R_i \qquad (6\text{-}34)$$

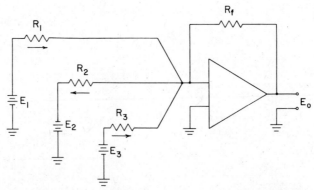

Figure 6-8 The currents entering the summing point need not all be in the same direction.

then

$$E_o = -R_f \left(\frac{E_1}{R_i} + \frac{E_2}{R_i} + \frac{E_3}{R_i} \right)$$

$$E_o = -\frac{R_f}{R_i} (E_1 + E_2 + E_3) \qquad \textbf{(6-35)}$$

If R_f equals R_i, the output voltage is just the sum of the input voltages with the sign inverted. In other cases, R_f/R_i represents the gain of the adder. To get accurate results from such an adder, it is necessary to use 1% or better precision resistors and to match them against each other in test circuits to be sure that they are effectively identical.

Section 6-7
INSTRUMENTATION AMPLIFIERS

In constructing laboratory instruments, it is frequently necessary to find the difference between two signals while not drawing significant current from either source. There are numerous ways to accomplish this, but one common approach is called the instrumentation amplifier and is diagrammed in Figure 6-9. The amplifier consists of three operational amplifiers. Two of these are used as voltage followers for the signal sources. In this way

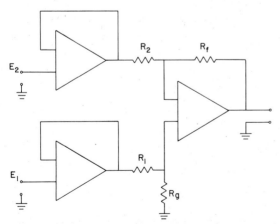

Figure 6-9 The instrumentation amplifier allows the comparison of two voltages without drawing significant current from either voltage source.

the sources can give their values without being significantly affected by the measuring device. Consequently, the key feature of these two operational amplifiers is that they have extremely high input impedance (10^8–10^{10} ohms). On the other hand, they need only moderate gain (10^3–10^4) because they are not amplifying the input signal.

The situation is completely reversed concerning the third amplifier. In order to get amplification, a high gain (10^5–10^7) is desired, but the input impedance is not so critical when other operational amplifiers are the sources of the current and will not readily be overloaded. The circuit around this amplifier is unusual because both inputs are actively being used. A mathematical analysis will show what is happening. As usual, we start with the operational amplifier equation:

$$E_o = A(E_+ - E_-) \qquad \textbf{(6-1)}$$

We may easily compute E_+, since it is merely a point on the voltage divider formed by R_1 and R_g.

$$I_+ = \frac{E_1}{R_1 + R_g} \qquad \textbf{(6-36)}$$

$$E_+ = I_+ R_g$$

$$E_+ = E_1 \frac{R_g}{R_1 + R_g} \qquad \textbf{(6-37)}$$

The point E_- is also on a voltage divider, but with a nonground voltage on both ends:

$$I_- = \frac{E_2 - E_o}{R_2 + R_f} \qquad \textbf{(6-38)}$$

$$E_- = E_o + I_- R_f$$

$$= E_o + \frac{E_2 - E_o}{R_2 + R_f} R_f$$

Putting everything in the same denominator:

$$E_- = \frac{R_2 E_o + R_f E_o}{R_2 + R_f} + \frac{E_2 R_f - E_o R_f}{R_2 + R_f}$$

$$E_- = \frac{R_2 E_o + E_2 R_f}{R_2 + R_f} \qquad \textbf{(6-39)}$$

By substituting Eq. 6-37 and 6-39 into Eq. 6-1, it is possible to solve for E_o in terms of E_1 and E_2 in the same way as was done before. The algebra is somewhat lengthy and complex. On the other hand, Eq. 6-2 is as valid as Eq. 6-1, if we have adequate gain, and substituting into it greatly simplifies the calculations:

$$E_+ = E_- \qquad (6\text{-}2)$$

$$\frac{E_1 R_g}{R_1 + R_g} = \frac{R_2 E_o + E_2 R_f}{R_2 + R_f} \qquad (6\text{-}40)$$

$$E_1 R_g \left(\frac{R_2 + R_f}{R_1 + R_g} \right) = R_2 E_o + E_2 R_f$$

$$E_o = E_1 \frac{R_g}{R_2} \left(\frac{R_2 + R_f}{R_1 + R_g} \right) - E_2 \frac{R_f}{R_g}$$

$$(6\text{-}41)$$

This equation is still too complex for everyday use, but fortunately it can be greatly simplified by the appropriate choice of resistors. That choice is to make the ratios of resistors on both inputs the same. This can be thought of as a sort of "constant amplification" condition. This condition is expressed as

$$\frac{R_f}{R_2} = \frac{R_g}{R_1} \qquad (6\text{-}42)$$

If we solve this equation for R_f and substitute into the bracketed term in Eq. 6-41,

$$E_o = E_1 \frac{R_g}{R_2} \left(\frac{R_2 + R_g R_2 / R_1}{R_1 + R_g} \right) - E_2 \frac{R_f}{R_2} \qquad (6\text{-}43)$$

$$= E_1 R_g \left(\frac{1 + R_g / R_1}{R_1 + R_g} \right) - E_2 \frac{R_f}{R_2}$$

$$= \frac{E_1 (R_g / R_1)(R_1 + R_g)}{R_1 + R_g} - E_2 \frac{R_f}{R_2}$$

$$= E_1 \frac{R_g}{R_1} - E_2 \frac{R_f}{R_2} \qquad (6\text{-}44)$$

Amazingly enough, we can substitute Eq. 6-42 once again into the E_1 term:

$$E_o = E_1 \frac{R_f}{R_2} - E_2 \frac{R_f}{R_2}$$

$$= \frac{R_f}{R_2} (E_1 - E_2) \qquad (6\text{-}45)$$

We have now obtained an equation that gives the output voltage in terms of a simple difference and the circuit gain. The restriction of equal gain (or constant amplification) is not a severe one and is usually implemented by choosing $R_2 = R_1$ and $R_f = R_g$.

The advantages of the instrumentation amplifier are that it takes the fewest operational amplifiers to accomplish the subtraction of two signals and, at the same time, draws negligible current from the input sources. Only one amplifier needs to be of high gain and only one variable resistor (R_1, for example) is needed to balance Eq. 6-42. Relative to other configurations, the instrumentation amplifier can be made inexpensively and is easy to use. The disadvantage is that it does not necessarily operate with inputs near ground, and the main amplifier must therefore have a very good common mode rejection ratio.

Section 6-8
INTEGRATORS

While calculus has been avoided in this text, it is necessary to cover two principles usually associated with calculus in the remainder of this chapter. To assist readers unfamiliar with calculus, algebraic explanations will be given and simple examples shown. The first of these principles is integration.

Figure 6-10A shows a constant current level in a circuit. Let us suppose that we want to collect all the charge flowing starting at a time t_0. After a short time t_1, we would have gathered an amount of charge q. After twice t_1, we would have twice q gathered. After three times t_1 we would have three times q. This could continue indefinitely. We can graph what is happening to give Figure 6-10B. We note that we have a ramp increasing at a constant rate. The equation for the current is

$$I = k \qquad \text{(since the current is constant)} \qquad (6\text{-}46)$$

The equation for the collection of charge is

$$Q = It = kt \qquad (6\text{-}47)$$

This equation is simply a revision of Eq. 1-5, which shows that if the current is constant, the

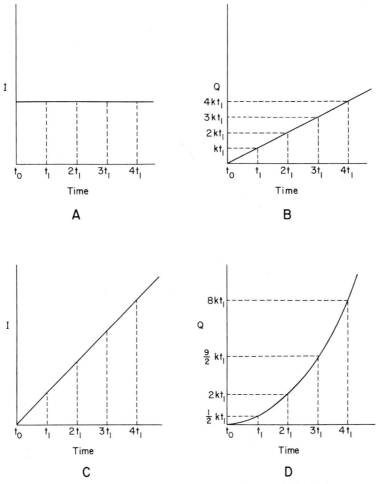

Figure 6-10 The integration of the current level in part A yields the ramp of growing charge in part B. The integration of the current ramp in part C yields the second-degree charge equation in part D.

charge will build up at a uniform rate. Equation 6-47 is called the integral of Eq. 6-46 because it is the equation for the sum of all charge that flows in Eq. 6-46 over a period of time.

Let us look at another example as shown in Figure 6-10C. Here we have a ramp with a constant rate. If we again start at t_0 with zero charge, we can then compute the total charge up to any point. The equation for the current is

$$I = kt \qquad \textbf{(6-48)}$$

At time t_1, the average flow has been

$$I = \frac{I_1 + I_0}{2}$$

$$= \frac{kt_1 + 0}{2}$$

$$= \frac{k}{2} t_1 \qquad \textbf{(6-49)}$$

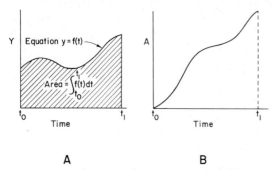

Figure 6-11 The integral of a function can be thought of as an equation that gives the area under its graph.

Since the charge is equal to the average current flow times the time

$$Q = It$$

$$= \left(\frac{k}{2} t_1\right) t_1$$

$$= \frac{k}{2} t_1^2 \qquad \text{(6-50)}$$

Because t_1 is an arbitrary point and can be any distance from t_0, this equation can be generalized:

$$Q = \frac{k}{2} t^2 \qquad \text{(6-51)}$$

This equation is graphed in Figure 6-10D. The integral of an equation is therefore another equation that gives the area between the x axis and the graph line of the first equation (Fig. 6-11). The function of an integrator then is to collect (or sum up) all the material as it flows through so it can tell how much has gone by in a certain time period.

The equation for a charge integrator is:

$$Q = \int_0^t I \, dt \qquad \text{(6-52)}$$

The integral sign as written indicates charge is collected between time equals zero and some arbitrary time t. When the current is constant, only time remains under the integral, and Eq. 6-47 results. If the current is a function of time, the charge will be a higher degree function of time, as in Eq. 6-51. Even with no knowledge of calculus, it should be possible to see that the integrator is act-

ing like a dam on a river. If no water is allowed out, then the whole stream is collected into a lake no matter how fast or slow it flows.

One device that collects electrical charge is a capacitor. The problem with a lone capacitor, however, is that it builds up a voltage that reduces the amount of current flowing. Consequently to be successful, we must arrange the circuit in such a way as to prevent the voltage of the capacitor from affecting the current flow. Figure 6-12 shows such an arrangement. A current source, perhaps a battery and resistor, shoves current into the summing point at the inverting input of an operational amplifier and onto the capacitor. This causes a charge build-up. The basic equation for the capacitor must remain true, $E = q/C$. The current cannot be reduced, as in the case of charging the simple capacitor, because this charge is being added to the capacitor at virtually zero potential, and that potential is not affected by the growing charge. The only way all these things can be true simultaneously is for E_o to change to generate the necessary voltage over the capacitor to hold the charge.

Let us go through that again. Assume that the current is flowing toward the inverting input. In that case, positive charge is moving onto the left capacitor plate. An equal amount of positive charge is leaving the right plate and heading toward the output of the amplifier. This separation of charge means that a voltage is created over the capacitor. Since the side of the capacitor receiving the positive charge remains effectively at ground, the voltage on the other side must grow more negative to

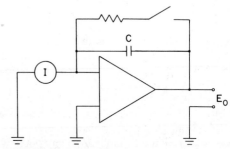

Figure 6-12 An integrator builds up charge on a capacitor as a result of the current coming into the summing point. A small resistor is needed to discharge the capacitor before starting measurement.

create a voltage difference large enough to satisfy the capacitor equation. The amplifier output therefore must produce this negative voltage. The equation for the output voltage is just the capacitor equation with the charge being that expressed in Eq. 6-52. The sign is negative because the output voltage must decrease to allow the capacitor to charge:

$$E_o = -\frac{q}{C}$$

$$E_o = -\frac{1}{C} \int_0^t I \, dt \qquad (6\text{-}53)$$

This equation will hold true until either the limit of the amplifier is exceeded or the capacitor breakdown voltage is reached.

Equation 6-53 can be refined for particular uses. If the current is a constant generated by a battery and resistor, Ohm's laws can be used to substitute for I:

$$E_o = -\frac{1}{C} \int_0^t \frac{E_s}{R} \, dt$$

When integrated, this is

$$E_o = \frac{-E_s t}{RC} \qquad (6\text{-}54)$$

If the input voltage is a ramp, where $I = E_r t / R$, then we get

$$E_o = -\frac{1}{C} \int_0^t \frac{E_r t}{R} \, dt$$

which, when integrated, is

$$E_o = \frac{-E_r t^2}{2RC} \qquad (6\text{-}55)$$

These equations are very similar to those plotted in Figure 6-10. The equation of any regular current source can be substituted into Eq. 6-53 for E_o. Irregular sources cannot be calculated beforehand and can only be determined by observation.

Integrations are essential parts of many instrumental measurements. When one runs a gas chromatograph, for example, one gets a series of peaks. The concentrations of the components are proportional to the areas under those peaks. Integrating the wave form as it passes allows one to readily

determine these areas. An integrator can be used to set the baseline in a noisy environment. When as much of the background noise is above the baseline as below, the integral remains constant. By adjusting to a constant integral value, the baseline can be accurately set to zero.

The use of an integrator requires a certain amount of circuitry that is not shown in the diagram. In addition to the "other circuit" of the operational amplifier, there is also a control circuit necessary to run the shorting switch to reset the capacitor. If the capacitor is not too large, the discharge can safely be done without a resistor in series to dissipate the energy. Under normal conditions, the switch is closed, and it is opened only when a reading is started.

EXAMPLE 6-4

What is the voltage ramp necessary to cause the voltage output to reach 3.1 V in 0.092 sec if the input resistor is 8.2 kΩ and the feedback capacitor is 6.1 μF?

Solution: Since we have a ramp

$$E_o = \frac{-E_r t^2}{2RC}$$

$$E_r = \frac{-2E_o RC}{t^2}$$

$$E_r = \frac{-2 \times 3.1 \times 8.2 \cdot 10^3 \times 6.1 \cdot 10^{-6}}{(0.092)^2}$$

$$E_r = -37 \text{ V/sec} \qquad \blacksquare$$

EXAMPLE 6-5

What is the input current after 0.142 sec in the previous example?

Solution: We start with the ramp circuit equation:

$$I = \frac{E_r t}{R}$$

$$= \frac{-37 \times 0.142}{8.2 \cdot 10^3}$$

$$I = -6.4 \cdot 10^{-4} \text{ A} \qquad \blacksquare$$

Section 6-9
DIFFERENTIATORS

The last operational amplifier circuit we will consider here is the differentiator. The derivative of a quantity (what one gets when one differentiates) is the opposite of the integral. If one integrates the equation plotted in Figure 6-10A, one gets the equation plotted in Figure 6-10B. If one differentiates the equation in Figure 6-10B, one gets the equation plotted in Figure 6-10A. A similar relationship exists between Figures 6-10C and 6-10D. While the integral of an equation is regarded as the area under the equation, the derivative is regarded as the slope of the graph of the equation at any point.

Let us consider the following examples. The derivative of a quantity x with time is written as dx/dt, the change in x with respect to the change in time. If we have a constant value for an equation, as in Figure 6-10A, the equation is

$$I = k \qquad (k \text{ being constant}) \qquad \textbf{(6-56)}$$

The value of the current equation does not change, since it is a horizontal line. Therefore, the slope is zero:

$$\frac{dI}{dt} = \frac{dk}{dt} = 0 \qquad \textbf{(6-57)}$$

If, on the other hand, we have an equation for the current such as shown in Figure 6-10B, we have a ramp.

$$I = kt \qquad \textbf{(6-58)}$$

The slope of the graph of this equation at every time is the same, namely, k.

$$\frac{dI}{dt} = k\frac{dt}{dt} = k \qquad \textbf{(6-59)}$$

The slope of the graph of the equation in Figure 6-10D is even more complicated because it is not constant, but increases with time. Its equation is unimportant for the following discussion.

The importance of the differentiator is that it reduces the dependence of a signal on time. A constant current will give a zero output. A linear current ramp will give a constant output. While the integrator flattens the response to noise, the differentiator is highly sensitive to sudden changes in the

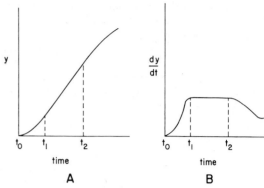

Figure 6-13 A differentiator highlights the changes in the slope of an equation or the rate of an input.

magnitude of the input. The result is the differentiator can be used to find at what point things change or where a certain signal first appears. If one wishes to measure a rate reaction consisting of an incubation period, a steady rate, and depletion region (Fig. 6-13A), one can get these regions clearly separated and the value of the rate calculated by use of a differentiator (Fig. 6-13B). This is one of the common uses of a differentiator in laboratory equipment.

A simple differentiator circuit is shown in Figure 6-14. The current that enters causes charge to pile up on the left plate of the capacitor. An equivalent amount of charge is forced off the capacitor and, since it cannot flow into the inverting input, it must flow through the resistor to the output. The inverting input acts as a virtual ground. This causes two effects. The voltage over the capacitor must all be

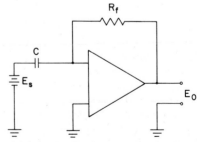

Figure 6-14 A differentiator builds up charge on a capacitor in the input circuit to the operational amplifier.

seen at the left plate of the capacitor because the right plate is at ground. The voltage of the output is $-IR_f$ because the voltage must be low enough at E_0 to permit the current to flow through the resistor while the other end is at virtual ground. The equation for a differentiator is calculated as follows:

$$E_o = E_- - IR_f$$

$$E_o = 0 - IR_f = -IR_f$$

$$I = \frac{dq}{dt} \quad \text{(definition of current)}$$

$$dq = C \, dE_s$$

(derivative of the definition of capacitance)

Therefore

$$E_o = \frac{dE_s}{dt} R_f C \qquad \textbf{(6-60)}$$

The output voltage is proportional to the time constant $R_f C$ and the *change* of the input voltage. If E_S is constant

$$\frac{dE_s}{dt} = 0 \qquad \textbf{(6-61)}$$

and

$$E_o = 0 \qquad \textbf{(6-62)}$$

If the input voltage is a constant ramp

$$\frac{dE_s}{dt} = E_r \qquad \textbf{(6-63)}$$

and

$$E_o = -E_r RC \qquad \textbf{(6-64)}$$

Those who are familiar with calculus will be able to apply the basic Eq. 6-60 to numerous different waveforms. For others, suffice it to say that the differentiator produces a zero value when the input is constant, a constant value when the input is changing uniformly, and a sharply changing value when the input is changing nonuniformly.

EXAMPLE 6-6

What is the value of the capacitor C_2 needed to make E_0 equal to E_i in Figure 6-15 if $R_1 = 4.1$ kΩ, $R_2 = 9.3$ kΩ, and $C_1 = 2.3$ μF?

Solution: For the integrator, we need constant voltage Eq. 6-54:

$$E_o' = \frac{-E_i t}{R_1 C_1}$$

To substitute into a differential equation, we need the rate of change of E, which we get by differentiating.

$$\frac{dE_o'}{dt} = - \frac{E_i dt}{R_1 C_1 dt} = \frac{-E_i}{R_1 C_1}$$

We insert this into the basic differentiator Eq. 6-60.

$$E_o = - \frac{dE_o'}{dt} R_2 C_2$$

$$E_o = - \left(\frac{-E_i}{R_1 C_1} \right) \times R_2 C_2$$

$$C_2 = \frac{E_o R_1 C_1}{E_i R_2}$$

If $E_o = E_i$

$$C_2 = \frac{R_1 C_1}{R_2}$$

then

$$C_2 = \frac{4.2 \cdot 10^3 \times 2.3 \cdot 10^{-6}}{9.3 \cdot 10^3}$$

$$C_2 = 1.0 \ \mu\text{F} \qquad \blacksquare$$

These two sections have been difficult because of the new concepts involved. Everything is there, however, and a careful rereading may be necessary. Do not fear the differentials and integrals.

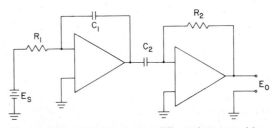

Figure 6-15 This integrator–differentiator combination gives an output signal in the same form as the input signal.

They are used here just like other numerical operations, such as addition or multiplication. No further detailed use of these concepts will be made subsequently, but you will do well to understand to this level of complexity because these terms and symbols frequently appear in the professional literature of clinical chemistry.

With the completion of this section on operational amplifiers, we have finished the last of the standard analog electrical components. Although no new analog components will be introduced, all the components seen so far will be used in future instrumentation discussions. In Chapter 7 we will use many of these analog components to explain the operation of power supplies.

REVIEW QUESTIONS

1. What is an operational amplifier?
2. What are the three circuits used in an operational amplifier?
3. Why is the power circuit called "the other circuit"?
4. What are some common values for the power circuit voltage?
5. What are the connections to an operational amplifier for the signal circuit called? What symbols are used to represent them?
6. Explain the gain of an operational amplifier. What are some typical values?
7. What is the principal equation of an operational amplifier? What is the secondary equation?
8. How is the working range of an operational amplifier determined?
9. Define "limit."
10. Why might the gain from the inverting and non-inverting inputs be different? How is this situation resolved?
11. What is the input impedance of an operational amplifier? Why?
12. What is the output impedance of an operational amplifier? Why?
13. Why can the output of an operational amplifier both emit and absorb current?
14. What is common mode voltage?
15. Define the common mode rejection ratio.
16. How are the effects of common mode minimized?

17. What is a voltage follower?
18. How does a voltage follower work?
19. Why can the $A/(A + 1)$ factor be dropped from the equations?
20. What is feedback? Why is it needed?
21. What is circuit gain?
22. What is the relationship between circuit gain and amplifier gain?
23. Why is amplifier gain unstable?
24. Why is the circuit gain of a follower with gain always greater than 1?
25. What are the conditions necessary for a follower with gain to work?
26. What is virtual ground?
27. What is another name which a virtual ground has in some circuits?
28. What part of the circuit determines the amount of current entering the point of virtual ground?
29. What part of the circuit determines the magnitude and nature of the output signal?
30. What part of the circuit determines what the current flow of the amplifier output will be?
31. What is an invertor?
32. How does the gain of an invertor differ from that of a follower with gain?
33. Why does a virtual ground electrically isolate the attached circuits?
34. What is a summing point?
35. How does an adder work?
36. What is the output voltage of an adder proportional to?
37. How does one subtract with an adder?
38. What is an instrumentation amplifier?
39. Why do the different operational amplifiers in an instrumentation amplifier need different properties?
40. What is the nature of the constant amplification condition in an instrumentation amplifier?
41. What are the advantages and disadvantages of the instrumentation amplifier?
42. What is integration? How does it relate to the graphic representation of an equation?
43. What effect does integration have in general on the independent variable?
44. How is signal integration accomplished?
45. Why is an operational amplifier circuit needed to integrate instead of just a capacitor?
46. Why does the output voltage change as the capacitor is charged?

47. What are some uses of an integrator?

48. How is an integrator initialized at time equals zero?

49. What is a derivative? How does it relate to the graph of an equation?

50. What effect does differentiation have in general on the independent variable?

51. How is signal differentiation accomplished?

52. Explain how the capacitor functions in a differentiator.

53. What are some common uses for a differentiator?

PROBLEMS

1. If the gain of an operational amplifier is 1,000 and the common mode rejection ratio is 10,000, what amount of common mode would produce 0.01 V of output signal?

2. If R is 20. kΩ and the output voltage is -3.0 V in Figure 6-16, what is the input current?

3. What resistance is needed to make an input current of -5.2 mA produce a voltage of 1.7 V in Figure 6-16?

4. If the input voltage in Figure 6-3 is 0.70 V while the ground resistor is 503 Ω and the feedback resistor is 5.98 kΩ, what is the output voltage?

5. If the output voltage in Figure 6-3 is 8.6 V while the ground resistor is 470 Ω and the feedback resistor is 560 Ω, what is the input voltage?

6. If the output voltage in Figure 6-3 is 1.91 V and the input voltage is 0.89 V, what is the feedback resistor if the ground resistor is 2.22 kΩ?

7. If the output voltage in Figure 6-3 is 3.42 V and the input voltage is 0.75 V, with a feedback resistor of 14.2 kΩ, what is the ground resistor?

8. If the output voltage in Figure 6-4 is 7.16 V, the feedback resistor 2.67 kΩ, and the input resistor 943 Ω, what is the input voltage?

9. If the output voltage in Figure 6-4 is 3.95 V, the feedback resistor 690 kΩ, and the input voltage -1.04 V, what is the input resistor?

10. In Figure 6-6, assume the values of the resistors left to right are 412 Ω, unknown, 677 Ω, and 384 Ω. If the input voltage is 1.025 V and the output voltage is -3.90 V, what is the value of the unknown resistor?

11. Assuming the following values for the appropriate components of Figure 6-7, what is the value of E_2? $R_1 = 25$ kΩ, $R_2 = 10.0$ kΩ, $R_f = 4.3$ kΩ, $E_1 = 6.1$ V, and $E_o = -2.87$ V?

12. In Figure 6-8, assume that R_2 is twice R_1 and that R_3 is three times R_1. If E_1 is three times minus E_o, E_2 is twice E_o, and E_3 is the negative of E_o, what is the value of the feedback resistor?

13. If the inputs E_1 and E_2 to the instrumentation amplifier in Figure 6-9 are 3.79 mV and 1.87 mV, respectively, and if both R_1 and R_2 are 1.68 kΩ and R_g and R_f are 220. kΩ, what will be the output voltage?

14. Assume that the values given below are the values for the instrumentation amplifier in Figure 6-9. What is the output voltage? (*Note:* Since the amplifier is unbalanced, the formula *will not* work, and other means must be used to find the answers.) $R_1 = 8.3$ kΩ, $R_2 = 12.0$ kΩ, $R_g = 5.0$ kΩ, $R_f = 28.2$ kΩ, $E_1 = -1.38$ V, and $E_2 = 2.51$ V.

15. What is the output of the operational amplifier in Figure 6-17B if $R_1 = 214$ Ω, $R_2 = 387$ Ω, $E_1 = 2.09$ V, and $E_2 = 4.14$ V?

16. In Figure 6-17B, the output voltage is 6.45 V

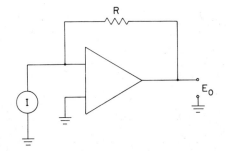

Figure 6-16 A current-to-voltage convertor.

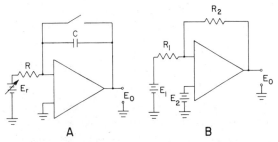

Figure 6-17 Circuits for Problems 15 through 18.

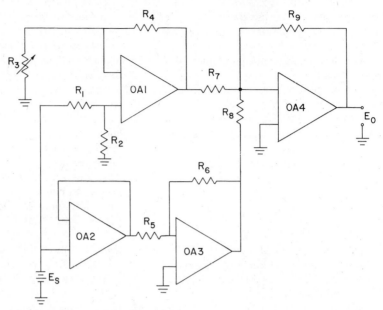

Figure 6-18 A complex amplifier circuit.

and E_2 is 3.71 V. If R_1 is 8.27 kΩ and R_2 is 4.97 kΩ, what is the value of E_1?

17. If the output voltage of the operational amplifier in Figure 6-17A is -7.52 V after 40. sec, what is the capacitance if the input voltage ramp is 0.031 V/sec and the resistor is 12.0 kΩ?

18. If the voltage ramp in Figure 6-17A increases at the rate of 0.0687 V/sec for 12.7 sec and then decreases at the same rate for the same period of time, what will be the output voltage of the integrator after 25.4 sec? (Assume that the resistor is 223 kΩ and the capacitor is 178 μF.)

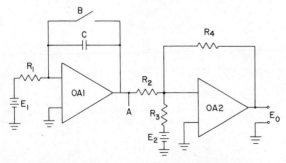

Figure 6-19 An integrator-amplifier circuit.

19. What is the output voltage of the amplifier network in Figure 6-18 if $R_1 = 7.00$ kΩ, $R_2 = 5.00$ kΩ, $R_3 = 10.00$ kΩ, $R_4 = 8.00$ kΩ, $R_5 = 22.0$ kΩ, $R_6 = 14.0$ kΩ, $R_7 = 6.20$ kΩ, $R_8 = 7.30$ kΩ, $R_g = 12.80$ kΩ, and $E_s = 1.000$ V?

20. All the resistors in Figure 6-18 have the value of their subscripts times 10 kΩ (except for R_3, which is variable) and are accurate to one part in 400. What value must R_3 be set at so that the output voltage is zero for any input voltage?

21. If the voltage ramp in Figure 6-14 increases at 1.28 V/sec, what is the output voltage after 4.62 sec if the capacitor is 14.9 μF and the resistor is 47.3 kΩ?

22. What voltage E_1 is needed in Figure 6-19 so that E_o will reach 5.3 V at 0.273 sec after switch B is opened? Let $R_1 = 47$ kΩ, $R_2 = 68$ kΩ, $R_3 = 56$ kΩ, $R_4 = 290$ kΩ, $C = 0.086$ μF, and $E_2 = 2.71$ V.

23. Assume that Figure 6-19 is modified by removing E_2 and attaching that end of R_3 to the output. If E_1 is 0.099 V, $R_1 = 56$ kΩ, $R_2 = 62.6$ kΩ, $R_3 = 82$ kΩ, $R_4 = 149$ kΩ, and $C = 0.104$ μF, what is the output voltage after 0.652 sec from when switch B is opened?

CHAPTER 7
POWER SUPPLIES

In order to make a laboratory instrument work, some source of reliable power is needed. In Chapter 3 we discussed how a battery is constructed. Various types of batteries are used in laboratory instruments, of which the carbon–zinc, mercury, nickel–cadmium, and alkaline batteries are most common. These batteries perform best as reference sources or when only a very small amount of current is drawn. Since operating laboratory instruments on very low power is seldom practical, it is necessary to get the power from some other source. This source is most commonly the alternating current (ac) available at a nearby wall outlet, although some instruments need unusual power input and require special power lines.

Section 7-1
TRANSFORMERS

Chapter 3 discusses the theory of alternating current generation. The same basic action occurs electrically whether the armature of the generator is driven by falling water or by steam produced by a coal-fired boiler or by a nuclear pile. The problem with ac is that it cannot be used directly in most analytical circuits. Looking back at the different effects of ac and dc on a capacitor, or considering what would happen to an operational amplifier if the supply voltage polarity were to change 60 times a second, it becomes obvious that something must be done to the ac to convert it to usable dc. Even the D'Arsonval meter becomes useless when ac is applied, as can be seen by trying to measure ac on a dc range of a VOM.

The first step in deriving dc for laboratory instruments from ac is to reduce the ac to a workable voltage. Electricity is normally transmitted from power stations at very high voltages. This is done to reduce power loss, which is proportional to the square of the current. Since the power transmitted is equal to the product of the current and the voltage (Eq. 1-8), one must increase the voltage as the current decreases in order to maintain the power level. While raising the voltage at the same time as lowering the current appears to defy Ohm's law, it can be accomplished by also raising the resistance in the circuit. Therefore, power lines, which have very high voltage applied to them, have very high resistances at the user end and transmit a relatively low current.

When the ac reaches a transformer, be it in a power station or an instrument, the mix of voltage and current is changed. This is accomplished in the following fashion. The incoming line is wrapped numerous times around a soft iron core. As the ac fluctuates, it causes a magnetic field to build and collapse, as was discussed in Chapter 3. The soft iron is highly permeable to magnetic lines and concentrates them in a loop as shown in Figure 7-1A. This is called the primary winding. Note that the wire must have a coating to prevent the whole device from shorting out, but that the coating must be very thin to permit the wire windings to be packed tightly together.

The same piece of metal that contains the primary winding also has another winding called a secondary winding. The secondary winding is similar to the primary winding, except that it is attached to a load instead of a power source. When a wire is moved in a magnetic field, a current is generated as the lines of magnetic flux are cut. Because nature is symmetrical, the same thing happens when the field is moved and the wire is stationary. Since the field in the transformer is continually increasing and de-

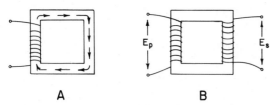

A   B

Figure 7-1 A soft iron core concentrates the magnetic lines of force generated by ac through the primary winding. A secondary winding receives an induced current from the magnetic field.

creasing in size, it is in essence a moving field created by the alternating current in the primary winding, and the secondary winding has a current generated in it as this magnetic field oscillates. Figure 7-1B shows the classic transformer design. Actual transformers use the same principle, but the windings may be in a different geometric configuration, including interspersed, to take advantage of the shape of the magnetic field.

It is best to consider this in a more mathematical context. The change in magnetic flux with time is equal to minus the voltage over the coil divided by the number of turns on the primary winding (Eq. 7-1). This is true for the primary winding:

$$\frac{\Delta \Phi}{\Delta t} = \frac{-E_p}{N_p} \qquad \textbf{(7-1)}$$

but since there is no inherent difference between the primary and the secondary windings (both are just coils of wire around a core), it is also true for the secondary winding:

$$\frac{\Delta \Phi}{\Delta t} = \frac{-E_s}{N_s} \qquad \textbf{(7-2)}$$

If one substitutes for the common quantity $\Delta \Phi / \Delta t$, Eq. 7-3 results:

$$\frac{E_p}{N_p} = \frac{E_s}{N_s} \qquad \textbf{(7-3)}$$

When this equation is rearranged as shown in 7-4, the output voltage, that is, the voltage on the secondary winding, is equal to the ratio of the number of loops in the secondary winding to that in the primary winding times the voltage on the primary.

$$E_s = \frac{N_s}{N_p} E_p \qquad \textbf{(7-4)}$$

If the number of loops in the secondary winding is less than the number in the primary winding, the transformer decreases the voltage out compared with the voltage in, and the transformer is called a step-down transformer. If the number of loops in the secondary exceeds the number in the primary, the voltage increases as the energy passes through the transformer, and it is called a step-up transformer.

The above facts lead to some erroneous conclusions. To step down from 200 volts ac to 100 volts ac appears to require only $N_p = 2$ and $N_s = 1$. This gives the correct ratio. Nevertheless, this will not work. To get a satisfactory magnetic couple between the two windings, one must have a uniform field at both the primary and secondary windings. This can only be accomplished by the use of a large number of loops (hundreds to thousands). Second, it appears that we are creating or destroying voltage with the transformer, which defies the conservation of energy. The key fact here is that voltage is not energy. The energy is, in fact, conserved. We use this fact to develop the second important relationship concerning transformers. The power (in watts) coming out can be no greater than the power going in. Since a transformer is not 100% efficient, some power is dispersed as heat and is not available to the secondary circuit. Nevertheless, for a good transformer the transfer of power from the primary winding to the secondary winding is sufficient for us to assume that it is 100% as a first approximation. Therefore we have

$$P_s = P_p \qquad \textbf{(7-5)}$$

$$E_s I_s = E_p I_p$$

$$I_s = \frac{E_p}{E_s} I_p \qquad \textbf{(7-6)}$$

We now have a relationship between the current and the voltage over the primary winding and that over the secondary winding. Note that as the voltage on the secondary winding decreases with respect to the primary winding, E_p / E_s grows larger and the current in the secondary circuit increases relative to the current in the primary circuit. This is clearer if we substitute for the ratio of the voltages from Eq. 7-3, which gives

$$I_s = \frac{N_p}{N_s} I_p \qquad (7\text{-}7)$$

The voltage of the secondary circuit varies directly with the ratio of the number of turns of wire in the secondary winding to the primary winding (N_s/N_p), but the current varies inversely with this ratio. When the voltage steps down, the current steps up; the converse is also true. This then is the reason for using the transformer. Electricity at high voltage and low current can be sent to a distant station, where the user transforms it to low voltage and high current for local use. It is neither current nor voltage itself that is important, but their product, which is energy.

There is still one thing amiss. Equations 7-6 and 7-7 tell us what the current in the secondary circuit is in terms of the current in the primary circuit. But what is the current in the primary circuit? Here we have the cart before the horse. It is the secondary, not the primary, circuit that dissipates the energy; consequently, it is the secondary, not the primary, circuit that determines the amount of current in both circuits. The relationship between I_s and E_s must be given by Ohm's law:

$$I_s = \frac{E_s}{R_s} \qquad (7\text{-}8)$$

If Eq. 7-8 is substituted into Eq. 7-6, we get

$$\frac{E_s}{R_s} = \frac{E_p}{E_s} I_p$$

$$I_p = \frac{E_s^2}{R_s E_p} \qquad (7\text{-}9)$$

Finally, if we then substitute for E_s from Eq. 7-4,

$$I_p = \frac{N_s^2 E_p}{N_p^2 R_s} \qquad (7\text{-}10)$$

The current in the primary circuit is a function of the primary circuit voltage, the ratio of turns between the two windings and the resistance in the secondary circuit. This is merely Ohm's law with a factor for the transformer included. Note that if the

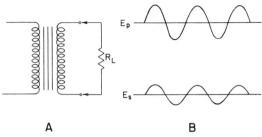

A   B

Figure 7-2 The representation of a transformer with a resistor as the load in the secondary circuit. The phase of the primary and secondary are the same, but the amplitude of the secondary voltage is affected by the ratio of the number of loops of wire in the windings.

resistance is infinite (i.e., the ends of the secondary winding are not connected in an external circuit) then, at least in theory, I_p is zero, even though the primary circuit is just a piece of wire with a high-voltage difference between the ends.

Figure 7-2 shows the basic transformer circuit. Also shown is the phase diagram of the input and output voltages. Note that the voltages are in phase between the primary and secondary circuits, but the amplitude is dependent on the stepping factor N_s/N_p. In addition to changing the current and voltage levels, a transformer isolates the secondary circuit from the primary. This is the case because there is no electrical connection. Only the magnetic flux connection ties the two circuits together. Isolation transformers, which take advantage of this fact, are sometimes used to prevent multiple grounds in different parts of an instrument from causing troublesome interactions between components.

One final fact about transformers is worth noting. It is possible to have more than one secondary winding with the primary. Each secondary winding acts completely independently, and the resultant current drawn from the primary is the sum of all the demands of the individual secondaries.

Section 7-2
RECTIFIERS

Reducing the amplitude of the ac voltage still does not solve the basic problem caused by the nature of

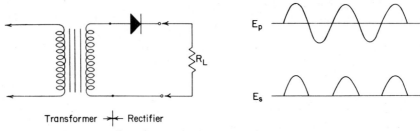

Transformer →|← Rectifier

Figure 7-3 Transformer, half-wave rectifier, and phase diagram.

the waveform. The sine wave is left unchanged by the transformer. To improve the situation, it is imperative that we at least eliminate the negative half of the wave. This can easily be accomplished by the use of a diode, as introduced in Chapter 5. The addition of a diode to the transformer circuit, as shown in Figure 7-3, removes the negative portion of the sine wave. This design is called a half-wave rectifier because only one-half of the wave remains after rectification by a simple diode. This signal is called "pulsed dc," because while it is dc (no negative voltage component), the power is delivered in a series of pulses rather than at a uniform level. As a consequence, one-half the available power is lost, never being drawn from the primary.

The half-wave rectifier is a beginning, but it is obviously not the whole solution to obtaining a uniform current level. The next step is to invert the missing half of the wave and to add it to what we already have. This is accomplished by the circuit in Figure 7-4, which is called a full-wave rectifier. To use such an approach, it is necessary to have a special transformer with a center tap, a third connection equidistant from either end of the second-

ary winding. As the voltage increases in the positive direction, the current flows through the top diode, through the load, and returns to the transformer through the center tap. No current can flow through the bottom diode in a backward direction. As the voltage increases in the negative direction, the current flows through the bottom diode, through the load, and returns to the transformer through the center tap. No current can flow through the top half of the secondary because it would have to flow through the top diode backward. As one can see, the current flows through the load in only one direction, regardless of the direction of current flow in the secondary winding. It is therefore rectified, the whole waveform contributing to the operation of the load. Note that the voltage over the load is only one-half that over the secondary winding. In either direction the voltage is measured relative to the center tap. As a consequence, the output voltage is only one-half that which would be expected on the basis of the number of turns on the secondary winding, because at any one time only one-half the secondary winding is contributing to the voltage over the load. The need for the center tap to be

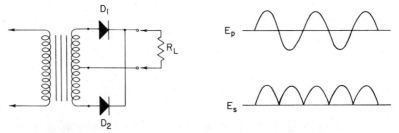

Figure 7-4 Transformer, full-wave rectifier, and phase diagram.

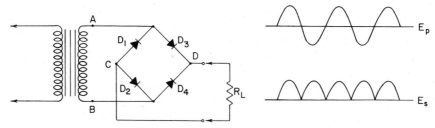

Figure 7-5 Transformer, bridge rectifier, and phase diagram.

precisely placed is evident; otherwise the two half-waves will not be of the same amplitude. A second important feature of a full-wave rectifier is that the frequency of the output is double that of the input. Frequency is defined as the number of identical waveforms passing a point in a unit of time. Since each full sine wave entering produces two identical half-waves leaving, the total number of these waves leaving is twice the number of sine waves in and therefore twice the frequency.

The fact that extra cost is involved in building a full-wave rectifier that results in only one-half the maximum output has caused engineers to devise another way to get full-wave rectification. This new device is called a bridge rectifier and is shown in Figure 7-5. Following the current through a complete sine wave is somewhat complicated but worth doing. As the voltage rises at point A, the current must flow through diode D_3 because it cannot go through diode D_1 backward. When it reaches point D, it must go through the load resistor because it cannot go through diode D_4 backward. It goes through R_L top to bottom and reaches point C. From here it must flow through diode D_2 to point B, since the potential on the other side of diode D_1 is

greater than at point C. As the voltage rises at point B, the current must flow through diode D_4 because it cannot go through diode D_2 backward. When it reaches point D, it must go through the load resistor because it cannot go through diode D_3 backward. It goes through R_L top to bottom, just as before, and reaches point C. This time it must flow through diode D_1, to point A, since the potential on the other side of diode D_2 is greater than at point C. As a result, the current must always flow in the same direction through R_L; therefore, it is rectified. Since the whole secondary winding contributes to the voltage over R_L, the voltage of a bridge rectifier is twice that of a full-wave rectifier with the same number of turns in the secondary winding.

It is possible to develop other rectifier configurations for special purposes. One of these is the voltage doubler rectifier shown in Figure 7-6. During the positive half of the sine wave cycle, C_1 is charged to the peak voltage of the transformer. During the negative half of the cycle, C_2 is charged to the peak voltage. Since C_1 and C_2 are in series, the voltages over them add to give a total voltage, demonstrated by the load. The approximate wave form is shown. It must be realized that there is

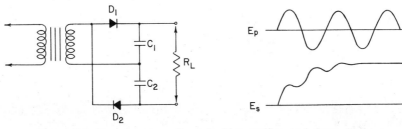

Figure 7-6 Transformer, voltage doubler rectifier, and phase diagram.

instability in this arrangement. Although the capacitors are charged to the peak of the input voltage, they leak this charge through the load resistor when the wave is not at its maximum. Without the capacitors, the circuit would not work at all. Even with them, it is necessary for R_L to be large to prevent significant loss of charge, and therefore loss of voltage, over the capacitors between peaks. While the voltage doubler rectifier is a full-wave rectifier because it draws power during both halves of the sine wave input, it is also a filter circuit because it reduces the size of the voltage fluctuation.

Section 7-3
FILTERS

The purpose of a filtering element is to reduce the amount of ripple that comes from a power supply. Figures 7-3 through 7-5 show that the voltage value, although always positive, varies between ground and some maximum value. So that we may describe this waveform quantitatively, we introduce the concept of the ripple effect. To define ripple, we need to identify some other components of a signal. The height of a voltage sine wave from the top of the crest to the bottom of the trough is called the peak-to-peak voltage E_{p-p} (Fig. 7-7). The difference between the height of the crest and ground is called the peak voltage E_p and is one-half of E_{p-p}.

$$E_p = \tfrac{1}{2}E_{p-p} \qquad (7\text{-}11)$$

(*Note:* The notation E_p is also used for voltage in the primary circuit of a transformer. Usage dictates which term is meant. Be careful.)

The voltage term used in power calculations and commonly referred to as the ac voltage is actually the root-mean-square (rms) voltage, defined as follows:

$$E_{rms} = \frac{1}{\sqrt{2}} E_p \qquad (7\text{-}12)$$

When an ac voltage is rectified, it has both a dc component, which is the average voltage, and an ac component, which is the ripple. The dc component is given by Eq. 7-13 and represents the area under the voltage line during a cycle divided by the length of the cycle.

$$\bar{E} = E_{dc} = \frac{2}{\pi} E_p \qquad (7\text{-}13)$$

The ac voltage is much more complicated to compute for a rectified signal because it requires a Fourier transform (an infinite series of sine and cosine functions) to represent the rectified ac. The ripple factor r is defined by Eq. 7-14 in terms of the ac and dc component voltages:

$$r = \frac{E_{ac}}{E_{dc}} \qquad (7\text{-}14)$$

To remove the ripple from the circuit, we can use capacitors and inductors. Figure 7-8 shows a simple capacitor filter. As the voltage rises at point A, the capacitor C charges rapidly because there is little resistance to the current in the rectifier, and RC is therefore small. When the voltage entering the rectifier begins to decrease, the capacitor cannot discharge back through the rectifier because the rectifier has one or more diodes that will not let the current flow backward. As a result the capacitor can only discharge through the load resistor. If R is large, then RC will be large, and the discharge will be slow. Figure 7-9A shows what happens when there is an open circuit or infinite resistance in

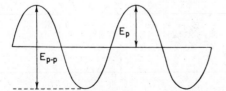

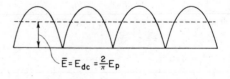

Figure 7-7 The representations of peak-to-peak voltage, peak voltage, average voltage, and dc voltage are shown. The ac voltage is just the peak voltage minus the dc voltage for this unfiltered current.

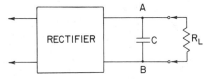

Figure 7-8 A simple capacitor filter attached to a rectifier.

place of R_L. The capacitor rapidly charges, but has no path through which to discharge. Therefore, it retains the peak voltage through the entire cycle of the input wave. In Figure 7-9B, R_L is finite, and the voltage of the capacitor decays until it is revitalized by the next E_p pulse. The smaller R, the smaller will be the time constant RC and the farther the voltage over the capacitor will fall. Hence, the greater the ripple will be.

A careful review of Figure 7-9B shows that there are two other factors besides the resistance that affect the amount of the ripple. One is the size of the capacitor. Increasing the size of the capacitor will also increase the time constant RC. However, rather than increasing the time constant, one can also decrease the time allowed for decay. This is done by increasing the frequency. The ripple factor can be computed from these three values, as shown in Eq. 7-15. No effort will be made to derive the equation from first principles.

$$r = \frac{1}{2\sqrt{3}fRC} \qquad (7\text{-}15)$$

Note that the units of the fRC term cancel, which is necessary since r is unitless, being defined as the ratio of two voltages in Eq. 7-14. Note that the frequency in this equation is that produced *by* the rectifier, *not* that input *into* the rectifier.

It should be apparent from Figure 7-9B that the average or dc voltage drops as a load is applied to a filter output. The amount of this drop is estimated

by Eq. 7-16. This equation gives good results until the ripple reaches 20% of the peak voltage:

$$E_{dc} \approx E_p \left(1 - \frac{1}{2fRC}\right) \qquad (7\text{-}16)$$

EXAMPLE 7-1

If the dc component is to be 95.0% of the peak voltage, what is the frequency needed to operate a filter with a capacitor of 27.1 μF and a load resistor of 3.04 kΩ?

Solution:

$$E_{dc} = E_p \left(1 - \frac{1}{2fRC}\right)$$

$$\frac{E_{dc}}{E_p} = 1 - \frac{1}{2fRC}$$

$$0.950 = 1 - \frac{1}{2fRC}$$

$$\frac{1}{2fRC} = 0.050$$

$$fRC = 10.0$$

$$f = \frac{10.0}{RC}$$

$$f = \frac{10.0}{3.04 \cdot 10^3 \times 27.1 \cdot 10^{-6}}$$

$$f = 121 \text{ Hz} \qquad \blacksquare$$

Figure 7-10A shows a simple inductor filter. An inductor is placed in series with the load resistor. During the rising portion of the input, the magnetic field of the inductor builds. As the input voltage drops, the field collapses, generating current to maintain an IR drop over the resistor. The voltage regulation capacity of inductors is very good, with the dc voltage given by Eq. 7-17. The voltage is almost independent of the resistance of the load resistor unless the resistor is very small. It is somewhat lower than that of a capacitor filter, however.

$$E_{dc} = \bar{E} = \frac{2}{\pi} E_p \qquad (7\text{-}17)$$

The best classic filters are composed of both capacitors and inductors in combination. Figure 7-

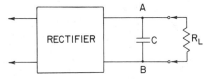

Figure 7-9 The output voltage of a capacitor without a load resistor (A) and with a load resistor (B).

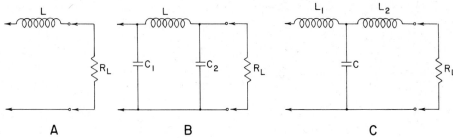

Figure 7-10 A group of commonly used filtering circuits.

10B,C shows such combinations that contribute the strengths of both methods to the final output. The former is called a capacitor input filter and the latter an inductor input filter, on the basis of the first element encountered by the current. Most filtering today is accomplished by large capacitors with suitable regulators as the next circuit elements.

Section 7-4
REGULATORS

The output of the filter in a circuit is a relatively smooth wave. Nevertheless, a small amount of ripple will remain, as shown by the equations in the previous section. How then does one get a steady dc voltage level? The solution to this remaining difficulty is a voltage regulator. Many different types of regulators exist, so we shall consider only the simplest. The purpose of all regulators, regardless of how simple or complex, is the same—a constant voltage level.

Figure 7-11A shows a simple circuit. It has a power supply producing a ripple, a resistive load that requires a constant voltage, and a regulator. Since the regulator is in series with the load, it has a tricky job. It must vary its resistance with the ripple of the power supply so that the voltage drop over the load stays constant. Equation 7-18 shows what the constraints on the regulator are because E_L must remain constant.

$$E_s = E_R + E_L \qquad (7\text{-}18)$$

While building a series regulator is possible using operational amplifiers and various feedback com-

ponents, the needed circuits are clearly not trivial. This approach is used in many available power supplies.

Figure 7-11B shows another method of controlling the voltage level. This method uses a regulator in parallel with the load. On the surface, such an approach would seem to hold out little hope because the voltage over R_L (and therefore the current through it) should be the same, no matter what the resistance of the regulator, unless the regulator is shorted. In that case, there would be no voltage and a burned-out transformer. As strange as it may seem, this parallel circuit is the approach to take in order to accomplish the easiest form of voltage regulation. What we want to do is not to short point A to point B under all conditions, but only for voltages over the desired voltage. In effect, if point A should try to rise to more than x volts above point B, then all that extra voltage generated by the transformer should be shorted to ground. While this may appear complicated, it can easily be accomplished by the use of a Zener diode. In Chapter 5 the unusual properties of this diode were dis-

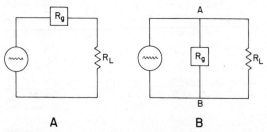

Figure 7-11 Two general approaches to regulation of voltage at a constant level (A = series, B = parallel).

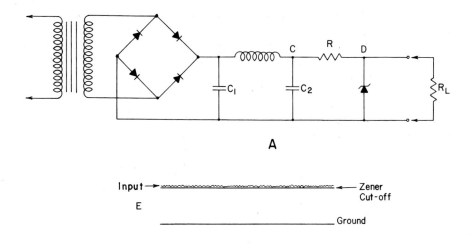

A

Input $\longrightarrow$ ———————————————— $\longleftarrow$ — Zener
Cut-off

E

——————————————————— Ground

B

Figure 7-12 A Zener diode as part of a power supply. Part B shows how clamping works.

cussed. At a particular potential, the current flowing backward through the diode increases drastically to prevent further voltage rise. Figure 7-12 shows the Zener diode in a power supply and how it cuts off the excess current. The appropriate size of diode must be selected for each application. If it has too high a breakdown voltage, it will not break down and will not remove the ripple. If it is too low, inadequate current will be driven through the resistive load. The key to the operation is the resistor R. As the voltage at point C rises, more current tries to pass through R to raise the voltage at point D. Since point D cannot exceed the voltage fixed by the Zener, the extra current will merely cause an *IR* drop over the resistor R equal to the excess ripple voltage and will leave through the Zener, thereby leaving the resistive load unaffected. This technique of cutting off the wave just below the ripple is called clamping.

Another circuit element that will accomplish the same thing as a Zener diode is a gas-filled diode. Figure 7-13 shows the electrical symbol for such a diode. Note that the presence of a free-standing dot in the circle indicates that the tube contains gas. This gas does not normally conduct current. When the voltage becomes high enough across the tube, the gas begins to ionize. The amount of ionization is a function of the applied voltage. Once ions have

formed they travel between the electrodes, carrying current. The more ions produced, the more current flows. Since the production of ions rises rapidly once the ionization potential of the gas is reached, a large amount of current will flow above this potential. This effectively shorts out any voltage above this level, just as occurs with the Zener diode.

The components of a power supply permit a high ac voltage to be changed into the appropriate dc voltage for internal use by an instrument. Many power supplies produce several voltage levels for use in different parts of the instrument, since different components frequently have different voltage demands. Some circuits require more uniform voltage levels than others, so the complexity of power supplies varies. Another factor in the construction of a power supply is the amount of current which will be drawn from the supply. All the components

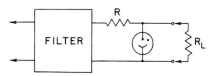

Figure 7-13 A gas-filled diode used for voltage regulation is attached to a filter.

come with various power and voltage ratings that must be matched appropriately to meet the demands placed on the power supply. The appropriate use of fuses is also necessary to protect the power supply components against excessive current demands.

The power supply is the last analog circuit device to be discussed as a separate entity. In Chapter 8 we will examine digital electronics and the role it plays in laboratory instrumentation.

REVIEW QUESTIONS

1. Why is a power supply needed between the wall outlet and the analytical circuits in most laboratory instruments?
2. Why is electrical power transmitted at high voltage?
3. What is the primary winding?
4. What is the secondary winding?
5. How does the transformer move power from the primary to the secondary winding? What links the two?
6. Why is a soft metal core used in a transformer?
7. What is the difference between a step-up and a step-down transformer?
8. To what is the voltage in the secondary circuit equal?
9. Why are numerous turns of wire needed in a transformer when the same voltage ratio could be attained by fewer loops?
10. Why can the voltage be lowered and the current be raised by a transformer without defying Ohm's law?
11. To what is the current in the secondary circuit equal? In the primary?
12. How much current flows through the primary circuit when the secondary circuit is open?
13. What is the stepping factor?
14. What happens when there are multiple secondary windings?
15. What is a rectifier?
16. Why is a rectifier used in a power supply?
17. What is half-wave rectification? Why does it cause difficulties?
18. What is pulsed dc?
19. What happens to the power of the other half of the wave with pulsed dc?
20. What is full-wave rectification?
21. Why is a special transformer needed for a full-wave rectifier?
22. Sketch a half-wave rectifier and explain how it works.
23. Sketch a full-wave rectifier and explain how it works.
24. Why is the voltage from the secondary only half as great as expected from the number of turns in a full-wave rectifier?
25. What is a bridge rectifier?
26. Sketch a bridge rectifier and explain how it works.
27. Sketch a voltage doubler rectifier and explain how it works.
28. What is an electronic filter?
29. What is electronic ripple? How is it defined?
30. Define the peak-to-peak voltage. Peak voltage. Average voltage. Root-mean-square voltage.
31. What is the dc voltage component of a rectified sine wave?
32. What is the ac voltage component of a rectified sine wave?
33. What circuit elements can be used as filters? How must they be installed?
34. What determines the success of a capacitor filter?
35. What are the units of the ripple factor?
36. Why does the output voltage of a filter decrease when the load resistor decreases?
37. What is a capacitor input filter and an inductor input filter?
38. What is the purpose of a voltage regulator?
39. What two general circuit approaches are available to create regulation?
40. How does a series regulator work?
41. How does a Zener diode regulate voltage?
42. How does a gas-filled diode work?
43. Why are fuses used?

PROBLEMS

1. If the voltage in the primary circuit is 490. V and the voltage in the secondary circuit is 185 V,

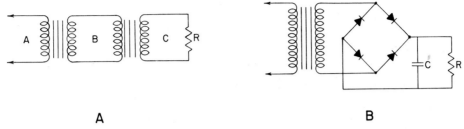

A   B

Figure 7-14 Circuits for Problems 5 through 9.

how many loops of wire are in the primary winding if there are 350. in the secondary?

2. If the peak-to-peak voltage is 283 V, what is the peak voltage, the average voltage and the root-mean-square voltage?

3. If the average voltage is 50.3 V, what is the peak voltage, the peak-to-peak voltage, and the root-mean-square voltage?

4. If the voltage in the primary circuit is 241 V, if the transformer has 941 turns in the primary winding and 379 turns on the secondary winding, and if the resistance in the secondary circuit is 1,694 Ω, what is the current in the primary and secondary circuits?

5. For the double transformer circuit illustrated in Figure 7-14A, the input voltage is 8,270 V. The following number of turns exist on the windings: $N_{p_1} = 1,947$, $N_{p_2} = 1,283$, $N_{s_1} = 394$, and $N_{s_2} = 405$. If the resistor R in the circuit is 28.9 kΩ, what is the current and voltage in all parts of the circuit?

6. If the ripple factor in Figure 7-14B is $0.183 \cdot 10^{-2}$, $C = 174 \ \mu F$, and $R_L = 3.97$ kΩ, what is the frequency in the rectified circuit?

7. What is the capacitance needed for a filter in Figure 7-14B to reduce the ripple factor to 0.0100 if $E_{p-p} = 340.$ V, $f = 60.0$ Hz, $R_L = 1.000$ kΩ, $N_p = 1,000$, and $N_s = 500.$?

8. What is the ripple voltage in Problem 7-7?

9. If the peak voltage for Problem 7-6 is 47.1 V, what is the dc voltage?

CHAPTER 8
DIGITAL ELECTRONICS

In the previous chapters we have examined the electronics necessary to make experimental measurements. These are called analog electronics because the properties of circuits, such as voltage, current, or capacitance, can have any real number value. A real number, as you will recall, can be an irrational number, such as π or e, as well as a rational number, which is just the quotient of two integers, such as 23/8. The real numbers are a continuum of values, any point on the number line having a real number value. The integers do not form such a continuum but are equally spaced points on the number line. The measurement of an analog quantity is best illustrated by the D'Arsonval meter. The value of the quantity can be equivalent to any position on the meter face.

The problem with transducers that map electrical quantities into the real numbers is that humans cannot absorb and remember these values directly. The human eye cannot see a meter position precisely, and the human mind cannot apprehend an irrational number. That is, in fact, why such numbers are called irrational. The human mind works in terms of increments of rational numbers, no matter how small such increments may be. Since nature, at least to the best of most instruments' ability to determine, has a continuum for all electrical properties, an approximation of the real number value by a rational number value must be made by the human observer in order to remember, record, or use the information.

The approximating of the real number representation of an electrical value by a rational number has always been a source of measurement error. The analog (D'Arsonval) meter not only affects the circuit into which it is placed, an effect that can be reduced by the use of operational amplifiers, but its reading is also subject to inaccuracies due to mechanical linkage and variations in temperature. The meter position itself is then subject to human approximation in the conversion to a rational number. Such approximation is nonreproducible and biased in favor of numbers divisible by 2 and 5. The recording of such measurements is a tedious process. The use of a servo-driven recorder, while creating a permanent record, does not diminish any of the aforementioned problems in transducing the value of the electrical property into the appropriate rational number.

To eliminate both the error and the tedium inherent in such analog measurements, modern electronics have increasingly embraced digital manipulation. This is clearly indicated by the way in which digital computers have rapidly relegated analog computers to practical oblivion. Digital electronics is based on the holding of a discrete rational number. All manipulations are accomplished by doing arithmetic operations on these numbers rather than obtaining results by the interaction of the quantities in analog circuits.

A second instrumental area in which digital principles are essential is that of experimental control. As an instrument proceeds through the various stages of a measurement, processes must be started and stopped at the appropriate times. Historically such control has been exercised by switches, cams, and timers. Newer instruments use microprocessors to supplement these devices. This chapter and the next discuss the use of digital electronics in the control of automation and in the numeric manipulation necessary to report the experimental results.

Section **8-1**
SWITCHES AND RELAYS

At various times in the previous material, switches were included that opened or closed circuits. Everyone is familiar with switches as a means of turning lights and appliances on and off. As we begin to examine digital control, we should look somewhat deeper into the nature and functions of switches.

Switches are primarily classified by the number of positions they can occupy and how many circuits they open or close when they go from one position to another. Figure 8-1 shows some switches. Figure 8-1A is the common single-pole single-throw (SPST) switch. It has two stable positions, one with the circuit open and one with the circuit closed. Other varieties of the SPST have only one stable position, as shown in Figure 8-1B,C. One is called normally open (N.O.), and the other, normally closed (N.C.). A spring forces these switches back

to their normal position when they are not activated by an outside agent.

Switches can have multiple throws for the same pole. The switch shown in Figure 8-1D is a single-pole double-throw switch (SPDT), which causes input to be switched between two leads. This switch can also be spring controlled so as to have one position normally closed and the other normally open (Fig. 8-1E). Since it is symmetrical, only one switch is needed to serve both normal state conditions. In addition, a "center off" condition can be added to the SPDT switch to give it a third, or neutral, position (Fig. 8-1F). This switch can also be spring controlled to return to off (Fig. 8-1G). Switches with even more throws can be made. These are called multiposition switches (Fig. 8-1H) and appear in many configurations. The letter before the T is replaced by the number of throws as in SP4T for the switch shown. These switches are seldom spring controlled.

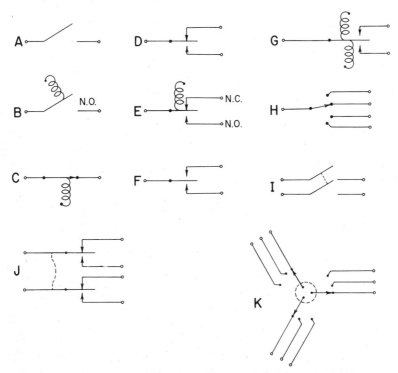

Figure 8-1 The switches are SPST (A, B, C), SPDT (D, E), SPDT-center off (F, G), SP4T (H), DPST (I), DPDT (J), and 3P3T (K).

It is also possible to build switches which have multiple poles. The most common of these are the double-pole single-throw (DPST) and double-pole double-throw (DPDT) switches (Figs. 8-1I,J). The dashed line indicates the poles are physically, but not electronically, attached. When the switch is operated, all poles move at the same time to the same relative position. Spring control is feasible, but is not shown in Figure 8-1. It is possible to have a larger number of poles in a stacked switch (one set of contacts above another) or interspersed as shown in Figure 8-1K. The letter in front of the P is replaced by a number to indicate the switch type (3P3T for the one in Figure 8-1).

The physical appearance of switches can vary greatly. Everyone is familiar with the light switch and the slide switch. The knife switch (a metal blade that slides between two contacts) is used for heavy current applications. The microswitch, a small push button switch, is used in many instruments to terminate mechanical motion when the moving part touches the switch and changes its position. Switches that must not "bounce" upon contact frequently use mercury on one of the contacts, so that once contact is made, it is not momentarily broken because of the irregular movement of the contact arm. Sometimes in a double throw switch, current must always flow to one contact or the other, and no interruption during the switching can be permitted. In these switches the second contact must be made before the first is broken. These switches are called "make-before-break" in contrast to the normal switch which is "make-after-break."

Switches are necessary at some point in most circuits. Let us study switch usages by first looking at the concept of switch logic. When the SPST switch in Figure 8-2A is open we have an "off" or "circuit false" condition. When the switch is closed, we have an "on" or "circuit true" condition. We can combine several switches together to get the information which is inherent in the position of all of them. The first example of this is Figure 8-2B, where two SPST switches are arranged in series. In this arrangement, both switches must be closed for the on or true condition to exist. This is referred to as the AND operation. Both switch A AND switch B must be closed for the circuit to be on. In Figure 8-2C we have two switches in parallel. In this case if either of the two switches is closed, the circuit will be turned on. This is the OR operation because either switch A OR switch B will activate the circuit.

The use of this type of switch logic is extremely common in laboratory instrumentation. Frequently, a particular thing is to be done if, and only if, several conditions are true. For example, the pump is turned on if reagent is present AND the reaction vessel is up to temperature. Each condition acts as one of the SPST switches in the AND circuit. Similarly, the SMAC should stop sampling if an error is detected OR the stop button is pushed OR someone gets their hair caught in the pumps. Each condition acts as one of the SPST switches in the OR circuit.

The SPST logic proves inadequate to handle more complex situations. For example, suppose we wish to wire a light which can be turned on and off independently from two switches. Neither arrangement shown in Figure 8-3A will work. In both cases the position of the one switch may have an effect on the second. Figure 8-3B shows two ways that a two-way switch can be wired using SPDT switches. Note that the lower one is preferred to the upper

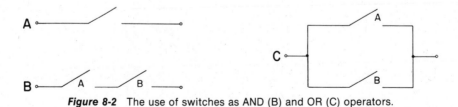

Figure 8-2 The use of switches as AND (B) and OR (C) operators.

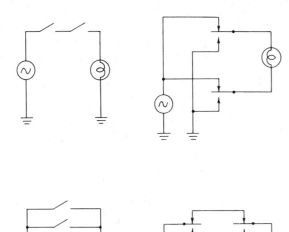

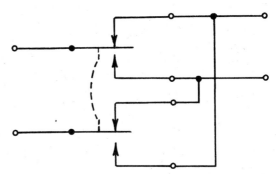

Figure 8-4 A reversing switch made from a DPDT switch.

A   **B**

Figure 8-3 Incorrect (A) and correct (B) ways of wiring a two-way switch.

one because when the light is off, no power reaches the bulb. This may or may not be true for the upper circuit.

EXAMPLE 8-1

Wire up a DPDT switch so that by changing the position of the switch, the polarity of the two input signals is switched between two output lines.

Solution: This is called a reversing switch and is shown in Figure 8-4. It is the central item in any circuit where the polarity of the circuit must be switched between two lines. Study this carefully as an example of a common switch usage. ∎

The concept of switching both leads of a circuit at the same time is important where more than one circuit can be used to power a particular device. In these cases, a DPNT switch (where $N \geq 2$) is necessary to prevent current from flowing from one circuit to another and causing an imbalance. A

common example of this is switching sections of track for an electrical train from one transformer to another.

A switch can be designed to be activated by electricity instead of physical force. Such a switch is called a relay. Examples of relays are shown in Figure 8-5. A relay differs from a regular switch in that it has two electronically isolated circuits, a coil circuit and a signal circuit. The relay remains in its rest (normal) position until current is applied to the coil circuit. The magnetic field of the coil then causes the contact arm of the relay's signal circuit

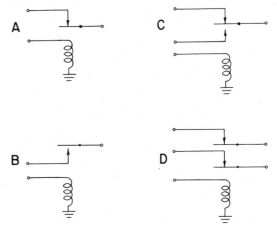

Figure 8-5 Relays come in many different types. Those shown are SPST (N.C.) (A), SPST (N.O.) (B), SPDT (C), and DPST (N.C.) (D).

to move from the rest position to the activated position. Relays come with various numbers of poles, but universally have only one or two throws. If a relay has a single throw, then it can be either normally open or normally closed when the coil is not activated. If the relay has two throws, then it will be normally closed to one and normally open to the other.

The relay we are interested in is the N.C. relay in Figure 8-6A. If switch A in front of the relay in the coil circuit (circuit 1) is open, then the coil is inactive and the signal circuit of the relay (circuit 2) is on. If the switch A is closed, then the coil is activated, the switch contact of the relay is opened, and no current flows in the signal circuit. The relay is, therefore, wired to cause negation and is called a NOT operator. It reverses the effective polarity of the switch A, since closing the switch causes the current to stop flowing.

This concept can be used in more complex relay circuits. In Figure 8-6B there are two switches in the coil circuit (circuit 1) of an N.C. relay. To activate the coil and turn off the signal circuit will require that both switch A and switch B be closed. This then is a simple combination of the NOT operation and the AND operation. It is called NAND. Another arrangement can be seen in Figure 8-6C. Here we have the switches in the parallel or OR configuration in the coil circuit of an N.C. relay. This has the effect of negating the OR operation and is called a NOR operator. There is one more logical operator to consider. It is called EXCLUSIVE OR because it gives an ''on'' or ''true'' condition only if either switch is closed but not if both switches are closed.

Figure 8-6D illustrates a switch circuit that does this operation. The dashed lines again indicate that the switches at either end must be opened or closed together. If both switches are open, no current flows into the signal circuit. If either switch A or switch B is on, current flows into the signal circuit and the circuit is on. If both switch A and switch B are closed, current tries to flow into the signal circuit, but it also flows into the coil circuit, opening the relay and preventing current flow in the signal circuit.

The above examples of relay combinations were chosen because they parallel the solid-state logic elements that we will look at later in the chapter. Clearly, many additional combinations can be made by the use of more complex relays. On the other hand, all the complex circuits can also be made from combinations of SPST switches and SPST (N.C.) relays. A few circuits using relays will be examined after other mechanical control elements are introduced.

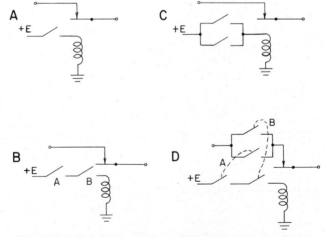

Figure 8-6 The representation of NOT (A), NAND (B), NOR (C), and EXCLUSIVE OR (D) using switches and relays.

Section **8-2**
CAMS, GEARS, AND TIMERS

Various instrument cycles are controlled by cams, gears, and timers. A cam is a misshapen circle, examples of which appear in Figure 8-7. As the cam rotates, an arm riding on or attached to the cam experiences linear motion or periodic motion, or a switch is opened or closed. On the other hand, linear motion can be used to force a cam to turn as does expanding steam in old railroad locomotives. To time different events in a cycle, a number of cams of different types and orientations can be placed on the same shaft. Since all rotate at the same speed, synchronization is maintained. Cams are used on the Fischer Autocytometer to count blood cells, for example.

Gears are another key element in the control of some automation. While cams can cause events to happen in a fixed time sequence, gears allow certain events to occur more or less frequently than others. The minute hand moves 12 times as fast as the hour hand on a watch. Like other mechanical components, gears have been extensively replaced by electrical timers, as will be discussed later.

The driver for cams and gears is a motor that rotates at a known speed. The gears divide that speed and the cams move switches and valves appropriately. Frequently such motors are reversible, such as syringe drivers, so that events can occur in both directions. A common device to be attached to a motor assembly is a spiral potentiometer, where the outer case holds the coil of wire, and the variable contact arm is attached to a central shaft turned by the motor. The relative motion of the motor can then be determined by the voltage between the contact arm and the end of the potenti-

ometer. This arrangement permits the generation of a uniform voltage ramp for comparison purposes. This voltage can be used to run equipment and relays. To understand how instruments are controlled, it is best to look at a few examples.

EXAMPLE 8-2

Design a turntable that will advance by one position every 60 seconds and which has a sampler that samples for 30 seconds from each cup.

Solution: Figure 8-8 gives the solution. It is important to look at the various parts to see what must be done. Motor A sets the time scale for the turntable. Everything is based on its speed. Gears B and C reduce the motor speed so that the camshaft D turns only once each minute. Several gear reductions may be necessary to accomplish this, but one will suffice in the drawing to show that gear reduction is necessary. The cam E controls the sampler position. If the sampler is not physically raised during the rotation of the turntable, it will be broken off. Cam F controls the sampling. It activates the vacuum motor I during the half rotation when cam E has the sampler sitting down in the cup. Cam F controls motor I because it causes microswitch G to be tripped during the raised part of the cycle. The microswitch activates N.O. relay H. The relay is used to prevent excessive current from flowing through the microswitch. Relays can be made to tolerate high signal current but run off low coil current. Also on camshaft D is cam J, which trips microswitch K when the sampler has been raised.

This causes N.O. relay L to close and motor M to start turning. As it does, cam N on the shaft of

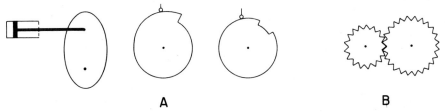

A   **B**

Figure 8-7 Cams come in various shapes. Gears rotate more rapidly if they have fewer teeth than their meshing partner.

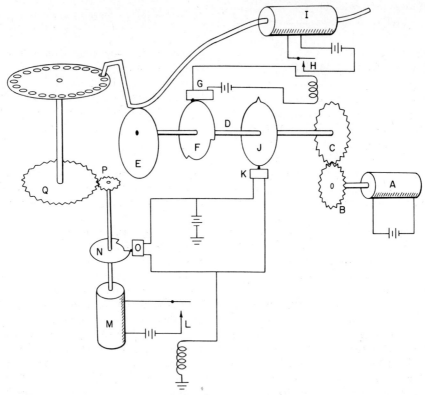

Figure 8-8 A turntable and sampler controlled by a cam drive and microswitches.

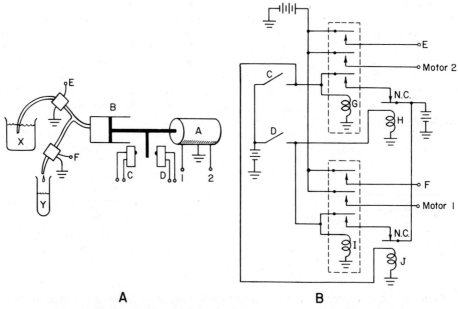

A   B

Figure 8-9 The pictorial and electrical diagram of a motor-driven syringe.

motor M turns on microswitch O, which is in parallel with microswitch K (OR arrangement). This action guarantees that motor M will stay on for a whole revolution, and the turntable will be properly positioned for the next sampling. Sometime during the motor revolution microswitch K will turn off. Gears P and Q gear down the rotation so only one position is turned per motor revolution. Microswitch O turns off when the revolution is complete, deactivating relay L and turning off the motor M. Thus every revolution of the camshaft causes the turntable to advance by one position and sampling to occur. ■

EXAMPLE 8-3

Design a device that will transfer a constant amount of material from reservoir *X* to reaction vessel *Y* every 30 seconds.

Solution: The heart of this device will be a motor-driven syringe set to give the desired volume. The syringe must draw the appropriate amount of liquid from the reservoir, change direction, push the solution into the reaction vessel and again change direction to repeat the cycle. Figure 8-9 shows the solution to the problem.

Part A is the physical equipment. A is a bidirectional motor that goes forward if contact 1 has voltage applied and backward if contact 2 has voltage applied. B is the syringe. The syringe plunger has a side arm used to trip microswitches C and D when it reaches them. These switches cause the direction to reverse. E and F are solenoid valves which are open when a current flows between the contacts and are closed otherwise. Solenoid valves are simply relays that control liquid current rather than electrical current. The one to the reaction vessel is closed during the intake part of the cycle, and the one to the reservoir is closed during the ejection part of the cycle.

The electronics are shown in Figure 8-9B. When N.O. microswitch C is momentarily closed by the contact arm, 3PST (N.O.) relay G is closed. Since SPST relay H is N.C., the current which runs through the lowest contact of the 3PST relay and to its coil will keep it activated even when microswitch C is no longer closed. Switch C and the lowest contact of switch G are in parallel. When

microswitch C is closed, SPST (N.C.) relay J is opened, interrupting the current to 3PST (N.O.) relay I and causing it to open. (Current can flow into the coil through neither switch D nor switch J, both of which are open.) When G closes, power is supplied to solenoid E to open to the reservoir and also to motor contact 2, causing the syringe to fill. When microswitch D is closed, the reverse happens, closing everything open and opening everything closed. Note while the solenoids and motor are driven by the same power supply here for simplicity, this might not be the case in actual practice. ■

Logic that depends on microswitches, cams, and relays is bulky and difficult to construct. As a result, solid-state methods were developed to accomplish the same effect. These approaches are introduced later in the chapter.

Section 8-3
NUMBER SYSTEMS

Before proceeding, we must further explore number systems. The basis for any number system is the human necessity to count objects and events. To count, one assigns names to the presence of objects. Each unit increase in the quantity of objects present requires a new name. It is this process that led to the integers. The difficulty with extending this process indefinitely is that the number of names is equal to the number of numbers, and the latter quantity can grow without bound. It therefore becomes necessary to organize the naming of numbers so that it is possible to remember the names or easily derive them, at least for any quantity of material one would be likely to count. Such an organization is called a number system. The primary feature of a number system is the cyclic arrangement of the names and symbols used. The number system in which we normally work is called decimal because it has 10 symbols and names to represent objects, as shown in Table 8-1. When these symbols are exhausted in counting, we resort to a bigger cycle by creating another digital place called the 10s digit. Consequently, the number system is said to have a base of 10. When the symbols for the tens positions have been exhausted, one progresses to the hundreds, thousands, and so on.

Table 8-1 Decimal and Binary Systems

Decimal		Binary	
0	Zero	0	Zero
1	One	1	One
2	Two	10	Onety
3	Three	11	Onety-one
4	Four	100	Hundred
5	Five	101	Hundred one
6	Six	110	Hundred onety
7	Seven	111	Hundred onety-one
8	Eight	1000	Thousand
9	Nine	1001	Thousand one
10	Ten	1010	Thousand onety
11	Eleven	1011	Thousand onety-one
12	Twelve	1100	Thousand hundred

Table 8-2 Binary Addition and Multiplication

+	0	1	×	0	1
0	0	1	0	0	0
1	1	10	1	0	1

The reason that 10 was chosen is a result of humans having ten fingers. Originally, counting consisted of equating the number of objects present to a certain number of fingers. There is nothing magic about ten, however, and any number could have been chosen as the base for the cycle of a number system. Number systems with odd bases lack symmetry and are harder to work with, while bases above thirteen require the memorization of such a large multiplication table as to be difficult for the average person to use. Two bases other than ten which we will examine more closely are binary (base two) and octal (base eight).

The use of binary for data representation is predicated on the idea that there are really only two discrete states for any nonanalog object. These can be yes–no, on–off, there–not there, and so forth. The binary representation is frequently thought of as a switch which is either closed or open. Such an approach readily relates the binary system to electrical circuits. Elements of a circuit, as we have seen, can be either on or off, depending on whether an appropriate switch is closed.

The first numbers in the binary counting scheme appear in Table 8-1, and the addition and multiplication tables are shown in Table 8-2. As can be seen, the cycle is very short, and the number of binary positions grows rapidly. Each of these is called a *binary digit* (or "bit"). Every number that can be represented in decimal can also be represented in binary. This means that a machine can store any decimal number we choose in a series of binary devices. While this representation may bear little resemblance to the decimal number as we conceive of it, it will have the same intrinsic value. It is only necessary that we convert from one representation to the other before we use it.

The conversion from decimal to binary is based on the concept that a number is just the summation of individual digits times the base to various powers. To go from decimal to binary one must change a summation of single digits times powers of 10 to a summation of single digits times powers of 2.

$$\Sigma a_j 2^j = \Sigma a_i 10^i$$

where

$$a_j < 2 \quad \text{and} \quad a_i < 10 \quad \text{for all } i \text{ and } j \quad \textbf{(8-1)}$$

An example might be helpful. The decimal number 147 can be written as $1 \cdot 10^2 + 4 \cdot 10^1 + 7 \cdot 10^0$. In binary the same quantity is represented by $1 \cdot 2^7 + 0 \cdot 2^6 + 0 \cdot 2^5 + 1 \cdot 2^4 + 0 \cdot 2^3 + 1 \cdot 2^1 + 1 \cdot 2^0$, or 1001011. One need only multiply out the binary expression to verify the equality. To accomplish the general conversion, however, a formula is needed that can be used for computation. There are two general approaches that can be used. The first requires that the mathematics be done in the base in which one is initially working and is called the method of division. For the conversion from decimal to binary, it can be expressed as

$$N = 2(2(2(2(\cdots(2(a_N) + a_{N-1})$$
$$+ \cdots) + a_3) + a_2) + a_1) + a_0 \quad \textbf{(8-2)}$$

This equation can be best understood by trying it on an example.

EXAMPLE 8-4

What is the binary equivalent of 279 decimal?

Solution: Begin by partitioning the number into a part divisible by 2 and a remainder.

$$279 = 2 \times N_1 + a_0$$

$$\begin{array}{r} 139 + \text{rem } 1 \\ 2\overline{)279} \end{array} \qquad N_1 = 139 \quad a_0 = 1$$

We repeat the process by defining a new N and a.

$$139 = 2 \times N_2 + a_1$$

$$\begin{array}{r} 69 + \text{rem } 1 \\ 2\overline{)139} \end{array} \qquad N_2 = 69 \quad a_1 = 1$$

and continue:

$$\begin{array}{r} 34 + \text{rem } 1 \\ 2\overline{)\ 69} \end{array} \qquad N_3 = 34 \quad a_2 = 1$$

$$\begin{array}{r} 17 + \text{rem } 0 \\ 2\overline{)\ 34} \end{array} \qquad N_4 = 17 \quad a_3 = 0$$

$$\begin{array}{r} 8 + \text{rem } 1 \\ 2\overline{)\ 17} \end{array} \qquad N_5 = 8 \quad a_4 = 1$$

$$\begin{array}{r} 4 + \text{rem } 0 \\ 2\overline{)\ 8} \end{array} \qquad N_6 = 4 \quad a_5 = 0$$

$$\begin{array}{r} 2 + \text{rem } 0 \\ 2\overline{)\ 4} \end{array} \qquad N_7 = 2 \quad a_6 = 0$$

$$\begin{array}{r} 1 + \text{rem } 0 \\ 2\overline{)\ 2} \end{array} \qquad N_8 = 1 \quad a_7 = 0$$

$$\begin{array}{r} 0 + \text{rem } 1 \\ 2\overline{)\ 1} \end{array} \qquad N_9 = 0 \quad a_8 = 1$$

As a result,

$$279_{10} = 1 \cdot 2^8 + 0 \cdot 2^7 + 0 \cdot 2^6 + 0 \cdot 2^5 + 1 \cdot 2^4$$
$$+ 0 \cdot 2^3 + 1 \cdot 2^2 + 1 \cdot 2^1 + 1 \cdot 2^0$$

or

$$279_{10} = 100010111_2$$

The subscript here indicates the base of the number. If written in the form of Eq. 8-2,

$$279 = 2(2(2(2(2(2(2(2(1)$$
$$+ 0) + 0) + 0) + 1) + 0) + 1) + 1) + 1 \quad \blacksquare$$

The conversion by the method of division is therefore accomplished by dividing the number in the old base by the new base and saving the remain-der. The process is then repeated until the quotient is zero. This process, in effect, changes the old cycle to the new cycle by the regrouping of the value of the number in terms of the new base. To prove that this will work between any bases, consider the next example.

EXAMPLE 8-5

What is the decimal equivalent of 100010111 binary?

Solution: We will follow the same procedure, except now we must do the math in the binary system. The value 1010 is 10 in binary.

$$100010111 = 1010 \times N_1 + a_0$$

$$\begin{array}{r} 11011 \text{ rem } 1001 \qquad N_1 = 11011 \\ 1010\overline{)100010111} \qquad\qquad a_0 = 1001 \quad \text{or } 9 \\ \underline{1010} \\ 1110 \\ \underline{1010} \\ 10011 \\ \underline{1010} \\ 10011 \\ \underline{1010} \\ 1001 \end{array}$$

We then repeat the process.

$$11011 = 1010 \times N_2 + a_1$$

$$\begin{array}{r} 10 \text{ rem } 111 \qquad N_2 = 10 \quad a_1 = 111 \quad \text{or } 7 \\ 1010\overline{)11011} \\ \underline{1010} \\ 111 \end{array}$$

$$\begin{array}{r} 0 \text{ rem } 10 \qquad N_3 = 0 \quad a_2 = 10 \quad \text{or } 2 \\ 1010\overline{)10} \end{array}$$

Therefore

$$100010111_2 = 279_{10} = 10(10(2) + 7) + 9 \quad \blacksquare$$

The second method of converting from one base to another is through multiplication. Each digital position in the old base has a value in the new base. One simply multiplies the number in that digital position by that position's value in the new base for each position and sums over all positions.

$$N = \Sigma a_i V_i \qquad (8\text{-}3)$$

where V_i is the position value in the new base. The disadvantage is that the position values in the new base must be known in advance. The arithmetic is done in the new base, rather than the old.

EXAMPLE 8-6

What is the value in binary of 314 decimal?

Solution:

$$100_{10} = 1100100_2$$
$$10_{10} = \quad\ \ 1010_2$$
$$1_{10} = \qquad\ \ 1_2$$

$$
\begin{array}{rlll}
300 = & 11 \cdot 1100100 = & 100101100 \\
10 = & 1 \cdot \quad 1010 = & 1010 \\
4 = & 100 \cdot \qquad 1 = & 100 \\
\hline
& 314_{10} & 100111010_2 \quad \blacksquare
\end{array}
$$

EXAMPLE 8-7

What is the value in decimal of 100111010 binary?

Solution: In binary, one has a 1s column, 2s column, 4s column, 8s column, and so on:

$$
\begin{array}{llll}
100000000_2 = 256_{10} & \times 1 & = 256 \\
10000000_2 = 128_{10} & \times 0 & = 0 \\
1000000_2 = 64_{10} & \times 0 & = 0 \\
100000_2 = 32_{10} & \times 1 & = 32 \\
10000_2 = 16_{10} & \times 1 & = 16 \\
1000_2 = 8_{10} & \times 1 & = 8 \\
100_2 = 4_{10} & \times 0 & = 0 \\
10_2 = 2_{10} & \times 1 & = 2 \\
1_2 = 1_{10} & \times 0 & = 0 \\
\hline
& 100111010_2 & 314_{10} \quad \blacksquare
\end{array}
$$

Since most people find doing arithmetic in base 10 easier than in base 2, the common practice is to convert from decimal to binary via the method of division but to convert from binary to decimal via the method of multiplication. Either method will work provided the arithmetic is done correctly. Calculators are available to do this type of conversion if it is frequently needed.

Table 8-3   Decimal, Binary, Octal

Decimal	Binary	Octal
00	000 000	00
01	000 001	01
02	000 010	02
03	000 011	03
04	000 100	04
05	000 101	05
06	000 110	06
07	000 111	07
08	001 000	10
09	001 001	11
10	001 010	12

Binary numbers are obviously difficult to work with. Trying to remember a specific pattern of ones and zeros is like trying to recall a pattern of random polka dots. The need to use binary information does arise with certain instruments in the clinical laboratory, so some simplification in the handling of binary coded information is essential. Some common instrumental uses of binary information in the laboratory are status registers on computer-controlled equipment, switches to examine or initialize internal states, and procedure identification lights.

The way the problem of this length of binary numbers is solved is by the introduction of another number system called octal. Octal has eight numeric symbols instead of two or ten. The manner of counting in octal is shown in Table 8-3. The octal system bears a special relationship to the binary system, because $8 = 2^3$. As the binary system counts from 000 to 111, the octal system counts from 0 to 7. When the binary system counts 1000, the octal system counts 10. Each octal position can hold exactly the same amount of information as three binary positions. Consequently, a binary number can be converted to an octal number by inspection and vice versa.

EXAMPLE 8-8

What is the value in octal of 1011100110 binary?

Solution: Separate the binary number into groups of three digits working from the decimal point:

$$1\ 011\ 100\ 110$$

Convert each group individually:

$$1 = 1, \ 011 = 3, \ 100 = 4, \ 110 = 6$$

Therefore,

$$1011100110_2 = 1346_8 \qquad ■$$

With a little practice, the interconversion between binary and octal becomes trivial. This allows one to rapidly read and set information for certain laboratory instruments. In addition to its easy interconversion with binary, octal has the advantage of being similar to decimal in the amount of information it can hold per digit. For example, 1024_{10} is 2000_8, but 10000000000_2. The same methods of interconversion that worked between decimal and binary will work between decimal and octal. In fact, octal is frequently the intermediate in the conversion process. Decimal information will be converted to octal, which is then broken up digit by digit to get binary. Since the decimal-to-octal interconversion requires fewer arithmetic steps, it is usually preferred when manual conversion is necessary.

While the use of binary may be acceptable for status registers and troubleshooting, it is clear that the reporting of laboratory results in binary or octal would not set well with the physicians, and most laboratory workers have small interest in converting these octal numbers to decimal manually. As a consequence, it is mandatory that the laboratory instruments convert binary representations to decimal representations before they feed the information to the output devices, which are usually some form of light display or series of print wheels or print hammers. Since the instruments do not have available any components with 10 states, they must retain the information in binary devices, but code them into decimal representation. This procedure is called *b*inary *c*oded *d*ecimal (BCD).

The most common form of BCD is the truncated binary or 8 4 2 1 code, as shown in Table 8-4. The code uses four bits for every decimal digit. The binary counting occurs as with normal binary until 9_{10} is reached. The next count sets the digital position (these four bits) to zero and generates a carry to the next most significant digital place. The representations from 1010 to 1111 are never used. Some computers in the past (e.g., the IBM 1620) have used this numeric representation to do internal arithmetic in place of binary. Most devices use it only to store information as it is readied for output to the user. Because each binary position in the representation of a decimal digit has value that is added in if the bit is set, this type of coding scheme is called a weighted code.

Other schemes can be used for special purposes. The second column in Table 8-4 has a variety of Gray code. In this scheme only one bit changes at each increment as one counts through the digits. This is important in devices such as position encoders which must have low error tolerance. As they move from one position to another, several bit positions that might change not quite simultaneously could cause incorrect position definition. Note that even the carry between 9 and 10 generates only one change per digit.

Some coding schemes use parity to prevent er-

Table 8-4   Binary-Coded Decimal Representations

Decimal	BCD[a]	Gray	2-out-of-5	Paritied BCD	ASCII[b]
0	0000 0000	0000 0000	00011 00011	10000 10000	10110000
1	0000 0001	0000 0001	00011 00101	10000 00001	00110001
2	0000 0010	0000 0011	00011 00110	10000 00010	00110010
3	0000 0011	0000 0010	00011 01001	10000 10011	10110011
4	0000 0100	0000 0110	00011 01010	10000 00100	00110100
5	0000 0101	0000 1110	00011 01100	10000 10101	10110101
6	0000 0110	0000 1010	00011 10001	10000 10110	10110110
7	0000 0111	0000 1011	00011 10010	10000 00111	00110111
8	0000 1000	0000 1001	00011 10100	10000 01000	00111000
9	0000 1001	0000 1000	00011 11000	10000 11001	10111001
10	0001 0000	0001 0000	00101 00011	00001 10000	10110000 + carry

[a] Binary coded decimal.
[b] American Standard Convention for Information Interchange.

rors from occurring. Parity means that either an even number or an odd number of bits must be on in each decimal digit representation, regardless of the position of the actual bits that are on. An extra bit is available to set or clear to fulfill this parity condition. If the correct parity condition (let us say odd) is not met for each digit in the system, then an error flag is generated to notify the user that there is a problem.

The next two entries in Table 8-4 are the 2-out-of-5 code and the paritied standard BCD. In both cases, five bits instead of four are used to represent each digit. For this extra cost, one gets extra security that the result is accurate. In the 2-out-of-5 case, each representation has exactly two of the five positions set for each digital representation. More or less than this number means that an error has occurred in the information set-up stage. This scheme is used on the SMAC (it is discussed later in this book). The paritied standard BCD has a fifth bit that is set or cleared to make the total number of bits set in the word an odd number. This basic approach is used on most magnetic data storage systems.

The final scheme shown is called the American Standard Convention for Information Interchange (ASCII). It is very similar to the paritied standard BCD except that it has some extra bits, making eight bits per digit. These are necessary because ASCII also has coding representation for all the alphabet letters (uppercase and lowercase), punctuation, and a group of printer control commands. Such a code can be used to store English words and sentences in an instrument. When a numerical answer is printed out by the instrument, the name of the procedure, its units and normal range, and perhaps even the patient's name can also be printed. This simplifies the work of the technologist who no longer has to struggle trying to match the data with the sequence the specimens were inserted into the instrument.

Section 8-4
DIGITAL LOGIC

The logical operators introduced with switches and relays earlier in this chapter permit manipulation with the binary representation of numbers because the binary 0 can be treated as the OFF state and the binary 1 as the ON state. All the operators introduced involve two operands, except for negation. These operators are frequently indicated with an arithmetic symbol. Several different sets of symbols exist, and we will use the following: $\bar{A} = $ NOT, $A \cdot B = A$ AND B, $A + B = A$ OR B, $\overline{A \cdot B} = $ NOT $(A$ AND $B) = A$ NAND B, $\overline{A + B} = $ NOT $(A$ OR $B) = A$ NOR B, and $A \oplus B = A$ EXCL. OR B. (Note that $\bar{\bar{A}}$ is NOT (NOT A). This is the same as A. $(A = \bar{\bar{A}})$.)

In an effort to see the effect of operators on various combinations of inputs, the representation called a truth table has been developed. The truth tables for the operators discussed above are given in Table 8-5. In reading the tables, **0** is read as false and **1** is read as true. R means the result of the

Table 8-5   Truth Tables for Logical Operators

NOT ($\bar{A}$)		AND ($A \cdot B$)			OR ($A + B$)			EXCL OR ($A \oplus B$)		
A	R	A	B	R	A	B	R	A	B	R
0	1	0	0	0	0	0	0	0	0	0
1	0	1	0	0	1	0	1	1	0	1
		0	1	0	0	1	1	0	1	1
		1	1	1	1	1	1	1	1	0

NAND ($\overline{A \cdot B}$)			NOR ($\overline{A + B}$)		
A	B	R	A	B	R
0	0	1	0	0	1
1	0	1	1	0	0
0	1	1	0	1	0
1	1	0	1	1	0

Table 8-6 Single Operand Logic Rules

AND	OR
$A \cdot 0 = 0$	$A + 0 = A$
$A \cdot 1 = A$	$A + 1 = 1$
$A \cdot A = A$	$A + A = A$
$A \cdot \bar{A} = 0$	$A + \bar{A} = 1$

operation on A and B. We will go through Table 8-5 for AND as an example of how these tables are used. If A is false AND B is false, the result is false. This is the case where both switches in series are open. Obviously, no current flows. If A is true AND B is false, the result is still false. No current flows with only one switch closed. If A is false AND B is true, the result is false. This is really identical to the previous case for the AND operator. If A is true AND B is true, then the result is true. If both series switches are closed, then current can flow. The reader should go through the rest of the tables to verify that they do work just as the switches and relays do and to become more familiar with the notation. Failure to work through these tables now will lead to confusion later.

In addition to these truth tables, certain rules of logic apply when A is the only named operand. These must be known because they are frequently encountered in the logical handling of expressions representing binary quantities. Let us go through these rules to verify their validity (Table 8-6). If A is ANDed with a false condition, the result is false because the corresponding series circuit has at least one open switch. If A is ANDed with a true condition, the result is whatever A is, because the corre-

sponding circuit will be completed only if switch A is closed. If A is ANDed with itself, that is A, obviously the whole outcome depends on A. If A is ANDed with NOT A, then whatever A is, NOT A is the opposite. Together they guarantee that one switch will be open and one closed in the corresponding circuit and no current can flow. Therefore, the circuit is false.

If A is ORed with a false, the corresponding parallel circuit will be open or closed depending on the value of A only. If A is ORed with a true, one of the switches of the corresponding circuit is already closed and current is flowing, so the result is always true. If A is ORed with A, the whole outcome is dependent on A. If A is ORed with NOT A, then one of the two parallel branches is always closed, hence the circuit will give a true result.

Logical rules also apply when there are several named operands (Table 8-7). These rules have properties similar to those of the operators in arithmetic. Because of the significance of these rules to an understanding of logic circuits, we will discuss these five rule pairs. The first rules deal with the property of commutativity and are identical to the arithmetic rules. They can be easily verified by inspection, by looking at the corresponding truth tables; this should be done before proceeding.

The same can be said about the property of associativity, which permits regrouping with the same operator. To verify this from the truth tables requires that the tables be extended to cover all the combinations of the three inputs. This means that there are 2^3 (or 8) rows. Table 8-8 shows how each side of the expression is developed and that the two sides are indeed the same for $A + (B + C) = (A + $

Table 8-7 Multiple Operand Logic Rules

Commutation	$A + B = B + A$	(A OR $B = B$ OR A)
	$A \cdot B = B \cdot A$	(A AND $B = B$ AND A)
Association	$A + (B + C) = (A + B) + C$	(A OR (B OR C) = (A OR B) OR C)
	$A \cdot (B \cdot C) = (A \cdot B) \cdot C$	(A AND (B AND C) = (A AND B) AND C)
Distribution	$A + (B \cdot C) = (A + B) \cdot (A + C)$	(A OR (B AND C) = (A OR B) AND (A OR C))
	$A \cdot (B + C) = (A \cdot B) + (A \cdot C)$	(A AND (B OR C) = (A AND B) OR (A AND C))
DeMorgan	$\overline{A + B} = \bar{A} \cdot \bar{B}$	(NOT (A OR B) = (NOT A) AND (NOT B))
	$\overline{A \cdot B} = \bar{A} + \bar{B}$	(NOT (A AND B) = (NOT A) OR (NOT B))
Absorption	$A + (A \cdot B) = A$	(A OR (A AND B) REDUCES TO A)
	$A \cdot (A + B) = A$	(A AND (A OR B) REDUCES TO A)

Table 8-8   Verification That $A + (B + C) = (A + B) + C$

B	C	(B + C)		A	(B + C)	A + (B + C)		A	B	(A + B)		(A + B)	C	(A + B) + C
0	0	0		0	0	0		0	0	0		0	0	0
0	0	0		1	0	1		1	0	1		1	0	1
1	0	1		0	1	1		0	1	1		1	0	1
1	0	1		1	1	1		1	1	1		1	0	1
0	1	1		0	1	1		0	0	0		0	1	1
0	1	1		1	1	1		1	0	1		1	1	1
1	1	1		0	1	1		0	1	1		1	1	1
1	1	1		1	1	1		1	1	1		1	1	1

$B) + C$. Note well how the columns for A, B, and C are developed. Be sure to work through this example before proceeding.

A third familiar arithmetic property is distributiveness. The logical operators are more thorough than the arithmetic ones, because not only does AND distribute over OR, but OR distributes over AND. This latter fact is verified in Table 8-9. This should be studied carefully.

The remaining two properties have no arithmetic equivalent. DeMorgan's theorem enables one to break up a NAND or a NOR operator into the more primitive OR and AND operators. These rules can be verified easily, and the reader should do so at this point to prevent future confusion over these equalities. The rules of absorption are also strange because they allow a part of the expression to be dispensed with, without further evaluation and without loss of information. Let us briefly examine how this works. If we have $A + (A \cdot B)$, and if A is true, then the result is true because a true on one side of an OR always gives a true result. If A is false, then $A \cdot B$ is false because a false on one side of an AND operator always gives a false. Consequently, we have falses on both sides of the OR, which means the result is false. Therefore, if A is true, the result is true, while if A is false, the result is false. It follows that the result is identical to A. If we have $A \cdot (A + B)$, and if A is false, then the result is false because one side of an AND is false. However, $A \cdot (A + B) = A \cdot A + A \cdot B$ by distributiveness. If A is true, $A \cdot A$ is true and the expression is true because one side of the OR is true. As before, the result is identical to A. Be careful with absorption because a variable will absorb another expression only if one of the two patterns shown exists.

These logic rules allow the combining of operands into one result. In digital electronics, these operands are data and control signals from various points. Recall the example in which an instrument would start a pumping operation if enough reagent were present and if the temperature had reached a certain value. We will next turn our attention to the actual digital circuit components.

EXAMPLE 8-9

Reduce the expression $\bar{A} \cdot \bar{C} \cdot B + (\bar{A} \cdot \bar{B} + B) \cdot \bar{C}$ to its simplest terms.

Solution:

By associativity

$$(\bar{A} \cdot B + \bar{A} \cdot \bar{B} + B) \cdot \bar{C}$$

By associativity

$$(\bar{A} \cdot (B + \bar{B}) + B) \cdot \bar{C}$$

$B + \bar{B} = 1$

$$(\bar{A} \cdot 1 + B) \cdot \bar{C}$$

$\bar{A} \cdot 1 = \bar{A}$

$$(\bar{A} + B) \cdot \bar{C}$$

$B = \bar{\bar{B}}$

$$(\bar{A} + \bar{\bar{B}}) \cdot \bar{C}$$

By DeMorgan

$$\overline{A \cdot \bar{B}} \cdot \bar{C}$$

By DeMorgan

$$\overline{A \cdot \bar{B} + C}$$

■

Table 8-9 Verification That $A + (B \cdot C) = (A + B) \cdot (A + C)$

B	C	(B · C)	A	A + (B · C)	A	B	(A + B)	A	C	(A + C)	(A + B)	(A + C)	(A + B) · (A + C)
0	0	0	0	0	0	0	0	0	0	0	0	0	0
0	0	0	1	1	1	0	1	1	0	1	1	1	1
1	0	0	0	0	0	1	1	0	0	0	1	0	0
1	0	0	1	1	1	1	1	1	0	1	1	1	1
0	1	0	0	0	0	0	0	0	1	1	0	1	0
0	1	0	1	1	1	0	1	1	1	1	1	1	1
1	1	1	0	1	0	1	1	0	1	1	1	1	1
1	1	1	1	1	1	1	1	1	1	1	1	1	1

Section **8-5**
LOGIC GATES

As originally introduced, logical operations were in terms of relays and switches. This type of an implementation is very slow and extremely bulky. Its application is limited to real systems which are very simple such as those shown in Section 8-2. Faster and smaller components, like transistors and diodes, are needed for more complex implementations. In laboratory instruments transistor logic circuits control much of the internal operations and do the computing. Because the logical circuits feed directly into one another, the circuitry is called *transistor-transistor logic*, or TTL.

In Figure 8-10A is the simplest element used in transistor logic—the NOT operator. The NOT operator can be built using one BJT transistor and two resistors. If the input is low, the output (R = result) is effectively connected only to the power supply and is high. If the input is high, the transistor turns on, there is an IR drop over the load resistor, and the output is effectively shorted to ground. The transistor representation of a logical operator is called a gate. This is exactly analogous to the SPST (N.C.) relay given in Section 8-1.

A NOT operator is also referred to as an invertor. Since very little current is drawn by the base of an n–p–n transistor, the output of this logical circuit gate can be used as an input by other logical circuit gates without having a significant effect on its out-put voltage. Attaching it to many gates, however, will cause significant current to be drawn from it. This means an IR drop will exist over the resistor, and the output voltage will fall. The number of gates that a transistor output can drive is called its fan-out.

The second easiest logical operator to construct is the NAND gate. Figure 8-10B shows that this is accomplished by placing two n–p–n transistors in a type of series arrangement. In order for the output to be pulled low, both the inputs must be high. In all other cases, the output will be high. This is the typical NOT AND situation. Trying to build an AND gate in a similar straightforward way can lead to instability in some applications; therefore, a more complex arrangement is used. This is shown in Figure 8-10C. An invertor is placed after the output of the NAND gate to create the effect of an AND, since NOT NAND is NOT NOT AND. The two NOTs cancel, and the AND results.

The design of the OR and NOR operators follows the same pattern. Figure 8-11A shows a NOR gate. If both of the inputs are low, the output is high. If either or both of the inputs are high, the output is low. The OR gate is obtained by inverting the output of the NOR gate as shown in Figure 8-11B. Both of these representations use the basic principle of ORing with a parallel circuit.

The EXCLUSIVE OR operation is somewhat harder to accomplish. One circuit for it is shown in Figure 8-11C. This representation takes advantage of the fact that $A \oplus B = (A \cdot \bar{B}) + (\bar{A} \cdot B)$. A num-

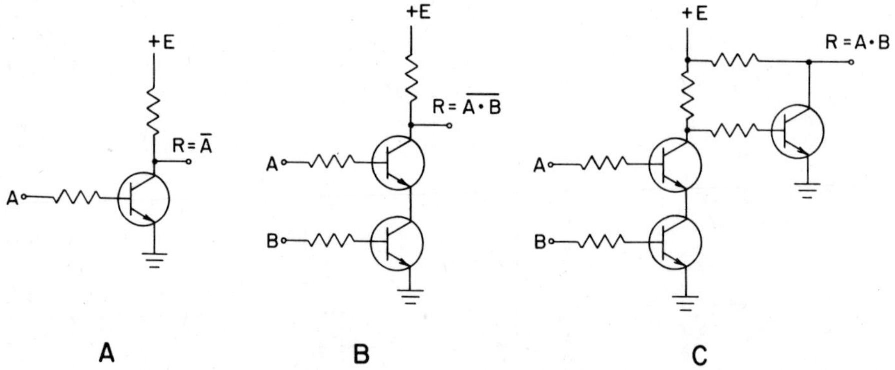

Figure 8-10 The NOT (A), NAND (B), and AND (C) gates are shown in terms of their resistor and transistor equivalents. (Resistor-transistor logic, RTL.)

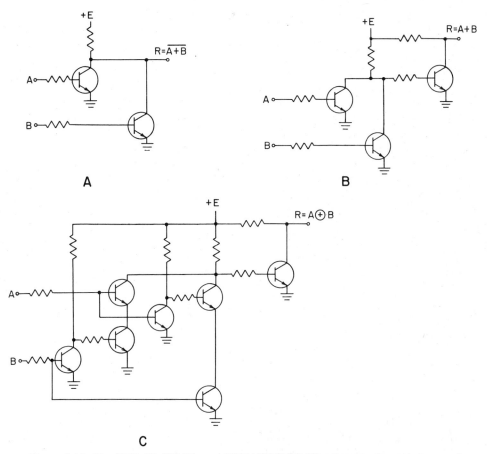

Figure 8-11 The NOR (A), OR (B), and EXCLUSIVE OR (C) gates are shown in terms of their resistor and transistor equivalents. Note well where the wires are connected and where they just cross in the EXCLUSIVE OR gate circuit.

ber of other arrangements of gates is possible if one derives a different, but equivalent, means of representing $A \oplus B$.

As should be evident from the transistor equivalent circuits, there is no reason to have only two inputs for most operators. One can, for example, add a third input to a NAND gate by placing it in series with the first two. This gives us a three-input NAND gate instead of a two-input NAND gate. This can be carried on to 4, 5, 6 and more inputs. Practical limits are the perfectability of the transistor gates as switches and the reduction of their base-emitter resistance. Logic gates with 1, 2, 3, 4,

6, and 8 inputs are commonly available. In the actual construction of logic gates, special solid-state devices, such as transistors with multiple emitters, are frequently used instead of individual components for each input.

While the logic gates are truly composed of resistor and transistor circuits, the drawings of these circuits are time-consuming and, as can be seen in the case of the EXCLUSIVE OR gate, frequently confusing, due to the large number of components. To circumvent these problems, electronic symbols for these gates have been created. Figure 8-12 shows these symbols, which will be used consistently in this text to simplify the circuit drawings. These symbols have several characteristics worth noting. The AND symbols have a flat input side while the OR components have a curved input side. The negated gates have a small circle just before the output line. This circle always means negation of the value present up to that point and can appear on inputs as well as outputs, although none does in Figure 8-12. An AND gate with two inverting inputs is the same as a NOR gate because $\bar{A} \cdot \bar{B} = \overline{A + B}$ by DeMorgan's theorum. Note that any negating gate can be used as an invertor by tying all its inputs together.

Having created gates that can do logic, it is worthwhile building a few circuits with them to see how they work. One problem that we might use these circuits to solve is when to launch a moon rocket. For the rocket to take off, all systems must be GO. The decision to launch is based on a large AND gate network where all positive factors must be at logic **1** while all negative factors must be **0** (negated on input). (See Fig. 8-13.)

On the other hand, let us suppose that we want to get $1000.00 out of a safe. We can do this if the safe is open (A) OR if we have the combination (B) AND if there is at least $1000.00 in the safe ($C$). The circuit for this decision is also shown in Figure 8-13. Large numbers of conditions can be arranged in these networks to produce positive outputs only when the appropriate combination of events has occurred.

In an effort to gain clarity, it is frequently necessary to reduce the interaction of the variables to the simplest terms. To accomplish this, first a logical reduction of the expression is made, and then the gates are laid out. At other times only a specified gate can be used for circuit construction. This happens because components come in packages of a number of gates, and there is not always room on the circuit board to have packages of each kind of gate available. When this happens, most frequently it is the NAND gate which is used as the basic building component. The following example shows these design considerations at work.

EXAMPLE 8-10

Using only 3-input NAND gates, construct a circuit that will produce the following logical expression: $\bar{A} \cdot (B + \bar{C} + \bar{B} \cdot D) + C \cdot (\bar{A} + B \cdot D)$.

Solution: First reduce the problem to its simplest representation.

Eliminate parentheses

$$\bar{A} \cdot B + \bar{A} \cdot \bar{C} + \bar{A} \cdot \bar{B} \cdot D + C \cdot \bar{A} + C \cdot B \cdot D$$

By commutativity

$$\bar{A} \cdot \bar{C} + C \cdot \bar{A} + \bar{A} \cdot B + \bar{A} \cdot \bar{B} \cdot D + B \cdot C \cdot D$$

By commutativity

$$\bar{A} \cdot \bar{C} + \bar{A} \cdot C + \bar{A} \cdot B + \bar{A} \cdot \bar{B} \cdot D + B \cdot C \cdot D$$

By associativity

$$\bar{A} \cdot (\bar{C} + C) + \bar{A} \cdot B + \bar{A} \cdot \bar{B} \cdot D + B \cdot C \cdot D$$

$\bar{C} + C = \mathbf{1}$

$$\bar{A} \cdot \mathbf{1} + \bar{A} \cdot B + \bar{A} \cdot \bar{B} \cdot D + B \cdot C \cdot D$$

$\bar{A} \cdot \mathbf{1} = \bar{A}$

$$\bar{A} + \bar{A} \cdot B + \bar{A} \cdot \bar{B} \cdot D + B \cdot C \cdot D$$

By absorbtion with $\bar{A}$

$$\bar{A} + \bar{A} \cdot \bar{B} \cdot D + B \cdot C \cdot D$$

By absorbtion with $\bar{A}$

$$\bar{A} + B \cdot C \cdot D$$

Now put everything into NAND format.

$$B \cdot C \cdot D = \overline{\overline{B \cdot C \cdot D}}$$

$$\bar{A} + \overline{\overline{B \cdot C \cdot D}}$$

By DeMorgan

$$\overline{A \cdot \overline{B \cdot C \cdot D}}$$

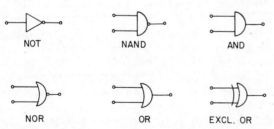

NOT   NAND   AND

NOR   OR   EXCL. OR

Figure 8-12 Symbols representing the logic gates.

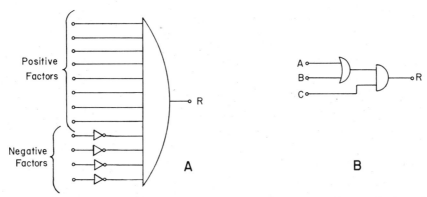

Figure 8-13 The use of logic gates to make decisions is illustrated by a rocket launch circuit (A) and a money retrieval circuit (B).

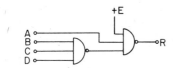

Figure 8-14 Solution to Example 8-10.

This is now drawn as a 3-input NAND gate representation in Figure 8-14. Note that unused inputs for AND function gates are tied up (to positive voltage) and for OR function gates are tied down (grounded).

Section 8-6
FLIP-FLOPS

All the digital circuitry discussed so far is based on the flow of the signal. The voltage, current, and so on, are assumed to be continuously varying. It is clear that there are many instances when we do not want this to be the case. We want to hold a value from a specific instant for an arbitrary length of time. To do this, we need a device that will not allow the value to escape, but will hold it captive until told to replace it.

A device that will enable us to hold data is shown in Figure 8-15. This device is a pair of NAND gates connected in a strange fashion. Such an arrangement is called "cross-coupled." Let us examine how this circuit works. In Figure 8-15A, we assume

that inputs A and B are high. We further assume that point C is high. If this is true, then both inputs to NAND gate 1 are high, and the output of NAND gate 1 is going to be low. This low not only appears at output 1, it also is applied to point D. Since one input of NAND gate 2 is low, then the output will be high. This means that output 2 is high and that point C will also be high. Because this was also one of the assumptions, everything is stable.

Now let us apply a low to input A. This means that one input of NAND gate 1 is low and the output 1 will be high. This will cause point D to be high. Since NAND gate 2 now has both of its inputs high, its output will be low. This will make point C low, as can be seen in Figure 8-15B. If input A now returns to high, the outputs of the cross-coupled NAND gates will remain the same because the low value at point C will keep the output of NAND gate 1 turned on.

What we have observed is the cross-coupled NAND gates flipping from one logical configuration to the other. Having changed states, they will remain in the new state even when the stimulus for the change has gone away. It will not change again until a stimulus appears on the other input. Because a cross-coupled NAND gate pair can flip back and forth between two states, it is called a flip-flop. The essence of a flip-flop is that it will hold information until appropriately pulsed.

The flip-flop is clearly a binary device since it only has two states, ON and OFF or HIGH and LOW. Note that both the value of the flip-flop (out-

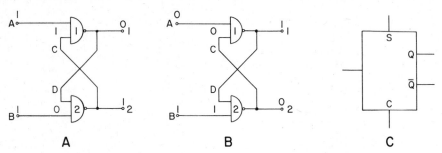

A   **B**   **C**

Figure 8-15 The cross-coupled NAND gates in a stable state (A) and as they would respond to a SET input (B). The electrical symbol is shown in Part C.

put 1) and the negation or opposite of the value (output 2) are available from the way that the flip-flop was created. In fact, the two halves of the flip-flop are identical. Which is the value and which is the negation are a matter of convention. The value is called Q and its negation Q̄. Flip-flops have numerous uses, but a common one is to keep on the indicator lights on a panel. The light bulb is driven from the Q output of a flip-flop. It is off until the flip-flop is pulsed. It then stays on, even though the set pulse leaves, until a clear pulse resets the flip-flop to off.

The two inputs to the flip-flop in Figure 8-15 have distinct names. The input A is called the SET because the flip-flop's output Q is set to 1 when A is made 0. The input B is called the RESET or CLEAR because the output Q is reset to 0 when this input is made 0. The flip-flop is called a SET–RESET flip-flop or an R–S flip-flop because of this property. Note that the inactive state of the input is 1, and the signal is a 0 state or pulse. If both inputs are grounded, the flip-flop will oscillate as both outputs are driven high and will not stabilize until one input is removed from ground. Figure 8-15C shows the electrical symbol for an R–S flip-flop.

The R–S flip-flop is not the only one available. There are at least several others that are worth looking at briefly. The D flip-flop has all the inputs and outputs of the R–S flip-flop plus two more. One new input is the data input, where the data enter the flip-flop. The second is a clock or trigger input. When the trigger input is 0, the data input is logically disconnected from the cross-coupled NAND gates that hold their previous value. When the trig-

ger pulse rises, the data (a 0 or 1) is forced into the flip-flop. The internal logic of this flip-flop is shown in Figure 8-16, and the reader should work through the procedure of loading data into the flip-flop. This type of flip-flop can be used to sample and hold the data of a rapidly fluctuating signal so that a number can be displayed in an instrument's readout register. Without this, the number might flicker back and forth so rapidly that the eye would see only a blur of light.

Another useful flip-flop is the toggle flip-flop. Unlike the D flip-flop, the toggle flip-flop has only one extra input, which is the CLOCK or TOGGLE (T). Everytime that the T input goes from the 1 to 0 state, the values of Q and Q̄ are interchanged. As can be seen in Figure 8-17, this means that there is one pulse generated at the output for each two pulses at the input. The NAND gate representation of this flip-flop has a mysterious block in it. This box is responsible for generating a very sharp pulse to cross-coupled NAND gates on the falling edge of

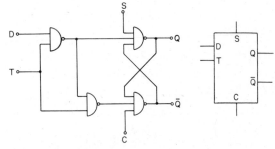

Figure 8-16 The data (D) flip-flop.

the input so that the state of the flip-flop is reversed. This box contains a number of logic gates and transistors of the type already seen, but these are not shown to reduce the complexity of the circuit. All the important signals are shown in Figure 8-17. A modification of the toggle flip-flop called a J-K flip-flop allows special conditions to be placed on the toggling function.

The ultimate in flip-flops is the master–slave concept. In these flip-flops the outputs of the master flip-flop are not accessible to the user. Instead the user sees only the slave outputs. Under normal conditions the master and slave are disconnected. This enables the master flip-flop to set up and stabilize while the slave holds the previous value. The value of the master is then transferred to the slave via two NAND gates which can be activated by a short clock pulse.

The input conventions for flip-flops are reasonably standard. The SET (S) and CLEAR (RESET) (C) inputs must be high when not active and can be activated by a short pulse. The TOGGLE, CLOCK, or TRIGGER (T) input is normally low. Some flip-flops trigger when the pulse is going high, but most do not react until the high-to-low transition occurs. This is called negative edge triggering. The DATA (D) input can be either level depending on the data.

The use of flip-flops and other binary state storage devices (such as magnetic cores, circulating charges, and magnetic bubbles) make possible digital calculations and control. Most of digital processing consists of making or changing the values of these binary state devices. It is even possible to have various patterns of information stored in flip-flops that can be used to instruct an instrument what to do. This permits the internal programming of laboratory instruments, allowing them to perform complex sequences of tasks without human intervention. The use of flip-flops also forces us into the binary number system discussed previously. A series of flip-flops can act as the digits in a binary number. It is on numbers of this form that computations are done.

In addition to the flip-flop, there are many other devices which can be constructed from simple NAND gates or other logic gates. Figure 8-18 shows three that are useful in laboratory instrumentation. The first one is a spike generator. When the input is low, the output is low. When the input rises the output rises very briefly, but then falls after a short interval (approximately 20 nsec) because the cross-coupled NAND gates change state. Another spike will not occur until the next positive input occurs. The reader should work through the sequence of events as the input goes from 0 to 1 to 0. A circuit of this type might appear in the undefined box in the toggle flip-flop in Figure 8-17.

Figure 8-18B shows a multiplexer. The function of a multiplexer is to allow multiple inputs of the same type to be brought alternately to the same output. An example of the use of a multiplexer is any multichannel laboratory instrument. The information from each channel must in turn be brought

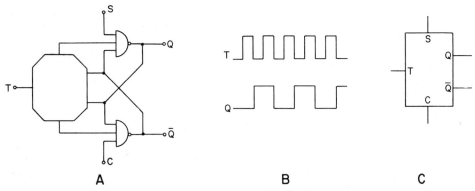

A   B   C

Figure 8-17 The toggle flip-flop.

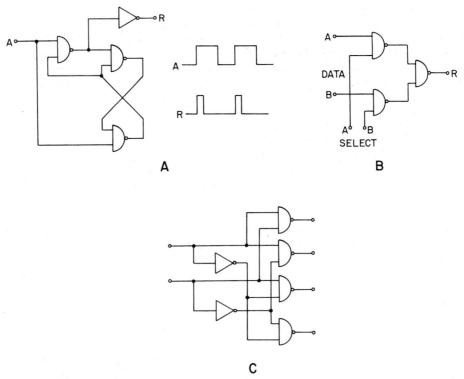

Figure 8-18 Part A is a spike generator with the associated timing diagram. Part B is a multiplexer. Part C is a 2-to-4 binary decoder.

to the printer to be output for the user, because although laboratory instruments may have many analytical channels, they usually have only one printer or display to serve them all. A considerable cost savings results from channeling together the various signals as early as possible to prevent having to duplicate electronics for each channel. Figure 8-18 shows that data, in the form of 0's or 1's, are always being applied to the data inputs of the multiplexer. The select inputs are normally low. This means that the outputs of the first NAND gates are normally high. All high inputs into the concentrator (multiplexing) NAND gate means a constant zero output. When one of the select lines is made high, the data from that data line begins to get through the first NAND gate, but the value is inverted in polarity by the gate. When it reaches the concentrator gate it can again get through (all the

other inputs are high), but it is again inverted. This means that the input has been inverted twice and appears at the output identical to the way it entered. The data which appears at the output will be whatever data is on the input of the NAND gate whose select line is high. Obviously, only one select line can be raised at a time or garbage results. Any number of input NAND gates may be tied into a concentrator NAND gate.

While the multiplexer allows the busing of data (different data traveling on the same wire) on output to the computation circuitry, it is also desirable to save cost on the transmission of control signals. This is accomplished by coding the select signals for channels of the instruments in binary. Each control point monitors a common cable (or bus) and responds to only those signals meant for it. The circuit allowing a device to identify the signal in-

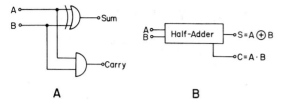

Figure 8-19 The half-adder circuit and symbol.

tended for it is a binary decoder, as shown in Figure 8-18C. If, for example, the input was $B = 1$ and $A = 0$, then all the output lines, except 2, would be high (not selected). Change the patterns to $B = 0$ and $A = 1$, and line 1 is selected. These decoders can be made more complex by the inclusion of additional binary positions. In addition to the 2-to-4 decoder shown, 4-to-16 and 6-to-64 are heavily used in instruments.

While previously discussed digital circuits would allow one to build the control electronics for numerous applications, a large application yet untouched is digital arithmetic. While it is not necessary to go into the complex calculating circuitry of a large computer, it is perhaps well if we look at just one arithmetic operation. Figure 8-19A shows the circuitry necessary to add two binary digits together. This circuit involves two distinct parts. The first is the formation of the sum bit. Here we discover a use for the EXCLUSIVE OR. If both the inputs are not high, then the result of the simple OR is correct. If both are high, the summing operation must generate a carry and set the sum for the current position to 0. Therefore, SUM $= A \oplus B$. The carry bit is only set if both inputs are true, so CARRY $= A \cdot B$.

Addition, however, is not so simple. We have added one bit of two potentially multibit numbers. To add the rest of the bits will mean that we have

carries that may propagate. We must, therefore, add in the carry at each stage as well as the two numbers. This requires a two-step process. What we really have in Figure 8-19A is not an adder, but a half-adder. It does only half the summing job. To do the whole addition at any position except the least significant, we need two half-adders and an OR gate, as shown in Figure 8-20. The sum of the two data bits is added to the carry from the previous bit to get the final sum for that bit position. The carries from the two half-adders are ORed together to get the final carry for that bit position. This latter operation is quite safe because both half-adders cannot generate a carry simultaneously, as will be obvious with a little thought of how the addition process works. This device is a sequential adder, which adds from right to left until all the bit positions are completed. This procedure is very slow and has been replaced for multibit numbers with more complex circuitry which does the addition asynchronously. Subtraction can be accomplished by inverting the subtrahend and adding. Multiplication and division are more complicated, but can be accomplished with the same basic logic gates that we have already seen.

Section **8-7**
COUNTERS

Since the goal we are striving for is the representation of analog data as digital numbers, it would be well for us to look at how flip-flops are used to contain, manipulate, and move numbers. It is, after all, flip-flops that will hold our data before output. We have already mentioned the use of flip-flops to keep panel lights on and to hold numbers. Let us now look at a grouping of flip-flops called a register. A register is defined as an ordered group of flip-flops having the same general purpose. If we have a group of equipment error status flags, for example, we could call them a register. A register may or may not have interconnected flip-flops. Since the case of the nonconnected register is just an ordered 1 by N array of R-S flip-flops, it is not very interesting, and we will not investigate it further.

Figure 8-21A shows one simple connection that can exist between adjacent flip-flops. In this case

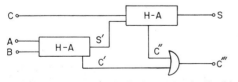

Figure 8-20 A full adder built from two half-adders and an OR gate.

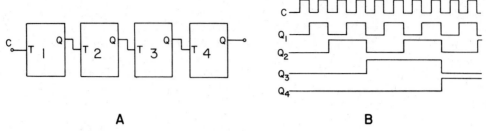

A **B**

Figure 8-21 An up-counter with a timing diagram showing clock division.

the Q output of one flip-flop is attached to the toggle input of the next toggle flip-flop. Let us assume that all the flip-flops are initially zero. When the input to the first flip-flop moves up and down once, the first flip-flop (Q output) will become 1. When it repeats the process, the first flip-flop will return to zero. This action by the first flip-flop will cause the toggle on the second flip-flop to see a rise and fall, and this flip-flop will now become a 1. A third pulse will set flip-flop 1 (FF1). A fourth pulse will clear FF1, which will clear FF2, which will set FF3. If we consider FF1 to be the 1's place, FF2 to be the 2's place, FF3 to be the 4's place, FF4 to be the 8s place, and so on, then what we are doing is counting up (1, 10, 11, 100, and so forth). We have created a binary counter which can be used to count events, such as nuclear disintegrations with a Geiger counter. However, we have considerably more than this. Figure 8-21B shows the output at each of the Q's as the pulses enter the register. The pulses at Q_1 are only half as numerous as those entering at T_1. The pulses at Q_2 are one-half as numerous as those at Q_1 and only one-fourth as numerous as those at T_1. If the input signal is some sort of high-frequency clock, this register is reducing the frequency of the clock in a precise fashion. A very accurately known clock, such as a crystal oscillator or the ac wall frequency, can be reduced in frequency so that it can be used to time reagent addition, wash and transfer cycles, and incubation periods automatically. The clock frequency can be divided by any multiple of two just by picking the output of the correct flip-flop. This is similar to gears reducing the speed of a motor.

The versatility of this general arrangement is tremendous. It is used for a vast variety of time and counting operations. It can be extended by making the counter able to go down as well as up. Making a counter go down is accomplished by using the $\bar{Q}$, instead of the Q to link with the toggle of the next flip-flop. Figure 8-22A shows the design of an up–

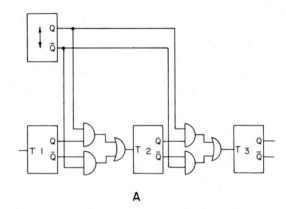

A

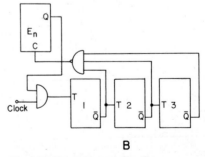

B

Figure 8-22 Part A shows an up-down counter with the direction controlled by another flip-flop. Part B shows a down-counter that will stop by disabling a clock-enable flip-flop when zero is reached.

down counter controlled by a directional flip-flop. If this flip-flop is set, the Q outputs are logically connected to the next toggle inputs, while if it is clear, the $\bar{Q}$ outputs are logically connected to the next toggle inputs. The up–down counter can count up for events, down for delay periods or change direction in integration sequences (see next section). Using J–K flip-flops allows this design to be simplified. Figure 8-22B shows how a counter can be stopped. When all the flip-flops are 0, the NAND of all the $\bar{Q}$ will be zero and the flip-flop that controls the counting (input of the clock signal) will be cleared. These types of modifications enable complex counters with many capabilities to be built.

The holding of data for a period of time is called data latching. A typical data latch is shown in Figure 8-23. The CLEAR line is used to remove the old data from the latch. The load data line is then pulsed to load the data at the data inputs. There are several things worth noting. The CLEAR pulse is a brief low. The load pulse is a brief high which causes data bits that are 1's to create 0 pulses as they go through the NAND gates. The 0's generate SETS of the corresponding flip-flops. This whole operation is done so quickly that devices responding to latch outputs see only the change from the old data to the new data.

Another common register activity is shifting. In a shift register, such as shown in Figure 8-24, the data are moved from a bit position to the one directly to its right or left. Naturally all the bits must be transferred at one time. The shift register in Fig-

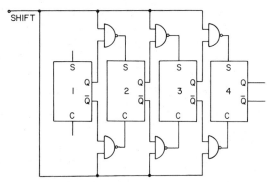

Figure 8-24 A simplified shift registor. Shifting is accomplished by a very short high pulse.

ure 8-24 is somewhat idealized. Unless the transfer pulse is very short and the internal timing of the flip-flops is perfect, the shift will not stop at one position. To prevent the continued propagation of the shift, a master–slave flip-flop is normally used. The master in each flip-flop sets up correctly and breaks contact with the previous slave before giving its own slave the new value. Shift registers are used in counting and in isolating parts of a data register.

One common use of a shift register is the propagation of ASCII. ASCII was introduced as a way of representing individual digits, alphabet letters, and punctuation within an instrument. For the instrument to get the appropriate letters and numbers printed, it must transmit them to the printer. It accomplishes this by loading them into a data latch called a *u*niversal *a*synchronous *r*eceiver–*t*ransmitter (UART). Although complex in internal design, a UART functions much as a shift register. It shifts one position to the right with every clock pulse. The output of the right-most bit is attached to the wire connected to the printer. When this bit is a zero, the printer sees a ground level; when it is 1, the printer sees a high level. As a result, the printer gets a series of high and low signals, as shown in Figure 8-25. The printer has its own UART which has its most significant bit attached to the connecting wire. It shifts to the right at the same rate as the instrument's UART and therefore shifts in the pattern of highs and lows coming over the line. When a complete digit or letter has been obtained, it is

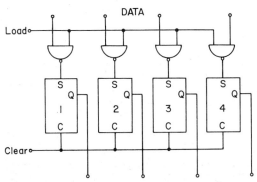

Figure 8-23 A data latch. A clear pulse (short low) is followed by a load pulse (short high).

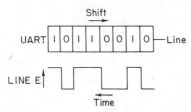

Figure 8-25 The UART will shift its contents to the right, creating the signal shown on the line.

transferred to the hammer driver and the character is printed. Information typed into an instrument follows the same procedure in the other direction. Common transmission speeds are 30, 120, 240, and 480 characters per second. These rates are commonly expressed as 300, 1,200, 2,400, and 4,800 baud (bits per second) because each character usually consists of 10 bits when control bits are counted.

Section **8-8**
ANALOG-TO-DIGITAL CONVERTORS

In previous chapters we have examined how to handle analog signals that have come from the measuring process. In this chapter we have looked at how the digital signals are manipulated to produce a final result that can be displayed or printed. One part of the process is still missing, however: the conversion of the analog signal to a digital signal.

The first important problem we will face in the conversion is how much the least significant binary digit is worth in terms of analog voltage, current, and so forth. This value is called the significance, for which there are several constraints. First, it is desirable to have the least significant bit correspond to some power of 10 of a recognized unit in which the answer is defined (e.g., millimoles, thousands of disintegrations per second, millions of particles per liter). Second, the stability of the analog signal will control the usefulness of the bit size. With a very stable signal, the bit size can be quite small and still have meaning. With a noisy signal, the last bits will change continuously if they represent a very small value and will not be able to be

read reliably. Finally, the speed necessary for the conversion may limit the number of bits, and therefore their relative size, because with certain techniques, as will be seen shortly, the conversion time is a function of the magnitude of the result.

The first general class of analog-to-digital convertors (ADC) that we will examine contains those that do quantum counting. The basic principle is that they count from zero, adding small voltage increments (called quanta), until they reach the desired value. The most common ADC of this type is the ramp ADC, shown in Figure 8-26. Although the circuit has numerous elements, it is relatively simple in operation. When a zero is applied to the start input, the RUN flip-flop is set and a spike is generated by a circuit (Fig. 8-18A) that clears the counter. Setting of the RUN flip-flop causes the clock pulses to be gated through into the counter (an up-counter). It also causes R_A to close and R_B to open. The operational amplifier I (OAI) is just an integrator of a constant current. As time passes, the output of OAI rises at a constant rate (Fig. 8-27). The output of OAI is fed into the noninverting input of OAC, called a comparitor because it compares the value of two signals. The analog voltage to be

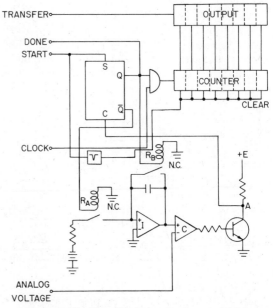

Figure 8-26 Simplified circuit of a ramp ADC.

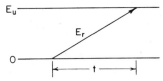

Figure 8-27 The measurement principle of a ramp ADC ($E_u = E_r t$).

converted is fed into the inverting input of OAC. At first, E_+ is 0 and OAC merely amplifies the voltage at E_- which, with no feedback, will drive the amplifier to limit in the negative direction. This gives a low signal to the base of the n-p-n transistor.

The transistor is off, point A is high, and the integration proceeds. When the value at E_+ rises to the level of E_-, the output of OAC jumps from the negative limit to zero and quickly on to the positive limit as E_+ rises. This causes the transistor to conduct, point A to drop to ground and the RUN flip-flop to be cleared. At this point the value in the counter is the digital equivalent of the analog voltage. The unknown voltage is just the rate of the voltage rise in volts per time (E_r) times the time (t) that the voltage ramp ran (Eq. 6-54):

$$E_u = \frac{E_s t}{RC} = E_r t \qquad (8\text{-}4)$$

The digital equivalent of the output voltage is then moved by a transfer pulse to a data latch for later use. Note that in real ADC, transistors would probably be used in place of relays to short the integrator and control the integrator input in order to improve the response time and reproducibility.

The ramp ADC is a very straightforward approach. It is basically easy to understand and implement, and the voltage is a simple function of one component. It has, however, two significant disadvantages. The first is stability. The comparator must have a high common mode rejection ratio for accurate work. The integrator circuitry and its voltage input must also be very stable or the size of a bit will vary with time. Second, the ramp ADC is very slow for large numbers because the counter must always run all the way from 0 up to the output value. The conversion rate is highly dependent on the magnitude of the data. The accuracy of the ramp ADC is 0.1–1%.

To eliminate the first, but not the second, difficulty of a ramp ADC, the dual-slope ADC was developed. The circuitry for this is shown in Figure 8-28. When the ADC is started, a value that is the negative of a fixed time t for which the integrator will integrate the unknown voltage is transferred to the counter. The counter will spend the first part of the operation counting from $-t_u$ up to 0. The $-t_u$ is usually permanently set either in a latch or by making the appropriate pattern of 0's and 1's hardwired to power and ground. When the RUN flip-flop is set, so is a DIRECTION flip-flop, causing the input to the integrator to be attached to the unknown analog voltage. The noninverting lead of the comparator is tied to ground to remove the common mode as a factor in the output. As a result, the integrator generates an increasingly negative voltage, driving the comparitor to the negative limit. When the counter reaches 0, an OR gate with inputs from each of the bits of the counter produces a zero, thereby clearing the DIRECTION flip-flop and causing the integrator input to switch to a reference voltage of opposite polarity. The counter continues to count upward, but the negative voltage on the integrator is now being reduced (Fig. 8-29). When it passes through zero, the comparitor will swing from the negative to the positive limit, the transistor will begin to conduct and the RUN flip-flop will be cleared, stopping the integration. The value of t can then be transferred to a data latch for further manipulation.

The calculations of the unknown analog voltage can be made readily from the data obtained above. The final voltage for both parts of its integration must be the same because of the way we set up the device. If we set these voltages equal and substitute from Eq. 6-54, we get the final voltage in terms of only the standard voltage (E_s), the fixed integration time for the unknown (t_u),

$$E_1 = E_2 \qquad (8\text{-}5)$$

$$\frac{E_u t_u}{RC} = \frac{E_s t_s}{RC}$$

$$E_u = \frac{t_s}{t_u} E_s \qquad (8\text{-}6)$$

and the variable integration time for the standard voltage (t_s). It is independent of the integrator pa-

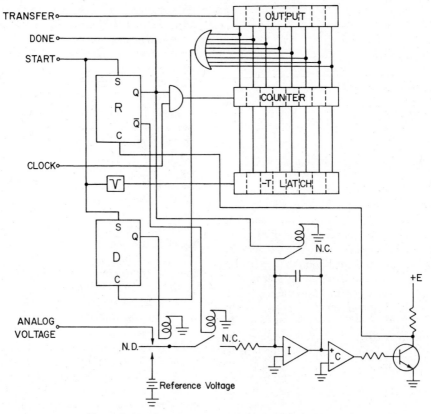

Figure 8-28   Simplified circuit of a dual-slope ADC.

rameters (R and C), as well as the common mode rejection ratio of the comparator. Since E_s and t_u are known quantities, they can be calculated beforehand to give the final equation a form similar to that shown in Eq. 8-4. It must be noted that the dual-slope ADC is even slower than the ramp ADC. Since it is more stable, however, there are times when the dual-slope ADC is preferred to other types of ADC. It is used extensively in digital panel meters and multimeters.

The second major class of ADC is called the "digital servo." The basic principle behind all these ADCs is the fact that the counter is converted from digital to analog to compare with the unknown voltage. Therefore, a part of every digital servo ADC is a *d*igital-to-*a*nalog *c*onverter (DAC). It is

necessary to investigate this device before we can proceed.

A rudimentary DAC is shown in Figure 8-30. While very simple, it illustrates the basic principles. A set of parallel resistors runs between a voltage line and the inverting input of an operational amplifier. Each branch of the circuit is controlled by a transistor (or other switch) driven from the

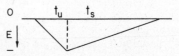

Figure 8-29   The measurement principle of a dual slope ADC. $E_u = (t_s/t_u)E_s$.

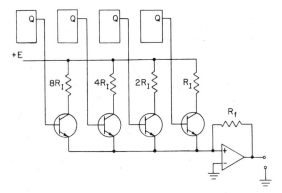

Figure 8-30 The circuit of a simple DAC.

digital register of the DAC. The flip-flops that are on cause the corresponding branches of the circuits to conduct. The resistors are arranged such that the resistance of each is twice as great as that of the previous more significant bit. Since the voltage is constant, the current in each branch is half as great as the previously more significant branch. Because all this current is coming into the summing point, it is added and passes through the feedback resistor, thereby causing an *IR* drop and creating the output voltage. The final voltage is therefore

$$E_o = R_f \Sigma I_i \qquad (8\text{-}7)$$

$$E_o = -R_f \Sigma \alpha_i \frac{E}{2^i R_I} \qquad (8\text{-}8)$$

Since E/R_I is constant

$$E_o = -\left(\frac{R_f}{R_I}\right) E \Sigma \frac{\alpha_i}{2^i}$$

$$= -E \frac{R_f}{R_I} \left(\frac{\alpha_0}{2^0} + \frac{\alpha_1}{2^1} + \frac{\alpha_2}{2^2} + \frac{\alpha_3}{2^3} + \cdots \right) \qquad (8\text{-}9)$$

$$E_o = -E \frac{R_f}{R_I} \left(\alpha_0 + \frac{\alpha_1}{2} + \frac{\alpha_2}{4} + \frac{\alpha_3}{8} + \cdots \right) \qquad (8\text{-}10)$$

The quantity α_i is 0 if the corresponding bit of the digital word is 0 and 1, if it is 1. This allows the production of an analog voltage that exactly represents the binary number in which α_0 is the most significant bit. It is imperative that the resistor values, particularly of the small resistors, be ex-

tremely accurate, or we cannot go from Eq. 8-8 to 8-9. In such a case, the conversion between digital and analog will be nonlinear and therefore inaccurate. The voltage drop over the transistor or other switching device must also be considered in the design to get the correct analog voltage for each digital number.

The digital servo concept can be used to create an ADC similar to the ramp ADC. This is called the staircase ADC. A circuit diagram and the principles of operation are shown in Figure 8-31. At the start, the RUN flip-flop is set and the counter cleared. The clock then causes the counter to start counting up. The DAC present in the instrument converts the count into the corresponding voltage which is fed into a comparator along with the unknown analog voltage. When the voltage of the DAC exceeds the voltage of the unknown input, the polarity of the comparator input changes and the RUN flip-flop is cleared. The value in the counter is the digital equivalent of the unknown voltage. This value can be transferred to a data latch and thereafter manipulated in subsequent circuitry.

The staircase ADC has many similarities to the ramp ADC. It suffers from the same slowness in reaching an answer and the common mode rejection problem. In place of the drift of the integrator, one has the drift of the DAC. All of this might tend to discourage the usage of the staircase ADC were it not for a feature inherent in the staircase ADC, which the ramp ADC cannot possess. The only way the circuitry of a ramp ADC knows what the unknown voltage is that is being fed into the comparitor is by the time that it has been counting. This limits the ramp ADC to unidirectional movement, always up toward the voltage. In a staircase ADC, the value of the standard voltage that is being fed into the comparator is always equal to the value in the counter, no matter how the value in the counter is obtained. Let us add to the circuit in Figure 8-31 a flip-flop that controls the direction of the counter, which must now be an up–down counter. Let us rewire the feedback from the output of the comparator so that it reverses the polarity of the DIRECTION flip-flop. When the ADC is started, it will count up to the unknown voltage. When that voltage is reached and surpassed by the counter, the

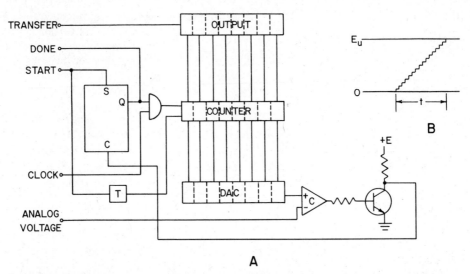

Figure 8-31   Part A shows a simple staircase ADC. Part B shows the principle on which it works. More complex models allow the signal to be tracked by counting both up and down once the initial value is found.

output of the comparator will change sign. Instead of stopping the counter, as in the previous case, it will merely reverse its direction, causing it to count downward. If the voltage is constant, this counting down will not last long, because the next clock pulse will cause the counter to fall below the unknown voltage. This will again cause the output of the comparator to reverse the polarity and to switch the DIRECTION flip-flop to the counting-up position. With such a stable voltage level, the ADC will oscillate back and forth from one count above to one count below the true voltage level. If, however, the input voltage varies, the staircase ADC will track the changing voltage, and the value in the counter will always reflect the input without having to restart the integration each time. This makes the staircase ADC much faster at finding the digital equivalent of the input than any of the previous ADCs once it has caught up with the signal initially. The human observer, however, cannot possibly follow the rapid changes of the ADC. As a consequence, the value of the counter is transferred to the data latch that controlled the display only a few times per second by appropriate pulsing of the

transfer line. This then adds more flexibility to ADC performance than previously seen.

The final type of ADC which we will examine uses the same general hardware as the staircase ADC. The difference is that the incrementation circuitry is much more complicated. Instead of counting up by adding one to the least significant bit, the first clock pulse sets the most significant bit to 1. If this produces a voltage on the DAC which is smaller than the unknown voltage, nothing further happens. If the voltage from the DAC is greater than the unknown voltage, the bit just set is cleared. At the next clock pulse, the next most significant bit is set and the process repeated. If there are n bits, it takes n clock pulses to set all the bits to their correct value. Figure 8-32 shows how the process zeros in on the correct value by successive approximation, which is what this ADC is called. A successive approximation ADC will always converge to the correct value in the same amount of time, regardless of the size of the input, providing that it is within range. The number 1750_8, for example, will require 1000_{10} clock pulses with a staircase ADC but only 10_{10} with a successive approximation

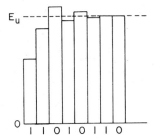

Figure 8-32 The successive approximation ADC closes in on an unknown voltage by halving the uncertainty with each step.

ADC. Because of the more complex circuitry in the latter, it is only of the order of 10 times as fast as the staircase ADC (10 versus 100 μsec). The successive approximation ADC solves the time of conversion problem, but does suffer from any instability in the DAC and from the common mode rejection limitation of the comparator.

All the ADCs discussed were presented as unipolar convertors (input voltage always has the same sign). This is usually adequate for biological systems since concentrations cannot be negative. The body cannot chemically be in debt. There are occasions, however, when a biochemical indicator, such as base excess in a blood gas calculation, can have a negative value. To handle this type of result, the ADC must be sensitive to the sign of the voltage and must either count down instead of up to get the digital voltage value or reverse the polarity of the input and later that of the result. The latter philosophy is more commonly used because of the way in which the standard voltage ramps and steps are generated. An ADC that can convert both positive and negative voltages is called a bipolar ADC convertor.

At this point, you should be able to follow the output signal for a chemical reaction all the way from where it is produced to where it is displayed or printed for a simple instrument. The control of instrumentation and the calculations used in many instruments, however, are so complicated that more extensive computing power is needed than is discussed here. As a result, we will examine a more powerful tool for digital calculation, the microprocessor, in Chapter 9.

REVIEW QUESTIONS

1. What is the difference between analog and digital electronics?
2. Why do people use digital numbers in preference to analog?
3. What are the problems related to measurement that one encounters when one uses a D'Arsonval meter?
4. How are digital numbers used in instrumental control?
5. Explain the switch notation XPYT.
6. What do N.O. and N.C. mean?
7. Draw a schematic for each of the following: SPST, SPDT, DPST, and DPDT.
8. Name several models of switches.
9. How does one prevent contact bounce?
10. What does "make-before-break" mean?
11. What do "circuit true" and "circuit false" mean?
12. Define how the following operators work: NOT, AND, OR, NAND, NOR, EXCLUSIVE OR.
13. Draw a schematic of an AND and an OR combination of switches.
14. What is the proper way to wire a two-way circuit?
15. What is a relay?
16. Explain how the two circuits of a relay work.
17. Draw a schematic of a NOT, NOR, NAND, and EXCLUSIVE OR.
18. What does the dashed line between switch parts mean?
19. What is a cam?
20. What is a gear?
21. What is a number system?
22. Why must a number system have a base and what is it?
23. Define decimal, octal, and binary.
24. What are the names of the positions in a decimal number?
25. What are the limiting restrictions on a base that is to be used for human computation?
26. Why was binary chosen for machine use?
27. Define bit.
28. What is the mathematical relationship between base two and base ten?

29. What are the two methods for converting between bases?
30. How are the mathematics done to convert from one base to another by each method?
31. Give the addition and multiplication tables for binary.
32. How are binary and octal interconverted?
33. Why is octal used?
34. What is binary coded decimal?
35. What is the principle of Gray code? The 2-out-of-5 code? ASCII?
36. What is parity and how is it implemented?
37. What are the symbols for the operators in question 12?
38. What is the effect of negation on a logical element? Double negation?
39. Define truth table.
40. What are the truth tables for the various operators in question 12?
41. How are truth tables constructed for more than two elements?
42. Define commutativity. Associativity. Distributiveness.
43. Why do DeMorgan's rules work?
44. How does absorbtion work?
45. Why are relays not used in digital logic in most laboratory instruments?
46. How does one construct the circuits for each of the logical operators in question 12 using n–p–n transistors?
47. How can more than 2-input gates be made?
48. What are the electrical symbols for the logic gates in question 12?
49. How is negation indicated in representing a logic gate?
50. What does one do with the extra inputs of an AND or OR gate?
51. Why is logical reduction performed *before* the circuit is laid out?
52. Define cross-coupled.
53. What is a flip-flop?
54. Explain in detail how a simple flip-flop changes state.
55. What is an R–S flip-flop and what are its inputs and outputs called?
56. How does one set and clear a flip-flop?
57. What is a D flip-flop and what are its inputs and outputs called?

58. When would a D flip-flop be used?
59. What is a toggle flip-flop? How does it work?
60. Why must the pulse generating the change of state in a toggle flip-flop be very short?
61. What is a master–slave flip-flop? How does it work?
62. What are the input conventions for signals into a flip-flop?
63. In what ways can flip-flops be used? Give examples.
64. How does a spike generator work?
65. How does a multiplexer work? When would it be used?
66. What is a binary decoder? How does it work?
67. What is a half-adder? How does it work?
68. How is a full adder made from a half-adder?
69. What is the drawback to synchronous addition?
70. Define register.
71. What is a counter? How does an up-counter work?
72. Give several uses of a counter.
73. What is the difference in circuitry between an up-counter and a down-counter?
74. What is a data latch, and how is it used?
75. What is a shift register?
76. What type of flip-flop is usually used in a shift register? Why?
77. What is a UART? How does it work?
78. What are some common transmission rates?
79. What is an analog-to-digital convertor?
80. How should the value of the least significant bit of an ADC be chosen?
81. What is quantum counting?
82. How does a ramp ADC work?
83. How is the counting in a quantum counting ADC terminated?
84. To what is the integrator voltage of a ramp ADC proportional?
85. What are the disadvantages of a ramp ADC?
86. How does the dual-slope ADC work?
87. On what principle is the dual-slope ADC based?
88. How do the digital servo ADCs differ from the quantum counting ADCs?
89. How does a DAC work?
90. Which resistors, the large or the small, cause the greatest error in a DAC?

91. How does a staircase ADC work?

92. Why is the staircase ADC more versatile than the ramp ADC?

93. How does the staircase ADC track a moving voltage?

94. How does a successive approximation ADC work?

95. What is the relative speed of a successive approximation ADC to other ADCs?

96. What is the difference between unipolar and bipolar ADCs?

97. How is the bipolar ADC usually implemented?

PROBLEMS

1. Design a three-way switch.

2. Design a circuit to switch three sections of electric train track between two transformers. Be sure not to short the transformers together.

3. Design an instrument which, once it has started, will fill a vat, stop the influx, and drain the vat.

4. Design a circuit to run a heating bath.

5. Design a device that, when it is turned on, will stay on for 12 seconds and then shut itself off.

6. Convert the following decimal numbers to binary.

a. 41	**d.** 1352
b. 214	**e.** 4721
c. 831	**f.** 12,530

7. Convert the following binary numbers to decimal.

a. 100110	**d.** 10001101100
b. 10111111	**e.** 111100111111
c. 1010000111	**f.** 100110100010000

8. Convert the following decimal numbers to octal.

a. 53	**d.** 1235
b. 310	**e.** 5107
c. 742	**f.** 11,188

9. Convert the following octal numbers to decimal.

a. 54	**d.** 2712
b. 245	**e.** 7471
c. 1127	**f.** 57,374

10. Convert the following octal numbers to binary.

a. 27	**d.** 1375
b. 135	**e.** 6734
c. 471	**f.** 25,710

11. Convert the following binary numbers to octal.

a. 11011	**d.** 1100010010
b. 1111000	**e.** 101110001100
c. 101000010	**f.** 11100001000001

12. Reduce the following logic expressions to simplest terms.

a. $A \cdot A + A \cdot \bar{B} + A \cdot B + B \cdot \bar{B} + A \cdot \bar{B} + \bar{B} \cdot \bar{B}$

b. $\bar{A} \cdot B + (\bar{A} + C) \cdot \bar{A} + B \cdot (C + \bar{B})$

c. $B \cdot (C + A) + (\bar{C} + B + \bar{A}) \cdot (C + B \cdot \bar{A}) \cdot B$

d. $A \cdot B + C \cdot (\bar{B} + A) + A \cdot (\bar{A} + A \cdot (\bar{B} + \bar{C})) + B \cdot C$

e. $\bar{A} \cdot (\bar{B} \cdot A) + (A \cdot \bar{B}) \cdot \bar{A} + \bar{A} \cdot \bar{B} \cdot (\bar{B} \cdot A) + \bar{A} \cdot \bar{A} \cdot B \cdot (\bar{B} + A) + \bar{B} \cdot A \cdot B$

f. $A \cdot A \cdot B + B \cdot D \cdot \bar{C} + \bar{D} \cdot (C + \bar{A})$

13. Using any logic gates, draw circuits for the following logic expressions.

a. $\overline{A \cdot B \cdot \overline{\overline{B \cdot \bar{C}}}}$

b. $(\bar{A} + \bar{B}) \cdot (\bar{A} \cdot \bar{B} + \bar{C})$

c. $(A + \bar{C}) \cdot B + \overline{(\overline{A \cdot B} + A) \cdot C}$

d. $(B \cdot C + \bar{A}) \cdot (B + \bar{C}) + \overline{A \cdot B} + A$

Table 8-10 Truth Tables

a.	A	B	C	R	b.	A	B	C	R	c.	A	B	C	R
	0	0	0	1		0	0	0	0		0	0	0	1
	0	0	1	1		0	0	1	0		0	0	1	1
	0	1	0	0		0	1	0	0		0	1	0	0
	0	1	1	0		0	1	1	1		0	1	1	1
	1	0	0	0		1	0	0	0		1	0	0	0
	1	0	1	1		1	0	1	1		1	0	1	1
	1	1	0	0		1	1	0	1		1	1	0	0
	1	1	1	0		1	1	1	1		1	1	1	0

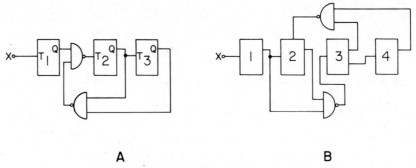

A   **B**

Figure 8-33 Two interesting counting circuits.

14. Draw a NAND gate network, using only 2-input NAND gates, which will satisfy each of the truth tables in Table 8-10.

15. Draw a NOR gate network, using only 2-input NOR gates, which will satisfy each of the truth tables in Table 8-10.

16. Design a counter that counts up to six and resets to zero using only toggle flip-flops, NAND gates, and an input clock.

17. Design a counter that will start counting up if all the flip-flops are zero but that will stop counting when seven is reached using only toggle flip-flops, NAND gates, and an input clock.

18. All the flip-flops in Figure 8-33A are initially zero. Give the value of each flip-flop after each of the first ten square waves input at point X. Remember that flip-flops change state on the trailing edge of pulses.

19. Solve Problem 18 for the circuit in Figure 8-33B.

20. In a dual-slope ADC, the known voltage is 2.893 V. If the unknown voltage is applied for 0.500 sec and the known voltage for 0.347 sec to reach a balance, what is the value of the unknown voltage?

21. In a dual-slope ADC, the known voltage is 0.872 V. If an unknown voltage of 1.086 V is applied for 0.649 sec, how long must the known voltage be applied to reach a balance?

CHAPTER 9
COMPUTER AND CONTROL

The intelligence controlling more and more laboratory procedures is coded into a computer, not supplied by a human operator. Because the computer can detect and compensate for instrumental drift more rapidly than can the human operator, it gives a more reproducible environment for the test to be performed and a more reliable result. In addition, computer-controlled analytical equipment can reduce repeats and downtime through early detection of sources of error. Since the computer, particularly in the form of the microprocessor, has become so important to clinical laboratory activity, it is necessary that we examine how it works and how it controls experiments.

Section 9-1
DATA REPRESENTATION

Before attempting to understand how a computer works, we must look at how a computer represents information. Some of the general concepts were presented in Chapter 8, but at this point we can get down to specific implementation of the concepts. There are several different items to be represented, and we will look at each in turn.

We must start with the concept of word length. A computer is composed of a large number of bits arranged in groups for easier reference. The basic unit of grouping is the "word." It contains a fixed number of bits, such as 12, 16, 32, or 48. Information is addressable by the word it is in. This word length is a basic property of a computer because all devices in the computer must accommodate word length. Devices that hold specific information, such as the location of the next instruction, are frequently called registers. Most registers have the same length as the word length of the computer. The terms "register" and "word" are sometimes used interchangeably.

The easiest item to visualize as the contents of a computer word is an unsigned binary number. Let us suppose that we have a 12-bit computer word that holds the number 100 011 110 111. Figure 9-1 shows the computer word as a series of boxes with bits being either on (1) or off (0). Any pattern of 1's and 0's in the 12 bits is permitted. Since there are 12 bits, there are 2^{12} bit patterns, ranging from 000 000 000 000 to 111 111 111 111. These bit patterns are hard to interpret at a glance, so the bits are frequently grouped by 3's and read as octal. The number in Figure 9-1 is 4367 in octal. Octal representation for a 12-bit machine is 0000 to 7777.

A second representation that can be applied to the pattern in Figure 9-1 is that of a signed number. Computers use the left-most bit to indicate if a number is positive (0) or negative (1). Positive integers are straightforward and translated as unsigned numbers. Negative integers require more work. To interpret a number with the left-most bit set, it is necessary to know whether the machine works in 1's complement or 2's complement arithmetic.

In the 1's complement, a negative number is the exact opposite of a positive number of the same magnitude. Each 1 is a 0, and each 0 is a 1. The number in Figure 9-1 when complemented is 3410. We then must attach a minus sign, and we say that 4367 in a 12-bit 1's complement computer is −3410. The 1's complement representation, however, leads to some unusual situations. If 0000 is zero, then 7777 (its complement) must be minus zero! By definition, −0 = 0, but having two quantities that mean the same thing can cause confusion. For ex-

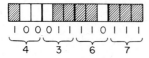

Figure 9-1 A computer word is a fixed number of bits that can have any pattern of 0's (blank) and 1's (shaded).

ample, let us add 50 to −50:

$$50_8 = 0050$$
$$-50_8 = 7727$$
$$\text{Answer} = 7777 = -0$$

Any number minus itself is −0, not 0. Obviously, this is not the way we learned mathematics, and the computer and programmers must be able to handle the situation. Another abnormality arises when adding a positive and negative number. For example, let us add 37 to −14:

$$37_8 = 0037$$
$$-14_8 = 7763$$
$$23_8 = 0022 \quad + \text{ a carry}$$

This is a pretty shocking result! Instead of the correct answer, 23, the computer gets 22 and a carry. To get the correct answer, the carry must be added into the least significant place.

$$\begin{array}{r} 0022 \\ +\quad 1 \\ \hline 0023 \end{array}$$

This process is called end-around carry and is essential to make 1's complement arithmetic work. The computer, of course, does this automatically, and the user never sees the problem.

The alternative to 1's complement arithmetic is 2's complement arithmetic. Here a negative number is interpreted to be the positive number subtracted from one more than the largest number that the computer can hold. Since a 12-bit machine can hold 7777, to translate the number in Figure 9-1, −1, we subtract it from 10000.

$$\begin{array}{r} 10000 \\ -\quad 4367 \\ \hline 3411 \end{array}$$

With this number, a negative sign is then associated, so that 4367 in a 12-bit 2's complement machine is −3411. Note that this is one less than in a 1's complement machine. This occurs because 7777 is now interpreted as −1, not −0, and each of the other negative numbers is shoved down one on the scale. The general means of finding the negative of a number is to complement the number and add one. For example, $4367 \Rightarrow 3410 + 1 = 3411$. If we do addition in this representation using the same numbers as before, we get

$$37_8 = 0037$$
$$-14_8 = 7764$$
$$23_8 = 0023 \quad + \text{ a carry}$$

In this case, the carry is discarded. If we now try to find the negative of 0, we find that $0000 \Rightarrow 7777 + 1 = 0000$ and a carry which is discarded. The negative of 0000 is 0000. Clearly both ways of representing negative numbers and doing arithmetic have their peculiarities. Both are used extensively in computers, and the one that is being used by a specific computer must be determined before the numeric representations can be interpreted.

Integer representation is extremely useful, but it lacks sufficient range to handle all the results that occur in a clinical laboratory. The largest unsigned number that can be represented in a single 12-bit word is 4,095 and in a single 16-bit word is 65,535. For signed numbers, the magnitude is cut in half. To increase the upper bound, two words can be used as one number, as shown in Figure 9-2. The sign bit (if a signed number) is the leftmost bit in the first word, and the second word acts as the continuation of the first and never has a sign bit. This representation is called double precision.

For a 12-bit machine, this means numbers up to 2^{24} ($\approx 1.68 \cdot 10^7$) unsigned and $\pm 2^{23}$ ($\approx \pm 8.4 \cdot 10^6$) signed can be represented. On a 16-bit machine, the values are $4.3 \cdot 10^8$ unsigned and $\pm 2.1 \cdot 10^8$ signed. Even greater precision can be gained by adding on a third word to give triple precision.

The types of numerical representation previously discussed include only integers where the decimal point is after the last bit. It is referred to as "fixed point" representation. Mixed numbers and decimal fractions cannot be handled by this convention. To

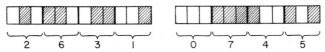

Figure 9-2 The double precision representation uses two words to hold one number, in this case, 26310745.

represent these numbers one must allow the decimal point to "float" to the appropriate position. It would be difficult to work with numbers with decimals at arbitrary positions, so an alternative has been developed. The number is split into an exponent (an integer power of 2) and a mantissa (binary representation of the value of the number). A number is converted to floating point by converting the whole number and fractional part of the number separately and joining them at the decimal, now a binary, point. The binary point is then moved left or right until it sits immediately to the left of the most significant bit. The exponent is incremented by 1 for each place to the left the binary point is moved and decremented by 1 for each place to the right. Since it is necessary to retain a sign bit, the binary point, for a normalized number, will always reside between the first and second bit from the left. Since the second bit of the word is the most significant bit, it must, by definition, be the opposite of the first bit or the number is not normalized as described above.

Figure 9-3 shows how floating point is implemented. On a computer with 12 or 16 bits, at least two words will be needed. The first word contains the exponent, which is just an integer that can be positive or negative. The second word has the sign

and the normalized mantissa. Additional words can be appended to make the floating point double or triple precision as needed. On machines with a long word length (32 or 48 bits), the exponent and mantissa may be in the same word in the single precision representation.

EXAMPLE 9-1

Convert 24.5 to binary floating point representation (assume 12 bits).

Solution: First convert 24 to binary:

$$8\overline{)24} \quad \dfrac{3}{} \quad R = 0$$

$$8\overline{)3} \quad \dfrac{0}{} \quad R = 3$$

Therefore, $24_{10} = 30_8 = 11000_2$.

To convert 0.5 decimal to binary, we must first transform it to octal. We can accomplish this by multiplying the decimal fraction by the new base in the old base notation to move the most significant digit into the units place and by then dividing it by the new base in the new base (shifting the decimal place) to restore it to the correct fractional value. In

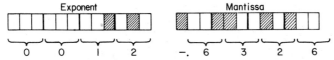

Figure 9-3 For a floating point number, the exponent is just a signed integer, which is a power of 2. The mantissa has a sign bit, followed by a binary point, followed by the number. To interpret, the octal digits must be grouped starting at the binary point and complemented if the sign is negative (as shown). There is one too few bits in the word, so the missing bit is assumed to be the same as the sign. The complete number is found by multiplying the mantissa by the exponent. The number shown is $-.11001101011 \cdot 2^{10} = -1100110101.1 = -1465.4_8 = -821.5_{10}$.

base 8, the places to the right of the octal point are 1/8, 1/64, and 1/512, respectively. By the process described, we change a cycle of 10 to a cycle of 8. For example, to convert 0.5 to octal we multiply by 8:

$$8 \times 0.5_{10} = 4.0$$

We then shift the octal point one place to the left.

$$4.0 \Rightarrow 0.4_8$$

Since the number to the left of the octal point is zero after the "4" is transferred to octal, no further steps are necessary. If the number were nonzero, as will be seen later, the above process is repeated with each new octal digit being placed to the right of the previous one:

$$0.5_{10} = 0.4_8 = 0.100_2$$

Summing the two parts and dropping trailing zeros gives

$$24.5_{10} = 30.4_8 = 11000.1_2$$

To make floating point, shift the binary point

$$11000.1_2 = 0.110001 \cdot 2^5$$

or

$$24.5_{10} = \text{mantissa } 0.11000100000 \quad \text{exponent } 101$$

or

$$M = 3040_8 \quad \text{and } E = 5_8 \qquad ■$$

EXAMPLE 9-2

Convert 1.00110110111 exponent 110 to decimal (assume 12 bits).

Solution: The reverse of the above process is necessary to convert to decimal. First note that the number is negative, because the sign bit is 1. We complement the mantissa (assuming 1's complement representation), but not the exponent:

$$M = -0.11001001000$$

$$E = 110$$

We next reposition the binary point to dispose of the exponent and drop trailing zero.

$$N_2 = -110010.01$$

Converting 110010 gives

$$110010_2 = 62_8 = 6 \cdot 8 + 2 = 50_{10}$$

Converting 0.01 gives

$$0.01_2 = 0.010_2 = 0.2_8 = \frac{2}{8} = 0.25_{10}$$

Combining gives us

$$-110010.01_2 = -62.2_8 = -50.25_{10} \qquad ■$$

EXAMPLE 9-3

Convert 0.000215 to binary floating point representation (assume 12 bits).

Solution: Convert the decimal to octal by successive multiplication by 8:

$$8 \times 0.000215 = 0.00172 \quad \text{Integer } 0 \quad N = 0.0$$

$$8 \times 0.00172 = 0.01376 \quad \text{Integer } 0 \quad N = 0.00$$

$$8 \times 0.01376 = 0.11008 \quad \text{Integer } 0 \quad N = 0.000$$

$$8 \times 0.11008 = 0.88064 \quad \text{Integer } 0 \quad N = 0.0000$$

$$8 \times 0.88064 = 7.04512 \quad \text{Integer } 7 \quad N = 0.00007$$

$$8 \times 0.04512 = 0.36096 \quad \text{Integer } 0 \quad N = 0.000070$$

$$8 \times 0.36096 = 2.88768 \quad \text{Integer } 2 \quad N = 0.0000702$$

$$8 \times 0.88768 = 7.10144 \quad \text{Integer } 7 \quad N = 0.00007027$$

At this point we can stop. Since we have only 12 bits to work with and the significant part of the number (7027) takes up all 12, any further digits would be later discarded. We round up if the decimal is more than one-half (it is not). To position the binary point correctly, we must convert to binary and move the point to the right.

$$0.00007027_8$$
$$= 0.000\ 000\ 000\ 000\ 111\ 000\ 010\ 111$$
$$= 0.111\ 000\ 010\ 111 \cdot 2^{-12}$$

We next retain 12 bits starting at the left. Since the bit we will drop is a 1, we must round the number up.

$$0.111\ 000\ 010\ 111 \leftarrow \text{dropped}$$
$$\underline{\qquad\qquad\qquad 1} \leftarrow \text{round}$$
$$0.111\ 000\ 011\ 00$$

The final result in 12-bit 1's complement notation is

$$mantissa = 0.11 \quad 100 \quad 001 \quad 100$$

$$exponent = 111 \quad 111 \quad 110 \quad 011$$

$$(M = 3414; \quad E = 7763) \quad \blacksquare$$

Conversions back and forth to floating point are indeed complex procedures for which programming or hardware exists. For the sake of brevity (and to preserve sanity) arithmetic with floating point numbers will be omitted.

Floating point representation offers a great advantage over multiprecision fixed point. In the clinical laboratory, the data seldom have more than two, and at most three, significant figures. One 12-bit word gives adequate precision. The problem is rather where the decimal point in the result will be placed.

Floating point allows the range to vary over many orders of magnitude so that cell counts in the millions and heavy metal concentrations in parts per billion can be both held in the same type of representation.

Computer words can be used to hold more than numbers. We have seen how the same pattern of bits can mean 4367 as an unsigned integer, −3410 as a signed 1's complement integer, and −0.7020 (−0.111000010000) as a 1's complement floating point mantissa. The same bit pattern can also be used to represent alphanumeric information. Since most computers have relatively long words, it frequently is desirable to be able to use only parts of them at times. The parts are called "bytes." A byte is any group of consecutive bits in a word. Most computers have a standard byte defined that the hardware is set up to handle directly. Most commonly, such bytes contain eight bits, although six bits are in standard bytes on some machines (Fig. 9-4). This explains why computers with 8-, 12-, 16-,

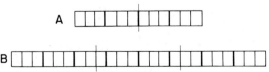

Figure 9-4 Standard bytes are six or eight bits. A is a 12-bit word with two 6-bit bytes, and B is a 24-bit word with three 8-bit bytes.

and 32-bit word lengths are common, especially in laboratory instruments.

By use of bytes we can store numbers as characters, instead of numeric values. The quantity "123" has a value, but it is also a collection of three characters "1", "2", and "3". If one codes these three characters as byte-long entities, then with three bytes one can represent 1 2 3. This may seem like the hard way to code a number which has straightforward binary representation, but this scheme will also permit the coding of upper case letters, lower case letters, punctuation, and control characters.

The most common coding scheme is called ASCII and was introduced in Chapter 8. ASCII requires 8-bit bytes and is ideal with 16-bit machines. For 12-bit machines, only 6-bit bytes are available, so the most significant bits are stripped off. This representation (called stripped ASCII) is more limited than regular ASCII and has restrictions on lower case letters and control characters. Table 9-1 gives the standard ASCII characters and indicates what is in the stripped ASCII set. In stripped ASCII, 43 = "#" and 67 = "7"; therefore, our previous representation as alphanumeric characters would be "#7". By combining consecutive words, one can form an alphanumeric or text message internally in the computer.

Table 9-1 is read by adding the number at the top of the column to the number at the left of the row. For example, "[" is 120 + 13 = 133 in ASCII and 33 in stripped ASCII. Symbols in italics are control characters.

EXAMPLE 9-4

What is the text equivalent of the following stripped ASCII message? 2324 0115 2040 1725 2440 2022 1706 0523 2317 2223 4141

Solution: To use Table 9-1 for stripped ASCII, we must add 100_8 to all numbers less than 40 and nothing to those above. The first byte is 23. To this we add 100 to give 123. In Table 9-1 we find this is the letter "S". The same process shows us that the next four letters are "T", "A", "M", and "P". We then encounter a byte of 40. Here we do not add 100, but go directly to the table. It is the char-

Table 9-1 Standard Seven-Bit (Nonparity) ASCII

	00	20	40	60	100	120	140	160
0	NULL		SPACE	0	@	P	'	p
1	SOH		!	1	A	Q	a	q
2	STX		"	2	B	R	b	r
3	ETX		#	3	C	S	c	s
4	EOT		$	4	D	T	d	t
5	ENQ	NAK	%	5	E	U	e	u
6	ACK		&	6	F	V	f	v
7	BELL		'	7	G	W	g	w
10			(	8	H	X	h	x
11	HT		)	9	I	Y	i	y
12	LF		*	:	J	Z	j	z
13	VT		+	;	K	[	k	{
14	FF		,	<	L	\	l	¦
15	CR		-	=	M	]	m	}
16			.	>	N	Λ	n	~
17			/	?	O	—	o	

STRIPPED ASCII

acter "space". If we finish the rest of the message in the same manner we discover it says:

STAMP OUT PROFESSORS!! ∎

The above representations are most common, although two others are also worth mentioning. If one has a 16-bit word, one has 65,536 (2^{16}) possible combinations of bits. If one takes the cube root of that number and discards the decimal fraction, one has the number 40. There are 26 alphabet letters and 10 digits. If one adds ".", ",", "-", and space to that set, one has 40 characters which are commonly used in addresses and other messages. If one gives each of these a representation between 0 and 39, one can then represent in one 16-bit word any three of these characters (X Y Z) as $X \cdot 40^2 + Y \cdot 40 + Z$. This allows 3 rather than 2 characters per word as in the ASCII coding. This coding is called RADIX 50, because $40_{10} = 50_8$.

Finally, instead of grouping 3 bits together to get octal, we can group 4 bits together to get hexadecimal (base 16). It has 16 symbols, including 0–9. The quantities from 10 to 15 are represented by the letters A to F (Table 9-2). A 12-bit word can therefore be represented by 3 hexadecimal digits as well as by 4 octal digits. Our old friend 4367_8 is $8F7_{16}$. Four hexadecimal characters are contained in a 16-bit

word. If the computer is built to disallow any representation other than 0–9, this allows the computer to handle decimal code material at two digits per 8-bit byte, rather than 1 per byte, as with ASCII. Some computers, like the IBM 1620, were built to do decimal arithmetic using this type of representation. Certain instruments, such as the Coulter S Plus and some Xerox machines, use hexadecimal to report status information.

To hold all the various data representations, a computer must have a memory. The memory is like a warehouse for data. It, in itself, has no intelligence or knowledge of the structure of the data it stores. To the memory, data are just a series of 1's and 0's grouped by words. The main memory is made from ferrite cores or semiconductors. Core memories have one miniature doughnut made of an iron alloy for each bit. These can be magnetized so that the field through the core is pointed either up or down. This direction is used to indicate 1 or 0.

Table 9-2 Hexadecimal Representation

0000	0	0100	4	1000	8	1100	C
0001	1	0101	5	1001	9	1101	D
0010	2	0110	6	1010	A	1110	E
0011	3	0111	7	1011	B	1111	F

The values are set and changed by pulses on wires running through the centers of the cores. These current pulses create magnetic fields which cause the magnetic fields of the cores to realign if they were oppositely aligned before. The cores are read by current pulses which are not large enough to cause the cores to change state. Instead a pulse is generated on a second wire which also runs through the core and is perpendicular to the first wire (this is a simplified explanation). Semiconductor memory can be thought of as miniature capacitors which are charged or uncharged, or as tiny flip-flops. More about memory structure will be mentioned in connection with microprocessors.

Main memories vary in size from 2^{10} bytes (= 1024 bytes and called "1K" bytes) to several million bytes (megabytes). Many computers also have auxiliary storage facilities for data that are slower in response than memories. These include disks, drums, tapes, and punch cards. While the response time of the memory (called "memory cycle time") is of the order of 0.2–1 μsec, other devices can take seconds or minutes to retrieve or store information. These will be discussed later with other peripherals.

The main computer memory is divided into words as previously mentioned to permit the storage and retrieval of information by word. Each word has an address. These addresses run sequentially, beginning with 0, the smallest unsigned integer that can be represented in the binary system. The memory size is usually determined by the highest address that can be stored in a memory word. For example, if a computer has a 16-bit word, the maximum memory size would likely be 2^{16} = 65,536 words. The words would be numbered 0 to 65,535 decimal or 000000 to 177777 octal (Fig. 9-5). Sometimes computers number the bytes instead of the words (byte-addressable). Some have a special register to allow a larger address to be held than what will fit into one word.

To access information in the memory, the address must be used. This address is placed into a control register called the *memory address register*. This register determines which part of the memory is pulsed to get information. The information to be written into the memory or which is received from the memory is placed in the *memory buffer regis-*

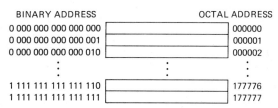

BINARY ADDRESS		OCTAL ADDRESS
0 000 000 000 000 000		000000
0 000 000 000 000 001		000001
0 000 000 000 000 010		000002
:	:	:
1 111 111 111 111 110		177776
1 111 111 111 111 111		177777

Figure 9-5 Addresses start at 0 and go to the largest number that can be held in the word length N, namely $2^N - 1$.

ter. These registers can be accessed by other parts of the computer, as will be described later.

Section 9-2
INSTRUCTION SET

A computer is a machine that executes instructions that result in the change of information from a previous state to a subsequent state. To carry out the instructions, the instructions must be in a specific general form. The first part of the instruction is the *op*eration *code* (OP CODE), which indicates what should be done (e.g., addition). Next come the addresses of the two operands on which the operation will be executed. A third address is needed to indicate where to place the result. A fourth address then tells the computer where to find the next instruction. An example of an instruction "word" is shown in Figure 9-6.

The part of the computer responsible for the execution of the instructions is the *logical control unit* (LCU). The LCU has two primary registers: the *instruction register* and the *instruction address register*. To perform an instruction, the contents of the instruction address register are transferred to the memory address register accompanied by a read request. The contents of the corresponding memory word are then placed into the memory buffer register and transferred to the instruction register. This word is then decoded by the LCU.

The LCU actually needs all the information in the word in Figure 9-6, but that word is too bulky to be used in a real computer. Another approach must be used to get this information for the LCU. This is done by fixing some of the four addresses as stan-

OP CODE	OPERAND ADDRESS	OPERAND ADDRESS	RESULT ADDRESS	INSTR. ADDRESS

Figure 9-6 A computer instruction containing all the fields needed by the LCU.

dard addresses so that they need not be indicated each time. The fourth address, that of the next instruction, can be set as that of the next location (word) after the current instruction. This address is the one being held in the instruction address register. While each instruction is being performed, therefore, this register is incremented by 1 so that the next instruction can be found when the current instruction is completed.

The second and the third fields can also be disposed of if they are set to a fixed register called the *accumulator*. This leaves only the OP CODE and the first operand address. When an operation is performed, one operand is taken from the operand address while the other is taken from the accumulator. The result is stored in the accumulator, and the next instruction address is taken from the instruction address register. Storage instructions take the contents of the accumulator and store them at the address specified by the operand address (Fig. 9-7).

Not all computers approach the addressing situation in the same way. Some computers do not have an accumulator. All instructions must, therefore, have fields to specify both operands. The address to store the result is the same as one of the operands. As a consequence, one of the operands is always altered by this process (Fig. 9-7).

Not all things a computer does require two operands. For example, to halt requires no operands. Some instructions require only one operand, which is also the result. For example, to set an operand to zero requires but one operand. For an accumulator-oriented machine, this one operand is the accumulator; for a two-address machine, the one operand

must be listed so as to be cleared. The forms of this instruction are shown in Figure 9-8.

When the computer gets a new instruction, it must decode it to find out what to do. This is accomplished by looking at the OP CODE. A fixed part of the instructions will always be included in the OP CODE. This is usually the first several bits and gives the family of the instruction. Figure 9-9 shows this concept for the Digital Equipment Corporation (DEC) PDP 11, a commonly used laboratory computer. The most general instructions are the two-operand instructions. These instructions have combinations of bits 12, 13, and 14 that are not equal to zero. Bit 15 is frequently used to indicate byte instructions and does not affect the instruction class. The second instruction group is the single operand class, in which bits 12–14 are 0, but at least some of the bits between 6 and 11 are nonzero. Finally there are the no-operand instructions, which have bits 6–14 equal to 0 and other bits appropriately set.

Within each class of instructions are sub-classes. A special type of subclass is one in which bits behave independently of each other. For the PDP 11, the codes 000240 to 000277 are such a sub-class. Bits 0–3 represent 4 separate 1-bit flag registers that can be set and cleared independently. If bit 4 of the instruction is 0, the flags indicated by the bits set between 0 and 3 are cleared. If bit 4 is 1, the flags indicated are set. Consequently, one can set or clear any or all of the flags with one instruction. This is an elementary example of a technique called microprogramming, which allows bits in instructions to indicate operations independent of other

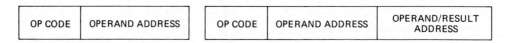

OP CODE	OPERAND ADDRESS

A

OP CODE	OPERAND ADDRESS	OPERAND/RESULT ADDRESS

B

Figure 9-7 Part A shows the structure of an instruction for a typical one-address machine (with an accumulator), while part B shows an instruction for a typical two-address machine.

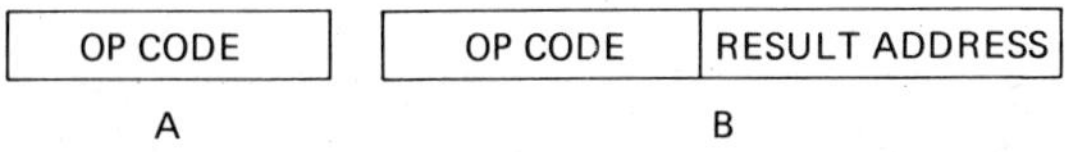

OP CODE

A

OP CODE	RESULT ADDRESS

B

Figure 9-8 Part A shows the structure of an instruction to clear the accumulator on a one-address machine, and Part B, to clear a designated register on a two-address machine.

bits. On the PDP 8, specific bits can bring about clears, complements, and rotations of the accumulator independently.

Whenever the instruction register receives a new instruction, the instruction address register is incremented by 1 to prepare for the next instruction. This new address frequently will not be the address of the new instruction for one of three reasons. First, the instruction may require an address so long that it will not all fit into the word with the OP CODE. In this case, the address must be placed somewhere else. A common place is in the word immediately after the instruction. Therefore, to interpret the instruction completely, the LCU must access the memory again and fetch this address. The instruction address register must be incremented by 1 a second time to skip this additional word. This type of instruction is called a two-word instruction because it takes two words to contain all of it. Some computers, like the PDP 8, have no two-word instructions. Others, like the PDP 11, have both two- and three-word instructions, be-

cause they are two-address machines. The second reason the next instruction may not be used is that the present instruction is a skip instruction. A skip instruction causes the instruction address register to be incremented by 1 another time, thereby ignoring the next instruction. Skip instructions can be either unconditional (always skip) or conditional (skipping only if some condition is met). These are also called branch instructions because they allow the program to change direction on the basis of some condition that is discovered. Finally, the instruction currently being executed may be a jump instruction. In such a case, the address field is transferred (absolute jump) or added (relative jump) to the instruction address register. The new address, rather than the old, is used to fetch the new instruction.

Through the process described above, the logical control unit permits a computer to operate from an internally stored program. This means that it is not necessary to give the computer the instructions one at a time, but instead they can be loaded at the start of the operation. Once started, the computer becomes master of its own fate until some instruction stops it.

To get data to and from memory, the LCU must have ways of determining the addresses in memory to access. We have already seen two ways of doing this. The first is the full-address instruction, in which the whole address is in the word with the OP CODE. The second is the two-word instruction

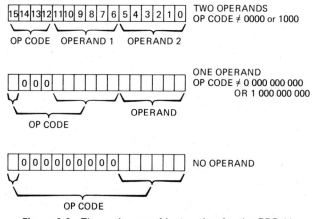

Figure 9-9 Three classes of instruction for the PDP 11.

where the address is in the word following the instruction. These approaches are called "direct address" methods because the address is directly available. Several other approaches are possible (Fig. 9-10). For example, if the operand, rather than its address, is in the word after the instruction, it is called "immediate" class addressing.

The major alternative to direct addressing, however, is indirect or deferred addressing. In this case, the instruction does not contain the address of the operand, but rather the address of the address of the operand. This means that the LCU must get the contents of the address it has and use those contents as an address to get the actual information desired. The address of the operand can be a memory address, but it is frequently more desirable to use a special register, frequently called an index or general register, to hold the address of the operand. The address field necessary to hold the address of an index register is short because only a few are included in a computer. Therefore, the use of an index register to hold the operand permits the OP CODEs to be longer, because the address field is shorter. This concept is used extensively on the PDP 11.

In addition to permitting indirect addressing, general registers frequently also increment and decrement. This means that when they are accessed by certain instructions, they automatically increase or decrease their values by 1. Consequently, if they are accessed again, their contents will be one address higher or lower. If one wants to perform the same operation on a series of numbers, a common programming practice, one can readily move through the numbers. To use a general register in this fashion, one loads the register with the initial

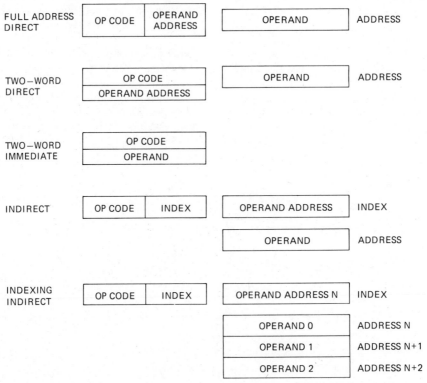

Figure 9-10 Five different ways to access a piece of data. The layout of the instructions and the addressed words are shown.

address and then enters a programming loop, where the general register is accessed indirectly and incremented numerous times. This process continues until some loop-ending condition is encountered. While general registers are sometimes the first few locations in memory, they are more commonly separate registers in the LCU, which reduces the time needed to access and increment them.

Since general registers are so important, let us look more closely at this operation. Let us assume a general register R2 has the contents 54. The word at address 54 contains 23 and the word at 55 contains 144 (Fig. 9-11). If the instruction is ADD I R2 (add to the accumulator indirectly the contents of word R2), the LCU will get the contents of index register R2, increase it by 1 and write it back (R2 is now 55), use this content (55) as an address to load the number sought (144), and add this 144 to the accumulator. The next time this same instruction is used, register R2 will be indexed again, this time to 56, and the contents of location 56 will be used as the operand. Registers used in this fashion are called pointers. These pointers can be used to store as well as retrieve information and are essential to the manipulation of data arrays. Since these index registers count up, they are referred to as autoincrementing registers. It is also possible to have

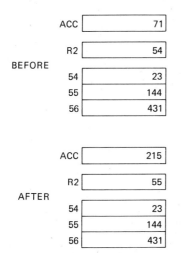

Figure 9-11 The execution of ADD I R2 causes the indexing of R2 and the addition of the contents of address 55 to the accumulator.

autodecrementing registers that subtract one after each operation. These latter registers are frequently used to determine when the end of the list is reached. An instruction called index-and-skip-if-zero (ISZ) is used to decrement a register until it reaches 0. Then, and only then, does the program skip and break out of the loop. Used in this manner, general registers are called counters. Counters and pointers are used extensively in all computer operations.

The LCU frequently assigns additional structure to the memory in the form of subdivision. This does not affect the physical property of the memory, but only the way the LCU looks at it. These logical divisions are frequently called pages, blocks, banks, or fields. The meanings of these vary somewhat between machines, but the underlying concepts are similar. A page is the part of memory that the computer can address directly with a one-word instruction. The PDP 8, for example, can address the 128 (200_8) words that include the memory location of the instruction. As the program crosses the page boundary, a new set of information can be accessed directly while the old set cannot. This means that the pages on the PDP 8 are fixed in location. On the PDP 11, the pages are twice as large and are centered on the current instruction. As the instruction address register is incremented, the page location of the accessable information (by a branch instruction) is also incremented. The page is not fixed, but floats. Memory blocks are the standard size of a disk transfer from a "blocked" disk. This is usually a power of 2, such as 256 or 512 words. A bank or a field is the amount of memory that can be jumped to by an instruction without doing a special field transfer operation. It is, in effect, the programming space of the machine. For example, the field in the PDP 8 is 2^{12} or 4096 words long. The PDP 8 may have up to 8 fields of memory.

The apparent structure of the memory can also be affected by the way the programmer represents the data. Information within memories can be arranged in many ways. Five common ways are arrays, lists, strings, trees, and stacks. These will be explained and compared to give some insight into why certain computer processes happen as they do. An array is a group of consecutive numbers of the same type (Fig. 9-12). For example, we could store

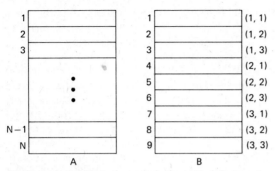

Figure 9-12 An array is a group of consecutive words. Part A shows a one-dimensional array (1 × *N*). Part B shows a two-dimensional array (3 × 3). Both arrays are stored linearly.

the temperature in the laboratory as an integer every hour for a week. This would give us 168 numbers. If these are stored in order, we can easily review this data. A general register set as a pointer to the beginning of this group of values allows them to be accessed sequentially. A general register set to 168 could act as a counter to indicate when we were through with the array. Some arrays have several subscripts, and these require several pointers and counters to handle them. Arrays are easy to use because the location of any item can be computed based on the start of the array, standard length of an item, and the number of the item sought.

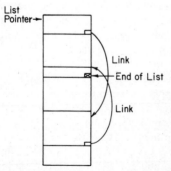

Figure 9-13 A linked list allows information to be stored in arbitrary sized blocks of arbitrary number and arrangement. The list parts may be randomly scattered in the file.

(BEFORE)	STRING A = "THE BOY IS GROWING."
REPLACE	"IS GROW" *WITH* "WAS LOOK"
(AFTER)	STRING A = "THE BOY WAS LOOKING."

Figure 9-14 Strings are used to manipulate text information.

Lists are very similar to arrays (Fig. 9-13). They differ in that the items on a list may be of different lengths, and a list can be of arbitrary length. To use an array, the size of the items and the array itself must be known and cannot vary because space is set aside for it. A list can be of indefinite length because its parts need not be consecutive, but can be linked together by pointers. When searching a list, one proceeds to search through it item by item until a pointer (link) is found. The search pointer is then set to the same value as the link, and the search resumes. The advantages of a list are (1) one does not have to know how big to make it at the beginning, and (2) one can store different types of data in it. The disadvantage of a list is that one cannot compute the location of the *n*th item, but must search for it from the beginning of the list.

Strings are lists of symbols that have the same purpose (Fig. 9-14). English text is a typical example. Whereas lists are usually manipulated by changing, adding, or deleting items, strings are manipulated by adding together (concatenating) strings, splitting strings, and replacing substrings with other substrings of greater or lesser length. Editing text on a word processor is an example of string processing.

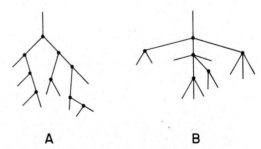

A　　　　　　　　**B**

Figure 9-15 Trees are lists that branch. Part A shows a binary tree (only two branches per node), while Part B shows a tree with multiple branching.

Trees are lists that are not linear, but have branches (Fig. 9-15). At various points in the tree structure, trees can branch into two or more paths, which in turn can branch as well. The game of tic-tac-toe illustrates the use of a tree structure. The first player has 9 possible moves (branches). Each of these branches has 8 possible branches (moves) for the second player, followed by each having 7 possible branches for the second move of the first player, and so on. Such trees allow very extensive expansion.

Finally, there is the stack (Fig. 9-16). A stack works like a plate holder in a cafeteria. As plates are added to the top, the stack sinks down so the last plate added is the first plate removed. This is called a *First-In-Last-Out* (FILO) buffer. To implement a stack conveniently, the LCU of the computer must have a stack pointer register (perhaps it uses a location in memory) that will index upward when items are added to the stack and index downward when items are requested from the stack. Special instructions are used to push (add to) and pop (remove from) the stack. Although the stack is nothing more than a group of sequential memory locations, its organization may be complex because of the type and order of its contents, which can only be found by tracing the activities of the program. The advantages of the stack are that it permits easy storing and retrieving of information in a systematic manner and allows a program to go arbitrarily deep in subprogram layers. The disadvantage is that each program must verify that the stack pointer is at precisely the same place when it leaves as when it entered.

The nature of the memory organization, then, is highly dependent on the instructions that the machine has available to handle it and the hardware of the LCU. For example, a machine with an instruction set that permits easy matching of an arbitrary series of bytes would be useful for string manipulation but might make stack manipulation difficult. Therefore it is not the physical structure of the memory, but the logical structure imposed on the memory by the LCU, that is the key to information management.

Section 9-3
THE ARITHMETIC-LOGICAL UNIT

To accomplish the manipulation of the information from memory, the computer must have an *arithmetic-logical unit* (ALU). This is the part of the computer that carries out the intent of the instructions as they are decoded by the LCU. By means of hardware, it can do arithmetic (add, subtract, multiply, and divide) and Boolean algebra (AND, OR, and NOT).

The main register of the ALU is called the accumulator, as discussed earlier in this chapter. This register may or may not be accessible to the user. It is on the PDP 8, for example, but not on the PDP 11. If it is not accessible, the various operations appear to happen between two memory locations. This, in fact, is not the case because the memory has no arithmetic capabilities. All the special arithmetic circuiting is attached to the accumulator. Invariably, arithmetic is accomplished by moving the contents of one memory location to the accumulator, loading the contents of a second memory location into the memory buffer register from which it is used to interact with the accumulator, and then transferring the new contents of the accumulator to the memory buffer register for return to the memory. This may happen in one instruction or may take numerous instructions, but the general scheme is the same regardless of the number of instructions involved.

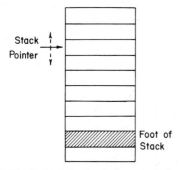

Stack
Pointer

Foot of
Stack

Figure 9-16 A stack is a set of consecutive memory locations. The top of the stack is the only word that can be accessed, and its address is held by the stack pointer. As items are added or subtracted from the stack, the pointer moves up and down to create the room or salvage the extra space.

It is easy to realize how complex the accumulator is if we look at the functions it must perform. For example, addition might seem straightforward, but what happens if there is a carry into the sign bit of a signed number?

$$
\begin{array}{rl}
\text{(User's intended } 2571 = & 2571 \text{ (Computer's} \\
\text{meaning)} \quad \underline{3421} = & \underline{3421} \text{ representation)} \\
6212 = & -1766
\end{array}
$$

Some sort of error must result from such an operation. Then there is the case of overflowing the word for an unsigned number.

$$
\begin{array}{rl}
\text{(User's intended } 4571 = & 4571 \text{ (Computer's} \\
\text{meaning)} \quad \underline{3421} = & \underline{3421} \text{ representation)} \\
10212 = & 0212 \text{ (2's complement)}
\end{array}
$$

This too is an error that must be flagged, yet it is different from the previous error. How does one distinguish between them when the same instruction is used to carry out both additions and is ignorant of the presence or absence of a sign? Overflow can also occur in the addition of two floating point numbers. In this case the overflow into the sign bit is also an overflow over the binary point. This is yet another complication which must be handled by the hardware. If one adds to these difficulties those that arise out of the other arithmetic operations, it becomes clear that the accumulator is a complex piece of hardware.

Although it may not at first seem obvious, the accumulator must be twice as long as other registers in the computer. This length is needed to accomplish multiplication and division. For example

$$
\begin{array}{r}
3427 \\
\times \quad 3105 \\
\hline
13071463
\end{array}
$$

Clearly, twice as much space is necessary to hold this answer as for the operands (Fig. 9-17). On the other hand, let us assume these are floating point numbers:

(Computer's representation)		(Computer's meaning)
3427_8	=	0.7056
$\times \quad 3105_8$	=	0.6212
$2616\ 3146_8$	=	0.54346314

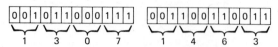

Figure 9-17 A double-length accumulator is needed to hold the product of a multiplication of two single-length integers.

The representations of the product of these two identical bit combinations are different. Which part of the representation to save for later use must be decided on the basis of the magnitude and format of the number. After all, 0005×0005 is $0000\ 0031$, and one would hardly want to retain the four most significant figures, all 0's, as the answer.

As well as performing arithmetic, the ALU can do logical operations (Boolean algebra), such as AND, NOT, or OR. These operations are done bit by bit. If a computer has 12 bits, then 12 parallel operations of the same type are performed at once. For example

$$
\begin{array}{rl}
& 2574 = 010\ 101\ 111\ 100 \\
\text{AND} & \underline{4361 = 100\ 011\ 110\ 001} \\
& 0160 = 000\ 001\ 110\ 000
\end{array}
$$

Only positions in which both words have 1's are retained as 1's in the final word. Logical operations permit "masking" of positions in a word while other parts are used. If the third bit of a word contains a flag, we can isolate it by ANDing it with 1000_8 (001 000 000 000). This will cause all the other bits to disappear, and we can then test if the accumulator is zero. To facilitate logical and arithmetic operations, accumulators can also roll their contents a number of positions to the right or left or swap contents between the parts of the accumulator.

Section 9-4
INPUT/OUTPUT

The parts of the computer previously discussed are shown in Figure 9-18. The final part of a computer proper is the *input/output* (IO) system. The primary component of the IO system is its bus structure. An electrical bus is a wire or group of parallel wires

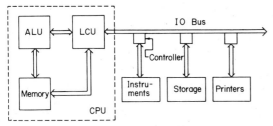

Figure 9-18 The relationship between the various parts of a computer is shown. The arrows indicate the buses.

that carries information to different places along its length. For example, a ground bus is a heavy-gauge piece of wire that ties numerous points to ground. Buses are controlled by bus driver gates and are frequently attached to binary coders and decoders. All the other parts of the computer are also tied together with buses so that information can be exchanged.

The IO bus itself runs from the rest of the computer, called the *central processing unit* (CPU), to the peripheral controllers. Common peripherals include terminals, line printers, tape drives, and cardreaders. In the clinical laboratory, the peripherals may include instruments; in fact, the computer may be part of an instrument as will be seen later. The bus runs only to the controllers of the peripherals and not to the peripherals themselves, because the traffic on the bus is very heavy and the bus is sensitive to noise. As the bus gets longer, more time and energy are required to raise and lower the voltage levels on the bus. This slows computer operation. The power radiated by many circuits, such as those that carry high current, can induce false signal changes on the bus, as mentioned in Chapter 4. To prevent this, the controller or interface for each instrument interacts with the bus to get and give information. Since this interface is physically located within the computer cabinet, the bus can be kept short and free of noise. The interface communicates with the peripheral at a slower pace, since the average peripheral is several orders of magnitude slower than the computer.

Let us look at a few items that might be part of a computer's bus (Fig. 9-19). One common item is an interrupt line. This is a wire which carries a signal if any peripheral wants the attention of the computer. When a peripheral wants attention, it puts a signal on the bus and the LCU jumps to its peripheral handling program, putting a bookmark into its current task. In effect, the computer is "interrupted." It tries to discover what interrupted it by asking each peripheral whether it is responsible. To do so, it places binary coded device addresses as signal levels on the device address lines and a query pulse on a device identification line. When the correct peripheral interface is pulsed, it places a pulse on a wire called a "skip" line, causing the LCU to skip an instruction. By appropriate programming, this new instruction can be made to jump to a service program that will determine why the peripheral interrupted the computer. In the process more information will probably be exchanged via the device address lines and various data lines. When the peripheral controller is satisfied, it will remove its signal from the interrupt line, and the computer can find its bookmark and resume what it was previously doing.

Peripheral controllers range from very simple to extremely complex. Simple controllers may do such things as translate a parallel character representation to a serial representation. Such a controller would be centered around a UART, which was discussed in Chapter 8. Other controllers may be extremely complex, such as a cardreader controller that reads a card into an external buffer and then transfers it to the computer's memory. Controllers can be plugged into the IO bus just as electrical appliances plug into the wall. This means the addition of new devices is usually very easy to imple-

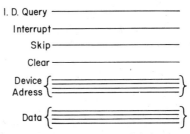

Figure 9-19 Signal lines compose the IO bus of computers.

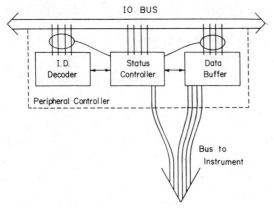

IO BUS

I.D. Decoder

Status Controller

Data Buffer

Peripheral Controller

Bus to Instrument

Figure 9-20 A peripheral controller consists of a circuit to decode its identity, a data buffer, and a status controller, which handles status signals and controls the information exchange with the IO bus and the instrument. From the status controller and the data buffer the bus goes to the instrument.

ment. Obviously software to tell the controller what to do must also be added. Figure 9-20 shows a block diagram of how a peripheral controller works.

Section 9-5
PERIPHERALS

Any number of peripherals can be attached to a computer. These devices allow information to be entered and returned and provide extra storage capability. We will briefly discuss those which are important in a clinical laboratory. Peripherals can be classified in numerous ways, but the easiest way for the student to follow is perhaps by function. To start many of the new laboratory instruments, it is necessary to insert a program. These programs are stored on cassette tapes or floppy disks. Cassette tapes are familiar as a storage medium for music and voice. They can also be used to store computer programs. These are stored as 1's and 0's on the magnetic surface of the tape. In effect, lines on the surface of the tape perpendicular to its length are magnetized in one direction or the other, one direction being interpreted as a 1 and the other as a 0.

When erased, the surface magnetism is randomized. Floppy disks appear to be small records in jackets, but are flexible. They always remain in their protective jacket while in use. The disk surface acts like that of a tape, but instead of being arranged in a linear fashion, the information is arranged in concentric circles. This permits any information to be accessed in one revolution of the disk rather than having to wait for the correct spot on the tape to be found. The analogy to the conventional tape and record players should be obvious. When used to start up a computer or instrument, these cassettes and floppies have certain fixed portions of their information read into a specific area of memory by a built-in device called a "bootstrap loader." Loading this information is, therefore, called "booting the system."

Before proceeding, it is perhaps well to look at tapes and disks in general. A tape contains its information on one or more magnetic rows of 1's and 0's called "tracks." The tracks can be used independently or in parallel. Large reel storage tape has nine tracks. The information on the tape is of a fixed density. Common densities on commercial storage tape are 800 and 1,600 bits per inch. In order for the tape to be read, the tape reader on the computer must have a read/write head for each track and must be able to absorb information as quickly as it appears on the tape. The more densely the information is packed, the more uniform the surface of the tape must be to prevent errors from occurring. Alignment of the reading heads over the tape tracks is also important to get reliable information transfer. Tapes may be of any length, as long as they fit into the physical space available when wound. Commerical 9-track tapes run up to 2,400 feet in length. The information is stored in consecutive words, and the word grouping is called a record. Special, otherwise illegal, combinations of bits mark the beginning and end of records. Between records are interrecord gaps, where the magnetism is randomized to prevent accidental reading. Some tapes are "blocked," that is, have fixed length records, while others have arbitrary length records, determined by the computer at the time of writing. Cassettes are the slowest and lowest quality magnetic tape in general use, but require little hardware space or expense to use.

Disks come in two varieties: fixed-head and moving-head. The fixed-head disk has a read/write head over every track of information. This allows rapid access to the information, but it also is very expensive for large disks with thousands of concentric data tracks. Few disks of this type are made anymore. The moving-head disk has relatively few read/write heads for the number of tracks it has. Therefore, it must move the appropriate head to the track that is to be read. This causes delay between when the information transfer request is issued and when it can be honored. Newer designs have reduced this latency time to a reasonable level. Floppy disk drives are moving-head devices. Information on disks can be packed much tighter than on a tape because the medium is much more stable. Disks are always blocked to eliminate the need to search them from the beginning. As a consequence, they are called "random access" devices, while tapes are "sequential access" devices. High-speed, high-density disks are operated in sealed, pressurized housing, whereas slower disks, such as floppies and cartridges, can be inserted and removed from the disk drives by the user.

Another means of entering bulk information into the computer is by punched tape or punched card. In this case a reader optically determines the locations of holes and nonholes and passes that information on to the computer. Paper tape has just about been replaced by magnetic tape, which is reusable and easier to handle. Punch cards are also being replaced by key-to-disk systems, but the computer readable card still has a place in many laboratories. It is generally the mark-sense card, rather than the punch card, that is used, however. Medical technologists can record the results of procedures such as cell differentials, urinalysis, and bacteriological tests on cards as they do them at the bench and then take the cards to a card reader to enter the information into the computer. The card reader has one optical channel, composed of a light source and a photodiode, for each row on the card. There are usually 12 information rows and a timing channel row on each card. Light from the black pencil marks is not reflected to the photodiode, and as a consequence, these are recorded as 1's while the rest of the card positions which do reflect are recorded as 0's. For repetitive, standardized procedures this is a quick way to enter large amounts of data.

Many laboratory instruments now have keyboards for data entry. Typing ability is becoming essential to laboratory work. The keyboard may be built into the instrument or be part of a terminal that sits next to it. When keys are depressed, the internal circuitry of the keyboard codes the key as a group of parallel pulses, frequently in ASCII, and sends it to a UART or similar device for transmission to the instrument's computer. If the keyboard is part of the instrument, such transmission is not necessary, but the information can be moved directly to the computer's memory. Each key struck, therefore, fills up a byte in the computer's storage. The computer will use this information as indicated by its program. Certain keyboard characters are called "control characters" (Table 9-1); they do not give a printable representation, but instead cause carriage returns, cursor movements, beeps, or other physical responses. Keyboards are frequently used to give the instrument instructions on how to proceed or to supply information to be printed out along with the laboratory data.

Paired with the keyboard is invariably a printer or a CRT. Even instruments without keyboards may have printers. Almost all newer instrumentation now converts information from analog to digital and further refines it to printable formated messages. These are output to the printer, which is called "hard copy" because a copy of the information can be retained. CRTs are, by contrast, called "soft copy" devices because the information they display is lost when it leaves the screen. Printers receive their information from the computer either coded as ASCII or as a series of pulses which can be recoded as ASCII. These are then converted with the help of a table to produce the pulses that drive the print head. Older printers used the impact printing of a ball or cylinder on paper. Most newer printers use solenoid-driven wires to give a dot matrix (Fig. 9-21) for the characters, charged ink droplet guns to spit in a pattern at the paper, or hot styluses to melt the characters on specially treated waxed paper. Printers commonly run at 30–180 characters per second. Some printers are bidirectional, printing every other line backward. This is possible because they have a character buffer that

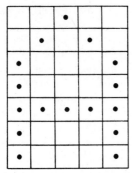

Figure 9-21 A 5 × 7 matrix represents the letter A. This pattern is typical of those created by solenoid-driven printers.

allows them to store a large number of characters at once. As a result, they already have the next line, which must be printed in the reverse order, before they start it. This saves the time necessary for the print head to move to the left margin (called a carriage return). The radical improvement in printers in recent years has made laboratory data much easier to read and preserve.

The CRT is an instrument generally used to query the technologist or report some problem requiring human intervention. Displaying messages that automatically disappear is pointless because the technologist may not be present to see them while they are on the screen. They are transmitted to the CRT from the computer in the way that information is transmitted to a printer. The information on the screen is stored in the memory associated with the CRT and is refreshed, much as a television screen, by a microprocessor from the memory. The information is placed on the screen as a dot matrix. Because the CRT can put information on the screen more quickly than a printer can put it on paper, the transmission rate is usually 240, 480, or 960 characters per second. When a key is struck on a keyboard and the character appears on a CRT or is printed, the transmission usually does not go directly between the two, even if both operations occur in the same terminal; it goes to the computer first and is then returned for printing. This is called full-duplex mode and is used to permit the human typist to detect transmission problems with the computer or instrument. If the printer receives the

signal directly from the keyboard, it is called half-duplex.

The printer attached to most instruments is a character printer because it prints one character at a time. Central laboratory computers frequently also have line printers that produce a whole line at one time. This is accomplished by sending a whole line to the line printer buffer and having the printer store it. As the character drum on the line printer revolves at high speed, a bank of hammers, one per character position, is triggered to hit the paper against the ribbon and the drum precisely as the correct character for that print position is facing forward. In one revolution of the drum, all the characters are printed. Line printers usually have pica type and print lines 80 or 132 characters in length. Speeds vary from 300 to 2,000 lines per minute. Because of its speed, the line printer is used to produce major laboratory reports.

The final peripheral that we must examine is the instrument itself. Since the computer may be part of the instrument, this might seem like putting the cart before the horse. Nevertheless, despite the physical bulk of the instrument, it is the computer that controls the operation and is, therefore, the central actor. The best way to examine the relationship is in terms of the functions the computer performs in the instrument. Before we do this, we will first introduce the microprocessor as a functioning computer because it is the computing power of so many instruments.

Section 9-6
MICROPROCESSORS

We saw a block diagram of the overall structure of a computer in Figure 9-18. The original commercial computers had only a few thousand words of memory, but these were long (more than 30 bits). Soon computer memories began to double in the number of words every two years, and commercial machines were financially out of reach of most researchers. To fill the computing void, minicomputers appeared in the 1960s. These had short word lengths (12–16 bits) and small memories (2–8 K bytes). These, too, began to grow in size as more applications developed. One can now get minicomputers with megabyte memories and peripherals that would have made the large computer users of the late 1960s envious. Many instruments incorporated "minis" as their computing power. As time passed, however, there was clearly a market for a still smaller computer. The technology of miniaturization that was necessitated by the space program produced the large scale integrated (LSI) circuits necessary to put a whole computer on a single chip. The tremendous market in hand-held calculators caused the production of these "microprocessors" to be commercially feasible. Manufacturers of thousands of instruments quickly recognized the usefulness of microprocessors in the operation of their instruments, and their use has proliferated. Microprocessors are almost exclusively used as parts of other instruments, not as stand-alone computers.

A microprocessor is actually a computer in a silicon chip (Fig. 9-22). It has numerous leads that allow signals to enter and leave. It frequently has only a few bits in its words and a very restricted instruction set. Because of its size and low power requirements, it can be placed in nearly any piece of equipment. While it may be relatively slow and inefficient as compared with a large computer, it can afford to be, since the procedures it is used to control are also relatively slow (a few hundred events per second or less). The microprocessor consists of the LCU and ALU in one unit or chip.

A printed circuit bus attaches the microprocessor to other LSI chips that contain the memory. The memory may be partly semiconductor *random-access memory* (RAM). This memory is used to store and manipulate information from the instrument being served. In addition the memory will probably be partly *read-only memory* (ROM). This memory is made from a specially designed RAM that has all the 1's and 0's permanently stored on the chip. Consequently, the computer cannot write any information to this memory, and it is "read only." Such memory is used to hold the key instructions on how the instrument is to run. Sometimes the whole program is there, eliminating the need for cassette tapes or floppy disks. Other times only the bootstrap and instrumental interface control are stored, so the user has more operational flexibility.

Also attached to the microprocessor via a bus are the interfaces to keyboard, printer, and CRT. These were previously described. Various wires to the parts of the instrument that must be controlled also are attached to the microprocessor. Some of these may come from an analog-to-digital convertor if an analog device such as an operational amplifier is being used. Others may run to digital counters or digital-to-analog convertors to carry information back to the various parts of the instrument to control it. Some are single lines that open and close switches that control valves, pumps, and heaters. Levels and pulses sent on these lines cause the instrument to go through its cycles. These are the means by which a microprocessor is attached to a laboratory instrument.

Section 9-7
COMPUTER CONTROLLED INSTRUMENTATION

Let us look at a hypothetical instrument (Fig. 9-23) and follow it through its operational protocol to see how it is controlled by a microprocessor.

The technologist who arrives in the morning turns the power on, inserts the cassette tape, and presses the load button. Part of the cassette tape is read into the computer's RAM, and the program is initiated by the bootstrap loader. A display appears on the CRT asking which procedure to run (Fig. 9-24A). The technologist types in a response on the keyboard. The microprocessor interprets the re-

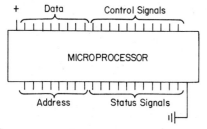

Figure 9-22 A typical microprocessor is a 40-pin chip. The general classes of connections are shown. Each of these pins is attached to a wire in one or another bus within the instrument. A typical control signal would be TRAP (enter trap mode), and a typical status signal would be READY (the processor is ready for data transfer).

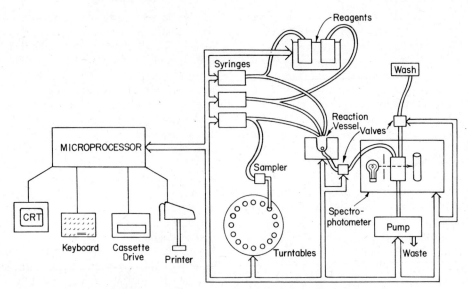

Figure 9-23 A hypothetical computer-controlled instrument.

sponse and looks it up in the table that was first loaded from the cassette tape. If the response is illegal, the computer returns an error message on the CRT (Fig. 9-24B) and the technologist must try again. If the response is legal, the microprocessor determines which procedural control program to load from the cassette tape, rewinds the tape, and looks for the procedure. This is loaded, if present, into the position of RAM set aside for the procedure. If absent, another error message occurs.

Once the procedure program is loaded, control is transferred to it. It first initializes any files or parts of the equipment necessary. It then inquires of the technologist any information needed to run the procedure (Fig. 9-24C). Such information might include experimental conditions, patient administrative data, the worksheet of test requests, or the output format. This information is then stored for later use as the experiment proceeds.

The computer next begins its checklist of items relevant to the procedure selected. It will turn on the heating bath, the radiation source, and the photomultipliers. It will set the reagent pumps to move wash solutions through the system. It will print test messages on the printer. It will then ask the user whether the correct reagents are in place. The mi-

croprocessor will continue to monitor the heating bath through an ADC. After a certain amount of time, it will change switch positions and begin pumping reagents. It will check the background color of the reagents at several different wavelengths by putting the right filters in place from the filter wheel. It will adjust the voltage on the radiation source and the photomultiplier tube to get the correct dark current and blank readings. All of this is accomplished by voltage pulses or levels sent on control lines. Occasionally a register will be set as a counter and incremented by a clock until zero is reached so as to time a process. Any problem with reaching temperature any place in the instrument or in setting up other experimental conditions will be reported by the microprocessor to the operator via the CRT.

When all is satisfactory, the computer tells the technologist via a panel light or the CRT that specimens may be entered. The specimens are placed around the edge of a plate, which is appropriately attached to the instrument. The technologist pushes the start button. The microprocessor detects this as an interrupt and initiates the sampling program. At regular intervals the microprocessor will transfer the amount of sample to be picked up

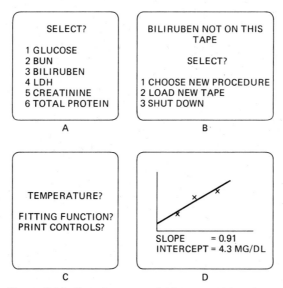

Figure 9-24 Sample screen displays on a laboratory instrument.

to the sampler mechanism, and will then pulse it to start the sample transfer. After the sampler has completed its work, it informs the microprocessor that it is done. The processor then pulses the plate drive to rotate the turntable one position. After waiting the appropriate amount of time, the processor restarts the cycle by transferring the sample amount to the sampler. When an empty specimen position is encountered, an optical detector, composed of a photodiode and an LED, signals the computer that the last sample has been picked up, and the computer shuts down the sampling process.

While controlling the sampler, the microprocessor is also controlling the addition of the other reagents. Here too, the amount or timing for each addition to the reaction mixture must be specified by the computer to the reagent pumps or syringes. Periodically the reaction vessel contents may have to be mixed with a stirrer. All this reaction timing is controlled by pulses and control levels sent out by the microprocessor based on the procedure program it read off the cassette tape.

The contents of the reaction vessel are transferred to the spectrophotometric cell for reading when the computer opens the appropriate valves. The re-

action vessel is washed. Readings taken may be for endpoint or reaction rate. In either case, multiple values for each point are taken via an ADC, and the values are averaged to remove the effects of transients. These are stored in the RAM for later calculations. When the last measurement is completed, the spectrophotometric cell is washed, and a reference measurement is made to compensate for any drift in the source or the P–M tube.

The specimen plate contains calibrators, controls, and samples. The location and value of calibrators and controls are contained in the procedure program from the cassette tape or are typed in by the technologist through the keyboard. As the readings are collected, they are preprocessed and tabulated. Any necessary offset is subtracted, and the average of the multiple readings is taken. When enough data have been gathered, results for the run are calculated. Working curves are prepared, if necessary, and the measured values of controls and samples are computed (Fig. 9-24D). The measured control values are compared against the actual control values, and erroneous readings are flagged. The test information is then combined with any available administrative data and printed on the printer

CUP#	READING	NAME	RESULT	UNITS	COMMENTS
1	1.02	STANDARD 1	76.5	MG/DL	
2	2.03	STANDARD 2	152.2	MG/DL	
3	2.99	STANDARD 3	224.2	MG/DL	
4	1.43	CONTROL ALPHA	107.2	MG/DL	CTL - IN RANGE
5	1.26	GOPHER A. HOMER	94	MG/DL	
6	0.78	RABBIT JACK	58	MG/DL	BELOW NORMAL
7	5.66	SMITH GEORGE	424	MG/DL	ABOVE SCALE
8	1.11	JACKSON JANE	83	MG/DL	

Figure 9-25 Sample printout from an instrument.

in an easily readable format with test names, units, and perhaps normal ranges (Fig. 9-25). The technologist must still review this information before releasing it. One of the options may be to transmit the data from the instrument to a central laboratory computer to prepare the integrated patient report.

When a new test procedure is desired, the operator must inform the instrument, which will load the new procedure from the cassette tape, and the whole episode will be repeated using the new parameters. When the day's work is done, the technologist tells the instrument to do its shut-down procedure. This instruction will cause the computer, step by step, to shut off and rinse the instrument so that it will be ready for another day's work.

The instrument described above does not exist as such. However, all the activities mentioned can be found in laboratory instruments. Increasingly, everyday instruments are incorporating various types of computer control over various operations or functions. The efficient laboratory worker must understand the methods and sequences of operation. Instruments are no longer just tools to be used in analysis. The growing knowledge (artificial intelligence) possessed by new instruments makes them real partners in laboratory analysis.

With the completion of the discussion of the microprocessor-controlled instrumentation, we leave our discussion of electronics and turn to the other methodology used in making laboratory measurements. We have come all the way from the simple resistor to the complex microcomputer. Each of the devices we have examined has its place in laboratory instrumentation. We will next review optics and explore optics-based measurements.

REVIEW QUESTIONS

1. Why have computers become common in laboratory instruments?
2. What are the advantages of computer-controlled instrumentation?
3. What is a computer word?
4. Define word length.
5. What is a register?
6. How are the contents of a computer word written?
7. How does one represent an unsigned integer in the computer?
8. How does one represent a signed integer?
9. Explain 1's complement.
10. Explain 2's complement.
11. What is end-around carry?
12. What is negative zero?
13. Explain double precision representation.
14. What is floating point?
15. Explain how floating point representation works.
16. What is a mantissa?
17. What does "normalizing a number" mean?
18. Where is the binary point in floating point notation?
19. What is the relationship between the sign bit and the most significant bit in floating point notation?
20. Why is floating point useful in the clinical laboratories?
21. What is a byte?
22. How long is a standard byte?
23. Why is information stored in alphanumeric notation?

24. What is stripped ASCII?
25. What is RADIX 50? How is it computed?
26. What is hexadecimal?
27. How can BCD be used for decimal computation?
28. What components are used to make a computer memory?
29. What is a core?
30. How is information written into a core? Obtained from it?
31. What is a "K"?
32. How large are computer memories?
33. What is memory cycle time?
34. How long is the memory cycle time of a main computer memory?
35. What is a memory address?
36. How are memory addresses assigned?
37. What is the limitation on memory size?
38. How is the memory address register used?
39. What is the memory buffer register?
40. What is an OP CODE?
41. How many address fields must be present to define an instruction completely? What do they contain?
42. How is the problem of excessively long word length overcome?
43. What are the contents of the instruction address register?
44. How do instructions get into the instruction register?
45. What is the LCU?
46. What is an accumulator?
47. Why are some computers two-address machines?
48. How are instruction classes differentiated?
49. What is microprogramming?
50. How is the address of a new instruction usually obtained?
51. Why might the next word not contain the next instruction?
52. How is a two-word instruction structured?
53. What is a conditional skip instruction?
54. What is a full-address instruction?
55. Define "direct address" mode.
56. What is "immediate class addressing?"
57. How does the computer do indirect addressing?
58. What is an index register?

59. In what two common ways are index registers used?
60. How can one use an index register to examine an array?
61. Define page, block, and field.
62. Why does the LCU subdivide the memory?
63. What is the difference between a fixed and floating page?
64. What is an array?
65. How do lists differ from arrays?
66. What is a "string"?
67. Explain how a tree is constructed.
68. How does a stack work?
69. How are lists tied together?
70. What do "push" and "pop" mean?
71. Define concatenation.
72. What is the ALU?
73. What two types of operation can an ALU do?
74. Explain the process of arithmetic as done in the accumulator.
75. What is arithmetic overflow?
76. List different types of overflow.
77. Why is the accumulator twice the length of other registers?
78. How is "masking" used?
79. What is a signal bus?
80. What is the CPU?
81. Why does the IO bus only run to the peripheral controllers, and not to the peripherals?
82. Where are the peripheral controllers located?
83. What types of signals are part of the IO bus?
84. How does a peripheral request service?
85. What two devices are commonly used to enter programs into laboratory instruments?
86. How is information stored on magnetic tape (physically and logically)?
87. What is a floppy disk?
88. What is a bootstrap loader?
89. What are common data densities on tape?
90. How is information stored on disks?
91. How does a fixed-head disk work?
92. How does a moving-head disk work?
93. Define random access.
94. For what are mark-sense cards used in a clinical laboratory?
95. How does a mark-sense reader work?
96. How does a computer keyboard work?
97. Why are some terminals called "soft copy"?

98. What is a control character?

99. List several ways of printing characters.

100. Why can a bi-directional printer print backward?

101. How are characters displayed on a CRT?

102. What are common transmission rates for a CRT?

103. What is full-duplex? Half-duplex?

104. How does a line printer work?

105. Why can a laboratory instrument be considered a computer peripheral?

106. What is a minicomputer?

107. Why was the microprocessor developed?

108. Why has the microprocessor become ubiquitous?

109. What is a RAM?

110. What is a ROM?

111. What type of devices are attached to a microprocessor within an instrument?

112. What type of information might an instrument request from a technologist?

113. What kind of instrumental processes might a computer control?

114. What information might an instrument output on its printer?

PROBLEMS

1. Convert the following octal numbers to 12-bit 1's complement representation.
a. −135   **b.** −2744   **c.** −1650

2. Convert the following 12-bit 1's complement numbers to signed octal integers.
a. 6371   **b.** 4413   **c.** 5670

3. Convert the following octal numbers to 12-bit 2's complement representation.
a. −3154   **b.** −2230   **c.** −1761

4. Convert the following 12-bit 2's complement numbers to signed octal integers.
a. 7037   **b.** 5112   **c.** 4060

5. Add the following 12-bit 1's complement octal numbers.
a. 6157, 2403   **b.** 7033, 0745   **c.** 5671, 6342

6. Add the following 12-bit 2's complement numbers.
a. 5447, 6311   **b.** 4255, 3700   **c.** 6265, 1513

7. Convert the following decimal numbers to 12-bit 1's complement floating point representation.
a. 641   **b.** 212.4   **c.** −71.8

8. Convert the following 12-bit 1's complement floating point numbers to decimal.
a. $M = 3571$, $E = 6$
b. $M = 5016$, $E = 4$
c. $M = 3147$, $E = -3$

9. Convert the following character strings to stripped ASCII.
a. THE SKY IS BLUE.   **c.** #4 IS < #12.
b. "OOPS!"   **d.** F(X)=4*X+5

10. Convert the following stripped ASCII to character strings.
a. 03-10-25-22-03-10-40-15-17-25-23-05
b. 24-10-05-40-04-17-17-22-40-11-23-40-22-05-04-56
c. 67-53-61-61-40-11-23-40-16-17-24-40-61-64-41
d. 43-41-50-30-55-53-41-50-32-41-41-17-56-13-54-24

11. Convert the following character strings to full ASCII.
a. Remember the Maine!
b. {[(INSIDE)]}
c. 101=~100 BELL LF CR

12. Convert the following full ASCII to character strings.
a. 116-145-167-040-131-157-162-153-040-103-151-164-171
b. 130-072-171-055-041-147-046-072-173-060-175
c. 002-013-013-014-000-000-123-124-117-120-012-015-003

13. Convert the following decimal numbers to hexadecimal.
a. 3572   **b.** 1974   **c.** 2057

14. Convert the following hexadecimal numbers to decimal.
a. A3F   **b.** 1B6   **c.** 987

CHAPTER 10

OPTICS

After electronic principles, the most widely used physical principles in laboratory instrumentation are optical. Many measurements are based on photometry and others on refractometry. Light for these measurements must be generated, dispersed, reflected, refracted, and detected. An understanding of the optical principles involved is essential to an understanding of how such instrumentation works and whether it is working properly. Improperly used and maladjusted optical systems account for a large number of laboratory errors.

Section 10-1
PLANE SURFACE REFLECTION

Except for the controversy of whether the chicken or the egg came first, the argument over whether light consists of waves or particles was the most hotly contested topic for more than a century. Because both approaches made so much sense, the proponents of each position were unwilling to yield. Finally, the situation was resolved when it was determined that light had both wave and particle properties, depending on the circumstance. Theoretical models of how these properties interacted were finally developed. As a consequence, we will use models of light as both waves and particles in the following discussion as is necessary to explain why the various natural phenomena occur.

The first interaction we will consider is that of light with a plane (flat) mirror. The ancient Greeks and Egyptians were already familiar with the two laws which describe how reflections of light occur at a plane surface. Let us first define that a line that is perpendicular to a plane at a point is called the normal to the plane at that point. There is, of

course, only one such line per point on the plane. We can now state the laws of reflection.

First Law of Reflection

The reflected ray, as it leaves the plane mirror, is in the same spatial plane as is the incident ray and the normal to the plane mirror at the point at which the incident ray strikes the mirror.

The incident ray (here light is acting like a ball thrown at the floor) and the normal to the mirror at the point of intersection are two intersecting lines. From geometry we know that these define a plane. The reflected ray is also in this plane. To represent what is happening graphically, we pick precisely this plane to draw as in Figure 10-1.

Second Law of Reflection

The angle that the incident ray makes with the normal to the plane mirror is equal to the angle that the reflected ray makes with the normal. (In other words, the angle of incidence equals the angle of reflection.)

If we apply the second law to Figure 10-1, we see that angle α is the same as angle β. Because of these two laws, we can determine exactly where a reflected ray will pass if we know the direction of the incident light and the location of the plane mirror.

It must be realized that not all reflection is what is called "specular reflection." Specular reflection occurs only off smooth polished surfaces. Rough surfaces cause "diffuse reflection." In specular re-

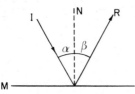

Figure 10-1 The reflected ray (*R*) makes the same angle (*β*) to the normal (*N*) of the mirror as the angle (*α*) made by the incident ray (*I*).

flection, all the incident rays of light that are parallel are reflected in parallel since all their angles of incidence and reflection are the same. The light appears to come from the other side of the plane mirror in a straight line rather than off the mirror's face. In diffuse reflection, each ray of light obeys the laws of reflection, but because the surface is irregular, the normals to the surface at the points the rays strike are not parallel. At each point the normal is affected by the local direction of the surface. As a result, parallel incident rays do not result in parallel reflected rays. The light is diffused. It is this phenomenon that allows us to see objects that are not sources of light.

The difference between a rough and a smooth surface is one of degree. Here the wave properties of light become significant. If the size of the irregularities (*d*) is small compared with the wavelength of the light (λ), specular reflection occurs. If the irregularities of the surface are large compared with the wavelength of the light, diffuse reflection occurs (Fig. 10-2). Obviously on the atomic scale, all surfaces are irregular. Because electromagnetic radiation (light) comes in many different wavelengths, an object can give specular reflection to radiation of longer wavelength and diffuse reflec-

tion to that of shorter wavelength. When we look at a mirror, we see many rays of light at the same time. All these rays of light, even if they come from the same object, are not parallel; hence the object we see assumes a shape.

Figure 10-3 shows the effect of light striking a plane mirror. Light from an object striking the mirror in different places will be reflected at different angles. The ray from the object striking the mirror along its normal (at right angles) will be reflected back on itself to the object. Rays striking progressively farther from the normal ray will be reflected through progressively larger angles to the normal. They will diverge as they leave the mirror's surface. Since detectors of light, such as an eye or a camera, assume that light always travels in a straight line, it appears to such detectors that the diverging light rays come from a source on the far side of the mirror. Using a simple geometric proof on Figure 10-3, we can show that the apparent source of the light, the image, is as far behind the mirror as the object is in front of it. (*Note:* ∠ means angle and Δ means triangle. Angles are named *XYZ*, with *XY* being one of the sides and *YZ* the other.)

$$\angle OAS = \angle PAS \tag{10-1}$$

Second law of reflection

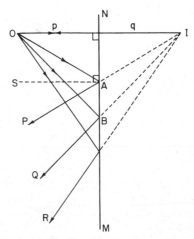

Figure 10-3 Light reflected off a plane mirror appears to emanate from a point that is the same distance behind the mirror as the object is in front of the mirror.

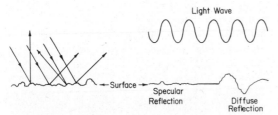

Figure 10-2 Specular reflection occurs when surface irregularities are small, and diffuse reflection occurs when they are large.

$$\angle OAN = \angle PAM \tag{10-2}$$

Complementary $\angle$'s to (10-1)

$$\angle PAM = \angle NAI \tag{10-3}$$

Opposite $\angle$'s are equal

$$\angle OAN = \angle NAI \tag{10-4}$$

$\angle$'s equal to the same $\angle$ are equal

$$\angle OBN = \angle NBI \tag{10-5}$$

Same as (10-1)–(10-4)

$$\angle OAB = \angle IAB \tag{10-6}$$

Supplementary $\angle$'s to (10-4)

$$AB = AB \tag{10-7}$$

Identity

$$\triangle OAB \cong \triangle IAB \tag{10-8}$$

Angle side angle

$$OA = IA \tag{10-9}$$

Corresponding parts

$$AN = AN \tag{10-10}$$

Identity

$$\triangle OAN \cong \triangle IAN \tag{10-11}$$

Side angle side

$$ON = IN \tag{10-12}$$

Corresponding parts

$$p = q \tag{10-13}$$

Renaming from (10-8)

$$\angle ONA = \angle INA \tag{10-14}$$

Corresponding parts

$$\angle ONA = 90° \tag{10-15}$$

Two equal supplementary $\angle$'s are 90°

Equation 10-13 tells us that the image is the same distance (q) as the object distance (p), while Eq. 10-15 states that the ray through the object normal to the plane also passes through the image. Thus the image will appear to be in the same relative position behind the mirror that it actually is in front of the mirror.

Several other facts about plane mirrors should be mentioned, all of which follow from the previous equations. First, the object does not need to be directly in front of the mirror; it can be off to one side and can still be seen, provided the observer is appropriately stationed. Second, the image will appear to be right side up (upright), but will actually be inverted left to right. Finally, the image will be virtual, that is, the rays of light never actually pass through it, and it cannot be captured on a screen.

Section **10-2**
SPHERICAL MIRRORS

We have seen that a flat surface gives specular reflection and a rough surface gives diffuse reflection or diffusion. These are not the only possibilities that exist. It is possible to create smooth surfaces that are not planar to reflect light in a regular manner. To be useful, these surfaces must concentrate or focus the light they reflect in order to form images. Very few surface designs will do this in a useful manner. Fun house mirrors have few analytical applications.

One surface that will produce useful reflection is a paraboloid. A paraboloid is a surface that consists of all points equidistant between a plane and a point not in the plane. If the paraboloid is cut by a plane perpendicular to the generating plane and through the generating point, a parabola results as the intersection (Fig. 10-4A). Another way of considering a paraboloid is as a parabola spun in the space on its axis. If light enters a paraboloid parallel to its axis, that light will be reflected off the parabolic surface and through the point used to generate the surface, which in this usage is called the focus. A parabolic mirror will rapidly heat up any object placed at the focus since all the energy of the radiation entering parallel to the axis is channeled to that point. On the other hand, if a source of light is placed at the focus of a parabolic mirror, the light will be reflected off the parabolic surface and form a beam parallel to the axis of the mirror. Light can travel either way along the path of a ray because the reflection process is symmetrical by the second law

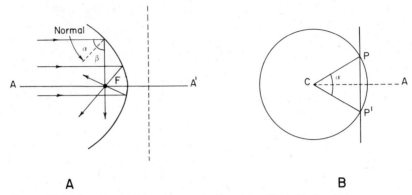

A

B

Figure 10-4 A cross-section of a parabolic mirror (Part A). Parallel rays are reflected through the focus. A spherical mirror is constructed from the portion of a sphere cut off by a plane (Part B).

of reflection. The use of a parabolic reflector is common in automobile headlights and searchlights. The portion of the paraboloid actually used in the mirror is arbitrary since every part of the paraboloid has the same property. A larger surface simply collects more light.

Most mirrors used in scientific work are not parabolic but spherical. For various reasons these have been more convenient to make. A spherical mirror can be considered to be created by a plane cutting a piece out of a sphere (Fig. 10-4B). The angle of the surface removed, as measured from the center of the sphere, is called the angle of aperture α. The distance across the mirror (PP') is called the linear aperture. If the inside surface of the sphere is used, the mirror is said to be concave, while if the outer surface is used, the mirror is said to be convex.

Spherical mirrors are not identical to parabolic mirrors since their shapes are different. If, however, the angle of aperture for a spherical mirror is very small, the difference in curvature between it and a similarly sized parabolic mirror cut perpendicular to its axis is very slight. The spherical mirror will focus parallel light very much like the parabolic mirror with only minor aberration (that is, distortion). The light will not be focused exactly to a point but to a very small sphere centered at the focus. By using small enough angles of aperture, spherical mirrors can be used in place of parabolic ones, as shown in Figure 10-5A. We shall do so in the subsequent discussions.

If one places a point light source on the axis through the center of a spherical concave mirror, as in Figure 10-5B, the rays of light will strike the mirror and be reflected back to another point. If the source of light is initially very far away, the rays will be almost parallel, and they will be reflected to the focus. As the light source approaches the mirror, the angles that the incident rays make with the normal of the mirror decrease and the reflected rays are bent through less of an angle. As a result, the point at which they meet is farther from the mirror. The point source of light is called the object, and the point at which the light rays meet is called the image. If one placed a screen at the point at which the rays meet, then one could see the image of the object. As a result, this is a real image, not a virtual one as in the case of a plane mirror.

From the above discussion, it should be clear that the focus is the closest point to the spherical mirror at which an image can form. This location is a fundamental property of each mirror, and its distance is called the focal length (f). A second major property of a spherical mirror is its radius of curvature (r). This is the center of the hypothetical sphere from which the mirror was cut. Both the focus and the center of curvature lie on the axis of the mirror. There is a relationship between them as shall be seen later. The focus always lies inside the radius, so we shall place it there in future drawings although we have not yet proven this.

If we place a one-dimensional object in front of

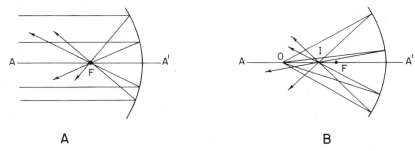

A   B

Figure 10-5 The spherical mirror reflects parallel light through the focus (Part A) and light from a point source through a point outside the focus (Part B).

the concave mirror, we create a one-dimensional image. Let us place the object, an arrow (AO), outside the radius of curvature with its tail on the axis of the mirror, as shown in Figure 10-6. In order to find the image, it is necessary that we follow the rays of light to the place where they converge. Since light can travel to the mirror along an infinite number of paths, this is a formidable job.

We can simplify our task if we recall that since all the rays converge at the image, any two of them must converge there after being reflected. We know that this position is the image because the rays of light are straight lines and straight lines can only cross once. If we pick two rays, we can find the location of the image.

The next question is which two rays to pick. Since it is difficult to sketch the direction of reflection off the curved surface for most of the rays

accurately, it will be very time consuming to pick rays at random. There are, however, several rays whose directions of reflection are known and that are easy to draw:

1. The ray that leaves the object parallel to the axis of the mirror is reflected through the focus F.
2. The ray that leaves the object and travels through the focus is reflected parallel to the axis of the mirror.
3. The ray that strikes the mirror at the axis is reflected back at an equal angle on the opposite side of the mirror's axis.
4. The ray that travels through the radius of curvature of the mirror strikes the mirror on its normal and is reflected back on itself.

These rays are referred to as the principal rays from the object.

We are now ready to locate the image in Figure 10-6. Since we do not yet know the location of the focus, we will use rays 3 and 4 to find the image (BI), as shown in Figure 10-6. The image is real, inverted, and inside the radius of curvature. It is also outside the focus since we have previously established that light from a source closer than infinity converges outside the focus. As a result, we have now shown that the focus truly is inside the radius of curvature.

It is possible for us to determine the relationship between the image distance and the object distance from Figure 10-6 by the application of plane geometry. We start with the fact that $\triangle$OAN and $\triangle$IBN are right triangles and that $\angle$ONA and $\angle$INB are equal by the second law of reflection (see Fig. 10-6). These right triangles are therefore similar. Since

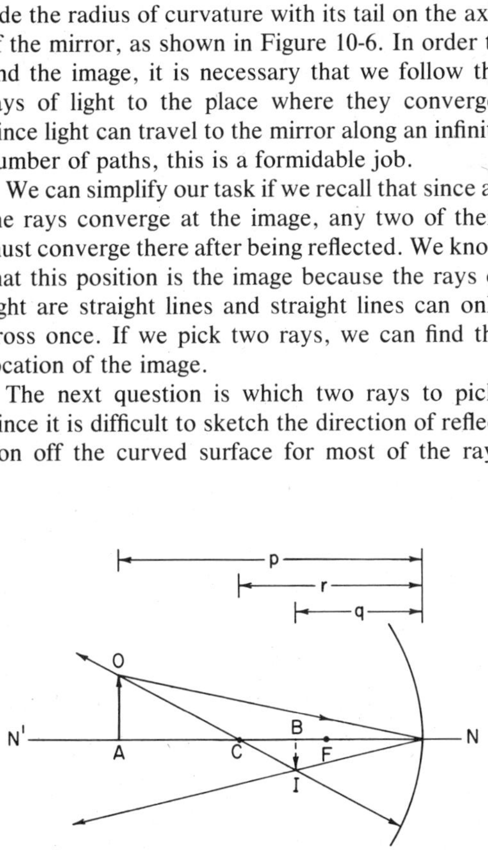

Figure 10-6 An object (AO) outside the center of curvature (C) of a concave mirror will produce a real, but inverted image (BI) between the focus and the center of curvature.

the ratios of corresponding parts of similar triangles are equal

$$\frac{OA}{IB} = \frac{AN}{BN} \qquad \text{(10-16)}$$

Since $\triangle OAC$ and $\triangle IBC$ are right triangles and $\angle OCA$ and $\angle ICB$ are equal because they are the opposite angles at an intersection, $\triangle OAC$ and $\triangle IBC$ are similar. By the corresponding parts rule,

$$\frac{OA}{IB} = \frac{AC}{BC} \qquad \text{(10-17)}$$

Since things equal to the same thing are equal to each other

$$\frac{AN}{BN} = \frac{AC}{BC} \qquad \text{(10-18)}$$

We can substitute for these in terms of object and image parameters. AN is the object distance p. BN is the image distance q. AC is the object distance minus the radius of curvature (r), or $p-r$. BC is the radius of curvature minus the image distance, or $r-q$. Therefore

$$\frac{p}{q} = \frac{p - r}{r - q} \qquad \text{(10-19)}$$

We now cross-multiply and regroup,

$$pr - pq = pq - qr$$

$$qr + pr = 2pq$$

Dividing by pqr

$$\frac{1}{p} + \frac{1}{q} = \frac{2}{r} \qquad \text{(10-20)}$$

A few points are worth noting about Eq. 10-20, referred to as the mirror equation. The position of the image is determined by the position of the object relative to the radius of curvature. If $p = r$, then q is also equal to r. If $p > r$, then $q < r$ and vice versa. The radius of curvature is that point about which the image and object balance. Second, the image and object are interchangeable. Note that p and q can be interchanged in Eq. 10-20 without any change in the equation. The straight lines called rays cross each other twice, once before reflection and once after. One of these crossings is at the

object and the other at the image. The geometry is the same no matter which is the object. Finally, the relative sizes of the image and the object are determined by the distances p and q. If we substitute p and q into Eq. 10-16, we get

$$\frac{OA}{IB} = \frac{p}{q} \qquad \text{(10-21)}$$

However, OA is just the object size S_o and IB is just the image size S_i. Therefore,

$$\frac{S_o}{S_i} = \frac{p}{q}$$

or

$$S_i = \left(\frac{q}{p}\right) S_o \qquad \text{(10-22)}$$

The size of an image is directly proportional to its distance from the mirror and the size of the object, but inversely proportional to the object distance.

We are now ready to derive the relationship between the focus and the radius of curvature. Let us move our object to an infinite distance. By definition, its rays will form an image at the focus. If we substitute these values into Eq. 10-20, we have

$$\frac{1}{\infty} + \frac{1}{f} = \frac{2}{r}$$

Since $1/\infty = 0$,

$$f = \frac{r}{2} \qquad \text{(10-23)}$$

The focus is just half the distance of the radius of curvature. As a result, the mirror equation can be written in its most common form:

$$\frac{1}{p} + \frac{1}{q} = \frac{1}{f} \qquad \text{(10-24)}$$

Equations 10-22, 10-23, and 10-24 establish the relationship between all the important properties for a concave mirror.

EXAMPLE 10-1

The sum of the image and object distances is 5.38 times the focal length of a concave mirror. If the focal length is 8.51 cm and the image is closer to the mirror than the object, what are the locations of the image and object?

Solution: We have two unknowns and therefore need two equations:

$$\frac{1}{p} + \frac{1}{q} = \frac{1}{f}$$

$p + q = nf$ where $n = 5.38$ and $f = 8.31$

Solve the second equation for p and substitute:

$$p = nf - q$$

$$\frac{1}{nf - q} + \frac{1}{q} = \frac{1}{f}$$

Multiply by $qf(nf - q)$

$$qf + nf^2 - qf = nqf - q^2$$

Regroup $q^2 - nfq + nf^2 = 0$
By quadratic formula

$$q = \frac{nf \pm \sqrt{n^2f^2 - 4nf^2}}{2}$$

$$q = \frac{nf}{2}(1 \pm \sqrt{1 - 4/n})$$

Since $p > q$

$$p = \frac{nf}{2}(1 + \sqrt{1 - 4/n})$$

$$p = \frac{5.38 \times 8.51}{2}(1 + \sqrt{1 - 4/5.38})$$

$$p = 34.5 \text{ cm}$$

and

$$q = \frac{nf}{2}(1 - \sqrt{1 - 4/n})$$

$$q = \frac{5.38 \times 8.51}{2}(1 - \sqrt{1 - 4/5.38})$$

$$q = 11.30 \text{ cm} \qquad \blacksquare$$

EXAMPLE 10-2

If the image height is 6.94 cm in Example 10-1, what is the object size?

Solution:

$$S_i = \frac{q}{p} S_o$$

$$S_o = \frac{p}{q} S_i$$

$$S_o = \frac{34.5}{11.30} \times 6.94$$

$$S_o = 21.2 \text{ cm} \qquad \blacksquare$$

We have thus far examined what happens when the object is outside the focus of a concave mirror. If the object is inside the focus, the complexion of the system changes dramatically. Figure 10-7 shows what occurs when one tries to trace the principal rays from an object inside the focus. Three of the four principal rays from an object have been drawn and, as can be seen, the rays do not converge at any point in front of the mirror. As a consequence, there is no real image. Instead, the rays appear to originate from a point behind the mirror. This point then is the image of the reflection. Because it is behind the mirror, it cannot be captured on a screen and is a virtual image just like that obtained from a plane mirror. A plane mirror can, in fact, be considered to be a concave mirror with the focus at infinity, so that all objects are inside the focus. The image is also erect like that of a plane mirror. The size and position of the image can readily be determined. Angle ONA is equal to angle INB by the laws of reflection. This means right triangles ONA and INB are similar. Since the corresponding parts of similar triangles are propor-

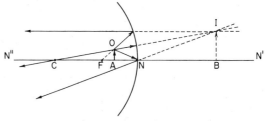

Figure 10-7 When the object is moved inside the focus of a concave mirror, the image becomes virtual, erect, and larger than the object.

tional, Eq. 10-16 is true. This immediately leads to Eqs. 10-21 and 10-22, which gives the size of the image in terms of the object distance, the image distance, and object size as seen before.

$$S_i = \left(\frac{q}{p}\right) S_o \qquad \text{(10-22)}$$

The distance of the image can be established from triangle IBC. Clearly by construction, triangle OAC is similar to it. Since the corresponding parts of similar triangles are proportional, Eq. 10-17 is true. On the basis of this equation and Eq. 10-16, the mirror equation (Eq. 10-20) is derived. Since the initial equations have been shown to be true here, Eq. 10-23 follows in the manner shown above. Therefore

$$f = \frac{r}{2} \qquad \text{(10-23)}$$

$$\frac{1}{p} + \frac{1}{q} = \frac{1}{f} \qquad \text{(10-24)}$$

EXAMPLE 10-3

If an object is 4.07 cm in front of a concave mirror of focal length 5.95, what is the position of the image?

Solution:

$$\frac{1}{q} = \frac{1}{f} - \frac{1}{p}$$

$$\frac{1}{q} = \frac{1}{5.95} - \frac{1}{4.07}$$

$$\frac{1}{q} = -0.0776$$

$$q = -12.9 \text{ cm} \qquad \blacksquare$$

The answer to this example gives us a negative number. A negative number in optics implies that the image is on the opposite side or behind the optical instrument. The position of the image should always be indicated in words such as "in front of" or "behind" a mirror or "to the left of" or "to the

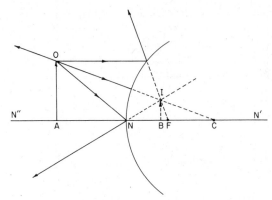

Figure 10-8 Reflection from a convex mirror always produces a virtual image inside the focus of the mirror.

right of" a lens. Note that since the image distance q is negative, it must always be larger in magnitude than the object distance p for the focal length f to be positive. Therefore, the image is larger than the object.

A concave mirror bows away from the viewer. One can also have a mirror which bows toward the viewer, called a convex mirror. Such a mirror is shown in Figure 10-8. If an object is placed in front of the mirror, a virtual image is formed. Figure 10-8 shows three of the principal rays from the object. Note that now we must make our drawing of the rays in respect to the center of curvature behind the mirror. The focus too is behind the mirror, because the outside rather than the inside surface is being used to reflect light. This means that the light striking the mirror parallel to its axis will leave the mirror as if it had come from the focus behind the mirror. Light heading for the center of curvature will be reflected back on itself without ever reaching that point. In fact, the entire diagram in Figure 10-8 is identical in geometry with that in Figure 10-7, but it is opposite in polarity. As a consequence, exactly the same geometric principles can be applied to Figure 10-8 as to Figure 10-7 to give precisely the same equations (10-22 and 10-24). How then does one differentiate between the two? In Figure 10-8 the focus is on the same side of the mirror as the image. Since the object is real, it must be on the positive side of the mirror, and the image distance and focal length must both be negative. .

Table 10-1   Various Images Formed by Reflection

Type of Mirror	Object Position	Image			
		Type	Location	Direction	Size vs Object
Plane	$p > 0$	Virtual	$p = -p$	Erect	Same
Concave, convex	$p = \infty$	None	$q = f$	None	Point
Concave	$\infty > p > r$	Real	$r > q > f$	Inverted	Smaller
Concave	$p = r$	Real	$q = r$	Inverted	Equal
Concave	$r > p > f$	Real	$\infty > q > r$	Inverted	Larger
Concave	$p = f$	None	$q = \infty$	None	Infinite
Concave	$p < f$	Virtual	$q < 0$	Erect	Larger
Convex	$p > 0$	Virtual	$f < q < 0$	Erect	Smaller

EXAMPLE 10-4

If the focal length of a convex mirror is 10.27 cm and the image is 8.14 cm behind the mirror, where is the object?

Solution:

$$\frac{1}{p} = \frac{1}{f} - \frac{1}{q}$$

$$\frac{1}{p} = \frac{1}{-10.27} - \frac{1}{-8.14}$$

$$\frac{1}{p} = 0.0255$$

$$p = 39.2 \text{ cm in front of the mirror} \quad \blacksquare$$

We discover two important points from this example. First, the image distance must be less than the focal length in order to make p positive. If all the numbers were negative, one could multiply by -1 and make them all positive, but this would give us the concave mirror situation. Second, from triangle OAC it should be clear that the image will always be smaller than the object. A convex mirror can never by itself give a real image or one as large as the object.

Let us review the important facts concerning spherical mirrors. The mirror equation (Eq. 10-24) holds for all spherical mirrors. The equation for the size of image (Eq. 10-22) also holds for all spherical mirrors. When all the distances (object distance, image distance, and focal length) are positive, we are dealing with concave mirrors with the object outside the focus. When the image distance is nega-

tive, we are dealing with either a concave or convex mirror. In such a case, either the object or the image is inside the focus, depending on which is on the same side of the mirror as the focus. If the focus is on the object side, the mirror is concave and the focal length positive. If the focus is on the image side, the mirror is convex and the focal length is negative. A plane mirror has its focus at infinity. Table 10-1 shows the various relationships between the image and object, depending on the position of the object and type of mirror.

Section **10-3**
NATURE OF LIGHT REFRACTION

When light strikes any surface, part of it is reflected. The amount reflected depends on the nature of the surface, the wavelength of the light and the angle of incidence of the light onto the surface. The light that is not reflected from the object is refracted (bent) into the object that the light strikes. This dual phenomenon lets us see through a window in the daytime when there is bright light outside but to see only our own reflection on a dark night. The reflection is present also in the daytime, but it is overwhelmed by the light refracted in from out-of-doors. The refraction of light is controlled by three natural laws.

First Law of Refraction

The refracted ray is in the plane determined by the incident ray and the normal to the plane at the point of incidence (this is the same plane that contains the reflected rays).

Second Law of Refraction

The sine of the angle of refraction is a constant times the sine of the angle of incidence, regardless of the angle of incidence. Both angles are measured from the normal. This is also called Snell's law, after Willebrord Snell, a Dutch astronomer of the early seventeenth century.

Third Law of Refraction

The path of a refracted light ray is exactly reversible; it can be traversed in either direction. This too is similar to the case of reflection.

Figure 10-9 shows what happens when light goes from one substance to another. As light goes from a less dense medium into a more dense medium, it is bent toward the normal. As it goes from a more dense medium into a less dense medium, it is bent away from the normal. The relative density of a material toward the travel of light is called the refractive index (μ). Therefore, Snell's law can be written as follows:

$$\sin \alpha = \mu \sin \beta \qquad (10\text{-}25)$$

where β is the angle of refraction, α is the angle of incidence, and μ is the relative index of refraction (a constant).

The index of refraction for a substance is calculated from the relative speed of light in vacuum versus that in the substance of interest. Vacuum was chosen as the reference value (assigned the value 1.00000) because light should travel no faster in any substance than in vacuum. Vacuum has no particles or fields to retard the movement of light. All substances are then referenced to vacuum by

$$\mu_S = \frac{c_V}{c_S} \qquad (10\text{-}26)$$

where c_S is the speed of light in substance S, c_V the speed of light in vacuum, and μ_S the index of refraction of S. This is called the absolute index of refraction. The indices of refraction for several common compounds are water = 1.333, ethanol = 1.360, air = 1.000, zinc crown glass = 1.517, light flint glass = 1.585, heavy flint glass = 1.650, and fused quartz = 1.458. These measurements were made at 589 nm, the sodium yellow light. Air is very close to vacuum in its ability to carry light, slowing light by only 0.03%.

To find the relative index of refraction, we divide the absolute index of refraction for the entering substance by that for the refracting substance. If we assume that angle α is in substance A and angle β is in substance B, then we have

$$\sin \beta = \frac{\mu_A}{\mu_B} \sin \alpha \qquad (10\text{-}27)$$

or

$$\mu_B \sin \beta = \mu_A \sin \alpha \qquad (10\text{-}28)$$

EXAMPLE 10-5

If light traveling through water strikes a piece of heavy flint glass at an angle of 28.3° to the normal, what will be the change in angle made by the light as it is refracted into the glass?

Solution:

$$\sin \beta = \frac{\mu_A}{\mu_B} \sin \alpha$$

$$\sin \beta = \frac{1.333}{1.585} \sin 28.3° = 0.3987$$

$$\beta = \arcsin 0.3987$$

$$\beta = 23.5°$$

$$\Delta\angle = \alpha - \beta = 28.3 - 23.5$$

$$= 4.8° \qquad \blacksquare$$

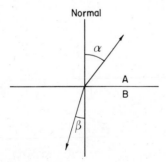

Figure 10-9 Light passing from a substance of lower refractive index (A) to one of higher refractive index (B) is bent toward the normal.

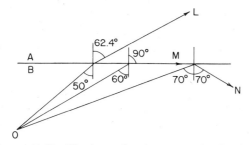

Figure 10-10 Whether refraction or total reflection will occur depends on the angle of incidence. Total reflection can only occur if substance B is denser than substance A.

Light can always pass from a less dense into a more dense medium. It is always possible to bend the light more sharply toward the normal. However, light cannot always travel from a more dense medium to a less dense medium. Let us look at the case when the ratio μ_B/μ_A in Eq. 10-27 is 1.157. This means that substance B is denser than substance A. Let us now find the value for α at three values for β: 50.0°, 60.0°, and 70.0°.

$$\alpha = \arcsin (\mu_B/\mu_A \sin \beta) \tag{10-29}$$

$$\alpha_1 = \arcsin (1.157 \sin 50.0°) = 62.40° \tag{10-30}$$

$$\alpha_2 = \arcsin (1.157 \sin 60.0°) = 90.0° \tag{10-31}$$

$$\alpha_3 = \arcsin (1.157 \sin 70.0°) = \arcsin 1.087 \tag{10-32}$$

It is clear that there is no problem with an incident angle of 50°. We get refraction as we would expect. In Eq. 10-31, the refracted angle is 90.0°, which means that light is being refracted along the surface of the interface rather than into substance

B. Equation 10-32 is impossible; we cannot have an angle whose sine is greater than 1. Therefore, refraction is impossible.

Figure 10-10 shows what is happening in the three cases. The first is regular refraction. The second case represents light at the critical angle, the angle that causes refraction along the surface. The final case is called total reflection. The light cannot obey Snell's law and therefore cannot be refracted. It must instead be reflected from the surface back into the substance of greater refractive index. Total reflection occurs for all light that strikes the interface at greater than the critical angle.

The use of total reflection is important in a number of applications in clinical laboratories. The most direct application is the refractometer, which is used to measure the density and concentration of substances based on the angle at which total reflection occurs. This creates a sharp light–dark interface on a ruled scale. (This instrument is discussed in Chapter 13.) The use of total reflecting prisms is common in optical instruments to change the direction of the light. Two common configurations are shown in Figure 10-11. Another application is that of optical fibers, which carry signals in the form of light down a flexible glass or plastic fiber. The principle involved is multiple total reflections with the angle of incidence always exceeding the critical angle, as shown in Figure 10-11.

Refraction is not limited to one interface but occurs whenever light passes from one substance to another. Figure 10-12 shows an example of what happens. Light passes through a piece of glass and back into the air. From the diagram one can see that angles β and γ will be the same, since they are opposite interior angles on a line cut by two parallel lines. By Snell's law, therefore, angles α and δ must

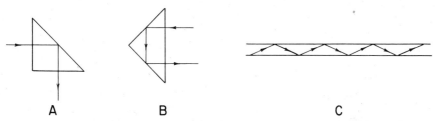

    A   **B**   **C**

Figure 10-11 Parts A and B show the use of the total reflection prisms. Part C shows the multiple total reflections in an optical fiber.

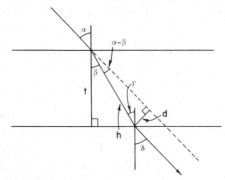

Figure 10-12 Light that goes through a glass plate with parallel sides is displaced in space, but emerges parallel to the incident beam.

be equal, since the sines of α and δ are only a constant times the sines of β and γ. This means that the light leaves the glass plate in the same direction as it entered, only displaced in space. This displacement can be calculated if the angle of incidence, the relative index of refraction, and the thickness of the glass are known. The displacement is one side of a right triangle whose opposite angle is the amount the light was bent $(\alpha - \beta)$. The hypotenuse (h) is the distance the light traveled through the glass. Therefore

$$\sin(\alpha - \beta) = \frac{d}{h} \qquad \text{(10-33)}$$

The distance h is also the hypotenuse of another right triangle formed by the normal to the glass at the point of intersection. In this case the thickness (t) of the glass is the adjacent side to the angle of refraction. As a result

$$\cos \beta = \frac{t}{h} \qquad \text{(10-34)}$$

We then solve for d.

$$d = h \sin(\alpha - \beta)$$

$$h = \frac{t}{\cos \beta}$$

$$d = \frac{t \sin(\alpha - \beta)}{\cos \beta} \qquad \text{(10-35)}$$

By the trigonometric formula for the difference of sines, we can reduce this equation.

$$\sin(\alpha - \beta) = \sin \alpha \cos \beta - \sin \beta \cos \alpha \qquad \text{(10-36)}$$

$$d = \frac{t}{\cos \beta}(\sin \alpha \cos \beta - \sin \beta \cos \alpha) \qquad \text{(10-37)}$$

$$d = t\left(\sin \alpha - \frac{\sin \beta \cos \alpha}{\cos \beta}\right) \qquad \text{(10-38)}$$

By the relationship between sines and cosines, we can replace the $\cos \beta$ term.

$$\sin^2 \beta + \cos^2 \beta = 1 \qquad \text{(10-39)}$$

$$\cos \beta = \sqrt{1 - \sin^2 \beta}$$

$$d = t\left(\sin \alpha - \frac{\sin \beta \cos \alpha}{\sqrt{1 - \sin^2 \beta}}\right) \qquad \text{(10-40)}$$

The $\sin \beta$ term can be replaced by $1/\mu \sin \alpha$ using Snell's law (Eq. 10-25):

$$d = t\left(\sin \alpha - \frac{\sin \alpha \cos \alpha}{\mu\sqrt{1 - (\sin^2 \alpha)/\mu^2}}\right)$$

$$d = t \sin \alpha\left(1 - \frac{\cos \alpha}{\sqrt{\mu^2 - \sin^2 \alpha}}\right) \qquad \text{(10-41)}$$

As can be seen, the displacement is only a function of the angle of incidence, the relative index of refraction and the thickness of the glass. A zero angle of incidence, a zero thickness of glass or no difference in the index of refraction all lead to no displacement.

A second example of multiple substance phenomena is shown in Figure 10-13A. After passing through several substances, the light reaches an interface where there is total reflection and proceeds to work its way back out of the object. In such a case it may be necessary to measure the horizontal displacement because the refracted light does not leave the object in a direction parallel to the entering light. To measure the horizontal displacement, one must use the tangent to the angle rather than the sine. For the first layer of the substance shown in Figure 10-13A

$$\tan \beta = \frac{d}{t} \qquad \text{(10-42)}$$

$$d = t \tan \beta$$

$$d = \frac{t \sin \beta}{\cos \beta} \qquad \text{(10-43)}$$

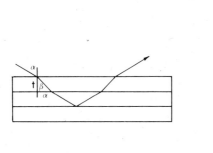

A

B

Figure 10-13 Solids of various densities and shapes cause light to be refracted at unusual angles.

By the interrelationship of sines and cosines (Eq. 10-39)

$$d = \frac{t \sin \beta}{\sqrt{1 - \sin^2 \beta}} \qquad (10\text{-}44)$$

If we substitute from Snell's law (Eq. 10-25)

$$d = \frac{t \sin \alpha}{\sqrt{\mu^2 - \sin^2 \alpha}} \qquad (10\text{-}45)$$

The same process can then be applied to all the substances until the total displacement is found.

EXAMPLE 10-6

A light ray enters the irregularly shaped glass prism in Figure 10-13B 5.8 cm from point A on side AB at an angle of 23.1° to the normal. Assuming the dimensions as given and a refractive index of 1.490, in what direction will the rays emerge from the prism?

Solution: First note that the prism is a right prism. Second, find angles β and B:

$$\sin \beta = \mu \sin \alpha$$

$$\sin \beta = \frac{1}{1.490} \sin 23.1°$$

$$\sin \beta = 0.2633$$

$$\beta = 15.3°$$

$$\sin B = \frac{AC}{AB} = \frac{5}{13}$$

$$\sin B = 0.3846$$

$$B = 22.6°$$

γ is a complimentary angle to β,

$$\gamma = 90 - \beta = 74.7°$$

The angles of a triangle add up to 180°

$$\delta = 180 - \gamma - B$$

$$\delta = 180 - 74.7 - 22.6 = 82.7°$$

ε is a complementary angle to δ

$$\varepsilon = 90 - \delta = 7.3°$$

By Snell's law,

$$\sin \zeta = \mu \sin \varepsilon$$

$$\sin \zeta = 1.490 \sin 7.3$$

$$\sin \zeta = 0.189$$

$$\zeta = 10.9° \text{ to the normal to side BC toward C}$$

∎

The bending and displacement of light is very important to the operation of instruments that use light in order to make measurements. Such instruments make up more than one-half the instruments in a typical clinical laboratory. Prisms will be discussed more extensively later in this chapter.

Section **10-4**
LENSES

Whereas mirrors use the principles involving the reflection of light, lenses use the principles of the refraction of light. A lens is a transparent substance with polished surfaces. At least one of the surfaces must be curved for the lens to be effective. The curvature of the lens surfaces in most cases is spherical. Lenses can be thought of as the intersection of two spheres, the intersection of a plane and a sphere, or the material left after either two spheres or a plane and a sphere cut away portions of a cylinder. The shapes of the six possible regular lenses are shown in Figure 10-14. Since these lenses are symmetrical about an axis, we can study their properties through the use of cross-sections through that axis as we did in the case of mirrors.

All lenses are divided into two classes. Lenses cause parallel light either to converge or to diverge. To cause light to converge, a lens must be thicker in the middle than at the edges. Convergence occurs because the light striking the lens at a greater angle (the edges) will be bent through a larger angle and will therefore gather on the far side of the lens with light that came through other positions of the lens.

To cause light to diverge, the lens must be thicker at the edges. Divergence occurs because light bent toward the normal at a greater distance from the center of the lens upon entrance will be directed further outward due to the direction of the normal at the surface on exit. The light then appears to come from an object on the near side (or entry side) of the lens. Figure 10-15 shows the effects of the two types of lenses.

All optical developments in this chapter assume that lenses are thin relative to their diameter and that they have a small angle of aperture (Fig. 10-14). This is necessary because spherical optics are not perfect and only approximately focus light. Various aberrations occur that yield a fuzzy image as the lens grows thicker and larger. These aberrations are discussed in detail in Chapter 11. For the present discussion, the assumption will be made that the aberration is insignificant.

The focal length of a lens, which is the distance at which entrant light parallel to the axis is focused, cannot be determined by the same means as those used for a spherical mirror. For a mirror, the focal length is half the radius of curvature. For a lens there are two radii of curvature, and both are bound to have an effect on the final image. As an additional difference, the light reflects off a mirror so

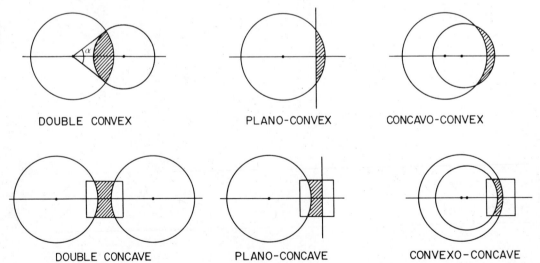

DOUBLE CONVEX   PLANO-CONVEX   CONCAVO-CONVEX

DOUBLE CONCAVE   PLANO-CONCAVE   CONVEXO-CONCAVE

Figure 10-14 The different types of spherical lenses. The shaded areas represent the lenses.

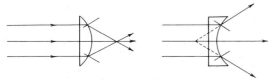

Figure 10-15 Lenses cause rays to converge or diverge, depending upon the relative thickness through a cross section.

the index of refraction has no effect on the position of the final image. Since the light passes through a lens, the effect of the index of refraction is very important.

It is possible by a complex derivation through the application of Snell's law to determine the focal length based on both radii of curvature and the refractive index. Since the equation is not used in future development, we give it here underived.

$$\frac{1}{f} = (\mu - 1)\left(\frac{1}{r_1} + \frac{1}{r_2}\right) \qquad \textbf{(10-46)}$$

The focal length is the same in both directions. This is consistent with the principle that the path of light rays is reversible. It does not matter which side is designated as the front and which side as the back for purposes of light travel. The index of refraction, of course, is always greater than 1. The radii of curvature may be positive, negative, or infinite, depending on the shape of the lens. The radius of curvature for a flat surface is infinite, for a double convex lens both radii are positive, while for a double concave lens both are negative. The other lens forms are left as an exercise for the reader to determine the relevant signs.

EXAMPLE 10-7

If the focal length is 60.1 cm, the index of refraction is 1.634, and one radius of curvature is 14.3 cm, what is the other radius of curvature?

Solution:

$$\frac{1}{f} = (\mu - 1)\left(\frac{1}{r_1} + \frac{1}{r_2}\right)$$

$$\frac{1}{r_2} = \frac{1}{f(\mu - 1)} - \frac{1}{r_1}$$

$$\frac{1}{r_2} = \frac{1}{60.1(1.634 - 1)} - \frac{1}{14.3}$$

$$\frac{1}{r_2} = -0.0437$$

$$r_2 = -22.9 \text{ cm} \qquad \blacksquare$$

Let us now turn to the converging lens. To discover what will happen, it is necessary to trace rays, as in the case of the mirror. Again, the task is simplified by using rays that can easily be sketched, the principal rays. For a lens, there are three such rays:

1. A ray that leaves the object and passes through the optical center of the lens is undeflected.
2. A ray that leaves the object and strikes the lens parallel to its axis will pass through the focus on the other side (F').
3. A ray that leaves the object and passes through the focus on the near side (F) will emerge parallel to the axis of the lens.

An example of what happens when an object is placed in front of a converging lens is given in Figure 10-16. The three principal rays are traced to determine the image, although only two are really needed. We can determine the relative position of the image if we do an analysis similar to the one we

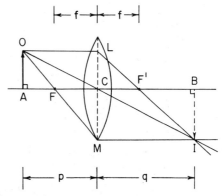

Figure 10-16 A converging lens forms a real, but inverted, image on the other side of the lens from an object outside the focus.

used for mirrors:

$$\angle OCA = \angle ICB \qquad (10\text{-}47)$$

Opposite angles

$$\triangle OCA \sim \triangle ICB \qquad (10\text{-}48)$$

Three corresponding angles

Therefore

$$\frac{OA}{IB} = \frac{AC}{BC} \qquad (10\text{-}49)$$

Ratio of corresponding parts

$$\angle LF'C = \angle IF'B \qquad (10\text{-}50)$$

Opposite angles

$$\triangle LF'C \sim \triangle IF'B \qquad (10\text{-}51)$$

Three corresponding angles

Therefore

$$\frac{LC}{IB} = \frac{CF'}{BF'} \qquad (10\text{-}52)$$

Corresponding parts

$$LC = OA \qquad (10\text{-}53)$$

Opposite sides of rectangle

$$\frac{OA}{IB} = \frac{CF'}{BF'} \qquad (10\text{-}54)$$

Things equal to the same thing are equal

From Eq. 10-49:

$$\frac{AC}{BC} = \frac{CF'}{BF'} \qquad (10\text{-}55)$$

Things equal to the same thing are equal

We can now substitute the same values for the distances: $AC = p$, $BC = q$, $CF' = f$, $BF' = q - f$. Therefore

$$\frac{p}{q} = \frac{f}{q - f} \qquad (10\text{-}56)$$

By cross-multiplication

$$pq - pf = qf$$

By division by pqf,

$$\frac{1}{p} + \frac{1}{q} = \frac{1}{f} \qquad (10\text{-}57)$$

This is precisely the same equation we obtained when we studied the mirror. Therefore, the mirror equation is also the lens equation. If we substitute into Eq. 10-49 for image (S_i) and object (S_o) sizes, we get

$$S_i = \frac{q}{p} S_o \qquad (10.58)$$

This is again the same equation as for the mirror. Note that the signs of all three items are positive in Eq. 10-56. The object distance is positive if it is on the front side of the lens. For lenses, object distances can be negative. The image distance is positive if the image is behind the lens. In such cases the image is real. The focal length is positive if the lens is a converging lens but is negative if the lens is a diverging lens. We will see examples of all these cases later.

Let us consider what happens to the image of a converging lens as the object approaches the lens. When it is far away, $1/p$ is small so $1/q$ is nearly $1/f$ (Eq. 10-57) and the image is close to the focus and relatively small (Eq. 10-58). As the object approaches the focus, the image moves further away and becomes very large. When the object reaches the focus, the image distance becomes infinite and no image is formed.

When the object moves inside the focus, we have the situation illustrated in Figure 10-17. The lens is no longer powerful enough to focus the diverging light from the object to form a real image. Instead, the best it can do is form a virtual image on the same side of the lens as the object. The tracing of the principal rays shows the location of the image.

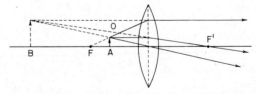

Figure 10-17 A virtual image is formed when the object is inside the focal length of a converging lens.

Table 10-2 Various Images Formed by Refraction

			Image		
Type of Lens	Object Position	Type	Location	Direction	Size vs Object
Converging	$p = \infty$	None	$q = f'$	None	Point
Converging	$\infty > p > 2f$	Real	$2f' > q > f'$	Inverted	Smaller
Converging	$p = 2f$	Real	$q = 2f'$	Inverted	Same
Converging	$2f > p > f$	Real	$\infty > q > 2f'$	Inverted	Larger
Converging	$p = f$	None	$q = \infty$	None	Infinite
Converging	$0 < p < f$	Virtual	$q < 0$	Erect	Larger
Converging	$p < 0$	Real	$0 < q < f'$	Erect	Smaller
Diverging	$\infty > p > 0$	Virtual	$-p < q < 0$	Erect	Smaller
Diverging	$0 > p > -f'$	Real	$f' < q < \infty$	Erect	Larger
Diverging	$p = -f'$	None	$q = \infty$	None	Infinite
Diverging	$p < -f'$	Virtual	$q < 0$	Erect	Smaller

For Eq. 10-57, it is clear that if $p < f$, then $q < 0$. This gives rise to the result shown. Because the image is outside the object, it is larger than the object.

If we examine a diverging lens, we again discover that we get a virtual image as shown in Figure 10-18. Here the image is always trapped between the object and the lens. No matter how close or far the object, the lens will always direct the light more outward so that it appears to come from a source closer to the lens. In a principal ray diagram for a diverging lens, the rays appear to be heading toward or away from a focus, although they do not actually pass through a focus. For the diverging lens, the focal length and image distance are both negative. Table 10-2 shows the various combinations of lens and object positions.

EXAMPLE 10-8

An object 18.35 cm in height produces a virtual image of 12.51 cm in height when placed before a lens. What is the focal length of the lens if the object was 42.3 cm from the lens?

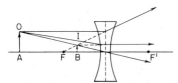

Figure 10-18 A diverging lens always produces a virtual image closer to the lens than the object.

Solution:

$$S_i = \frac{q}{p} S_o$$

$$q = \frac{S_i}{S_o} p = \frac{-12.51}{18.35} \times 42.3$$

Note that since the image is virtual, S_i has a negative sign.

$$q = -28.84$$

$$\frac{1}{f} = \frac{1}{p} + \frac{1}{q} = \frac{1}{42.3} - \frac{1}{28.84}$$

$$\frac{1}{f} = -0.01103$$

$$f = -90.6 \text{ cm} \qquad \blacksquare$$

The simple lens does have some uses. A magnifying glass is nothing but a converging lens held so the object is just inside the focal length. More complex applications require the use of lenses in combination. Figure 10-19 shows such a combination of lenses. The light passes through the first lens to form an image. The image, however, is just a point in space. The light rays continue to travel in a straight line and pass through a second lens that focuses them to form another image. In effect, the image of one lens has served as the object for another lens. Several facts must be considered concerning such an arrangement. An image is not a real object, so the lenses must be aligned for light to pass through the second lens and form a second

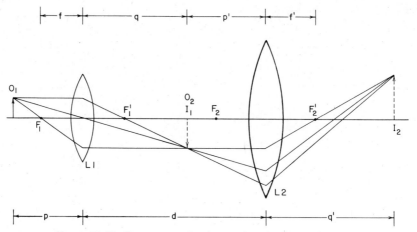

Figure 10-19 Two converging lenses form consecutive images.

image. The lenses must be along the same axis or distortion will occur. The relative positioning of the lens is important to get the final image at the correct place. Let us look at an example of two converging lenses used together.

EXAMPLE 10-9

The focal length of lens L1 is 24.2 cm and that of lens L2 is 19.60 cm. If these lenses are 78.9 cm apart and an object is placed 52.0 cm in front of lens L1, where will the object be?

Solution: For L1,

$$\frac{1}{f} = \frac{1}{p} + \frac{1}{q}$$

$$\frac{1}{q} = \frac{1}{f} - \frac{1}{p} = \frac{1}{24.2} - \frac{1}{52.0}$$

$$\frac{1}{q} = 0.02209$$

$$q = 45.3 \text{ cm}$$

Since $I_1 = O_2$, the object distance of the second lens will be the distance between lenses minus the image distance:

$$p' = d - q = 78.9 - 45.3$$

$$p' = 33.6 \text{ cm}$$

For L2,

$$\frac{1}{f'} = \frac{1}{p'} + \frac{1}{q'}$$

$$\frac{1}{q'} = \frac{1}{f'} - \frac{1}{p'} = \frac{1}{19.6} - \frac{1}{33.6}$$

$$\frac{1}{q'} = 0.02126$$

$$q' = 47.0 \text{ cm beyond L2}$$

Both images in Figure 10-19 are real.   ∎

It is possible to generate a general form for the image sizes created by multiple lenses, because at each lens the size of the image is a function only of the object size, the image, and object distances, as seen in Eq. 10-58. Since the image of one is the object of the next, we can substitute Eq. 10-58 into itself.

$$S_i' = \left(\frac{q'}{p'}\right)\left(\frac{q}{p}\right) S_o \qquad \textbf{(10-59)}$$

This process can be carried out indefinitely to give the overall object size. By substituting for p' in terms of q and d, we get the following for Figure 10-19.

$$S_i' = \left(\frac{q'}{d - q}\right)\left(\frac{q}{p}\right) S_o \qquad \textbf{(10-60)}$$

This expression is called the magnification factor.

Since the image is only a point in space and since it is the light rays that are actually being captured, it is not even necessary for the first image to form in order to form the second. Figure 10-20 gives an example of this phenomenon. A converging lens would cause an image to form at distance q if the light were not intercepted by a diverging lens. In this case, we have assumed that the diverging lens is relatively weak and is only capable of postponing the convergence of light. A more powerful diverging lens could have prevented a real image from forming. Note that for the second lens, the object is virtual because it is on the wrong side of the lens. Objects formed by previous lenses then do not have to be real to be used. It must be remembered that we are manipulating light rays with lenses and that objects and images are simply points in space.

Finally, let us look at the case where a mirror is inserted into the light path. This causes the light to change direction, but does not alter the relative geometry of the light rays to each other. As a consequence, converging light will continue to converge while diverging light will continue to diverge. Figure 10-21 shows an example of what happens as light is reflected. The events are measured along the line, which is the reflected axis of the lens. Such manipulation of the light beam is common in analytical instruments as a means of increasing the length of the light path without increasing the size of the instrument. Spherical mirrors as well as total reflection prisms and front surface mirrors (defined later) are used.

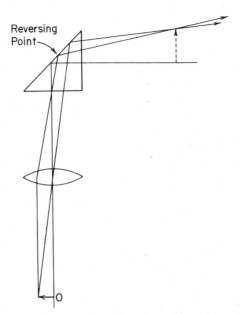

Figure 10-21 Light passing through a converging lens is reflected by a prism before it can form an image.

Section **10-5**
DISPERSION AND DIFFRACTION

When light enters a substance, refraction occurs as has been previously discussed. The light rays have previously been treated as if they moved through each substance as a unified quantity. This, however, is not really the case, although under many conditions such an approximation is adequate. In other cases it becomes obvious that white light is not a simple entity. Refraction can cause white light to break up into a rainbow of colors called the spectrum.

The reason that refraction can cause light to disperse into a spectrum is that the speed of light through a substance is not the same for each wavelength of light. White light is made up of a large cross section of the electromagnetic spectrum. In a vacuum all these wavelengths propagate at the same speed. When they are refracted, their different relative speeds through the inhibiting substance appear as differences in the refractive index of the

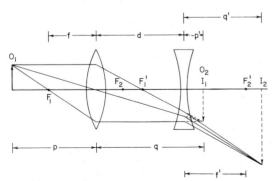

Figure 10-20 A diverging lens is shown delaying the formation of the images of a converging lens.

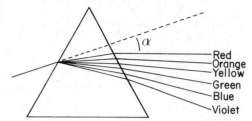

Figure 10-22 A prism disperses white light into its component colors.

substance. Since the refractive index is a factor in Snell's law, the angle through which the light is bent is directly affected by this difference.

Fig. 10-22 shows how the light is split into various colors by a prism. Violet, which has the short-

est wavelength, is retarded the most by the prism and therefore is refracted the most toward the normal and away from the line of entry. Note how the angle (usually near 60°) between the entering and departing faces of the prism causes the effect of the different refractive indices to be compounded instead of canceled as the light emerges from the prism.

Many laboratory instruments require that only a specific wavelength of light be used for the measurement of an unknown concentration. The need for a single wavelength arises from Beer's law and the absorption spectra of the various compounds in the reaction mixture, as discussed in Chapter 15. To measure a variety of substances with the same analytical instrument may require the use of many different wavelengths. To obtain them, one could

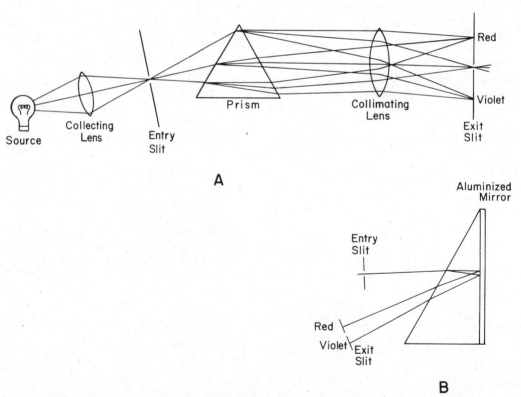

Figure 10-23 Part A is the Cornu-type mounting for a prism. Part B is the Littrow-type mounting for a prism. Collecting lenses are also used with it to increase the amount of radiation, but are omitted to simplify the drawing.

use different light sources. Since this is usually impractical, it is desirable to get the various wavelengths from the same white light source by splitting the white light into its component wavelengths. A prism can be used to do such dispersion.

Figure 10-23A shows a prism mounting that will disperse light into a spectrum. This arrangement is called the Cornu-type mounting. The light from the source is collected by a converging lens and focused on a narrow entry slit. The collecting lens enables a high proportion of the light from the source to enter the measuring chamber of the instrument. The entry slit assures that all the light originates from one point. If it does not, then destructive interference will make it impossible to get a spectrum. The light, following various paths as directed by the first converging lens, passes through the prism and is dispersed. The various light paths then pass through a second converging lens that causes the various colors to be focused along the blackened back of the prism housing. At one point along the back is a narrow exit slit. The exit slit selects only a small portion of the spectrum for use in making the measurement. By making the entrance and exit slits relatively narrow, a band of light that is nearly uniform in wavelength can be obtained. The limitations are the minimum amount of radiation needed to make the measurement and interference from diffraction as the slits get very small. Another lens, after the exit slit, may be used to collimate the light beam before it passes through the specimen.

The prism in Figure 10-23A is on a wheel that permits it to be rotated. As the prism rotates, different areas of the spectrum are focused on the exit slit. This allows the desired wavelength of light to be selected. The major disadvantages of this type of dispersion mounting are the limitation on the narrowness of wavelength bundle (called band pass) that one can get due to the slit size, the nonlinearity of the spectrum that one obtains as one rotates the prism, and the size of the instrument needed to carry out the dispersion.

The latter problem is solved by use of the Littrow-type mounting, as shown in Figure 10-23B. In this case, the prism is only one-half the Cornu-type prism, but the light passes through it twice. The same type of dispersion occurs, but the size of the

dispersion unit is much smaller. Note that the mirror on the back of the prism is, in effect, a front-surface mirror. Light is not allowed to enter the mirror, as it does a bathroom mirror, because this would cause refraction at the mirror surface, reflection at its back and refraction again at its surface. Such additional changes in the direction of light only make a complicated situation worse. Front-surface mirrors are created by using highly polished metal which, in this case, is bonded to or sprayed on the back of the prism.

Refraction is not the only means by which the breaking up of light can be accomplished. A second means uses the principle of diffraction. A diffraction grating is illustrated in Figure 10-24. Diffraction is a result of the wave properties of light. It occurs when numerous parallel surfaces are spaced at distances which are close to the incident wavelength of light. Under this condition the reflections from individual planes are not in phase with each other in all directions. Instead, the wavefronts for each wavelength coincide only at certain angles to the diffraction grating. Consequently, different wavelengths are seen at different angles.

A diffraction grating has numerous parallel planes which make an angle to the flat surface called the blaze angle β. This angle is the same for all the planes. The cut-outs that form the planes are called lines and run straight and parallel for the whole height of the grating. Approximately 4,000–20,000 lines/cm are in common commercial gratings. The grating is usually made of an epoxy resin with a polished aluminized surface to cause surface reflection.

In order to see how the grating works, let us follow two parallel rays of light in a wavefront destined to strike the grating at the corresponding spot on two adjacent planes. When A reaches the grating, B is still a distance off. As can be seen in Figure 10-24, this distance is d_1. Moreover, we know from trigonometry

$$\sin \alpha = \frac{d_1}{d} \qquad \textbf{(10-61)}$$

Angle α is the same as angle ϕ, the angle the wavefront makes with the normal to the grating because angle α is supplementary to the angle opposite an-

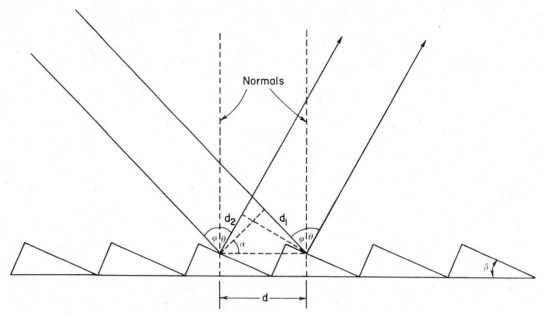

Figure 10-24 Light striking a grating is reflected as from a mirror. Since the surface is a series of parallel planes, only those wavelengths of light that are in phase will emerge. The rest will be destroyed by interference.

gle ϕ in a right triangle. Therefore

$$\sin \phi = \frac{d_1}{d} \qquad \textbf{(10-62)}$$

and

$$d_1 = d \sin \phi \qquad \textbf{(10-63)}$$

When ray A is reflected from the grating, it must travel a larger distance than ray B. That extra distance, d_2, can be computed in the same way.

$$d_2 = d \sin \theta \qquad \textbf{(10-64)}$$

The difference in the path length is then the difference between these two distances.

$$\Delta d = |d_1 - d_2| \qquad \textbf{(10-65)}$$

$$\Delta d = d|\sin \phi - \sin \theta| \qquad \textbf{(10-66)}$$

If we now recognize that wavefronts are nothing more than specific points on the light waves and occur once per wavelength, then constructive reinforcement will occur every time Δd in Eq. 10-66 is equal to a whole number of wavelengths. We

therefore have

$$m\lambda = d|\sin \phi - \sin \theta| \qquad \textbf{(10-67)}$$

In this expression m is a positive integer, indicating the order (harmonics) of the reflection and λ is the wavelength of the light.

Several factors relating to the grating equation (10-67) should be noted. First, one will get no reflection off the grating if angle ϕ is equal to angle θ. Second, the angles are measured from the normal to the grating surface plane, not the normal to the actual surface point where the light impinges. If angles ϕ and θ are both on the same side of normal (which is possible), then angle θ is taken to be negative. In such cases, Eq. 10-67 is frequently written with a plus sign and angle θ substituted as positive. Finally, the number of lines per centimeter, and therefore d, affects the wavelength. For good results over a wide area of the spectrum, several gratings with a substantially different number of lines per centimeter are most effective. Several mounts are available for gratings. These will be discussed in Chapter 14.

The light that emerges from a diffraction grating has several component wavelengths. These are harmonics of the first-order wavelength and cannot be removed by the grating. Filters can be used to remove these undesired wavelengths, as will be described in later chapters.

EXAMPLE 10-10

If the incident light makes a 74.2° angle to the normal and the resultant light leaves at an angle of 64.3° on the other side of the normal, what are the wavelengths of the first three orders of diffraction if there are $1.50 \cdot 10^4$ lines/inch in the grating?

Solution: Convert the dimensions to metric.

$$D = 1.50 \cdot 10^4 \text{ lines/inch}$$
$$\times 39.37 \text{ inch/meter}$$

$$D = 5.91 \cdot 10^5 \text{ lines/meter}$$

$$d = \frac{1}{D} = \frac{1}{5.91 \cdot 10^5}$$
$$= 1.69 \cdot 10^{-6} \text{ meter}$$

$$m\lambda = d|\sin \phi - \sin \theta|$$

$$\lambda = \frac{1.69 \cdot 10^{-6}}{1} |\sin 74.2 - \sin 64.3|$$

$$\lambda_1 = 103 \text{ nm}$$

If $m = 2$ $\lambda_2 = 52 \text{ nm}$

If $m = 3$ $\lambda_3 = 34.4 \text{ nm}$ ∎

The use of optics will be discussed in more detail as we examine specific instruments. The principles of reflection, refraction, diffraction, and dispersion are all extensively used in analytical machinery. The limitations inherent in optical design or when competing optical principles are involved will be discussed as necessary. The first instrument to be examined will be the microscope.

REVIEW QUESTIONS

1. Give some examples of light as waves and light as particles.
2. What are the two laws of reflection?
3. What is a normal to a plane?
4. What is specular reflection? What is diffuse reflection?
5. How can specular and diffuse reflection occur from the same surface?
6. Why does the image appear behind a plane mirror?
7. Why can an object not directly in front of a mirror be seen in the mirror?
8. What is the difference between a real and a virtual image?
9. What is a paraboloid? How does one create one?
10. Why is a paraboloid useful as a mirror?
11. Give some uses of parabolic reflectors.
12. How are spherical mirrors formed?
13. How do spherical mirrors differ from parabolic mirrors?
14. What are the two types of spherical mirrors?
15. Define focus.
16. Define radius of curvature.
17. What is the relationship between the focus and the radius of curvature for a spherical mirror?
18. What are the four principal rays of a spherical mirror?
19. Why are the object and image interchangeable?
20. What determines if an image is real or virtual?
21. What is the mirror equation?
22. How are the sizes of the image and object of a mirror related?
23. Around what point do the image and object of a mirror balance?
24. Where is the image for a concave mirror when the object is outside the radius of curvature? Inside the radius of curvature? Inside the focus?
25. What does a negative image size imply?
26. What are the properties of a convex mirror?
27. Why is the image of a convex mirror always smaller than the object?
28. Where is the focus of a convex mirror? Why?
29. Where is the focus of a plane mirror? Why?
30. Define refraction.
31. What are the three laws of refraction?
32. What is the equation for Snell's law?
33. Define index of refraction.
34. What is the difference between the relative and absolute index of refraction?
35. Define total reflection.

36. What is necessary to have total reflection?
37. What are some laboratory uses of total reflection?
38. If light enters a pane of glass, in which direction will it emerge?
39. What geometric shapes are the faces of a lens?
40. What are the six types of lenses possible?
41. Into what two classes are lenses divided? What are the properties of each class?
42. Why must lenses be thin? What else is this property called?
43. What is the lensmaker's equation?
44. How does the focal length of a lens differ from that of a mirror?
45. What are the principal rays for a lens?
46. What is the lens equation?
47. How are the sizes of the images and objects related?
48. For a converging lens, what is the image position if the object is outside the focus? Inside the focus? On the back side of the lens?
49. Where do real and virtual images appear for a lens compared to for a mirror?
50. Where is the image for a diverging lens if the object is real?
51. What is the relative size of the image in question 50?
52. How can a real image be formed with a diverging lens?
53. How does a magnifying glass work?
54. What are important things to remember when combining lenses?
55. How is the size of the image formed by multiple lenses determined?
56. Why can some lenses in a multilens combination form an image from a virtual object?
57. What effect does a mirror have on a converging beam of light?
58. Why are total reflection prisms used in analytical instruments?
59. Define dispersion.
60. Why does dispersion occur?
61. Why are dispersing devices used in analytical instruments?
62. How does a prism work?
63. Why are entry and exit slits used?
64. Explain the Cornu-type mounting.
65. How does the Littrow-type mounting work?
66. What is diffraction?
67. Define blaze angle.
68. What is a line on a grating?
69. How does a grating work?
70. What is a wavefront?
71. What is the formula for the wavelengths from a grating?
72. Why do harmonic wavelengths come off the grating?

PROBLEMS

1. If an object 14.0 cm high is 71 cm in front of a concave mirror of focal length 13.0 cm, where will the image be and what will be its size?
2. If the image appears 32.4 cm in front of a concave mirror having a radius of curvature of 43.6 cm and the image is 12.7 cm tall, where and how big is the object?
3. If the object is 28.2 cm in front of a concave mirror and the image is 67.1 cm in front of the mirror, what is the focal length of the mirror?
4. An object of 9.83 cm produces a real image of 6.91 cm when placed in front of a mirror with a focal length of 34.4 cm. Where are the object and the image?
5. If an object is placed 7.82 cm from a concave mirror of focal length 11.26 cm, it produces a virtual image 12.13 cm tall. What is the object size and where is the image located?
6. The image produced by a concave mirror of focal length 21.6 cm is 14.3 cm behind the mirror and 1.82 cm tall. Where and how big is the object?
7. An object 17.3 cm tall is located 87.3 cm in front of a convex mirror of focal length 31.9 cm. Where and how big is the image?
8. If the object is 71.4 cm in front of the mirror and the image 8.91 cm behind the mirror, what is the focal length and the type of the mirror?
9. Light enters a material with a relative refractive index of 1.643 at an angle of 53.2° to the surface. What angle will it make to the surface in the material?

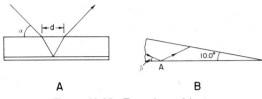

Figure 10-25 Two glass objects.

10. Light leaving a material with an index of refraction of 1.442 at a 42.6° angle to the normal enters another material and is bent at 34.7° to the normal. What is the index of refraction of the second material?

11. Light enters a pane of glass at an angle of 57.7° to the surface. If the glass has a relative index of refraction of 1.587 and a thickness of 1.702 cm, what will be the displacement of the light?

12. Light follows the path indicated in Figure 10-25A. If angle α is 46.1°, what is d if the glass plate is 3.89 cm thick and has a relative index of refraction of 1.511?

13. Light strikes the wall of the prism in Figure 10-25B at point A and experiences total reflection. If angle $\beta = 14.6°$ and the relative index of refraction is 2.073, how many times after point A will the light be reflected before leaving the prism?

14. If the radii of curvature for a lens are 64.3 cm and 51.1 cm and the focal length is 41.6 cm, what is the refractive index of the lens?

15. If one radius of curvature for a lens is 47.5 cm, if the index of refraction is 1.498, and if the focal length is 42.8 cm, what is the other radius of curvature?

16. The focal length of a converging lens is 22.0 cm. If an object 4.9 cm high is placed 31.3 cm in front of the lens, where will the image be? How big will it be?

17. If the focal length of a converging lens is 30.2 cm and an image is produced 61.3 cm beyond the lens, where is the object? If the object is 21.6 cm tall, how big is the image?

18. The object is on one side of a converging lens and the image on the other. If the object distance is 18.6 cm and the image distance 91.7 cm, what is the focal length of the lens?

19. An object 6.4 cm tall is placed 17.1 cm in front of a converging lens of focal length 22.5 cm. Where is the image and what is its size?

20. The object is 31.3 cm in front of a converging lens and the image is 57.2 cm in front of the lens. What is the focal length?

21. An object of 14.7 cm is placed 81.4 cm in front of a diverging lens of focal length 35.0 cm. What is the image size and distance?

22. An object placed 63.1 cm in front of a diverging lens produces an image 38.7 cm in front of the lens. What is the focal length?

23. In Figure 10-19 the focal length of L1 is 25.5 cm and the focal length of L2 is 16.9 cm. If an object 9.6 cm tall is placed 62.1 cm to the left of lens L1, where and what size will the final image be if the lenses are 61.4 cm apart?

24. Assume that lenses L1 and L2 in Figure 10-19 have focal lengths of 14.0 cm and 27.3 cm, respectively, and are 33.2 cm apart. Assume that a third lens, a diverging lens of focal length 44.0 cm, is placed 38.0 cm to the right of L2. If an object 1.87 cm tall is placed 20.0 cm to the left of L2, where and how big will the image be?

25. In Fig. 10-20, the focal length of the converging lens is 29.7 cm and that of the diverging lens is 86.9 cm. If the lenses are 36.0 cm apart and a 12.5-cm-high image forms 47.2 cm beyond the diverging lens, where and how big was the object?

26. Where should a second lens of focal length 25.0 cm be placed in Figure 10-21 to focus the image on a plate 60.0 cm beyond where the light is bent by the prism? Assume the first lens has a focal length of 30.0 cm and is 20.0 cm in front of the prism. Also assume that the object is 40.0 cm in front of the first lens.

27. A converging lens of focal length 20.1 cm sits 31.6 cm in front of a plane mirror. An object is placed in front of the lens so that the light passes through the lens and strikes the mirror and passes through the lens again to form an image twice the distance from the lens that the object is. If the object is outside the focus, where is it?

28. Light strikes a grating ruled at 687 lines/mm at

an angle of 68.3° and is diffracted at an angle of 47.1°. What are the wavelengths of the first three orders of light that are in phase coming from the grating?

29. Light strikes a grating at an angle of 57.6° and is diffracted at an angle of 44.8°. If the first-order

wavelength is 436 nm, what are the number of lines per millimeter?

30. When the incident light strikes a grating at 61.4°, light of first-order wavelength 381 nm emerges. If there are 1,194 lines/mm, at what angle does the light emerge?

CHAPTER 11
MICROSCOPES

Lenses and lens combinations must be arranged not only to produce an image, but to produce an image at a place and of a size that will facilitate its study. One of the common applications of lenses is in the making of microscopes. This is important for examination of cellular material and crystalline structures found in the body fluids and tissues.

Section 11-1
NATURE OF THE MICROSCOPE

The most elementary microscope, frequently called a simple microscope, uses only one converging lens. To obtain magnification, the object must be placed just inside the focal length. This creates an image that is virtual and erect, as shown in Figure 11-1A. This is the configuration of the magnifying glass. In order for the simple microscope to work, it must have a rather short focal length. If it is large, the image, which is beyond the focal point, will be too distant for the eye to view clearly. The average eye works best at 25 cm from the image being observed.

One can calculate the magnification if one first defines some terms and makes some simplifying assumptions. Magnification can be expressed as the tangent of the angle subtended by the image of the lens divided by the tangent of the angle subtended when the object is at the optimum viewing distance (Fig. 11-1B). This is written as

$$M = \frac{\tan \iota}{\tan \omega} = \frac{S_i/|q|}{S_o/E} \tag{11-1}$$

or, by rearranging,

$$M = \frac{S_i}{S_o} \times \frac{E}{|q|} \tag{11-2}$$

From Eq. 10-58, we can substitute for the ratio of the sizes to get

$$M = \frac{|q|}{p} \times \frac{E}{|q|}$$

$$M = \frac{E}{p} \tag{11-3}$$

The reason the object distance must be small is now apparent. If p is large, M will be small unless E, the distance from the eye, is very large. If we now substitute the lens equation for $1/p$, we get

$$M = \frac{E}{f} - \frac{E}{q} \tag{11-4}$$

We can now make a simplifying observation. Let us define the distance of the image to the eye as D. If the eye is close to the lens, this distance is effectively the distance of the lens to the image $(-q)$. We therefore have

$$D \approx -q \tag{11-5}$$

$$M = \frac{E}{f} + \frac{E}{D} \tag{11-6}$$

If one recalls that E, the optimum viewing distance, is about 25 cm for the average eye, one can appreciate the amount of magnification that can be obtained. To get strong magnification, f must be short, usually only a few centimeters. Distortion of the image by the lens is hard to prevent as the focal length approaches zero. Increasing M beyond 5× or 10× by this means is difficult. ("×" means times.) Increasing M by changing the ratio E/D is even more difficult. To make $D < E$ creates serious eye strain. If the image is moved toward infinity, the eye can continue to hold the image in focus if there is no distortion by the lens. Therefore, E/D

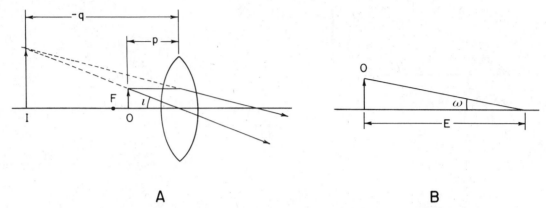

A   **B**

Figure 11-1 The relationship of the image to the object is shown in Part A and the angle subtended by the object without the lens present in Part B. *E* is the distance from the eye to the object.

contributes little to the magnification once D is several times E. E, and therefore the magnification, will vary with the eye characteristics of the viewer. Lenses are rated based on $E = 25$ cm.

EXAMPLE 11-1

A magnification of $6.7\times$ is obtained if someone with an optimum viewing distance of 28 cm looks through a simple microscope at an image 53 cm away. What is the focal length of the lens?

Solution: Use Eq. 11-6.

$$M = \frac{E}{f} + \frac{E}{D}$$

Solve for f:

$$\frac{E}{f} = M - \frac{E}{D}$$

$$\frac{1}{f} = \frac{M}{E} - \frac{1}{D}$$

$$\frac{1}{f} = \frac{6.7}{28} - \frac{1}{53} = 0.220$$

$$f = 4.5 \text{ cm} \qquad \blacksquare$$

The simple microscope is most effectively used when it magnifies an image that has already been

enlarged from the original. Such a microscope has two stages of magnification and is called a compound microscope. The diagram of such a microscope is shown in Figure 11-2. The simple microscope portion of it is the piece the viewer looks through, and is, therefore, called the eyepiece. The other lens is very close to the object and is called the objective.

For a compound microscope to work, the object must be just outside the focal length of the objective. This will cause a real image to form at a large distance beyond the objective. This area is referred to as the barrel of the microscope. The image must be real because it will act as the object for the second stage of the microscope, namely the eyepiece.

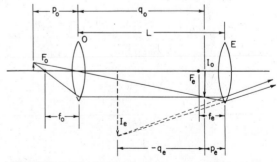

Figure 11-2 The compound microscope features two lenses, an objective and an eyepiece.

For the eyepiece to be of use, the first image must fall just inside the focal point of the eyepiece. The real image of the objective will be inverted; therefore, the virtual image of the eyepiece will also be inverted and will be pushed back up the barrel of the microscope toward the objective. Accuracy of placement is essential to obtaining an image of appropriate magnification and clarity. Characteristics of good objectives and eyepieces are discussed later in this chapter.

The magnification attained by a compound microscope is the product of the magnification of the objective and the eyepiece. If the objective lens produces an image twice the size of the object and the eyepiece doubles the size of the image, logically the final image is four times the size of the object. We therefore have

$$M = M_o M_e \qquad \textbf{(11-7)}$$

In common microscopes the magnifications are stamped onto the eyepiece and objective, and calculations are trivial using this equation. To find it in terms of more elementary quantities, we substitute from Eq. 10-58,

$$M_o = \frac{S_i}{S_o} = \frac{q}{p} \qquad \textbf{(11-8)}$$

Substituting this and Eq. 11-6 into Eq. 11-7 gives

$$M = \left(\frac{q_o}{p_o}\right)\left(\frac{E}{f_e} + \frac{E}{D}\right) \qquad \textbf{(11-9)}$$

This equation can be simplified if three assumptions are made:

1. p_o is almost the same as f_o ($p_o \approx f_o$). **(11-10)**
2. If D is large compared with f_e, then
   E/D is small relative to E/f_e
   ($E/D \approx 0$). **(11-11)**
3. If f_e is short, then q_o is almost the distance between the two lenses ($q_o \approx L$). **(11-12)**

Making these substitutions, one gets

$$M \approx \frac{LE}{f_o f_e} \qquad \textbf{(11-13)}$$

If E is 25 cm, then the magnification of a compound microscope can be found, at least to a first approximation, by Eq. 11-13. Note that greater magnification is obtained by lengthening the barrel

(L) and shortening the focal length of the lenses. These factors will be important in the description of real microscopes such as those used in the clinical laboratory.

EXAMPLE 11-2

Find the length of a microscope if the magnification is 143X, the focal length of the objective is 4.7 cm, and the focal length of the eyepiece is 3.4 cm.

Solution:

$$M = \frac{LE}{f_o f_e}$$

$$L = \frac{M f_o f_e}{E}$$

$$L = \frac{143 \times 4.7 \times 3.4}{25}$$

$$L = 91 \text{ cm} \qquad \blacksquare$$

Section **11-2**
STRUCTURE OF A BINOCULAR LABORATORY MICROSCOPE

Figure 11-3 shows the general layout of a binocular microscope such as is commonly used in the clinical laboratory. In this section we will examine the four sections of the microscope as indicated in Figure 11-3. These are the illumination system (A), the objective (B), the redirecting (zooming) system (C), and the eyepiece (D), all of which are complex, multilens systems in commonly used microscopes.

It all starts with the illumination system. In order to see the specimen, every point of the specimen must act as a source of light. As you will recall from Chapter 10, rays of light leave the object in all directions. The various parts of the object will have different abilities to act as sources of radiation depending on how well they can transmit light. Those areas that are less able to transmit radiation will appear darker to the viewer. To cause this differentiation in coloration to occur evenly is the goal of the illumination system.

The most common type of illumination is called Koehler illumination (Fig. 11-4). The source of the

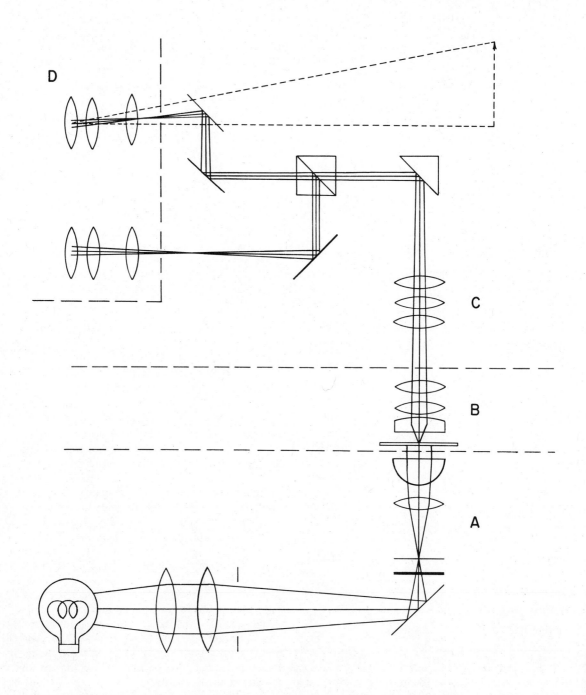

Figure 11-3 The overall diagram of a complex binocular microscope. The parts are the illuminating system (A), objective (B), redirecting system (C), and eyepiece (D).

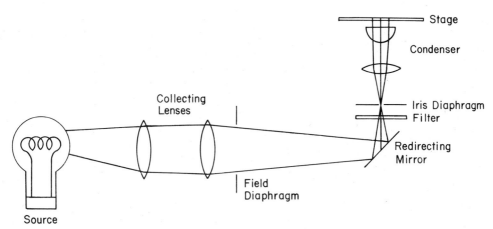

Figure 11-4 The Koehler illumination method. (Courtesy of Bausch & Lomb Instruments and Systems Division. Redrawn with permission.)

radiation is an incandescent filament bulb, such as tungsten, which gives high intensity over the visible range (see Chapter 14). The radiation is focused by collecting lenses to form a point image just in front of the condenser in the iris diaphragm. One or several collecting lenses are used, depending on the quality of light beam desired. The light beam can be restricted by a field diaphragm which serves to control the intensity of the light that reaches the specimen. (Excessively bright light is hard on the eyes.) The same effect can be accomplished by the application of a variable voltage to the light source. A variable-voltage divider, called a rheostat, is used for such control.

To reduce the size of the microscope, the light path is usually bent by means of a plane mirror. A color filter may be placed above the mirror to increase the contrast. Usually the filter is made of colored glass and allows a relatively wide band of light radiation to pass through. Interference filters can be employed to get narrower wavelength bundles, but these are not commonly used in the clinical laboratory. (The operation of these filters is discussed in Chapter 14.) If certain areas of the object are of a certain color, removing that color with a filter will cause those areas to appear dark, while the rest of the specimen will appear bright. This can be helpful where different colored areas overlap or partly obscure one another.

After traversing the filter, the light forms an image of the source in the aperture (iris) diaphragm. The purpose of this diaphragm is to control the size of the light cone that impinges on the specimen and is available to the objective. An objective has a certain light gathering ability called numerical aperture (N.A.), which will be discussed shortly. If the illumination system illuminates a larger area of the specimen than the objective can gather light from, the excess light is wasted, and the field is brightened to the point that details of the specimen are washed out. By use of the iris diaphragm, the numerical aperture of the illuminating radiation can be reduced until it is less than that of the objective. Continued closing down of the iris diaphragm will increase contrast, but it will also decrease resolution, the ability to distinguish two adjacent points. A balance must be struck between contrast and resolution for each specimen to get the most usable viewing field.

The final element of the illuminating system is the condenser, often called the substage condenser. This device is composed of two or more lenses that create the illuminated area on the specimen slide from the incident radiation. The lens closest to the specimen is abnormally shaped to give a flattened top surface in close proximity to the specimen slide. It bends light sharply to create the cone of illumination. One or more lenses prepare the light before it enters the final lens to permit correct focusing. In a more complex condenser, these lenses may compensate for spherical and chromatic aberrations of the light to improve viewing conditions. In the microscopes more commonly used in the clinical laboratory, the condensers are much simpler and do not correct for these aberrations. The typical condenser will produce a numerical aperture of 1.3–1.4, which can be reduced by use of the iris diaphragm.

After the light passes through the specimen on the microscope stage, it enters the objective. The objective is the first of the two lenses in a compound microscope. In laboratory microscopes the objective is itself composed of two or more lenses (Fig. 11-5). The purpose of the objective is twofold.

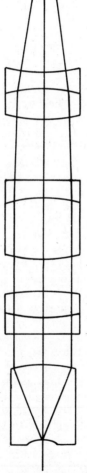

Figure 11-5 An objective may be composed of numerous lenses, all along the same axis. This is a typical flat field objective. (Courtesy of Bausch & Lomb Instruments and Systems Division. Redrawn with permission.)

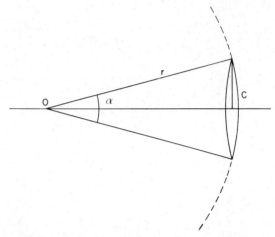

Figure 11-6 The fraction of the diameter of the circle (from which the front surface of the lens was cut) that is illuminated is 2C/d or C/r. C is half a chord and r is the radius of the circle. From trigonometry, we know that this is the sine of one-half alpha.

First, it must gather light from the specimen. Second, it must perform the initial magnification to create a real image to serve as the object for the eyepiece. The light-gathering function is the main duty of the first lens of the objective. The ability of the lens to accomplish this function is quantitated as numerical aperture, as previously mentioned. Figure 11-6 shows how numerical aperture is calculated. The angle of aperture is α (see Chapter 10 for discussion). To find what fraction of the diameter of the sphere from which the front surface of the lens was cut is illuminated, the sine of one-half this angle must be taken. This calculation assumes that light came to the lens in a straight line, that is, through a substance with a refractive index of one, such as air. If a denser material, such as oil, is used to connect the specimen with the objective, the refractive index of this material must be multiplied times the value of the previous calculation because the oil will increase the amount of light pulled into the lens. This gives the equation

$$\text{N.A.} = \mu \sin \frac{\alpha}{2} \qquad \textbf{(11-14)}$$

The use of immersion oil is indeed important in trying to improve the light gathering ability of an objective, since without oil, the maximum N.A. is

1.000, the sine of 90°. At this point, the front surface of the lens is a hemisphere. Moreover, the sine of an angle increases only about 5% between 70° and 90°. The use of oil is therefore necessary to get beyond a N.A. of 0.95. Immersion oil has an index of refraction of 1.5. This is better than water at 1.33, but not as good as some other organic liquids that reach more than 1.6. The practical limit of the numerical aperture for general usage is about 1.4, although higher values have been obtained. In order for the condenser to light the entire numerical aperture of such an objective, it too must be in oil contact with the bottom of the slide. The importance of a high N.A. to the resolving power of the lens will be discussed later.

In order to gather as much light as possible, the first lens in the objective must be far from the theoretical ideal of a thin lens for which we developed the laws of lenses. As a consequence, many types of aberrations are introduced by this first lens of the objective. These will be discussed in detail later. Before the viewer sees the image, the aberrations must be compensated for and minimized. This is accomplished by the rest of the lenses in the objective and the lenses of the eyepiece. For example, the first lens may cause the light to be dispersed in a spectrum by bending red and violet light to different extents. Successive lenses must compensate by making red and violet light coincide or at least be parallel. This may require different shaped lenses and lenses made of different types of glass. When all the corrections have been made, an intermediate image must still be formed at the appropriate place so it can be picked up by the eyepiece. Because of the critical relationship among the lenses, it is best if the objective is sealed to prevent misalignment. Simple objectives have two lenses and do little compensation, while complex compensation schemes may require eight or ten lenses.

The magnifying power of the objective is the ratio of the image distance to the object distance (Eq. 11-8). The distance of the physical object will be very short and is made to appear even shorter by effective lens combinations within the objective. It is, however, desirable to make the image distance as long as possible to increase this ratio. The length of the barrel of the microscope is fixed and must be reasonably short to permit convenient use. The effective lengthening of the barrel, and therefore the image distance, may be accomplished in two ways without increasing the microscope size. First is by the use of reflection as will be discussed in a few paragraphs. The second is through redirecting lenses which will cause the light to appear to be coming from a more distant place and, therefore, to form a larger image. Lenses at various positions in the light path can be used in this effort.

Another advantage that can be obtained through the redirection of light between the objective and eyepiece is to permit "zooming." A zoom lens system has several lenses that are movable by precision cams. As the zoom control is turned, the image becomes larger or smaller smoothly, rather than in increments, as by changing the objective or eyepiece. Usually a factor of 2 can be gained from the minimum to maximum zoom position. By changing objectives and using the zoom feature, a continuous range of magnification can be obtained. For example, all magnifications between 100× and 1000× could be obtained using the appropriate objectives. Details requiring various degrees of magnification can be brought into optimum viewing conditions because the cams in the system keep the specimen continuously in focus during the zooming process.

The concept of the use of reflection to increase the effective barrel length and to make the microscope easier to operate was an important development. The first reflection occurs when the light is bent away from the condenser–objective axis. If the light is not so bent, the eyepiece must be linearly above the objective, which makes the microscope hard to use. This bending is usually accomplished by a total reflection prism to minimize other optical effects that would reduce image quality. All prisms and mirrors used for light redirection have to be made precisely to prevent artifacts from being introduced into the image.

For most convenient viewing, it is best to use a binocular microscope where the image is presented to both eyes. This is accomplished by a beam splitter, a half-silvered, half-transparent surface, which reflects some of the radiation while allowing the rest to pass through it (Fig. 11-3). The two resulting beams are then supplied to separate but matched eyepieces. Special microscopes for teaching include more beam splitters to permit a number of people to see the same slide simultaneously.

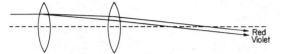

Figure 11-7 The Huygenian eyepiece compensates for the diverging spectrum by making the light parallel again.

The final portion of the microscope is the eyepiece. The purpose of the eyepiece is to compensate for the aberration introduced by the previous optical elements and to create the final image for the viewer. Like the other optical elements of the microscope, the eyepieces of common laboratory microscopes are composed of several lenses. In the simple two-lens combination, the first lens that the light encounters is the field lens and the one closest to the eye is the eye lens. The most common of these eyepieces is the Huygenian eyepiece, which is diagrammed in Figure 11-7. The field lens will tend to disperse the light into colors to some extent and the eye lens must compensate for this by redirecting the light to again make the different colors parallel. If the eye is focused at infinity, there is no color problem. If the lenses do not compensate for the dispersion, the edges of the items in the specimen appear as a spectrum, a phenomenon known as lateral color. The relative position of the eyepiece lenses must be carefully set to ensure compensation. To get optimum color compensation with a complex objective or a zooming system requires a more complex eyepiece with diverging as well as converging lenses.

The final image produced by the eyepiece is seen directly in front of the viewer, even though this is not the location of the object, because the eye and brain assume that light travels in a straight line. The image is diverted as was seen in Figure 11-3. To get the best view of the specimen, the eyepieces of a binocular microscope should be matched because, in reality, two images are formed, one for each eye, and the brain must combine the information.

Section **11-3**
ABERRATION OF LIGHT

If perfect images were formed by lenses obeying all the rules of thin lenses as they were derived in Chapter 10, microscopes would be easy to design and build. Unfortunately, numerous aberrations occur because of the nature of light and the way it passes through interfaces. Seven common optical problems will now be discussed.

Spherical aberration (Fig. 11-8) results from the fact that the outer portion of a spherical lens causes light to be bent more sharply than the inner portion. This light, therefore, has a shorter focal length. When the image is in focus based on the light through the center of the lens, the light from the lens edge is stray radiation, illuminating the general area of the image but not contributing to defining the image. As a consequence there is loss of contrast between the parts of the image, causing the image to be washed out. Naturally this problem becomes more severe as the numerical aperture increases, particularly with a dry objective. To minimize these effects the objective must be the precisely intended distance from the specimen. To compensate for spherical aberration, combinations of converging and diverging lenses are incorporated into the objective to get the short-focused radiation recombined with that through the lens center.

Curvature of field means that the field, that is, the specimen, appears to be curved when examined through the microscope. As a result, the whole field cannot be focused simultaneously. When the center is in focus, the rest of the specimen is blurry, with conditions getting worse the closer to the edge that one goes. This situation is a consequence of designing objective lenses with high light-gathering ability. It occurs because of the optical shortening of the object distance to the objective. To have a flat image, outer parts of the object must be moved proportionally closer to the objective, which becomes nearly impossible if other constraints are also to be met. Consequently, to eliminate curva-

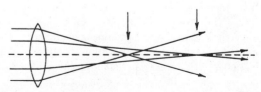

Figure 11-8 Spherical aberration is caused by the edges of the lens having a shorter focal length than the center.

ture of field at higher magnifications requires very complex objectives.

Distortion (Fig. 11-9) is the curving of straight lines in a specimen because magnification of the outer portion of the specimen is different from that of the center portion. This is caused by light from the edges of the specimen following paths that redirect it so that the initial relative position of the edges to the objective appears closer or farther than that of the center, causing edge magnification to differ from center magnification. If straight lines bow toward the center, the result is cushion distortion, while if they bow toward the edges, it is called barrel distortion. Distortion is generally easy to control in microscope design.

Astigmatism occurs when a point appears to be separated by the lens into two perpendicular lines (a ''plus''), but with one line appearing closer to the viewer. This is caused by lenses where the radius of curvature in one plane cutting the lens through its axis is different from that of the radius of curvature in its perpendicular plane. This results from poor workmanship in the manufacture of the lens or improper alignment of the optical elements. A slight astigmatism may exist in some lens designs. The user cannot correct for this since an astigmatic image cannot be focused.

A lens defect related to distortion and spherical aberration is coma. It is caused by the lens producing different magnifications depending on which part of the lens is traversed. While this is usually minimal for the center of the specimen, the effect can be pronounced in a poorly designed or treated microscope as one moves farther off the axis. Off-axis images are smeared toward the edge of the field, with a point distorted to appear as a comet and with loss of contrast.

Two types of aberration affect the color integrity of the specimen. Lateral color has previously been mentioned and is caused by greater magnification of one color of light as compared with that of another color. This aberration results from the different speeds of the various wavelengths of light through lenses, as discussed in Chapter 10. Consequently, off-axis objects will have indistinct edges marked by a spectrum, and detail will be lost in the color confusion. All lenses suffer from this aberration to a certain degree, thereby requiring that combinations of lenses be employed. In particular, it may be necessary to match the eyepiece to the objective or use a more complex eyepiece with a zoom system to eliminate lateral color.

Chromatic aberration is a result of different colors of light being focused at different distances from a lens, violet light being focused nearest the lens. Rather than images with multicolored edges, distinct colored images are formed, with further optics potentially increasing the spread to give a 3-D movie effect. This problem can be readily eliminated by the use of appropriate converging and diverging lens elements.

The problems that lensmakers must solve to manufacture a quality microscope become even greater as the magnification increases. To gather as much light as possible for resolution and to redirect light to shorten the effective object distance require lens properties that introduce numerous light aberrations. These must then be removed by later optical elements to give a final accurate image of the original object.

Section **11-4**
PHENOMENA AFFECTING THE OBJECTIVE

Magnification, as expressed by Eq. 11-9, can be increased indefinitely. There is no limit as to how small a geographical area can be blown up to visible size. There is, however, a limit to the useful magnification that can be obtained. As images get larger, they do not necessarily become more distinct. To be resolvable, features must be adequately lighted,

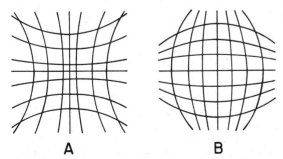

A　　　　　　　**B**

Figure 11-9 Cushion distortion (A) causes lines to bow in, while barrel distortion (B) causes them to bow out.

which is why the light gathering ability of the objective is so important. When enlargement increases the size without improving the clarity, it is called empty magnification. The ability of a microscope to show the detail of a specimen is called its resolving power.

The resolving power of a microscope depends on the quality of the objective and on the nature of the radiation used for illumination. The important factor is the distance that two objects must be apart in order to appear as separate entities. This is called the resolving distance and is given by Eq. 11-15, where λ is the wavelength of the radiation used.

$$d = \frac{0.61\,\lambda}{\text{N.A.}} \qquad \textbf{(11-15)}$$

This equation arises from the fact that the light from a point will not appear as a point but, because of constructive and destructive interference caused by diffraction, it will appear as a circle with a halo around it called an Airy disk, after an English astronomer. The closer this halo is to the circle, the smaller the resolving distance, and the more useful the magnification obtainable. As can be seen from Eq. 11-15, both the wavelength and numerical aperture are important, hence the emphasis on increasing the numerical aperture. The wavelength effect occurs because in order to see something, the wave reflected from the object cannot be significantly larger than the object. An ocean wave will bounce back from a huge rock but show no distortion from a pebble. As a consequence, light of shorter wavelengths gives the best resolution. In the visible spectrum this is violet light, which accounts for the blue and violet filters sometimes used. Ultraviolet light and x-rays are even shorter and give better resolution, but detection must be made by photographic or electronic means because the human eye cannot see them. As the wavelength becomes shorter, the energy becomes larger, as discussed in Chapter 14, and this can cause damage to sensitive specimens. These techniques are not commonly used in the clinical laboratory.

A final consideration of microscope operation is the depth of focus. When one focuses on a point in the specimen, a certain area above and below the object will also appear in focus. The thickness of this area decreases as the magnification of the microscope increases. The depth of focus has two components, one as a result of the power of the optics and the other as a result of the compensation by the eye.

$$d_\text{f} = d_\text{p} + d_\text{e} \qquad \textbf{(11-16)}$$

The optical component is called the depth of field for photomicrography and is given by the equation

$$d_\text{p} = \frac{\lambda\sqrt{\mu^2 - (\text{N.A.})^2}}{(\text{N.A.})^2} \qquad \textbf{(11-17)}$$

By substituting Eq. 11-14 and simplifying we obtain

$$d_\text{p} = \frac{\lambda\sqrt{\mu^2 - \mu^2 \sin^2(\alpha/2)}}{\mu^2 \sin^2(\alpha/2)} \qquad \textbf{(11-18)}$$

$$d_\text{p} = \frac{\lambda\mu\sqrt{1 - \sin^2(\alpha/2)}}{\mu^2 \sin^2(\alpha/2)}$$

Since $\sin^2 x = 1 - \cos^2 x,$ $\qquad \textbf{(11-19)}$

$$d_\text{p} = \frac{\lambda}{\mu} \frac{\sqrt{\cos^2(\alpha/2)}}{\sin^2(\alpha/2)}$$

$$d_\text{p} = \frac{\lambda}{\mu} \frac{\cos(\alpha/2)}{\sin^2(\alpha/2)}$$

$$d_\text{p} = \frac{\lambda}{\mu} \frac{\cos(\alpha/2)}{\sin(\alpha/2)} \cdot \frac{1}{\sin(\alpha/2)}$$

Since

$$\frac{\cos x}{\sin x} = \cot x \qquad \textbf{(11-20)}$$

and

$$\frac{1}{\sin x} = \csc x \qquad \textbf{(11-21)}$$

$$d_\text{p} = \frac{\lambda}{\mu} \cot \frac{\alpha}{2} \csc \frac{\alpha}{2} \qquad \textbf{(11-22)}$$

The ability of the eye to compensate is a function of the best viewing distance of the eye and of the magnification.

$$d_\text{e} = \frac{E}{M^2} \qquad \textbf{(11-23)}$$

For the average eye, as previously mentioned, this is 25 cm. If all the equations are combined (11-16, 11-17, and 11-23) we discover that we can calculate the depth of focus if we know the wavelength of light, the numerical aperture (or the angle of aperture), the index of refraction of the contact medium, the magnification of the microscope, and the best viewing distance for the observer.

$$d_f = \frac{\lambda \sqrt{\mu^2 - (\text{N.A.})^2}}{(\text{N.A.})^2} + \frac{E}{M^2} \qquad \textbf{(11-24)}$$

EXAMPLE 11-3

A farsighted viewer (32.4 cm) is looking through a $450\times$ microscope with a depth of focus of 2.06 μm using light at 514 nm without oil immersion. What is the numerical aperture of the objective?

Solution: Start with the depth of focus equation.

$$d_f = \frac{\lambda \sqrt{\mu^2 - (\text{N.A.})^2}}{(\text{N.A.})^2} + \frac{E}{M^2}$$

Rearrange algebraicly to permit squaring:

$$\frac{(d_f - E/M^2)}{\lambda} = \frac{\sqrt{\mu^2 - (\text{N.A.})^2}}{(\text{N.A.})^2}$$

$$\frac{(d_f - E/M^2)(\text{N.A.})^2}{\lambda} = \sqrt{\mu^2 - (\text{N.A.})^2}$$

$$\frac{(d_f - E/M^2)^2(\text{N.A.})^4}{\lambda^2} = \mu^2 - (\text{N.A.})^2$$

Substitute for known quantities to simplify:

$$\frac{\left(2.06 \cdot 10^{-6} - \dfrac{32.4 \cdot 10^{-2}}{(450)^2}\right)^2 (\text{N.A.})^4}{(514 \cdot 10^{-9})^2}$$

$$= 1^2 - (\text{N.A.})^2$$

Rearrange and solve the quadratic:

$$0.801 \, (\text{N.A.})^4 = 1 - (\text{N.A.})^2$$

$$0.801 \, (\text{N.A.})^4 + (\text{N.A.})^2 - 1 = 0$$

By the quadratic formula

$$(\text{N.A.})^2 = \frac{-1 \pm \sqrt{1 - [4 \times 0.801 \times (-1)]}}{2 \times 0.801}$$

The negative root is an artifact of squaring:

$$(\text{N.A.})^2 = 0.656$$

$$\text{N.A.} = 0.81 \qquad \blacksquare$$

Section **11-5**
SPECIAL TECHNIQUES

Sometimes the traditional way of looking at a specimen fails to show the detail desired. This may hap-

pen due to the lack of contrast between the parts of the specimen, the inability to stain, or overlapping features. These difficulties can frequently be overcome by the use of special techniques.

The most common special technique is dark field illumination, as illustrated in Figure 11-10. The light from the illuminating source is blocked in the center so that it cannot enter the objective directly. Instead the light is reflected from the periphery to form a hollow cone which is focused on the stage of the microscope. When the specimen is completely transparent, the light misses the objective and is not seen by the viewer. Hence the background is black, and the term "dark field" is used to describe the process. If the specimen contains areas of different refractive index or densities, light will be refracted and reflected at different angles and some of it will enter the objective. This light will be processed through the microscope and cause the areas deflecting the light to appear bright against the dark background.

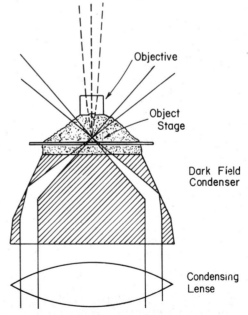

Figure 11-10 Dark-field illumination depends on a hollow cone of light focused on the specimen. (Courtesy of Bausch & Lomb Instruments and Systems Division. Redrawn with permission.)

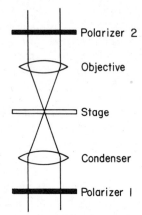

Polarizer 2

Objective

Stage

Condenser

Polarizer I

Figure 11-11 The use of cross-polarized filters will remove all light not rotated by crystalline material.

To be effective, the dark-field condenser must produce light at the correct angle of aperture with no scattering of light. The bottom of the slide must be in oil contact with the condenser. The numerical aperture of the lens must be restricted to 1.0 to prevent gathering the source radiation. The incoming beam of light must be intense, since most of it will not be deflected into the objective, and enough radiation must be deflected to make the details distinct.

One kind of material that can be isolated by a special type of light is the crystal. The crystal lattice of many minerals and chemical salts causes light to rotate. By looking at the rotated light, only the crystalline material is visible. Figure 11-11 shows the layout for such observation using polarizing filters. Light is composed of transverse waves that can be thought of as having a horizontal and vertical component. A plate of glass called a polarizer is made so that only one component of the light can pass through and all the component perpendicular to it is removed. If such a plate is placed in a light beam, the light wave becomes polarized, that is, transmitted in only one plane, and its intensity is reduced by one-half. If this light then encounters another polarizer set 90° to the previous plate, its progress is blocked because it has no component that can move through the second obstacle. This is called cross-polarized.

By placing a polarizer in the condenser, polar-ized light is directed onto the specimen. If nothing in the specimen rotates light, then the second polarizer, placed after the object and rotated 90° to the plane of the first, will remove all the radiation, leaving a dark field. If crystalline material is present, then the light passing through it will be rotated so that it is no longer perpendicular to the second polarizer's transmission plane. As a consequence, part of it will pass through the second polarizer to give a light object against the dark background. The closer to 90° that the crystal rotates the light, the brighter it will appear. Polarized light can, therefore, be used as a means of isolating and identifying crystalline substances.

Another technique that is frequently useful is phase-contrast microscopy. Here we are dealing with a bright field and attempting to see darkened areas against it. Phase-contrast microscopy is used when the specimen does not vary in density (which could be seen by bright field), has no significant edge effect (for which dark field would be of use), and has no crystalline properties (which would rotate polarized light), but instead has variations in refractive index. Phase contrast is accomplished by use of a cone of light created by a clear annular diaphragm in the condenser (Fig. 11-12). This light is focused to enter the objective and to be refracted so as to pass through a second annular diaphragm. This second diaphragm is composed of material designed to slow the light so that the resultant beam is one-quarter wavelength out of phase with the incident beam. This has no net effect unless some of the light is diffracted by the specimen. In this case the diffracted light will not pass through the delaying ring and will reach the image plane a quarter wavelength ahead of the undiffracted light. Partial destructive interference will occur between the misphased light coming through different paths. Areas from which the light was diffracted will therefore appear darker than other areas. The light–dark contrast, which is normally a result of density difference, occurs in this case due to the phase cancellation of the light resulting from variations in the refractive index.

While microscope lens systems may be quite complicated, the microscope basically uses light in a rather simple manner. Other measuring devices that rely on more complex properties of light will be discussed in the succeeding chapters.

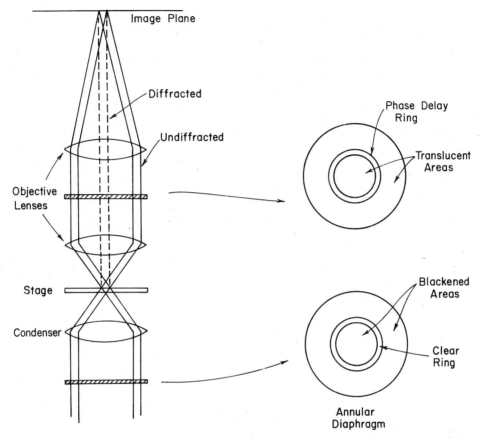

Figure 11-12   Phase contrast microscopy relies on delaying some of the light by a quarter of a wave length. (Courtesy of Bausch & Lomb Instruments and Systems Division. Redrawn with permission.)

REVIEW QUESTIONS

1. What is a simple microscope? How does it work?
2. What is the general equation for magnification?
3. What factors affect the magnification of a simple microscope?
4. What is the optimum viewing distance of the average eye?
5. Why is the magnification of a simple microscope so limited?
6. How does a compound microscope work?
7. What are the two lenses of a compound microscope called?
8. How is the magnification of a compound microscope calculated?
9. What physical properties of the compound microscope affect its magnification?
10. What is a binocular microscope?
11. List the four parts of a complex microscope.
12. What is the purpose of the illumination system?
13. List the components of a Koehler illumination system.
14. Give the function for each lens in the illumination system.
15. Why would a filter be used in the illumination system?
16. Give two ways to control the light intensity.

17. What is numerical aperture? How is it calculated?
18. What affect does reducing the numerical aperture of the illumination system have?
19. What are the two purposes of the objective lens system?
20. Why is oil immersion used?
21. Why does the objective cause aberration of the image?
22. How is aberration compensated for?
23. What is the purpose of a redirecting or zooming system?
24. How does zooming work?
25. Why are total reflection prisms used instead of mirrors?
26. How is the binocular effect accomplished?
27. How does a Huygenian eyepiece work?
28. What functions does an eyepiece perform?
29. Describe why spherical aberration occurs.
30. How is spherical aberration compensated for?
31. What is curvature of field?
32. Name and describe the two types of "distortion."
33. Explain astigmatism.
34. What effect is observed when coma is present?
35. Describe the physical phenomenon that causes lateral color.
36. Explain chromatic aberration.
37. What is empty magnification?
38. Define resolving distance.
39. Why does the wavelength of light affect resolution?
40. What is the Airy disk?
41. What wavelengths of light give the best resolution?
42. Define depth of focus.
43. What two factors affect the depth of focus?
44. Describe how dark-field illumination works.
45. Why is the background dark in dark-field illumination?
46. When is dark-field illumination used?
47. Explain polarized light.
48. Why can polarized light be used to study crystals?
49. How is polarized light used in a microscope?
50. What is phase contrast microscopy?
51. How is the phase-contrast accomplished?
52. For what kind of specimens is phase-contrast useful?

PROBLEMS

1. What angle does the image of a simple microscope of magnification $6.3\times$ subtend with the eye if the object subtends an angle of $9.8°$?
2. What is the optimum viewing distance for someone if a magnification of $5.61\times$ is obtained when the person views an image 26.2 cm away through a lens of focal length 4.38 cm?
3. If the lens of a simple microscope has a focal length of 7.1 cm and gives a magnification of $5.04\times$, what is the distance from the eye that a viewer with average eyesight would observe the image?
4. A manufacturer chooses to make a compound microscope with both lenses of the same focal length and the barrel 10 times that length. If the average viewer gets a magnification of $46.7\times$, what is the length of the microscope?
5. The focal length of the objective is 1.83 times that of the eyepiece in a compound microscope. If the barrel is 31.6 cm, the optimum viewing distance is 22.3 cm and the magnification is $152\times$, what is the focal length of the objective?
6. What is the relative error of dropping the E/D term for a compound microscope if $f_e = 3.91$ and $D = 60.4$ cm?
7. If the numerical aperture is 1.29 and the refractive index is 1.47, what is the angle of aperture?
8. What is the resolving distance of an objective if light of 483 nm is used and the objective has an angle of aperture of $134°$? (The refractive index of the oil used in the immersion is 1.53.)
9. What is the depth of field for photomicrography for the objective in Problem 8 under the conditions listed?
10. At what magnification will the eye generate a depth of focus of 235 nm when its best viewing distance is 40.5 cm?
11. A nearsighted viewer (21.6 cm) is looking through a microscope whose objective has a numerical aperture of 1.25. If the depth of focus is 2.24 μm using light of 790 nm with immersion oil of refractive index 1.57, what is the magnification?

CHAPTER 12
ELECTROCHEMICAL MEASUREMENTS

Electrodes are transducers that convert chemical concentrations directly into quantities in the electronic domain. As such, they can easily be used in conjunction with the electrical analysis and reporting hardware previously introduced. Electrodes are commonly used to measure pH, blood gases, and serum electrolytes. We will begin our study of electrodes with a brief review of the role of the Nernst equation in electrochemical measurement.

Section 12-1
NERNST EQUATION

In Chapter 3 we looked at a battery that was formed by using copper and zinc plates as electrodes. The elementary copper–zinc cell is shown in Figure 3-5. The key to the operation of this cell is the existence of two half-reactions. One of these reactions occurs at each electrode and involves the transfer of electrons at the electrode surface between the electrode and the corresponding solution species. As shown in Eqs. 12-1 and 12-2, the electrode reaction is a reversible process. While the reagents on the right side of the reaction are driven to form the products on the left side, the products on the left side are driven to form the reagents on the right side.

$$Zn \rightleftharpoons Zn^{2+} + 2e^- \qquad -0.763 \text{ V} \qquad \textbf{(12-1)}$$

$$Cu \rightleftharpoons Cu^{2+} + 2e^- \qquad +0.337 \text{ V} \qquad \textbf{(12-2)}$$

An equilibrium constant exists for such reversible reactions and is expressed in a general form as follows:

$$K_T = \frac{\Pi a_p}{\Pi a_r} \qquad \textbf{(12-3)}$$

In this equation, K_T is the thermodynamic equilibrium constant, Πa_p is the product of the activities of the products in the reaction, and Πa_r the product of the activities of the reactants in the reaction. (Remember, Π is to product as Σ is to sum.)

If we attempt to write the reaction in Eq. 12-1 in this form, we obtain Eq. 12-4. The term a_e^2 is the activity of the electrons, which is squared because there are two of them. To use this equation we must define the activities of terms of measurable quantities:

$$K_{Zn} = \frac{a_{Zn^{2+}} \, a_e^2}{a_{Zn}} \qquad \textbf{(12-4)}$$

For such a definition, it is necessary to return to the meaning of activity. Activity is the "effectiveness" of a species in solution, sometimes referred to as the "effective concentration." For a solid this will be a constant, because whether there is more or less solid in contact with a solution has no influence on the equilibrium within the solution. By adjusting (multiplying or dividing) K_T by the appropriate constant, the activity of the solid can be made 1. Therefore, we define the activity of any solid present as 1. This allows the solid terms to be dropped from the equation and gives rise to Eq. 12-5 for the case presented in Eq. 12-1.

$$K_{Zn} = a_{Zn^{2+}} \, a_e^2 \qquad \textbf{(12-5)}$$

Although there are none present in the zinc example, activities can also be defined for gases and liquids in terms of their effective concentrations. For a gas, its concentration is proportional to its partial pressure within the solution. The partial pressure value is normalized by appropriate adjustment of the equilibrium constant so that a gas with a partial pressure of 1 atmosphere (760 torr)* has an activity of 1. For a liquid, the activity can be defined as the mole fraction, which is the fraction of the solution that is the liquid of interest (a simplification of the actual thermodynamic expression). If only one liquid is present, it has a mole fraction of 1 and, therefore, an activity of 1. Hence for aqueous solutions the activity of water can be absorbed into the reaction constants.

If we return to Eq. 12-5, we have yet to define the activities of an ion in solution and of an electron. The activity of an ion is defined as the product of an activity coefficient and the concentration of the species. The activity coefficient is a function of the matrix effects of the solution and the particular ion with which we are dealing. Matrix effects are primarily determined by ionic strength and intermolecular forces. Various methods for calculating those coefficients have been derived, the most commonly used being known as the Debye-Hückel limiting law, given by Eqs. 12-6 and 12-7. Equation 12-7 is only the first term of a more complex expression.

$$I = \tfrac{1}{2}\Sigma Z_i^2 C_i \qquad \textbf{(12-6)}$$

$$\log \alpha_i = -0.509 Z_i^2 I^{\frac{1}{2}} \qquad \textbf{(12-7)}$$

The term I denotes the ionic strength, and Z_i is the charge of an ionic species (in atomic charge units). The ionic strength is therefore one-half the sum of the concentration of *all* ions present times their charges squared. Note that a change in any one ion concentration affects the ionic strength, which in turn determines the effective concentration of all ions. The activity coefficient is then calculated from Eq. 12-7, where Z_i is the charge of the ionic species of interest. As the solution becomes more dilute, the value of the ionic strength becomes very small, the right side of Eq. 12-7 approaches zero, and the activity coefficient approaches 1. Because the right side of this equation is always negative, the activity coefficient, as calculated, can never exceed 1. This value of the activity coefficient is only an approximation, however, because it does not take into consideration forces between solution species other than charge.

While our measurements and the reactions of

* Or 760 mm Hg.

ionic species in solution are dependent on activity, not concentration, for pedagogical purposes we will assume that the activity coefficients are sufficiently close to 1 for concentration to be used for activities. Note that except for dilute solutions or for special cases in which everything is at the same ionic strength, this is generally not true, but is usually not too inaccurate if the ionic strength is held constant between specimens.

We have now simplified the zinc equilibrium as follows:

$$K_{Zn} = [Zn^{2+}]\, a_e^2 \qquad \textbf{(12-8)}$$

The activity of the free electron has been determined by thermodynamics to be a function of potential applied to the electrons of the species involved. For zinc, that activity is as follows:

$$a_e = K_{Zn}^{\frac{1}{2}} \exp\left(\frac{F(E_{Zn}^{o} - E_{Zn})}{RT}\right) \qquad \textbf{(12-9)}$$

Where K_{Zn} is the equilibrium constant, T is the absolute temperature, R is the universal gas constant (8.314 joule/mole degree), F is Faraday's constant ($9.65 \cdot 10^4$ coulombs/mole), and exp implies that the expression in parentheses is the exponent of the natural constant e (2.71828). E_{Zn}^{o} is the standard potential associated with zinc and E_{Zn} is some other potential. If $E_{Zn} = E_{Zn}^{o}$, the exponent equals zero, $e^0 = 1$, and $a_e = K_{Zn}^{\frac{1}{2}}$. If this is substituted into Eq. 12-8, we have

$$K_{Zn} = [Zn^{2+}](K_{Zn}^{\frac{1}{2}})^2$$

or

$$[Zn^{2+}] = 1 \qquad \textbf{(12-10)}$$

When $E_{Zn} = E_{Zn}^{o}$, then $[Zn^{2+}] = 1$, and vice versa. This then becomes the definition of E_{Zn}^{o}; it has the value of E_{Zn} when $[Zn^{2+}]$ is 1.0000 M.

If we substitute Eq. 12-9 into 12-8, we get

$$K_{Zn} = K_{Zn}[Zn^{2+}] \exp\left(\frac{2F(E_{Zn}^{o} - E_{Zn})}{RT}\right) \qquad \textbf{(12-11)}$$

If we solve this equation for E_{Zn}, we have

$$E_{Zn} = E_{Zn}^{o} - \frac{RT}{2F} \ln \frac{1}{[Zn^{2+}]} \qquad \textbf{(12-12)}$$

In this form it is clear that what we have is just the Nernst equation, defined in more general form as

$$E = E^{\circ} - \frac{RT}{nF} \ln \frac{\text{[reduced]}}{\text{[oxidized]}} \qquad \textbf{(12-13)}$$

The way in which we derived the Nernst equation is very important to how it affects reactions. The difference in the potential $(E - E^{\circ})$ controls the availability (concentration) of electrons, one reactant in electrochemical reactions. Changing the activity of the electrons affects a reaction just as does changing the activity of any of the chemical species.

Section **12-2**
HYDROGEN ELECTRODE

Although we have derived a relationship among the potential of a half-reaction, the value of its equilibrium constant, and the concentration of the ions in solution, we are still hanging in air to some extent. Although we know that E° is equal to E when the operand of the log term is 1, we cannot assign a numerical value to it. In fact, it can only have value relative to other E° values, that is, other standard potentials of half-reactions.

This situation necessitates defining a standard against which to compare other half-reactions. The standard is the hydrogen reaction defined as follows:

$$\tfrac{1}{2}H_2 \rightleftharpoons H^+ + e^- \qquad \textbf{(12-14)}$$

For this reaction, the potential is defined as exactly 0.0000 V. This half-reaction was chosen many years ago for several reasons. It is near the center of the electromotive series; that is, there are many reactions of both higher and lower potential. Hydrogen is readily available all over the world and is easily made. The hydrogen ion concentration is important to many reactions.

Before we proceed to the measurement of the hydrogen ion, let us first simplify the Nernst equation. Let us recall that the natural logarithms can be expressed in terms of base 10 logarithms as

$$\ln X = 2.303 \log X \qquad \textbf{(12-15)}$$

Since F and R are natural constants, one can obtain Eq. 12-16 from Eq. 12-13 by setting T as 25°C (298°K) and combining the constants. Note that n,

the number of electrons, is dependent on the half-reaction and cannot be absorbed into the constant term.

$$E = E^{\circ} - \frac{0.0591}{n} \log \frac{\text{[red]}}{\text{[ox]}} \qquad \textbf{(12-16)}$$

At 37°C, this constant is 0.0614.

The Nernst equation for the hydrogen half-reaction is

$$E_H = -0.0591 \log \frac{P_{H_2}^{\frac{1}{2}}}{\text{[H}^+]} \qquad \textbf{(12-17)}$$

Since E_H° is 0, it has been dropped. Because only one electron is present, n is 1 and disappears. The concentration of H_2, a gas, is given by its partial pressure, but the square root is taken because only one-half molecule is used in the reaction as written.

To measure the hydrogen ion concentration, one can employ some device which will produce a potential as a result of the presence of both hydrogen and the hydrogen ion. Such a device is called a hydrogen electrode, as shown in Figure 12-1. It is, of course, not possible to make a plate out of hydrogen as one can out of zinc, but one can achieve the same effect by using a platinum black wire, which is an inert electrode, in contact with both hydrogen gas and a solution of hydrogen ions.

The potential of the hydrogen electrode can be determined by inserting the values of the partial pressure of hydrogen and the concentration of hy-

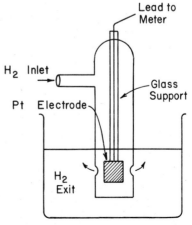

Figure 12-1 A hydrogen electrode.

drogen ions into Eq. 12-17. If we set both the partial pressure of H_2 and the $[H^+]$ to 1, then in Eq. 12-17 we have the log of 1 as a factor on the right side of the equation, and $E_{H_2} = 0$. An electrode with those conditions is called a standard hydrogen electrode (SHE). Such an electrode can serve as the reference against which to measure an unknown solution.

If we place a hydrogen electrode in an unknown solution and connect that solution to an SHE by a salt bridge, then the potential difference is

$$\Delta E = E_2 - E_1 \qquad \text{(12-18)}$$

The value of the SHE (E_1) is 0, while that of E_2 is given by Eq. 12-17.

$$\Delta E = -0.0591 \log \frac{P_{H_2}^{\frac{1}{2}}}{[H^+]} - 0$$

$$\Delta E = -0.0591 \log \frac{P_{H_2}^{\frac{1}{2}}}{[H^+]} \qquad \text{(12-19)}$$

If the partial pressure of H_2 for this electrode is set as 1, then

$$\Delta E = -0.0591 \log \frac{1}{[H^+]}$$

or

$$\Delta E = -0.0591 \, (-\log [H^+]) \qquad \text{(12-20)}$$

This gives the value of the potential difference as a direct function of the hydrogen ion concentration and vice versa.

To reduce the use of exponents for species like hydrogen ion, which vary over many orders of magnitude, the ''p'' notation was invented, defined as follows:

$$pX = -\log[X] \qquad \text{(12-21)}$$

When this is applied to Eq. 12-20, we get

$$E = -0.0591 \, pH \qquad \text{(12-22)}$$

Each increase of one pH unit will cause a voltage decrease of 0.0591 V.

EXAMPLE 12-1

Calculate the potential difference between two hydrogen electrodes if one electrode is in a solution of

$1.63 \cdot 10^{-5} \, M \, H^+$ and under a hydrogen pressure of 0.851 atmosphere and the other is in a solution of $4.33 \cdot 10^{-3} \, M \, H^+$ and under a hydrogen pressure of 0.675 atmosphere.

Solution:

$$\Delta E = E_2 - E_1$$

The general equation for E is

$$E = -0.0591 \log \frac{P_{H_2}^{\frac{1}{2}}}{[H^+]}$$

$$E_2 = -0.0591 \log \frac{(0.675)^{\frac{1}{2}}}{4.33 \cdot 10^{-3}} = -0.1346 \text{ V}$$

$$E_1 = -0.0591 \log \frac{(0.851)^{\frac{1}{2}}}{1.63 \cdot 10^{-5}} = -0.2809 \text{ V}$$

$$\Delta E = -0.1346 - (-0.2809)$$

$$\Delta E = 0.146 \text{ V} \qquad \blacksquare$$

Section 12-3
OTHER ELECTRODES

The hydrogen electrode might seem perfect for the measurement of pH, but it has many serious drawbacks. It is easily poisoned by proteins, it is bulky, it is an explosion hazard, and maintaining constant H_2 pressure is difficult. It is never found in a clinical laboratory.

Two other electrodes are used instead of a hydrogen electrode/standard hydrogen electrode pair. These two electrodes are referred to as the working (measuring) electrode and the reference (standard) electrode. In the above case, the hydrogen electrode is the working electrode and SHE is the reference electrode. Unfortunately, there is no one type of other electrode that can act as both the reference and working electrodes for a pH measurement. Therefore we will have to examine reference and working electrodes separately.

There are three classes of electrodes. The common electrode has a metal component in direct contact with the unknown solution or that contacts it through a salt bridge. The glass electrode has a surface area sensitive to the solution matrix. The membrane electrode has semipermeable coverings that allow only certain substances to reach the re-

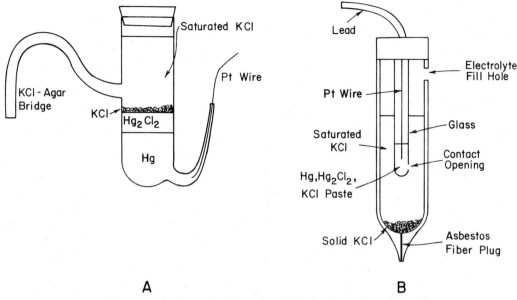

Figure 12-2 Two saturated calomel electrode configurations.

acting surface of the metal electrode. Each of these electrode types is used in the clinical laboratory and is discussed below. We will start with several common electrodes used as reference electrodes.

The classic replacement for the standard hydrogen electrode has been the saturated calomel electrode (SCE). Two configurations of this electrode are given in Figure 12-2. This electrode contains a suitable wire, frequently platinum, immersed in a mercury pool. The pool is in contact with mercurous chloride (called "calomel"), which is in turn in contact with a saturated solution of potassium chloride. Crystals of excess KCl guarantee saturation. The reference electrode is placed in contact with the unknown solution by use of a salt bridge, a sintered glass frit, or an asbestos plug.

The reaction at the calomel electrode is

$$2Hg + 2Cl^- \rightleftharpoons Hg_2Cl_2 + 2e^- \quad \textbf{(12-23)}$$

The potential (E°_{SCE}) for this reaction is 0.244 V at 25°C. This number comes from the Nernst equation for the half-reaction:

$$E = E^\circ_{Hg_2Cl_2} - \frac{RT}{2F} \ln \frac{a^2_{Cl^-} - a^2_{Hg}}{a^2_{Hg_2Cl_2}} \quad \textbf{(12-24)}$$

Since Hg and Hg_2Cl_2 are solids, their activity is 1 and they drop out. The activity of chloride is a constant at saturation, so the equation becomes

$$E^\circ_{SCE} = E = E^\circ_{Hg_2Cl_2} - \frac{RT}{F} \ln a_{Cl^-_{sat}} \quad \textbf{(12-25)}$$

Note that in this case E°_{SCE} already includes the concentration term and this must not be included again when doing calculations. The potential of the SCE is always precisely E°_{SCE}. Note also that while the last term is not affected by the concentration of any species, it is affected by temperature. Not only does T appear in the equation, but the solubility of KCl (and therefore its activity) is affected by temperature. As a consequence, it is imperative that the temperature be held constant at 25°C for the value of E°_{SCE} to be correct. Other temperatures imply other E°_{SCE} values.

The advantages of this electrode are considerable. The unique properties of the liquid metal element mercury and the diatomic mercurous ion permit the construction of a system with a very stable potential. Its potential is near the center of the electromotive series. It is easy to construct. These reasons have led to its widespread use as a reference electrode.

There are also some disadvantages. Temperature dependence has already been mentioned. The electrode becomes unstable as the boiling point of water is approached due to the disproportionation of mercurous ion into mercury and mercuric ion. To alleviate this temperature problem, calomel electrodes of $\leq 1\ M$ in KCl are sometimes used. This means that extreme care must be taken to avoid evaporation or osmosis of the electrolyte. The saturated calomel electrode is difficult to miniaturize, due to its complex structure. If damaged, the danger of mercury contamination exists.

Another commonly used reference electrode is the silver–silver chloride electrode. Its basic equation is

$$Ag + Cl^- \rightleftharpoons AgCl + e^- \qquad \textbf{(12-26)}$$

The $E^\circ_{Ag-AgCl}$ is 0.222 V at 25°C. The electrode is made by plating a layer of silver chloride onto a silver wire or plate (Fig. 12-3). If the appropriate substitutions are made in the Nernst equation, we get

$$E = E^\circ_{Ag-AgCl} - 0.0591 \log [Cl^-] \quad \textbf{(12-27)}$$

As in the case of the SCE, the potential depends upon the chloride concentration. If the electrode is to be used as a reference, then it is imperative that the concentration of the chloride ion be accurately known. Otherwise, the Ag–AgCl electrode becomes a chloride electrode, and pH measurement is

impossible. Usually KCl is used to set the chloride concentration. The situation is further complicated by the solubility of AgCl in concentrated chloride solution in the form of $AgCl_2^-$. This phenomenon can lead to the destruction of the electrode. To prevent it, the electrolyte should be saturated with AgCl with some excess AgCl present. In order to have the expected potential, the electrode must be prepared carefully.

The advantages of the Ag–AgCl electrode over the SCE are thermal stability and the ability to be miniaturized. It can be used for in vivo measurements in a biological system and as a reference standard inside a more complex electrode.

EXAMPLE 12-2

What is the chloride concentration if the potential of a Ag–AgCl electrode is −0.030 V versus a saturated calomel electrode?

Solution: We start with the basic difference equation and substitute those values that are known.

$$\Delta E = E_{Ag-AgCl} - E_{SCE}$$

$$\Delta E = E^\circ_{Ag-AgCl}$$

$$- \frac{0.0591}{1} \log [Cl^-] - E^\circ_{SCE}$$

$$-0.0591 \log [Cl^-] = \Delta E - E^\circ_{Ag-AgCl} + E^\circ_{SCE}$$

$$-0.0591 \log [Cl^-] = -0.030 - 0.222 + 0.244$$

$$\log [Cl^-] = \frac{-0.008}{-0.0591} = 0.135$$

$$[Cl^-] = 1.4\ M$$

Most of the significance is lost because of the 0.008 numerator, which has only one significant digit. ∎

While the SCE or the Ag–AgCl electrode can replace the SHE as the reference electrode in pH measurement, another type of electrode is needed to replace the working hydrogen electrode. The most popular electrode used for this purpose is a glass electrode, a representative of a whole family of surface sensitive electrodes.

"Glass electrode" is a misnomer, because glass cannot function as an electrode. The name has en-

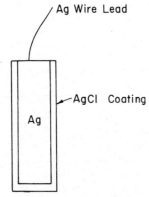

Ag Wire Lead

AgCl Coating

Ag

Figure 12-3 A silver–silver chloride electrode.

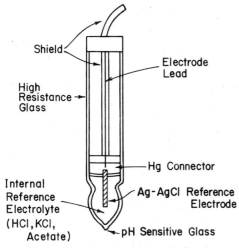

Shield

Electrode Lead

High Resistance Glass

Hg Connector

Internal Reference Electrolyte (HCl, KCl, Acetate)

Ag-AgCl Reference Electrode

pH Sensitive Glass

Figure 12-4   A typical glass electrode.

dured, however, because of the importance of the glass membrane to the operation of the electrode. A typical glass electrode is shown in Figure 12-4. The key to the operation of the glass electrode is a piece of glass which is sensitive to pH. The whole electrode functions in the following manner. A wire lead enters the stem of the electrode from the top. It is shielded to prevent it from acquiring a potential from the upper portion of the electrode. The wire is attached to an internal reference electrode, such as a silver–silver chloride electrode. The potential on this electrode is fixed because it is immersed in a solution of constant chloride concentration. In fact, the solution is a buffer solution in which the activity of chloride and the pH are carefully fixed. This is essential to the operation of the electrode.

The situation at the glass interface of the electrode is complex. It is not totally understood, but basically the following happens. The glass membrane is very thin and porous. Ions of the solutions on either side of the membrane migrate into the pores. The structure and composition of the glass determine the amount of the various ions entering the glass. For a pH electrode, the glass is designed to have a negative matrix with pores suitable for holding hydrogen ions. The extent to which the surface of the glass electrode absorbs the hydrogen ions in a solution is a function of how many hydrogen ions are present. The result is that a potential

difference develops over the glass membrane based on the extent to which each side of the membrane is charged. That glass can hold such a charge difference should be clear if one recalls the high school physics experiment in which glass and rubber rods were rubbed with cloth and then used to move the leaves on an electrometer. The potential which appears at the lead to the glass electrode is the sum of the potential of the internal reference electrode and the potential across the glass membrane.

We can express the difference in potential across the glass membrane as the difference in the activities of the hydrogen ion on each side of the membrane plus a function F_a peculiar to each membrane. F_a is dependent on temperature, aging, structure, composition, and perhaps other considerations.

$$\Delta E_{glass} = E_{outside} - E_{inside}$$

$$\Delta E_{glass} = -\frac{RT}{nF} \ln(a_{H^+})_O$$
$$- \left[-\frac{RT}{nF} \ln(a_{H^+})_I \right] + F_a \quad \textbf{(12-28)}$$

Since $n = 1$,

$$\Delta E_{glass} = \frac{RT}{F} [-\ln(a_{H^+})_O - (-\ln(a_{H^+})_I)] + F_a$$

$$\Delta E_{glass} = 2.303 \frac{RT}{F} (pH_O - pH_I) + F_a \quad \textbf{(12.29)}$$

Using the electrode in a reproducible manner, F_a can be held constant and its effect removed by circuitry. The activity of the hydrogen ion inside the glass electrode is also fixed by the composition of that solution which is constant. Therefore, it too can be removed electronically for the final measurement, leaving the net effect across the glass membrane only a linear function of the pH of the outside solution. For the final equation we can then gather up the terms that are effectively constant for any particular electrode and set of conditions:

$$\Delta E_{glass} = 2.303 \frac{RT}{F} pH + K \quad \textbf{(12-30)}$$

Because of the sensitivity of the glass surface, the glass electrode must be handled carefully. The portion of the electrode which is placed into the unknown solution can be damaged in numerous ways. If the electrode is allowed to dry out under uncontrolled conditions, the molecular structure can be altered to such an extent that the pores are no longer the correct size to hold hydrogen ions. If the electrode is placed in strong reagents, the glass surface may be chemically altered, thereby destroying its activity. If the electrode is placed in a strongly acidic or basic solution for too long, it may acquire a memory. For example, with a strong acidic solution, the hydrogen ions work their way far into the electrode, displacing Na^+ or other counter ions that were placed there in the manufacturing process to insure electrical neutrality. This can cause bleeding of hydrogen ions into the interior of the membrane (or from the interior in the case of alkaline exposure), which gives rise to the memory effect. In making a pH measurement, we will use a glass electrode as the working electrode and a saturated calomel electrode as the reference electrode.

A sketch of such a measurement device is shown in Figure 12-5. If one could read the potential difference between the two electrodes in their circuit with a voltmeter in the same manner as one can between zinc and copper electrodes, pH meters would be very simple; however, getting an accurate, usable value is much more complicated. First, the glass electrode cannot produce enough current to move the meter. While a Ag–AgCl electrode and a SCE can tolerate some electron transfer and still maintain their potentials, current cannot flow effectively through the glass membrane, because the resistance is 50–500 MΩ. Attempts to draw significant amounts of current will polarize the electrode and destroy the surface of the membrane.

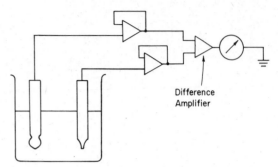

Figure 12-6 A refined circuit to measure pH.

To overcome this difficulty, one can use operational amplifiers. Figure 12-6 revises Figure 12-5 using several operational amplifiers to compare the values on the electrodes. If the input amplifiers have a high input impedance, then the potential of the electrodes will not be affected by the rest of the circuit.

A second source of trouble is the junction potentials. Every time that different materials are brought into contact, a small voltage develops over the interface, much as in the case of n-type and p-type semiconductors, owing to the difference in electron affinity of the two materials. This potential will be measured as part of the various voltage sources in series. Figure 12-7 shows the circuit as a series of potential sources representing the various elements of a pH measurement. To eliminate the junction potential from our readings, we need to have the ability to feed an adjustable signal (bucking voltage) into the measuring device to compensate for it. This allows us to adjust the reading for a known pH sample to the correct value and cancel the junction potential from the output. Naturally the unknown must have the same junction potential as the known, or a systematic error will be introduced when measuring the unknown.

Other factors also contribute to the nonideal nature of the pH measurement. The electrodes gradually deteriorate with age. The surfaces undergo decay, and the chemical interfaces become contaminated. The electronics drift with time because of temperature changes and microscopic irre-

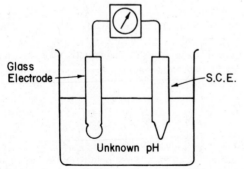

Figure 12-5 An elementary pH measurement configuration.

versibility. The temperatures of the solutions being measured may vary. All these things must be taken into consideration in making a successful pH measurement.

We can now determine what the design of our meter will be if we work through the mathematics involved. We start by writing the potential measured in terms of all the potentials present:

$$\Delta E = D(E^o_{Ag-AgCl} + \Delta E_{glass} - E^o_{SCE} + E^o_{junction}) \tag{12-31}$$

(*Note:* D is the scaling factor of the operational amplifier circuit.) If we substitute for ΔE_{glass} and regroup the constant terms, we have

$$\Delta E = 2.303 \frac{RTD}{F} \text{ pH}$$
$$+ D(K + E^o_{Ag-AgCl} - E^o_{SCE} + E^o_{junction}) \tag{12-32}$$

This equation can be simplified if we combine the standard electrode potentials and junction potentials into one constant E^o and replace the coefficient of the pH with the symbol S for scaling factor.

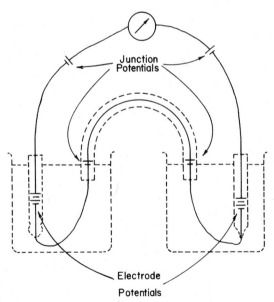

Figure 12-7 The actual circuit in a pH measurement is indicated by the solid line. Junction potentials exist every time two dissimilar materials adjoin, and potentials also exist at each of the electrodes.

This yields

$$\Delta E = S \text{ pH} + E^o \tag{12-33}$$

The pH can be measured in terms of ΔE if we know the values of E^o and S. Unfortunately, we do not know their values, but we can design our meter so it is unimportant to know them. If we can fix the values of E^o and S, we can still make the measurement. E^o is a potential that will remain constant for a specific set of conditions. S is a function of the electrode and the absolute temperature. The first two will not change over a short time, and the temperature can be controlled. As a result, we get a simple linear equation for the potential change and the voltage. This line can be determined by two point standardization.

Figure 12-8 shows an example of circuitry that can solve all the problems identified. Each electrode is protected by a high-impedance, low-gain voltage follower. One input is then inverted with no gain. An offset voltage (bucking voltage), for the purpose of canceling E^o, is fed into the summing point of the final amplifier which can have low impedance, but must have high gain. The feedback resistor in this amplifier is variable and is used to compensate for temperature and scale expansion drift.

To use such a meter, one must standardize with two buffer solutions of similar activity to the unknown solution. These are the two points that determine the straight line. At least two control knobs are needed, and frequently three are present. Controls affecting the offset are called calibrate, standardize, temperature, balance, or bucking, while those affecting the gain are called range or slope. For best results the calibration solution values should bracket the expected sample values. This is because the glass electrode is not linear with pH over the whole range, and extrapolation can rapidly become inaccurate. For the same reason, it is desirable to use standards no more than three pH units apart. Commonly used standards are at pH 4, 7, and 10.

The glass electrode used in the pH meter to measure the hydrogen ion concentration is only one of a number of ion selective electrodes that have been developed. To measure other ions, glass electrodes must be made with different pore structures. Total

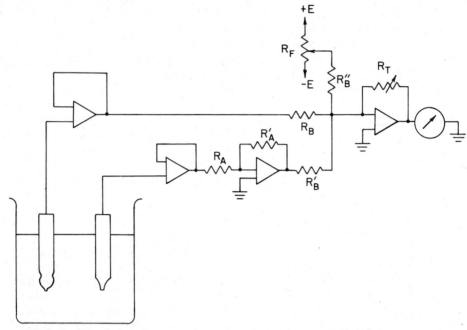

Figure 12-8 The electronics of a hypothetical pH meter including necessary control adjustments. R_F is the offset control and R_T is the slope control. Internal controls might allow R'_A, R'_B, and R''_B to be adjusted to get the best possible overall balance.

differentiation is not possible, however. For example, pH electrodes are also responsive to a lesser extent to sodium and potassium. High salt concentration will make the pH measurement invalid. Sodium electrodes are somewhat sensitive to pH, but this effect can be eliminated by buffering. Potassium is present in too low a concentration in the body to interfere with sodium measurements.

Membranes can be made of other materials than glass. Another common type of electrode uses a liquid membrane (Fig. 12-9). The central shaft of the electrode is filled with an aqueous solution of the ions of interest saturated with AgCl. Into this is inserted a Ag–AgCl electrode as a reference. In the outer chamber is a non-volatile immiscible organic liquid that can exchange the ions of the element of interest with aqueous solutions. The bottom of the electrode consists of a thin porous membrane that becomes permeated with the organic liquid. The ions in the aqueous solution interact with the organic liquid in a process called ion exchange to an

extent proportional to the logarithm of their concentration.

$$RH_2 + M^{2+} \rightleftharpoons RM + 2H^+ \qquad \textbf{(12-34)}$$

This reaction creates a potential at the aqueous–organic interface between the internal solution and the membrane as well as at the interface between an external solution and the membrane. The differ-

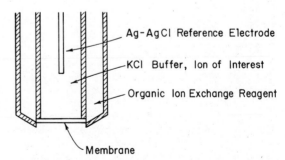

Ag–AgCl Reference Electrode

KCl Buffer, Ion of Interest

Organic Ion Exchange Reagent

Membrane

Figure 12-9 A liquid membrane electrode.

ence in these potentials can be measured between the internal reference electrode and an external reference electrode dipped into the unknown solution. The immiscible organic agent prevents contact between the internal and external aqueous solutions and therefore any transport of the ions of interest. This is analogous to the glass electrode. In the clinical laboratory ion membrane electrodes are commonly used for the measurement of calcium.

It is also possible to use neutral organic molecules in the ion exchange processes. The antibiotic valinomycin can be dissolved in diphenyl ether to create a membrane 10^4 times more sensitive to potassium than sodium. Due to the 40-fold excess of sodium to potassium in serum, this electrode is very important for such determination. Due to their specificity and the ease of use compared with other measurement methods, ion-selective electrodes are growing in popularity.

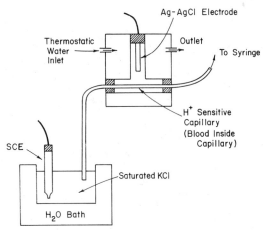

Figure 12-10 The pH of blood is measured in a capillary that is made of glass sensitive to the hydrogen ion concentration. The whole device is kept at a constant temperature. Note the path of the electrical circuit through the various liquids.

Section 12-4
MEASUREMENT OF BLOOD pH AND P_{CO_2}

The measurement of the gases in blood is concerned with oxygen and carbon dioxide, as well as the pH, which has an effect on the CO_2 concentration. The equations for the bicarbonate system equilibria are

$$CO_2 + H_2O \rightleftharpoons H_2CO_3 \qquad \textbf{(12-35)}$$

$$H_2CO_3 \rightleftharpoons HCO_3^- + H^+ \qquad \textbf{(12-36)}$$

$$HCO_3^- \rightleftharpoons CO_3^= + H^+ \qquad \textbf{(12-37)}$$

The production of CO_2 and the consumption of oxygen is a result of the metabolism of carbohydrates to generate energy for the body's activities:

$$C_nH_{2n}O_n + nO_2 \rightarrow nCO_2 + nH_2O \quad \textbf{(12-38)}$$

The measurement of oxygen will be deferred until Section 12-5. The measurement of pH has already been discussed in principle. An actual electrode configuration used for blood pH is shown in Figure 12-10. The measurement is made in capillary tubing with glass that is sensitive to the H^+ concentration. Because the pH of blood does not vary over a wide range (<1 pH unit), the accuracy of the

electrode over large pH changes is unimportant. The sensitivity of the electrode to small pH changes is critical. Due care must be exercised to protect the electrode from solutions with a pH differing dramatically from that of blood to prevent a bias from being created in the electrode due to the memory effect. Because of the sensitivity which is desired from the electrode, it is imperative that the thermostat in the measuring device hold the temperature very accurately ($\pm0.2°C$).

The measurement of CO_2 concentration is accomplished using an indirect technique. The blood passes through a chamber having a membrane which is permeable to CO_2, but not to the ions or the larger molecules in the blood (Fig. 12-11). Such membranes can be made from Teflon (tetrafluoroethylene resin), polyethylene, nylon, glass, or silicone rubber. The membranes are very thin, on the order of $10–50$ μm.

The solution on the other side of the membrane is composed of small amounts of sodium carbonate (0.01 M) in a sodium chloride solution (0.02 M). Two electrodes are present in the solution. One electrode is a Ag–AgCl electrode, which acts as the reference electrode. Because of this, sodium chloride must be present so a reference potential is set,

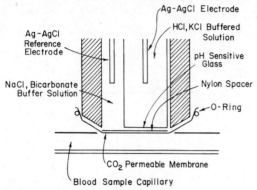

Figure 12-11 The P_{CO_2} electrode uses a semiperme-able membrane to allow the CO_2 to diffuse from the blood into the measuring chamber. The CO_2 concentration is then determined from the hydrogen ion created by its reaction with water.

but care must be taken in preparation so that the electrode's coating does not dissolve as $AgCl_2^-$. The other electrode is a glass electrode used for measuring the pH. This is the working electrode in the CO_2 measurement.

When the CO_2 crosses the membrane, some of it reacts with the water to form carbonic acid.

$$CO_2 + H_2O \rightarrow H_2CO_3 \qquad \textbf{(12-39)}$$

Some of this acid then dissociates to give hydrogen ion:

$$H_2CO_3 \rightarrow HCO_3^- + H^+ \qquad \textbf{(12-40)}$$

It is this hydrogen ion that is measured by the glass electrode. Note that this measurement is not that of the pH of the blood nor does it have any direct relationship to the pH of the blood. It is related only to the CO_2 concentration in the blood, because only gases can pass through the membrane. The concentration of CO_2 can then be determined based on the following derivation. We start with the first dissociation reaction, for which the equilibrium constant is given by

$$K_1 = \frac{[H^+][HCO_3^-]}{[H_2CO_3]} = 3.5 \cdot 10^{-7} \qquad \textbf{(12-41)}$$

and then substitute for $[H_2CO_3]$ from the association reaction of CO_2 and water:

$$K_s = \frac{[H_2CO_3]}{P_{CO_2}} = 3.4 \cdot 10^{-2} \qquad \textbf{(12-42)}$$

to give

$$K_1 = \frac{[H^+][HCO_3^-]}{K_s P_{CO_2}} \qquad \textbf{(12-43)}$$

Taking the negative logarithm of both sides, we get

$$-\log K_1 = -\log [H^+] - \log \frac{[HCO_3^-]}{K_s P_{CO_2}} \qquad \textbf{(12-44)}$$

If we put the reaction constant and $[H^+]$ in "p" notation and rearrange we get the famous Henderson-Hasselbach equation.

$$pH = pK_1 + \log \frac{[HCO_3^-]}{K_s P_{CO_2}} \qquad \textbf{(12-45)}$$

If instead we combine the constants in Eq. 12-43 ($K' = K_1 K_s$) and rearrange,

$$P_{CO_2} = \frac{[H^+][HCO_3^-]}{K'} \qquad \textbf{(12-46)}$$

If we take the negative logarithm of this equation, we get

$$-\log P_{CO_2} = pH - \log [HCO_3^-] - pK' \qquad \textbf{(12-47)}$$

P_{CO_2} can readily be calculated from this equation. The pK' is a constant. The log $[HCO_3^-]$ is also a constant for any particular electrode once the bicarbonate concentration has been set. This is the reason for the addition of sodium bicarbonate to the electrolyte in the measuring chamber. Since these are constants, they can be eliminated electronically by an offset control. Any change in log P_{CO_2} will then be just the negative of the change in pH.

$$\Delta \log P_{CO_2} = -\Delta pH \qquad \textbf{(12-48)}$$

The conditions needed to operate a P_{CO_2} electrode are very similar to those required to operate a pH electrode. Temperature is very important. Care must be taken not to expose the electrode to strong reagents or solutions with high concentrations of materials, which can penetrate the membrane. It takes approximately two minutes for the electrode to reach 99% of equilibrium.

A common source of confusion about the measurement of the CO_2 concentration is thinking of P_{CO_2} (the partial pressure of CO_2) as pCO_2, the negative logarithm of the carbon dioxide concentration. The CO_2 is originally measured as the negative logarithm of the hydrogen ion concentration, but this is then converted by an antilogarithm amplification device into units of partial pressure of CO_2. The device would be placed just before the meter in Figure 12-8. Such a device is basically a transistor with an emitter current that increases exponentially when the base current increases linearly for some range of inputs. Its detailed structure is beyond the scope of this text.

Section 12-5
MEASUREMENT OF P_{O_2}

The principles used to measure the pH and P_{CO_2} cannot be used to measure the P_{O_2}. The oxygen in water does not naturally react with the water to produce a species easily measured potentiometrically at an electrode or elsewhere. It is, therefore, necessary to force a reaction to occur that can then be measured. This is accomplished by use of an electrochemical technique called polarography.

Polarography is based on the measurement of the current that flows through a solution as an increasingly larger potential (usually negative) is applied to an electrode. The electrodes needed for polarogra-

phy must have special properties. The reference (positive electrode) must be nonpolarizable; that is, the electrode potential must remain the same even when a reaction is occurring at it. The reaction must not change the composition of the solution around the electrode and thereby "polarize" it. Suitable anodes are calomel electrodes, Ag–AgCl electrodes, and large mercury pool electrodes.

The cathode or working electrode must be polarizable, but not corrodible. This means that the electrode must be able to decrease the concentration of some solution species in its neighborhood as the reaction occurs. On the other hand, the electrode surface should not become contaminated with the products of the reaction so that its electron transfer properties deteriorate. As the voltage on the working electrode becomes more cathodic (negative), the current through the solution begins to rise very slowly (Fig. 12-12A). This is due to the charging of the electrical double layer of ions around the electrodes and the diffusion of the ions of water under the influence of the electrical field. This continues until a potential of -1.7 V is reached. At this point, water itself is decomposed. (Actually water can decompose at a lower potential, but various factors

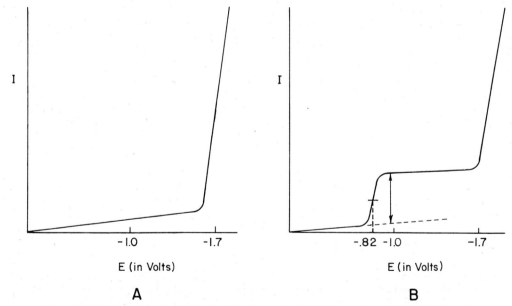

Figure 12-12 The polarogram in Part A shows the breakdown of pure water. In B, cadmium ion is present and therefore a "wave" can be seen at -0.82 V.

contribute to prevent this from happening under ordinary circumstances.)

$$2e^- + 2H_2O \rightleftharpoons 2OH^- + H_2 \qquad \text{(12-49)}$$

With a mercury pool anode, the other reaction is

$$2Hg \rightleftharpoons Hg_2^{2+} + 2e^- \qquad \text{(12-50)}$$

This breakdown of water is shown as a large increase in current in Figure 12-12A.

Certain elements are easier to reduce than hydrogen in aqueous solution. One that is commonly used by electrochemists is cadmium which is reduced at -0.82 V.

$$2e^- + Cd^{2+} \rightleftharpoons Cd \qquad \text{(12-51)}$$

If the solution is free of oxygen and contains only cadmium cations, then as the potential of -0.82 V is approached, the current begins to rise and continues to rise until some point past the -0.82 V value. Then the current levels off and continues to increase slowly, as before, until water breakdown is reached (Fig. 12-12B).

Both the voltage at which the cadmium wave appears and the height of the wave are significant. The height is proportional to the amount of cadmium present. This is true because of the way in which electrode reduction affects the neighboring solution. When the potential of a reducible species is reached, any of that species adjacent to the electrode is reduced. This, however, depletes that part of the solution of the reducible species. More ions of the species must work their way to the electrode before more reduction can occur. This process is called diffusion. The current is therefore limited by the rate at which reducible ions can diffuse to the electrode from the bulk of the solution. This rate is proportional to matrix effects of the solution and the concentration of the reducible species. By keeping the matrix effects constant for the standards and unknowns, the concentration can be found from the waveheight.

The voltage at which the reduction occurs is a fundamental property of the reducible species. The actual point used to measure the potential is when the wave has risen to one-half its final height. This is called the "half-wave potential." These are tabulated and can be used to identify unknown species. The reason this part of the line is a smooth curve

rather than an abrupt rise is that electron transfer is a microscopically reversible equilibrium. The probability of the process happening to a measurable extent becomes significant before the half-wave potential is reached, but does not approach unity until after it has been overrun by some margin.

Polarography is useful in identifying unknowns. Since we know what we want to measure, oxygen, we can simplify our approach. The reaction of interest is

$$4e^- + O_2 + 2H_2O \rightleftharpoons 4OH^- \qquad \text{(12-52)}$$

Oxygen will be reduced at a potential of a few tenths of a volt. The measurement of oxygen in blood can be accomplished by holding the potential at -0.6 or -0.7 V, well onto the plateau of the oxygen wave, but not so negative as to cause other reactions to occur. Note that this is a consumptive measurement process. The electrode is extremely small in area, resulting in reduction of a negligible but proportional amount of oxygen.

The name of the actual process used to measure the partial pressure of oxygen in blood is called amperometry and is carried out by a device such as the one shown in Figure 12-13. The oxygen passes from the blood through the semipermeable membrane into the buffer solution. The membrane excludes other reducible species. The buffer is composed of KCl to set the potential of the reference electrode and phosphate buffer to prevent the hydroxide generated by the reaction from affecting

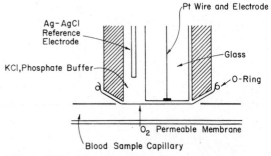

Figure 12-13 The P_{O_2} electrode uses a semipermeable membrane to allow the O_2 to diffuse from the blood into the measuring chamber. The O_2 concentration is measured through its reduction at a very small platinum electrode at a constant potential.

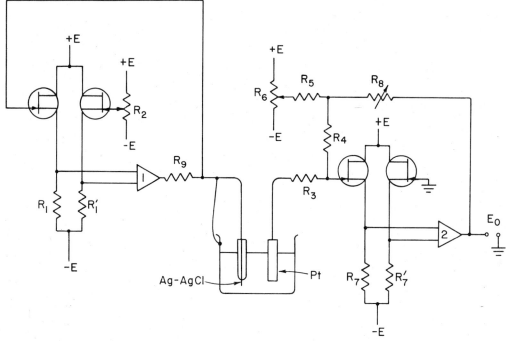

Figure 12-14 A simplified circuit of the electronics of a P_{O_2} electrode. It is important that the measurement cell be electrically isolated from the rest of the instrument so that other potential differences do not cause current to flow.

the chemical composition of the solution. Unlike in the P_{CO_2} and pH measurements, the potential of the electrodes is set by an external circuit to the appropriate voltage (in this case, -0.6 to -0.7 V). The measurement made is of the current flowing.

The simplified electronics for the oxygen measurement are shown in Figure 12-14. While they at first appear formidable, they can be readily segmented into components seen before. At the left is just a FET differential amplifier. If a voltage is set on the potentiometer, R_2, then operational amplifier OA1 must produce the same voltage to go into the other input of the differential amplifier to balance OA1. It is just a more complex feedback element than previously seen. If 0.70 V is set on R_2, then OA1 will produce this output, which is then applied to the reference electrode (and the measurement cell). The platinum electrode used for making the measurement is therefore -0.70 V with respect to the environment and will begin reducing

oxygen. The circuit on the right is composed of three basic elements. The differential FET amplifier allows the input signal to be compared with ground. The R_4–R_8 combination acts as the feedback resistor of an inverter with gain. Variable R_8 allows the gain to be adjusted. The R_5–R_6 combination allows an offset from zero to balance the differential amplifier. The output of OA2 is fed into the conversion and reporting circuitry.

While Figure 12-14 may not even appear to be a circuit, it is one in operation. The positive and the negative voltage supplies are common to all components, as is the ground. One can show this by connecting the relevant wires, but this only makes the circuit more confusing. The advantage of this type of circuit is that since the reference electrode is on the output of an operational amplifier, it can produce any amount of current the circuit may need. Because the other electrode is on the input of an operational amplifier, the voltage or current it produces can be readily absorbed. As a result, this general arrangement can be used for all of the electrode configurations used for blood gas measurements. Of course, for potential measurements, the feedback loop of the right hand part of the circuit would have to be altered to some extent. The output of all these electrodes can then be fed alternately into the same conversion electronics to reduce cost.

Because the electrochemical technique used to measure the O_2 concentration is linear in the unknown species, it is not necessary to do any additional manipulations as was the case for CO_2. This results from the fact that we are measuring diffusion, which is a linear function of the concentration, rather than reduction potential, which is a linear function of the logarithm of the concentration. The result of the measurement then is the partial presence of oxygen, P_{O_2}, expressed in torr.

A typical blood gas instrument is capable of calculating other information such as total CO_2 and bicarbonate concentrations from the species measured. If the hemoglobin is measured by the instrument or inserted manually, is also possible to calculate the base excess. With the advent of microprocessors, the blood gas instruments have become much easier to use. Previously, laboratory workers had to draw nomograms that related the various measured and calculated quantities to each other in order to come up with reportable answers.

Section 12-6
COULOMETRY

Another form of electrochemical measurement is coulometry, which arose out of the use of electricity to purify metals through replating. If a solution of metal salt has two electrodes inserted into it of sufficiently different potential, the metal will plate out at the more cathodic electrode while the other electrode dissolves. The net effect is to allow current to flow through the solution at some fixed potential. Because the plating is a transport-limited process, the rate of metal reduction is limited by diffusion and convection to the electrode surface. The effective resistance of the solution remains nearly constant because the metal ions of interest

are replenished from the dissolving anode. By measuring the current and the length of time the metal is plated out, one can determine how many coulombs of charge were used to reduce the metal.

The number of coulombs (q) is linearly proportional to the amount of metal ion present:

$$q = nFV[M] \qquad \text{(12-53)}$$

where q is the charge, n is the number of electrons, F is the Faraday constant (96,487 C/eq. wt), and V is the solution volume. Since the charge is just the product of time and current (Eq. 1-5), the concentration of the metal ion is

$$[M] = \frac{It}{nFV} \qquad \text{(12-54]}$$

The factor I/nF can be calculated or determined by a standard.

The metals present in the body are there in too minute concentration or are nonreducible in aqueous solution and cannot be measured by this method. By modification of the method to some extent, however, we can use it to measure chloride, the only halide present in the body to a significant extent. Silver chloride is insoluble, with a solubility constant of only 10^{-10}. If one could generate Ag^+ electrochemically, one could precipitate all the chloride. The amount of Ag^+ required would be equal to the amount of Cl^- present.

The apparatus to accomplish such measurements is diagrammed in Figure 12-15A. A large silver anode ionizes to generate Ag^+, while a platinum cathode serves as the counter electrode:

$$Ag \rightleftharpoons Ag^+ + e^- \qquad \text{(12-55)}$$

The Ag^+ precipitates the chloride:

$$Ag^+ + Cl^- \rightleftharpoons AgCl \qquad \text{(12-56)}$$

This process continues until all the chloride is precipitated. At that point the other two electrodes in the solution come into play. This pair of silver electrodes is used to monitor the silver ion concentration by the measurement of the current flowing between them at a fixed potential. When the amount of Ag^+ generated from the primary anode exceeds the amount of chloride present, the Ag^+ concentration rises abruptly. This permits Eq. 12-55 to proceed in the reverse direction at the nega-

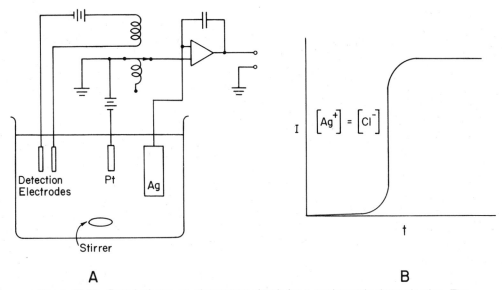

$$I \quad \left[Ag^+\right] = \left[Cl^-\right]$$

$$t$$

A   B

Figure 12-15 Part A shows an elementary circuit for a coulometric determination. The amplifier is shorted until the measurement starts. Part B shows the current through the monitoring circuit. More complex circuits allow the endpoint to be approached more slowly after the bulk neutralization has occurred.

tive monitoring electrode (Fig. 12-15B) and causes a current surge between the silver-monitoring electrodes. This current switches off the circuit generating the Ag^+. The amount of current that flowed in the generating circuit is determined by an integrator in series with the solution being measured. In more sophisticated instruments, additional circuitry allows the amount of current to be reduced as the equivalence point approaches to reduce the overrun error. Naturally the positioning of the electrodes is important to prevent intercircuit interaction. Keeping the ionic strength constant and the reaction vessel clean between samples is necessary to maintain calibration of the system. Other halides and anions that are easily reduced or precipitated interfere with this measurement. Such interferences are commonly present in urine. The standard deviation of replicates is 1–3%.

With the inclusion of chloride, we now know how to measure Na^+, Ca^{2+}, K^+, Cl^-, and CO_2 in blood. These constitute the electrolytes of the body which are frequently analyzed for. We shall encounter them again when we study flame photome-

try. Before that, however, we will look at some other basic laboratory technology.

REVIEW QUESTIONS

1. Explain the statement that a half-reaction is reversible.
2. What happens at an electrode's surface?
3. What is the equation for the thermodynamic equilibrium constant?
4. Define the activity of a solution species.
5. How is the activity defined for solids? Liquids? Gases? Ions? Free electrons?
6. Define partial pressure.
7. Define mole fraction.
8. Define activity coefficient. What is the upper limit of its value?
9. Define ionic strength.
10. Under what conditions is the activity coefficient near unity?
11. On what factors does the activity of the free electron depend?

12. Under what conditions does the reaction potential equal the standard potential?
13. What is the standard formulation of the Nernst equation?
14. What controls the availability of free electrons?
15. How are the potentials of half-reactions assigned?
16. Why was the hydrogen reaction chosen as the standard reaction?
17. What is the Nernst equation constant at 25°C? At 37°C?
18. Sketch and label the parts of a hydrogen electrode.
19. How does a hydrogen electrode work?
20. What is a standard hydrogen electrode? What are the values of the standard concentrations?
21. What are the disadvantages of the hydrogen electrode?
22. What is "p" notation?
23. What two types of electrodes are necessary to make a measurement? Explain how each works.
24. Sketch and label the parts of a saturated calomel electrode.
25. How does an SCE work? Why is its potential relatively stable?
26. In what two ways does temperature affect the potential of an SCE?
27. What are the advantages and disadvantages of an SCE?
28. Why are nonsaturated calomel electrodes sometimes used?
29. Sketch and label the parts of a silver–silver chloride electrode.
30. How is the potential on the Ag–AgCl electrode set?
31. What are the advantages and disadvantages of a Ag–AgCl electrode?
32. Sketch and label the parts of a glass electrode.
33. How does a glass electrode work?
34. What are the disadvantages of a glass electrode?
35. Why is it necessary to use operational amplifiers with glass electrodes?
36. What is a junction potential? How are its effects eliminated?
37. What instrumental factors contribute to the difficulty of making pH measurements?

38. How is standardization of a pH meter accomplished chemically? Electronically? Why?
39. Sketch and label the components of a liquid membrane electrode.
40. Describe how a liquid membrane electrode works.
41. From what reaction does the human body derive its energy?
42. What are the basic reactions of the bicarbonate equilibrium system?
43. Sketch and label the parts of the electrode chamber used to make pH measurements in blood.
44. What is the memory effect of glass electrodes?
45. How is the measurement of P_{CO_2} accomplished?
46. From what can the semipermeable membrane be made?
47. What factors determine the chemical composition of the electrolyte in the electrode chamber?
48. What is the relationship between the pH measured in the P_{CO_2} electrode and the pH of blood?
49. How long does it take for P_{CO_2} to reach equilibrium?
50. What is the difference between P_{CO_2} and pCO_2? Which is measured by the electrode? Which is reported?
51. What principle is used to measure P_{O_2}?
52. How does the measurement of P_{O_2} differ from that of pH and P_{CO_2}?
53. What are the two types of electrodes needed to measure P_{O_2}?
54. Define polarizable. How does it differ from corrodable?
55. How does polarography work? What solution property does it measure?
56. What is a half-wave potential? What determines it?
57. What determines the height of the current wave?
58. How was the potential used for oxygen selected?
59. Sketch and label the parts of a P_{O_2} electrode.
60. Explain how the circuit in Figure 12-14 works.
61. Contrast the circuit in Figure 12-8 with that in Figure 12-14.

62. What other parameters can newer blood gas instruments calculate?
63. What is the basic reaction in coulometry?
64. How does one determine the concentration in a coulometric measurement?
65. How is a chloride measurement made by coulometry?
66. What is the function of each electrode in coulometry?

PROBLEMS

1. Balance the following equations:
   a. $O_2 + Ag + HCl \rightleftharpoons H_2O + AgCl$
   b. $H_2 + Hg + HClO_3 \rightleftharpoons Hg_2Cl_2 + H_2O$
   c. $HCl + AgNO_3 \rightleftharpoons$
      $AgCl + NO + Cl_2 + H_2O$
   d. $H_2O + Hg_2Cl_2 + O_2 + Ag \rightleftharpoons$
      $Hg + AgCl + AgOH$
2. What is the ionic strength of the following?
   a. $2.67 \cdot 10^{-3} M$ NaCl
   b. $8.40 \cdot 10^{-4} M$ Na_2SO_4
   c. $1.042 \cdot 10^{-5} M$ $Al_2(SO_4)_3$
   d. $2.14 \cdot 10^{-3} M$ $BeCl_2$, $1.69 \cdot 10^{-3} M$ Na_3PO_4
   e. $0.0379 M$ $AgNO_3$, $0.0216 M$ $BaCl_2$
3. Calculate the activity coefficient of the following species in the solutions given in Problem 2.
   a. Na^+
   b. Na^+, SO_4^{-2}
   c. Al^{3+}, SO_4^{-2}
   d. Be^{2+}, Cl^-, PO_4^{-3}
   e. NO_3^-, Ba^{2+}
4. If one solution is $2.45 \cdot 10^{-3} M$ in $ZnCl_2$ and another solution is $1.843 M$ in $Cu(NO_3)_2$, what is the voltage between them at $25°C$ when they are placed in the appropriate sides of the apparatus shown in Figure 3-5?

5. If the concentration of the zinc solution in Figure 3-5 is $0.947 M$ and the potential is 1.271 V, what is the concentration of the copper solution at $25°C$?
6. A hydrogen electrode is in an acid solution. If the pH of the solution is increased by 1.84 units and the hydrogen pressure is increased by 112%, what is the change in the electrode potential?
7. What is the hydrogen ion concentration if the potential of a hydrogen electrode with hydrogen pressure of 1.243 atm is 0.0992 V versus an SHE?
8. What is the voltage between a hydrogen electrode and an SCE if the $[H^+] = 5.70 \cdot 10^{-4}$ and the pressure is 1.000 atm?
9. What is the difference in potential between a hydrogen electrode in a $3.89 \cdot 10^{-5} M$ $[H^+]$ solution under 0.742 atm of hydrogen and a Ag–AgCl electrode in a $6.44 \cdot 10^{-2} M$ $[Cl^-]$ solution?
10. If the chloride ion concentration is $8.79 \cdot 10^{-4} M$, what is the potential of a Ag–AgCl electrode immersed in the solution?
11. At what $[Cl^-]$ will the Ag–AgCl electrode have the same potential as that of an SCE?
12. How many grams of solid NaOH must be added to 100. ml $0.0128 M$ HCl (completely dissociated) to increase the pH by 1.00 unit?
13. How many grams of solid NaOH must be added to 89.3 ml $0.0206 M$ H_2SO_4 (completely dissociated) to increase the pH by 0.71 unit?
14. How long must a current of 6.34 mA flow to generate enough Ag^+ to precipitate 8.42 ml of $0.0725 M$ Cl^- solution?
15. How many moles of $BaCl_2$ were in solution if 4.79 mA were applied for 112.7 sec to generate enough Ag^+ to cause complete precipitation of the chloride?

CHAPTER 13
SIMPLE INSTRUMENTS

In this chapter we will investigate how elementary principles can serve as the basis for instrumentation. Because of the simplicity of these approaches, they have been used for many years in clinical laboratories. The first of these is refractometry, which uses the optical principles described in Chapters 10 and 11. The second is osmometry, which will tie together some freshman chemistry with electronic data measurement techniques. Finally, densitometry will set the stage for the light measurements in subsequent chapters.

Section 13-1
REFRACTOMETRY

In Chapter 10 we examined what happens when light passes from a less optically dense to a more optically dense material. The entering light is bent at a lesser angle to the normal than is the incident beam. When the incident light is parallel to the surface, a critical or maximum angle is reached, and light cannot be bent into the remainder of the prism (Fig. 10-10). The critical angle can be determined if the refractive indices of the two substances are known. On the other hand, if we can measure the critical angle (α) and know the index of refraction of one of the substances (a), the refractive index of the other substance can be calculated (b) (Section 10-3):

$$b = a \sin \alpha \qquad (13\text{-}1)$$

An instrument that can make this type of measurement is a refractometer. Several different types of refractometers exist because the phenomenon of the critical angle can be exploited in several ways.

We will examine two of the types most commonly used in the clinical laboratory, the Abbe and immersion models.

Figure 13-1 shows the general layout of the Abbe refractometer. White light from a source such as an ordinary tungsten filament bulb is reflected by a plane mirror into the specimen-containing prism pair, shown in Figure 13-2A. The light enters the illuminating prism perpendicular to its base and therefore suffers no refraction. When it reaches the upper surface of this prism, it is scattered in all directions because this surface is rough ground glass. Refraction at any point possesses no relationship to that at any other point, although Snell's law is obeyed at every point. This surface is therefore a nondirectional radiation source. Between the two prisms is the hinged sample compartment containing a few drops of specimen which have been spread to a 100 μm layer by the closing of the prisms. As the light traverses this liquid, most of it encounters the refracting prism. Since the liquid sample is of lower refractive index than this upper prism, the light bends toward the normal as it enters the upper prism. The light is traveling in all directions, however, so all angles of incidence to the normal in a full 360° circle are formed at any one point. In contrast, the light leaving the point into the refracting prism can travel only in pathways that have an angle to the normal equal to or less than the critical angle. This creates a cone of light proceeding from each point (shaded area in Fig. 13-2A). An observer in area B looking toward point I would see no light, whereas an observer in area A would see light.

To measure the angle α accurately, it is necessary to concentrate the numerous light paths. Each

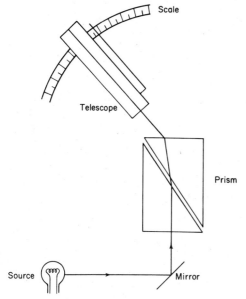

Figure 13-1 Block diagram of Abbe refractometer. (Courtesy of Bausch & Lomb Instruments and Systems Division. Redrawn with permission.)

point on the interface of the sample-refracting prism is, after all, the source of a cone of light. This results in light traveling in different directions through the various points of the prism. Since the light cannot be measured in the prism, it is allowed to emerge from the top and to enter a telescope. This telescope has lenses that allow close observation of the emerging parallel light paths in the vicinity of the critical angle, which appears as a light–dark boundary. To accomplish this, the telescope must be moved relative to the refracting prism (Fig. 13-2B). This complicates matters because there is now a second refraction to worry about as the light leaves the prism and enters the air. Fortunately, the critical angle at the sample-illuminating prism interface (α) is a function of the angle which we can measure (γ). This relationship can be calculated using Figure 13-3A. Snell's law for the light leaving the prism is

$$\mu_A \sin \gamma = \mu_P \sin \beta \qquad (13\text{-}2)$$

where μ_A and μ_P are the refractive indices of air and the prism, respectively.

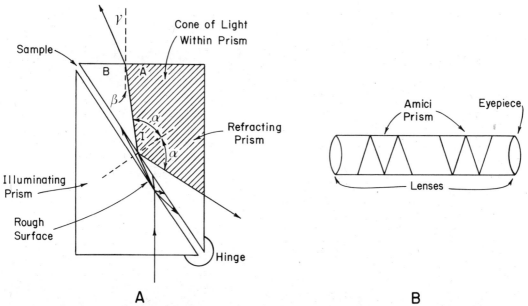

Figure 13-2 The refracting prism of an Abbe refractometer (A) and the telescope used for refractometry (B). (Courtesy of Bausch & Lomb Instruments and Systems Division. Redrawn with permission.)

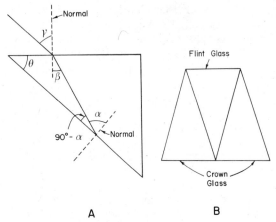

Figure 13-3 Part A shows the geometry of the refracting prism. Part B shows the Amici compensator.

Solving for the angle of incidence gives

$$\sin \beta = \frac{\mu_A}{\mu_P} \sin \gamma \qquad (13\text{-}3)$$

$$\beta = \arcsin \left(\frac{\mu_A}{\mu_P} \sin \gamma\right) \qquad (13\text{-}4)$$

Since there are 180° in a triangle,

$$(90° - \alpha) = 180° - \theta - (\beta + 90°) \qquad (13\text{-}5)$$

$$\alpha = \theta + \arcsin \left(\frac{\mu_A}{\mu_P} \sin \gamma\right) \qquad (13\text{-}6)$$

Applying Snell's law at the critical angle of the sample-prism interface gives

$$\sin \alpha = \frac{\mu_S}{\mu_P} \qquad (13\text{-}7)$$

$$\mu_S = \mu_P \sin \alpha \qquad (13\text{-}8)$$

Note that μ_S is the refractive index of the sample. Substituting Eq. 13-6 for α gives us the index of refraction of the sample as a function of γ and some constants.

$$\mu_S = \mu_P \sin \left[\theta + \arcsin\left(\frac{\mu_A}{\mu_P} \sin \gamma\right)\right] \qquad (13\text{-}9)$$

Fortunately, the user of the instrument does not have to do these calculations for every sample. A

pointer attached to the telescope moves relative to a scale. This scale is calibrated in terms of the index of refraction of the sample. A magnifier improves the ability to read the scale, allowing accurate reading to ±0.0002 units.

The telescope is equipped with crosshairs to allow precise positioning of it with respect to the light–dark interface. The situation is complicated by the fact that not all wavelengths of light have the same index of refraction. This causes a rainbow effect at the light–dark interface and prevents accurate measurement. This problem is circumvented by choosing a standard wavelength, which has historically been the sodium *D* line (589 nm). This wavelength, which is referred to as monochromatic (one-color) light, can be obtained in one of three ways. First, sodium radiation can be used instead of white light by employing a sodium arc lamp source. Second, a monochromator of the type described in Chapter 14 can be employed before the light reaches the prism. Most commonly, however, a device called an Amici compensator is placed within the telescope. This device, shown in Figure 13-3B, is made from two types of glass having different indices of refraction. Due to the nature of the geometry of this compound prism, light of longer or shorter wavelength than that of the sodium equivalent radiation is bent strongly away from the path of the incident light. In the Abbe telescope, two Amici compensators of opposite orientation are employed to further enhance wavelength isolation (Fig. 13-2B).

The range of the Abbe refractometer is limited by its components and geometry to a refractive index range of 1.30–1.84 (unitless). The lower limit is based on the geometry of light paths from the sample through the refracting prism to the telescope, while the upper limit is caused by the fact that the refractive index of the sample must be less than that of the refracting prism. Different prisms may be necessary to cover the range indicated.

The immersion or dipping refractometer is extremely simple, having only the refracting prism (Fig. 13-4). Light is reflected by a plane mirror onto the bevelled face of the prism which is immersed in a container of the liquid of interest. The light strikes the prism surface parallel to the surface or at slightly smaller angles to the normal. Inside the prism the light is bent toward the normal, and again a portion of the prism will not be lighted from a given point of light entry because the light cannot be bent enough to traverse it. Consequently, a light–dark interface develops that can be observed with a telescope. The Bausch and Lomb immersion refractometer is very accurate with a change of 0.01 division on the scale corresponding to the change of 0.000037 in refractive index.

The major problem with using a refractometer is the dependence of the refractive index of a solution on the temperature. A change of 1°C causes a decrease in the refractive index of nearly 0.0005 unit. Temperature control of 0.1° or 0.2°C is therefore necessary to yield usable readings. Samples for the

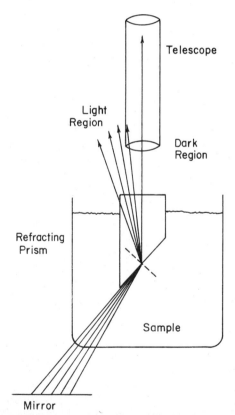

Figure 13-4 Block diagram of the immersion refractometer. (Courtesy of Bausch & Lomb Instruments and Systems Division. Redrawn with permission.)

immersion refractometer can be placed directly into a waterbath, while an Abbe refractometer must be kept in a highly controlled environment or be thermostated by circulating water through the instrument. Careful temperature control yields good reproducibility from this relatively simple physical measurement.

Refractometry can be used to estimate the total protein, total dissolved solids, and specific gravity of body fluids. In actuality, refractometry is a measure of the optical density of a liquid. By controlling conditions, however, a relationship can be established between optical and physical density. Because water is defined as having a specific gravity of 1, the relative density of body fluids which are primarily aqueous can readily be expressed as specific gravity. A principal contributor to specific gravity of body fluids is the protein present. With proper calibration a refractometer can be used to approximate the total protein concentration. By controlling all but one variable affecting the refractive index, any contributing factor to the index can be measured in theory, although in practice most are so small as to be difficult to quantitate.

Section **13-2**
OSMOMETRY

In a pure liquid each molecule interacts uniformly with every other molecule. This results in sharp phase transitions between solid and liquid and between liquid and vapor. When introducing any other molecules into the liquid, a solution is formed in which each molecule no longer interacts uniformly with its neighbors. Because solute molecules disrupt the structure and orderliness of a liquid, the liquid will try to minimize the concentration of the solute whenever possible. Solvent molecules already present will resist leaving. This will lower the vapor pressure, which in turn will raise the boiling point. Similarly, solvent will resist freezing out, which will lower the freezing point. If the solution is separated from a less concentrated solution by a semipermeable membrane, it will attract solvent through the membrane to dilute the solute. This causes osmotic pressure upon the membrane. These four affected attributes—

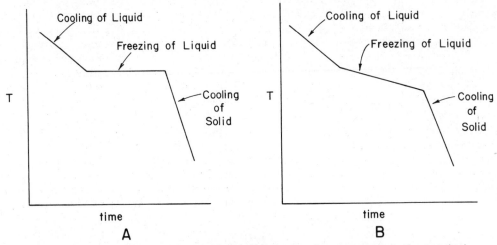

Figure 13-5 When materials are cooled uniformly, they lose temperature at a constant rate, depending on their specific heat, except when they cross a phase boundary. Part A represents the freezing of a pure liquid, while Part B represents a solution.

freezing point, boiling point, vapor pressure, and osmotic pressure—are collectively called the colligative properties.

It is the osmotic pressure that has clinical importance. The passive transport of fluid across cell membranes is dependent upon the osmotic pressure. The measurement of this osmotic tendency is made in terms of the solute concentration. This concentration is expressed in terms of moles per 1,000 g of solvent. In undergraduate chemistry courses such units were called a measurement of molality and were usually used to express the dissolution of a single compound in water. In the body many compounds and ions contribute to the total solute concentration, and the units are called a measurement of osmolality.

Contributors to the osmolality in body fluids include whole molecules, such as glucose, and ions, such as sodium and chloride. Undissociated molecules contribute one unit to the osmolality, while dissociated salts contribute one unit per ion released. The osmolality is then a measure of the total number of solute particles of all species, although the greatest contributors are sodium and chloride. The measured values in body fluids are expressed in milliosmoles.

The approach used most widely in the clinical laboratory to determine the osmolality is freezing point depression. While several milliliters of specimen are needed, the equipment is relatively simple in design and can be coupled with sample handling hardware to process numerous specimens automatically. Figure 13-5 shows how the dissolution of solute affects the freezing point. The freezing point of water is depressed at the rate of 1.86°C per mole of solute. But more than just depressing the freezing point, the presence of solute causes it to become diffuse, spreading over a range of temperature. As the liquid reaches its freezing point, those liquid molecules actively encountering solute molecules or ions cannot crystallize with other solvent molecules, so they remain in the liquid phase. Those liquid molecules not immediately encountering solute molecules or ions do crystallize and start to fall from solution. This crystallization involves almost pure solvent, which makes the remaining solution more concentrated. This in turn makes further freezing even more difficult. As the temperature is lowered, more areas of the solution reach the conditions necessary to crystallize. This further concentrates the remaining solution. Finally, the temperature reaches the point where all the solution must solidify. This freezing range can be spread over several degrees for a solution, while being precisely one temperature for a pure liquid.

Naturally the above scenario of a solution crys-

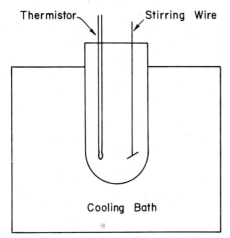

Figure 13-6 Cross section of an osmometer.

tallizing complicates freezing point measurements. The true freezing point will be obscured. Fortunately, we can overcome this adverse situation by playing a trick on nature. To freeze, a liquid must not only be cold enough, it must be given a chance to coalesce. By stirring a liquid we can prevent freezing until we have reached a temperature several degrees below the true freezing point. Such a process is called supercooling. When the liquid does begin to freeze, energy is given off because a solid has less entropy than a liquid. Since entropy

can never decrease, but must either remain constant or increase, the motion lost by the liquid during crystallization must be assumed by its environment. This released energy is called the heat of fusion, and it warms the rest of the supercooled liquid to the freezing point of the solution, where both the liquid and solid can exist in equilibrium. By continuing our attempt to extract heat from the solution, we will force the temperature to fall once again as the whole solution becomes solid. Meantime, however, we have a plateau that is indeed representative of the freezing point of the solution. By calibrating the method using standards, it is possible to accurately determine the osmolality to within 1%.

Figure 13-6 shows the configuration of the equipment used to make the measurement. The specimen is placed in a cuvette with a stirring wire and a thermistor (temperature-sensitive resistor). The cuvette is lowered into a cooling bath with an electrically controlled temperature of $-6°$ to $-7°C$. The stirring wire keeps the solution well mixed so the cooling is uniform, and no crystallization occurs. When point A in Figure 13-7 is reached, the stirrer momentarily is turned to a higher speed to induce freezing to start. The solution then begins to freeze and warms to the plateau temperature due to the heat of fusion. At this point the reading is taken and the specimen can be withdrawn.

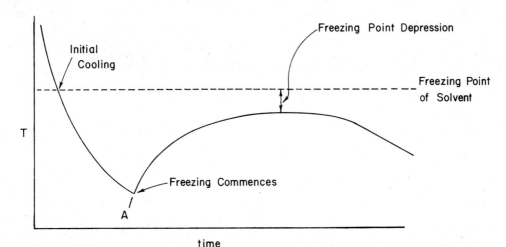

Figure 13-7 The graph of the temperature of a specimen versus time in an osmometer as cooling occurs.

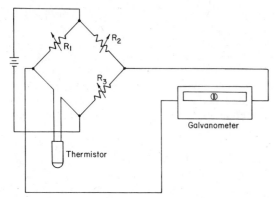

Figure 13-8 The basic circuit of a classical osmometer. In modern devices a differential amplifier replaces the galvanometer.

The reading electronics are shown in Figure 13-8. The thermistor forms one leg of a Wheatstone bridge. The current meter of the bridge has historically been a galvanometer. The other three legs of the bridge are variable resistors used to adjust the galvanometer to the zero position. The instrument is calibrated by using two standards of known osmolality. The value of each is set sequentially into R_3 (which is calibrated in milliosmoles) and R_1 and R_2 are adjusted until the galvanometer is in the zero position at the respective freezing points. Unknowns are then run, and the light beam of a reflecting galvanometer is allowed to move first in one direction and then the other, until it settles down at the freezing point. R_3 is adjusted until the galvanometer reads zero. The reading on the R_3 dial is the value of the unknown osmolality.

Newer electronics allow for more automation. The galvanometer can be replaced with a differential amplifier. The voltage difference across the bridge can be directly translated into a number of milliosmoles. This reading is then displayed on the instrument panel after being converted to the digital form by an analog-to-digital convertor as discussed in Chapter 8. If the instrument is designed to automatically handle a tray of specimens, then a printer is needed to record each specimen's sequence number and result. In such a case a timing circuit is also needed to determine how much time must elapse before the reading is to be taken for printing after

the insertion of the specimen in the cooling bath. In more sophisticated instruments this point is determined by examining the differences at small fixed time intervals and assuming the plateau is reached when the variation between sequential points is below a specified threshold.

Section 13-3
DENSITOMETRY

A number of methods are used in the laboratory to separate specific components of blood serum and urine. Electrophoresis and paper chromatography are two methods commonly covered in physiological chemistry. Such gradient methods produce spots, bands, or lines on the paper or plate that contain the different components that were separated by the application of the electrical field and/or by the movement of solution. These plates or strips must then be developed with chemicals to bring out the presence of the bands and then dried. Finally, the amounts and types of the various materials must be determined.

One means of analyzing these stripes of materials is called densitometry, because the density of the color development is measured as a function of its position on the strips. The rest of this chapter is devoted to the general approaches to densitometry, because the details of the components will be covered in our analysis of more sophisticated instrumentation in later chapters.

The block diagram of a densitometer is shown in Figure 13-9. A light source shines through a strip that contains varying densities of materials. Part of the light is blocked by the darkened areas on the strip. The transmitted light is detected and graphed, as shown in Figure 13-10. Finally the areas of the various bands, which have now been translated into peaks, are determined.

The source may be as simple as an incandescent light or it may be more sophisticated, depending on the nature of the materials being measured. Sources are discussed in Chapter 15 and monochromators in Chapter 14. The slits in Figure 13-9 restrict the light path so stray radiation does not reach the detector. The specimen, or alternately the reading mechanism, must be movable so that

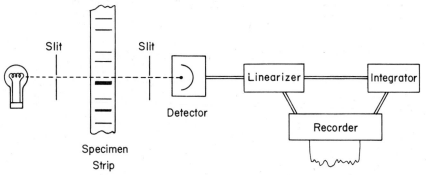

Figure 13-9 Block diagram of a densitometer.

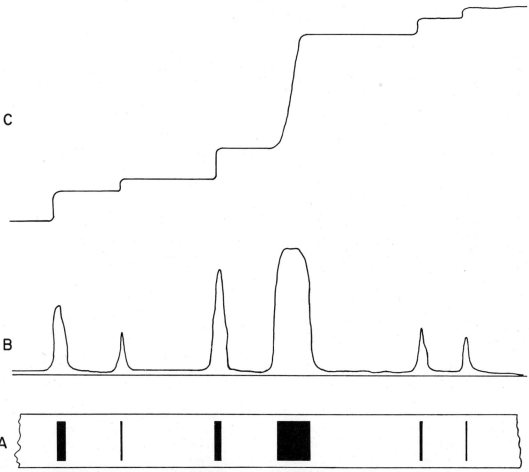

Figure 13-10 Part A shows a typical strip for analysis. Part B shows the densitometer chart record of this strip. Part C shows the integrated area under the various peaks of the recording.

the whole strip can be brought past the detector and recorded. The detector can be a photodiode or one of the more complex devices discussed in Chapter 14. Once the signal is gathered, it must then be interpreted in terms of the quantity of substance present.

Such interpretation is not trivial, and the most important part of the densitometer is the circuitry that analyzes the output of the detector. Formerly the output of the detector was directly recorded on a strip chart. The concentration of the species present is not proportional to the light detected, however, but rather to the logarithmic function of the light absorbed. This means that a circuit is necessary to linearize the signal in terms of absorbance before the data are plotted. At this point, the results can be recorded and the quantities manually calculated from the areas under the curves. Chapter 22 describes such manual methods to determine the areas. New instruments are able to do such calculations automatically by use of the integrating circuitry described in Chapter 6. The result of such integration is a second trace, which is also shown in Figure 13-10.

Densitometers have been coupled to microprocessors in the most recently developed equipment. This means that the results of the analysis can be digitized and stored in the RAM of the microprocessor by using the analog-to-digital convertor discussed in Chapter 8. The processor can then do such complex operations as remove the baseline, tentatively identify the peaks, and calculate their true concentrations based on a series of stored standard readings. Additional features such as CRT display before graphing and alternative peak analysis procedures can easily be implemented. Such computing power permits the study of secondary effects (e.g., peak shape and peak overlap) in specimens in which it was previously tedious just to get the basic data. A more detailed example of such computer data reduction techniques will be discussed in Chapter 19.

The densitometer is a fitting introduction for optical methods. These may rely on more sophisticated components and principles, but all must contain a source, a specimen, a detector, and a method of reporting the result. Chapters 14–17 discuss the general implementation of photometric methods and develop the components briefly introduced here.

REVIEW QUESTIONS

1. Upon what physical principle is refractometry based?
2. What is the equation for Snell's law?
3. Sketch and label the parts of an Abbe refractometer.
4. Explain how the Abbe refractometer works.
5. How does the illuminating prism create nondirectional light?
6. Why is a telescope needed to view the light–dark interface?
7. What complicates the measurement of the critical angle?
8. How is the critical angle read with an Abbe refractometer?
9. Why is monochromatic light needed in a refractometer?
10. What is the range of the Abbe refractometer?
11. Sketch and label the parts of an immersion refractometer.
12. What is the relative volume of specimen needed to use the two refractometers described?
13. What effect does temperature have on refractometry? Why?
14. What are several clinical quantities measured by refractometry?
15. How can monochromatic light be obtained for a refractometer?
16. Sketch and explain how an Amici compensator works.
17. What are the four colligative properties?
18. Upon what principle is osmometry based?
19. What is an osmole?
20. What contributes to the osmolality? How much?
21. How is osmolality measured most frequently?
22. Why is it difficult to measure the freezing point of a solution?
23. How does a laboratory osmometer circumvent the freezing point range problem?

24. Explain how a laboratory osmometer works.
25. How precise is osmometry?
26. Sketch and label the detection circuit of a classical osmometer.
27. Explain how an osmometer is calibrated.
28. Why are more sophisticated electronics needed when the osmometer is designed to handle numerous specimens automatically?
29. When is densitometry used?
30. Sketch and label the parts of a densitometer.
31. What problems complicate the interpretation of densitometry readings?
32. What types of enhancements are available to interpret densitometry readings?

PROBLEMS

All problems are based on Eq. 13-9. Assume that the index of refraction of air is 1.0000. Find the missing value in each problem below. You will have to use successive approximation for one of the quantities.

	μ_S	μ_P	θ	γ
1.		1.707	55.61°	24.65°
2.		1.582	56.94°	28.14°
3.	1.531	1.645	50.00°	
4.	1.526	1.609		18.50°
5.	1.606		52.71°	26.34°
6.	1.565		54.88°	23.13°

CHAPTER 14
EMISSION MEASUREMENTS

The most common method of measuring the concentrations of solution species in the clinical laboratory is by use of light. Both methods where light is absorbed and methods where light is emitted are common. Since the emission of light is simpler in concept and instrumentation than the absorption of light, we will look at it first. We will then consider absorption measurements in Chapter 15.

The most common light-emission method used is flame photometry. In flame photometry we monitor monochromatic light, a feature which was introduced in the discussion of refractometry. To understand why elements give off light at distinct wavelengths, we must examine the structure of the atom. After we have learned how atoms generate light, we can then explore the instrumentation needed to measure such radiation.

Section 14-1
ATOMIC RADIATION

For many years a fierce battle was carried on in the scientific community over whether light was really wave motion or particles. Both sides had strong evidence for their positions but also faced phenomena they could not explain by their models. The details of the history of the development of the theory of light are very interesting, but we need not review them here in order to understand the resolution of the controversy. The resolution is, of course, that light is both wave and particle. It is a particle called a photon, which has zero rest mass and which moves so as to propagate an electromagnetic wave. Since photons always travel at the speed of light, rest mass is naturally irrelevant. The speed of light in vacuum is designated as c and is

equal to $2.998 \cdot 10^8$ m/sec. A wavelength λ is associated with any portion of the light. We can define a quantity ν, the frequency, from these two:

$$\nu = \frac{c}{\lambda} \qquad (14\text{-}1)$$

The frequency is usually given in reciprocal seconds. It happens that the energy associated with a photon of light is directly proportional to its frequency:

$$E = h\nu \qquad (14\text{-}2)$$

The proportionality constant h is called Planck's constant, $(6.6262 \cdot 10^{-27}$ erg sec) after the German physicist Max Planck. The photons that compose light have a momentum (p) like any other particle. From the theory of relativity, this turns out to be

$$p = \frac{E}{c} \qquad (14\text{-}3)$$

Substituting Eq. 14-2 gives

$$p = \frac{h\nu}{c} \qquad (14\text{-}4)$$

If we substitute Eq. 14-1 into 14-4 and solve for the wavelength, we get

$$\lambda = \frac{h}{p} \qquad (14\text{-}5)$$

Note that this equation makes no specific reference to light. In fact, according to the theory of relativity, every object has a wavelength associated with its movement that can be calculated from this equation. An electron, therefore, has wave properties when it is moving, just as it has particle properties. This fact has deep implications regarding the structure of the atom.

In the early twentieth century, the structure of the atom was much in dispute. Scientists had determined that an atom was composed of a central core called the nucleus and a cloud of electrons. The nucleus contained most of the mass of the atom and a positive charge equal to the atomic number of the element of which it was a sample. In a neutral atom the number of electrons was equal to the number of positive charges in the nucleus. Some scientists held that the atom must be like a miniature solar system, but various laws of nature argued against such an analogy.

In 1913, Niels Bohr, a Danish physicist, proposed the model in which an atom has fixed locations, called orbitals, in which electrons can exist. The reason that the orbitals are fixed is due to the wave properties of the electron. In order for a wave to exist in a confined space, such as in water in a tank, it must assume a wavelength such that there is an integral number of waves between the ends of the confinement. If this is not the case, the wave motion will cancel itself out as peaks fall into troughs. The same is true of the electron wave moving around the nucleus. If it is at such a distance from the nucleus that the circumference of the orbit, $2\pi r$, is equal to a whole number of wavelengths, then the position should be stable. These positions are the Bohr orbitals and can be easily derived.

We start by setting the circumference of an orbital equal to an integer number of wavelengths.

$$2\pi r = n\lambda \tag{14-6}$$

If we substitute Eq. 14-5 and rearrange, we get

$$p = \frac{nh}{2\pi r} \tag{14-7}$$

From elementary physics, we know the angular momentum $p_\angle$ is the vector product of the momentum and the radius of the circle.

$$p_\angle = pr \tag{14-8}$$

By substituting we get

$$p_\angle = \frac{nh}{2\pi} \tag{14-9}$$

This means that only certain values of angular momentum can be present in stable orbitals. These values are the products of integers and the quantity $h/2\pi$. This $h/2\pi$ value is the quantity or "quantum" of momentum that must be added to go from one orbital to the next higher orbital. The coefficient n is therefore called the "quantum number" because it is the number of quantums (quanta) present. In fact, because several quantum numbers are all based on n, it is called the principal quantum number. For simplicity, we normally use $\hbar$ in equations:

$$\hbar = \frac{h}{2\pi} \tag{14-10}$$

Bohr orbitals exist for integer values of n beginning at 1. These orbitals exist whether or not electrons are present to fill them. They are located at distances from the nucleus of the atom that are a common factor times the square of an integer (n), which is simply the principal quantum number:

$$r = n^2 a_0 \tag{14-11}$$

This common factor a_0 (called the Bohr radius) was determined to be a combination of natural constants:

$$a_0 = \frac{1}{mZ}\left(\frac{\hbar}{e}\right)^2 \tag{14-12}$$

In this expression, e is charge on the electron ($1.6021 \cdot 10^{-19}$ C), m is the electron mass ($9.1094 \cdot 10^{-28}$ g), and Z is the number of positive charges in the nucleus. For hydrogen ($Z = 1$), the value is $0.5292 \cdot 10^{-10}$ m, or about one-half Angstrom (1 Angstrom $= 10^{-10}$ m). Because the quantum numbers are squared, the radius increases rapidly as n becomes larger (Fig. 14-1).

The Bohr orbitals are referred to as shells. When $n = 1$, the electron is in the K shell. When $n = 2$, the electron is in the L shell. This labeling continues with successive alphabet letters indicating the successive values of n. Each shell has a maximum number of electrons that it can hold. When it is filled, electrons are forced into the next higher level. This approach explained the structure of the periodic table, with the filled orbitals being the very stable inert gases, and the shells with only 1 electron being the highly reactive alkali metals. Further assumptions about the properties of partly filled shells allowed the Bohr model to explain the first three periods of the periodic table rather well, but

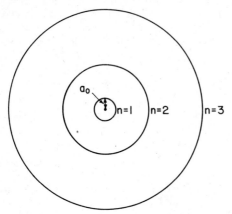

Figure 14-1 The Bohr model of the atom.

the transition metals caused severe problems. The lanthanide series caused even more complications. Clearly, there must be more to the atomic structure.

Explaining the existence of the transition metals and lanthanides is not difficult if, instead of a flat atom that is similar to the solar system, we assume that the atom is three-dimensional. Such an assumption is required by other physical evidence concerning the atom.

If we rigorously derived the equation for the momentum of an electron in a three-dimensional atom, we would find that the total angular momentum L would be dependent on a quantum number l and the factor $\hbar$.

$$L = \sqrt{l(l + 1)}\, \hbar \qquad (14\text{-}13)$$

The quantum number l is related to the roundness of the orbital. If the orbit is a sphere, then l is zero. These orbitals are called s orbitals. For the electrons in the K shell, only spherical orbitals are possible, so l must equal zero. As we go to higher shells, l can have larger values. The limit of l is set by n because l is always at least 1 less than n:

$$l = 0, 1, 2, \ldots, n - 1 \qquad (14\text{-}14)$$

For $n = 1$, l must equal 0. Hence we have only s electrons in the K shell. If $n = 2$, then l may be 0 or 1. In the L shell we have both s electrons with spherical orbitals and p electrons with eliptical or-

bitals. For the M shell, we have $n = 3$ and $l = 0, 1,$ or 2. This gives s, p, and d orbitals. While n determines the shell, l determines the type of electron orbital in the shell. Another quantum number can be introduced which is related to the direction of the orbitals. This is the quantum number m, and it indicates the angular momentum in the z direction (perpendicular to the $x-y$ plane).

$$p_z = m\hbar \qquad (14\text{-}15)$$

This quantum number is limited by the size of l (Fig. 14-2).

$$-l \leq m \leq +l \qquad (14\text{-}16)$$

Let us refer to Table 14-1. For the K shell, we have $n = 1$, $l = 0$, $m = 0$. There is only one configuration possible, which we call $1s$, and there are only two electrons in the shell. For the L shell, we can have $n = 2$, $l = 0$, $m = 0$, which are the $2s$ electrons in the shell. For the L shell, we can also have $n = 2$, $l = 1$, $m = -1$, and $n = 2$, $l = 1$, $m = 0$, and $n = 2$, $l = 1$, $m = 1$, which are the $2p$ electrons, of which there are six. If we look at the M shell, there are $10d$ electrons ranging from $m = -2$ to $m = +2$, but all having $l = 2$. For each set of quantum numbers there are always two electrons.

Since there are two negative charges traveling in the same orbital, there must be some accommodation between them. Such accommodation is accomplished by the electrons rotating in the opposite direction about their axes. This spin causes them to have individual angular momentum which is separate from that of their orbitals and gives rise to a new quantum number called "spin" (s), designated as $\pm\frac{1}{2}\hbar$, depending on the direction of rotation. Because the spin for the electron pair in each orbital is not identical, each electron is therefore uniquely specified by the four quantum numbers $n, l, m,$ and s.

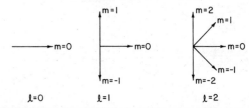

Figure 14-2 The relationship between quantum numbers l and m.

Table 14-1 Quantum Number by Electron Shells

Shell	n	l	m	Electron
K	1	0	0	1s
L	2	0	0	2s
		1	−1, 0, 1	2p
M	3	0	0	3s
		1	−1, 0, 1	3p
		2	−2, −1, 0, 1, 2	3d
N	4	0	0	4s
		1	−1, 0, 1	4p
		2	−2, −1, 0, 1, 2	4d
		3	−3, −2, −1, 0, 1, 2, 3	4f
O	5	0	0	5s
		1	−1, 0, 1	5p
		2	−2, −1, 0, 1, 2	5d
		3	−3, −2, −1, 0, 1, 2, 3	5f
		4	−4, −3, −2, −1, 0, 1, 2, 3, 4	5g

EXAMPLE 14-1

Give the quantum numbers for the electrons of sodium.

Solution:

K shell:	$n = 1$	$l = 0$	$m = 0$	$s = \frac{1}{2}$
	$n = 1$	$l = 0$	$m = 0$	$s = -\frac{1}{2}$
L shell:	$n = 2$	$l = 0$	$m = 0$	$s = \frac{1}{2}$
	$n = 2$	$l = 0$	$m = 0$	$s = -\frac{1}{2}$
	$n = 2$	$l = 1$	$m = 1$	$s = \frac{1}{2}$
	$n = 2$	$l = 1$	$m = 1$	$s = -\frac{1}{2}$
	$n = 2$	$l = 1$	$m = 0$	$s = \frac{1}{2}$
	$n = 2$	$l = 1$	$m = 0$	$s = -\frac{1}{2}$
	$n = 2$	$l = 1$	$m = -1$	$s = \frac{1}{2}$
	$n = 2$	$l = 1$	$m = -1$	$s = -\frac{1}{2}$
M shell:	$n = 3$	$l = 0$	$m = 0$	$s = \frac{1}{2}$ ∎

There is one more quantum number to mention that we will use later. This is the quantity j, the total angular momentum, which is the vector sum of l and s and which must be positive. The j values for l values are given in Table 14-2. Although we could go deeper into this structure, it is not necessary for our study of emitted radiation.

In the Bohr model, all the electrons with the same principal quantum number have the same energy. This is the energy required to free the electron from its bound orbital and give it zero velocity in the free state.

$$E = -\left(\frac{Z^2 e^2}{2a_H}\right)\left(\frac{1}{n}\right)^2 = -2.18 \cdot 10^{-11}\left(\frac{Z}{n}\right)^2 \quad (14\text{-}17)$$

The negative sign indicates that it will require energy to free the electron. As n gets larger, the electron moves farther away from the nucleus, and the attractive forces grow weaker. Consequently, the energy is less negative because the electron is less tightly bound. E is sometimes referred to as the binding energy of an electron. (*Note:* a_H is the Bohr radius for hydrogen and is not affected by the change in Z.)

If an atom undergoes a collision, it is possible for some of the collision energy to be dissipated by an electron moving from the orbital where it would normally reside (ground state) to a higher orbital (excited state). Excited states are unstable and will tend to decay, with the electron returning to its original ground state. While electrons may be excited by collision, it is unusual for them to return to the ground state by another collision. Another

Table 14-2 Table of j and l Values

$l = 0$	$j = \frac{1}{2}$
$l = 1$	$j = \frac{1}{2}, \frac{3}{2}$
$l = 2$	$j = \frac{3}{2}, \frac{5}{2}$
$l = 3$	$j = \frac{5}{2}, \frac{7}{2}$
$l = 4$	$j = \frac{7}{2}, \frac{9}{2}$

mechanism commonly comes into play. This allows the excess energy to be given off as radiation, with Eq. 14-2 giving the frequency of the light emitted. By combining Eqs. 14-2 and 14-1, we can get the wavelength directly.

$$\lambda = \frac{hc}{E} \qquad (14\text{-}18)$$

Since the energy of each orbital is always the same, the energy change between orbitals is always the same; therefore the wavelength for any particular orbital change is always the same. Consequently, if an electron goes from an $n = 2$ to the $n = 1$ orbital of hydrogen, one and only one wavelength of light will always result, and it will always be the same. It is characteristic of that orbital transition. We can compute that energy using Eq. 14-17. The value of e is always the same, and the values of Z and a_H are the same for two orbitals of one atom. For orbitals n and m, the energy difference is

$$\Delta E = E_n - E_m$$

$$\Delta E = -\left(\frac{Z^2 e^2}{2a_H}\right)\left(\frac{1}{n^2} - \frac{1}{m^2}\right) \qquad (14\text{-}19)$$

For hydrogen, the constant value is $2.18 \cdot 10^{-11}$ ergs.

$$\Delta E_H = -2.18 \cdot 10^{-11}\left(\frac{1}{n^2} - \frac{1}{m^2}\right) \qquad (14\text{-}20)$$

For each value of n, m can take on an infinite number of values as long as $m > n$. This fact leads to a family of wavelengths for each n as shown in Figure 14-3. For $n = 1$, transitions from $m = 2, 3, 4$, etc. form a sequence of wavelengths that approaches a limit when $m = \infty$. This is called the Lyman series. Similar series exist for $n = 2$ (Balmer series) and $n = 3$ (Paschen series). All these series are named after early physicists who studied atomic structure.

Together, these series, as well as others of higher n, form the spectrum of hydrogen. It is called a line spectrum (Fig. 14-4) because it is composed of a series of very sharp lines. Line spectra are characteristic of atoms because an exact energy change is needed to move from one orbital to another.

There are two more principles concerning atomic spectra that we must consider. First, within an atom not all possible transitions between orbitals occur. Some transitions are allowed, while others

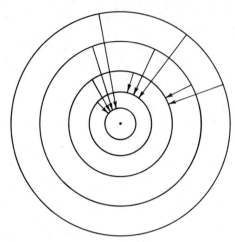

Figure 14-3 For each orbital n, there is a family of decay transitions that ends at n.

are forbidden by the quantum mechanical rules governing changes in angular momentum. To be allowed, a transition must cause the l value to change by 1 and the j value to change by ± 1 or 0. These restrictions prevent $2s$ to $1s$ transitions, for example. These rules account for the principal lines we will encounter when we try to measure atomic spectra later in this chapter.

A major complication to the structure of the electron shells occurs due to the shielding effect of electrons in the lower orbitals. If all the orbitals were spherical, this would be highly predictable because the screening action of the lower shells would merely reduce the effective Z value of the nucleus. Unfortunately, the nonspherical orbits (e.g., p, d, f) cut through the space occupied by the lower orbitals, causing them to experience various degrees of shielding at various points in their orbits. Consequently, a splitting of the orbitals of the same quan-

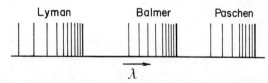

Figure 14-4 Part of the line spectrum of the hydrogen atom.

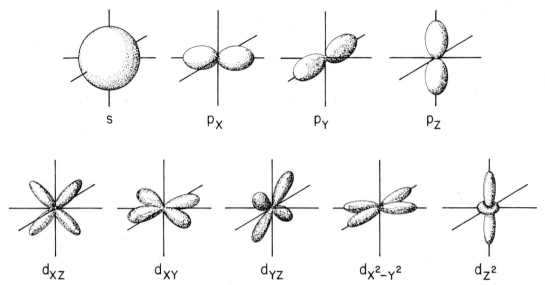

Figure 14-5 A pictorial representation of the configurations of the *s*, *p*, and *d* orbitals.

tum number into different energy levels occurs. All electrons in the *L* shell, for example, do not have the same energy predicted by the Bohr model once an atom has more than one electron. This result should follow rather logically if one recalls the general structure of atomic orbitals (Fig. 14-5).

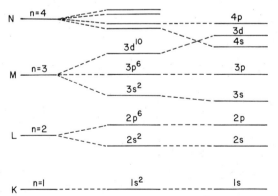

Figure 14-6 Orbitals are divided in energy by their principal quantum number *n*. The angularity of the orbitals (*L*) causes a splitting of the principal levels. The effects of shielding cause orbitals from neighboring principal quantum levels to cross in energy (witness 3*d* and 4*s*).

Figure 14-6 shows the effect of shielding on the energy of the orbitals. The effects are so strong as to invert the order of some levels. This explains why the *N* shell starts to fill before the *M* shell is complete. A further fine structure is imposed by the spin-orbital coupling that results in the *j* quantum numbers. This produces nearly as many energy levels as orbitals in heavier atoms and gives them incredibly complex spectra. More of this will be discussed later.

Section 14-2
THEORY OF FLAME PHOTOMETRY

Since atoms give off distinct wavelengths of light, measuring elements by their light emissions would seem to be quite straightforward. One excites an element in the absence of other emitting species and measures the radiation emitted at some wavelength. The intensity of the radiation should be proportional to the amount of the element present, and the wavelength of the light should be characteristic of the element being measured.

The actual implementation of emission measurements is far more difficult than just described.

First, we must have a means to excite the atoms to get them to emit radiation. This can be done most effectively by heating. Such heating can be done by electrical discharges, such as sparks or arcs, or by flames. In the clinical laboratory, the later are much more common, and we will restrict discussion to them. Even so, flames have numerous problems associated with them which have to be overcome to get good results, as will be seen in the next section.

One problem this approach to measurement is certain to have is the presence of other elements in addition to the one being measured. Combustion will almost surely require the presence of oxygen, carbon, and hydrogen. Naturally, these also emit radiation, which will be measured by the detector. To prevent this from happening, methods of removing or compensating for such background radiation will be necessary. Monochromators, auxiliary detectors, and internal standards are approaches we will consider the negate the effects of the flame.

The flame itself is not the only source of undesir-able light. Other compounds in the specimen also contribute radiation. These substances may be difficult or impossible to remove. Moreover, such compounds may also interfere through chemical means, thereby altering the amount of light emitted by a given quantity of the element being measured. The effect of these contaminants must somehow be minimized.

The sought-for element may itself be a problem. Few elements have but one excited state to which they totally proceed when activated by heat. On the contrary, heat will drive atoms to many excited states (Fig. 14-7) based on the Maxwell-Boltzman equation:

$$N_j = N_o(g_j/g_o) \exp\left(\frac{-\Delta E_j}{kT}\right) \qquad \textbf{(14-21)}$$

In this equation, N_j is the population of excited state j, N_o is the population of the ground state, g_j and g_o are statistical factors based on the multiplicity of the states (Eq. 14-22), ΔE_j is the energy differ-

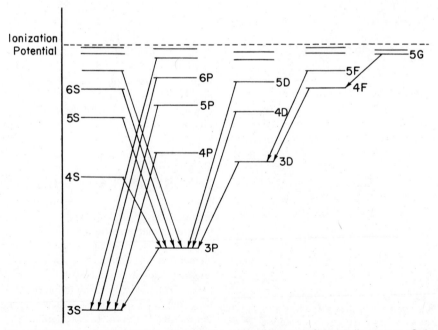

Figure 14-7 Numerous orbitals exist for the outer electrons of the sodium atom. Only certain transitions to return the electron to the ground state are allowed by the exclusion rules.

ence between the ground state and state j, k is the Boltzmann constant $1.3805 \cdot 10^{-16}$ erg/°K, and T is the absolute temperature:

$$g_j = 2j + 1 \qquad \textbf{(14-22)}$$

Equation 14-21 tells us many things. First, because there are a lot of potential excited state js, a large number of different radiation transitions is possible. Second, since the number of atoms in an excited state is proportional to the exponential of the energy difference between levels, the lower excited states will be much more highly populated than will the higher excited states. The temperature is also in the exponential term, which means that the population of the excited states will not vary linearly but rather exponentially with temperature. Moreover, since the temperature is in the denominator of the exponential term, it will not affect all excited states to the same extent. A change in temperature will have a greater effect on the population of the higher-energy excited states than on the lower-energy excited states.

Two other important factors about Eq. 14-21 are not as apparent. N_o is the concentration of the atoms in the ground state when the measurement is made. This is *not* equal to the total number of atoms present since some of the atoms are in the various excited states. If T remains relatively constant for a series of measurements, however, N_o can be assumed to be a constant fraction of N_T, the total concentration, and can be compensated for through calibration. Secondly, at flame temperatures of 2000°C, the percentage of atoms in the ground state is better than 98 or 99%. The population of a particular excited state is very small, even for those of lower energy. Frequently such a population is only a few hundredths or tenths of a percent of the total atomic concentration. This means that N_o is almost N_T, and the calibration of flame methods should be stable. It also means that any radiation observed will not be a sensitive measurement of the element since so little of the element is radiating from the corresponding excited state.

EXAMPLE 14-2

What percentage of the sodium atoms have excited electrons in a $4p$ orbital ($j = \frac{3}{2}$) at 2200°C? (The

energy difference is $3.3716 \cdot 10^{-12}$ erg.) (*Note:* the normal ground state of sodium is $3s$ ($j = \frac{1}{2}$.)

Solution: We find the percentage by dividing Eq. 14-21 by N_o and multiplying by 100%:

$$\%4p = \frac{N_j}{N_o} \times 100\% = \frac{g_j}{g_o} \exp\left(-\Delta E_j/kT\right) \times 100\%$$

$$g_j = 2j + 1 = 2 \times \frac{3}{2} + 1 = 4$$

$$T = 2200 + 273 = 2473$$

$$g_o = 2j + 1 = 2 \times \frac{1}{2} + 1 = 2$$

$$\%4p = \left[\frac{4}{2} \, exp \left(\frac{-3.3716 \cdot 10^{-12}}{1.3805 \cdot 10^{-16} \cdot 2473}\right)\right] \times 100\%$$

$$= [2 \exp(-9.876)] \times 100\%$$

$$= 200 \times 5.139 \cdot 10^{-5}\%$$

$$= 0.0103\% \qquad \blacksquare$$

Section **14-3**
THE FLAME

It is now time to turn our attention to the instrumentation itself. A block diagram of a flame photometer is shown in Figure 14-8. The purpose of the flame is both to atomize the specimen and to excite it. The flame is, in effect, a gaseous solution in

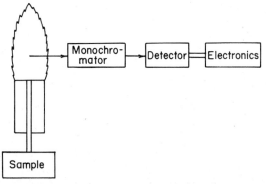

Figure 14-8 Block diagram of a simple flame photometer.

which the components of the sample are dispersed. Such a heated gaseous mixture is sometimes called a plasma. Within the flame, the original solvent is evaporated, leaving a crystalline salt. This salt is then decomposed by the heat into single atoms. The conditions and temperature of the flame must be adjusted to cause the atomic rather than the ionic form of the atoms to predominate. The atoms are excited by collision within the plasma and then decay to give the radiation measured. In the clinical laboratories the atoms of interest are the metal ions.

The flame itself is of familiar composition. Such fuels as natural gas, propane, acetylene, butane, and hydrogen are burned in air, oxygen, or nitrous oxide. The temperature is controlled by the burner design and the choice of fuels and fuel–oxidizer proportions. Cooler temperatures favor the less energetic excited states, which are the ones commonly measured. For this reason, and to prevent side reactions, flame temperatures are usually kept low.

The more difficult aspects of the process are the insertion and incorporation of the specimen into the flame. The customary manner of specimen introduction is through the use of the Venturi principle. The solution is pulled by capillary action from a reservoir into a capillary inlet (Fig. 14-9). The rush of gas past the upper end of the capillary causes a partial vacuum which sucks the sample into the base of the flame. Here the droplets are sheared off by the rush of the gases and evaporated by the heat of the flame.

The burner design shown in Figure 14-9 is called the total consumption burner. All of the sample is eventually pulled into the flame and consumed. The advantages of such a burner are low cost due to the simplicity of design, ease of maintenance, and good sensitivity, because a large number of atoms are present to be excited. As a consequence, small samples are adequate for making measurements. There are major disadvantages, however. The relatively large droplets cause some regions of the flame to be specimen rich, while others are specimen poor. This means the radiation from the flame is not uniform and therefore less stable, affecting precision. The large droplets also cause localized cooling of the flame, which affects the number of

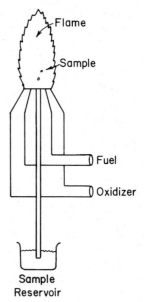

Figure 14-9 Total consumption burner using the Venturi principle.

excited atoms in that area of the flame through Eq. 14-21. Finally, the length of time required to vaporize the droplets is relatively long. During that time interval, the droplets become incredibly concentrated solutions in which side reactions can occur that will distort the final measurement. These facts indicate the need for another approach.

The alternate approach is the premix burner. In this burner, as shown in Figure 14-10A, the sample is introduced by means of the Venturi principle, but it is not introduced directly into the flame, rather into a mixing chamber. Here the droplets, after they are sheared off by the flow of oxidant, are buffeted by the gas stream and broken into a fine mist. Baffles or wire mesh eliminate the larger droplets which condense and are drained away. The fuel is also added to this mixture, which is forced by the gas pressure through the burner head. Here the mixture is consumed to excite the atoms of interest.

The advantage of the premix burner is that the droplets are very small and uniformly scattered throughout the flame. This restricts local cooling of the flame and ensures that the radiation from the flame will remain relatively constant. Flame sputter is minimized. On the other hand, only 2–5% of the specimen ever gets into the flame. The specimen must, therefore, be larger and the optics and the detector must be better to compensate for this loss of sensitivity. The premix burner is more expensive, since it has a more complex design. The problem of removing the previous specimen is also encountered because some of the previous specimen will be retained by the walls of the mixing chamber and may become renebulized to contaminate the current measurement. Since both fuel and oxidant are present before the flame, it is possible for combustion to occur within the burner itself if the gas pressure is too low. This is called flashback and is an explosion hazard due to rapid gas expansion in a confined space.

The premix burner is used almost exclusively in clinical laboratory equipment. The burners are usually made of metal, but they can also be made of glass or quartz. Metal burners suffer from corrosion and from plugging by salt deposits from the vaporized solutions. Quartz burners are harder to manufacture, while glass burners deteriorate at high flame temperatures. Appropriate burner choice is dependent upon the substances being measured and the precision necessary in the measurements.

Finally, the control of the fuel and the oxidant are necessary for successful flame measurements. Variation in the pressure of the gases will cause the temperature of the different portions of the flame to change by altering the nature of the combustion mixture. These variations can also affect the shape of the flame and the location of the most intense emission through pressure effects at the burner head (Fig. 14-10B). The gas supplies are normally derived from cylinders under high pressure (several hundred to thousand pounds per square inch) and reduced to a few pounds per square inch in two or more steps. Gas pressure from such sources is very stable as long as the lines are not plugged by foreign material. Gases can also be obtained from piped-in supplies, but since these supplies are at relatively low pressure and have numerous users on the line, special care must be taken to prevent pressure fluctuations. Gas purity is also of concern. Dirt can clog small passages in the gas lines and will cause spurious radiation in the flame. Water vapor, particularly from compressed air, can make the flame noisy (flickering) through localized cooling. Traps are sometimes used to remove impurities before they reach the burner. Safety valves that automati-

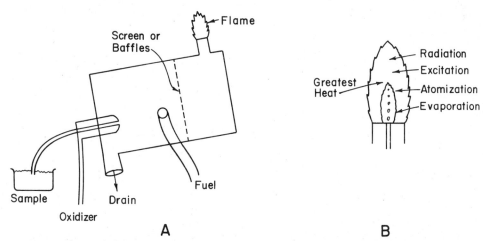

Figure 14-10 Part A shows a premix burner in which the fuel, oxidant, and sample are mixed before reaching the base of the flame. Part B shows what happens in the various areas of the flame.

cally shut off the fuel and oxidant flow if the flame goes out are important to reduce to chance of explosion or gas inhalation.

Section 14-4
THE MONOCHROMATOR

After examining the burner assembly that composes the first block of Figure 14-8, it would seem that we should be ready to study the detection of our radiation. Since the light from any transition between orbitals is monochromatic, it consists nominally of only 1 wavelength. Therefore, it would seem that a monochromator, a device to eliminate all but a narrow portion of the spectrum, would be unnecessary to isolate the radiation of the element of interest. Alas, this is not the case. Background radiation from the flame and other transitions of the element of interest, besides the one being used for the measurement, contribute radiation as has already been mentioned, and this must be removed. Since monochromators are necessary in flame photometry, and even more essential for the absorption methods discussed in the next chapter, we will examine them here and use them in the rest of this text.

The easiest way, in principle, to get monochromatic light is by filtering out all the light of other wavelengths than the one desired. Colored glass filters perform this function but are far from ideal. While such simple filters absorb radiation, they do so in the characteristic pattern shown in Figure 14-11A. At no point is all the incident radiation transmitted; much is either reflected or absorbed. Even at the point of maximum transmission, as little as 5% of the incident light may get through the filter. This obviously reduces the sensitivity because the absorbed radiation merely excites molecules in the filter and is not available to the detector. In addition, more than one wavelength is permitted to traverse the filter. Common glass filters will allow a band of radiation wavelengths 30–50 nm or more to pass with at least half of the peak intensity. This bundle of wavelengths is called the bandpass. As the bandpass of such an absorption filter is reduced, so is the maximum percentage of light transmitted. This means that absorption filters are good for excluding major radiation that is highly dissimilar to the radiation of interest, such as harmonics, but ineffective against isolating one wavelength from those closely adjacent. A similar type of filter transmits radiation almost entirely above or below a certain wavelength and then quickly drops to zero transmission at longer or shorter wavelengths (Fig. 14-11B). This is called a ''cut-off'' filter.

A more effective means of removing undesirable radiation while retaining the maximum usable radiation is the interference filter. This filter uses the

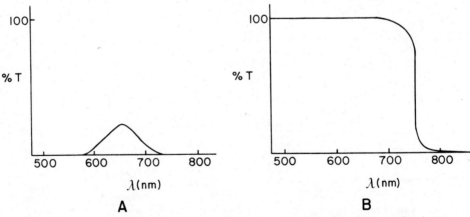

Figure 14-11 Part A shows the bandpass of a typical glass filter. Part B shows the characteristics of a cut-off filter.

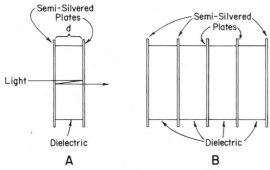

Figure 14-12 A simple (Part A) and a multiple (Part B) interference filter.

wave properties of light to retain some wavelengths while rejecting others. The basic concept is shown in Figure 14-12A. Light entering the filter passes through a glass or quartz plate coated on the inside with a thin semitransparent film. It then passes through a transparent spacer (frequently magnesium fluoride) and strikes the semisilvered surface of a second plate. Part of the light is able to pass through these semitransparent surfaces, while the rest is reflected. The light that is reflected will travel through the spacer again, where it will encounter the first semitransparent surface. If it is again reflected, it will traverse the spacer a third time and again encounter the second semitransparent surface. Light that emerges after this double reflection will be traveling through the same space as light which arrived later and was not reflected. If this light is in phase, no difference can be seen between the light waves, and they will proceed as if the filter were absent. If they are not in phase, interference between the waves will reduce the amplitude of the composite propagation. The wavelengths that will be in phase are those which required a whole number of wavelengths to be reflected through the filter. These wavelengths can be identified by an equation based on the properties of the filter and the direction of the incident light:

$$n\lambda = 2d\mu \sin \theta \qquad \text{(14-23)}$$

Where n is the order of the reflection, d is the distance between the semitransparent plates, μ is the refractive index (1.38 for MgF_2), and θ is the angle

to the surface of the filter made by the light. Normally, θ is 90°, and the sine term is unity.

Interference filters are not ideal. Absorption cannot be totally eliminated and much radiation is still lost. As a consequence the single interference filter has a bandpass of about 15 nm and a peak transmission of roughly 50%. Moreover, cut-off filters may be needed after an interference filter because harmonics of the primary wavelength survive the damping process.

Improvement in performance can be obtained by the use of multilayers of spacer and semitransparent materials (Fig. 14-12B). The result is that multiple reflections and interferences occur as the light moves through the filter. Only the wavelengths extremely close to those given by Eq. 14-23 will be passed. Typical multilayer filters have 5 to 25 layers of spacer and semireflective materials interleafed. Uniformity in layer thickness is imperative and contributes to the costliness of these filters. Typical multilayer filters have a bandpass of 5–8 nm and will transmit 60–90% of the radiation. Since the wavelength band is fixed by the manufacturing process for each filter, filters are not versatile, and a separate filter will probably be needed for each method used in the laboratory. Since the filters are expensive and require careful handling, using them for an instrument that performs many different analyses becomes impractical.

While filters have numerous applications, extensive use is also made of older methods of creating monochromatic light, namely the prism and the grating. The basic principles of these methods were discussed in Chapter 10. The different mountings of the prism, combined with the appropriate slits, lenses, and mirrors, permit the effective generation of a small band of wavelengths. In Figure 14-13, the

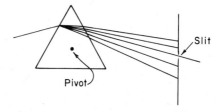

Figure 14-13 Rotatable prism permits different wavelengths to fall on the exit slit.

prism can be rotated so as to make the appropriate wavelength fall on the exit slit. There is really no limit, in theory, to the narrowness of the bandpass that can be obtained from the dispersion by a prism provided one has an intense enough light source. This bandpass width reduction cannot, however, be accomplished simply by narrowing the slit. Because light is composed of waves, diffraction becomes too great when the slit is reduced beyond a certain point. Instead of this approach, the length of the light path is increased so that other wavelengths drift far enough away from the one of interest to be readily excluded by a reasonable sized slit. This naturally leads to an increase in size for the instrument, which is not especially desirable. The folding of the light path by the use of precision optics is necessary to eliminate this difficulty, but will increase the instrument's cost. The nonlinearity of the light dispersion is also a problem, and it is frequently addressed by the use of appropriately cut cams that permit a uniform change in dial position to yield a uniform change in wavelength.

The use of gratings closely parallels that of prisms in laboratory instrumentation. The amount of space required for light separation is somewhat less, however, and the wavelength distribution is nearly linear. The wavelength from the grating that passes through the exit slit is changed by rotating the grating face compared with the incident radiation. Since the wavelength of the emergent light is determined by the difference in the sines of the angles of incidence and reflection, the gear that linearizes the movement of the grating is sometimes called a sine bar. One common means of extending the light path for a grating is the Ebert mounting, shown in Figure 14-14. This is effective both at removing stray light and spreading the spectrum before it reaches the exit slit. Because gratings produce harmonics of the primary frequency, cut-off filters are needed to eliminate these from the final beam.

Any of the above monochromators can be used as the second block in Figure 14-8. Since flame methods are frequently used on several elements at once, however, monochromatic light at several wavelengths may be needed simultaneously. Figure 14-15 shows two ways in which the light path can

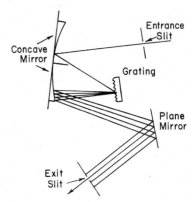

Figure 14-14 The Ebert mounting of a grating.

be manipulated to accomplish this. In part A, the light passes through a wheel containing several filters. In the clinical laboratory these would most commonly be for sodium, potassium, lithium, and calcium. The wheel rotates so that the various filters in turn are in the light path and allow only the corresponding element-specific wavelength to pass. The electronics must then credit the different radiation readings to the correct element. Such an approach is possible because the elements mentioned have relatively simple spectra at lower flame temperatures, which means that simple filters are adequate. Background radiation can be compensated for if the flame is well controlled. This is accomplished by using an internal standard (Section 14-7) and by measuring the level of radiation through each filter when distilled water is aspirated into the flame.

In Figure 14-15B, a grating with multiple slits is used to produce three monochromatic beams. These beams are used to measure lithium, sodium, and potassium in this case. Because a grating produces different wavelengths at different angles to its surface, this method can be employed by finding the appropriate places to put the slits once the light has left the grating. With this approach it is not possible to readily convert the instrument to measure other species because of the relative position of the emergent light beams. Such flexibility is not needed for routine clinical laboratory measure-

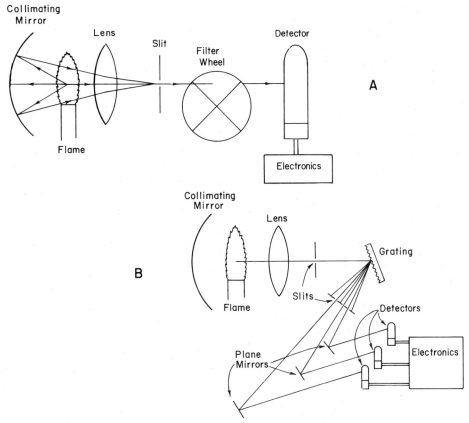

Figure 14-15   Part A shows a single beam with a rotating filter wheel, while Part B shows a grating used to create three beams, which represent the optimum wavelengths for three different elements.

ments. A separate detector is used for each channel. This eliminates the need for timing circuitry.

Both parts of Figure 14-15 show a collimating mirror and lens around the flame. This is a common approach for gathering as much radiation as possible into the entrance slit. More radiation means more sensitivity, and one can ill afford to capture only the miniscule amount that originally heads in the direction of the slit. Unfortunately, this introduces a new complication, since ground state atoms of high concentration, such as sodium in serum, can absorb this reflected radiation and thereby limit the linearity of the measurement.

Section 14-5
THE DETECTOR

Once the radiation has emerged from the monochromator (Fig. 14-8), it must be measured. To make such a measurement, three types of detectors, in addition to the photodiodes, are available to us. The first is called the barrier layer cell (photovoltaic cell) and is shown in Figure 14-16A. Its base is an iron plate and spring. The former is coated with a semiconductor, such as selenium, which is in turn coated with a thin transparent film of a good

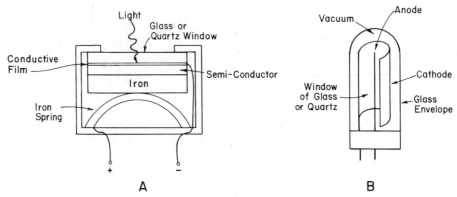

Figure 14-16 A barrier layer cell (Part A) and a phototube (Part B).

conductor such as silver or gold. The assembly is covered with a glass or quartz window and packaged in a plastic case. Leads from the iron spring and surface metal run to terminal connectors on the case. The cell works because a barrier to the transfer of electrons exists at the silver-selenium interface due largely to the difference in the electronic structure of the materials at this junction. Light entering the window penetrates to this interface where it excites electrons in the selenium. These electrons find the conduction band of the silver more energetically favorable than the valence band of selenium and do not readily recross the interface. If given an external path to the iron plate, however, they will move there and then cross the iron–selenium interface to return all parts of the apparatus to electrical neutrality. The amount of current that flows is proportional to the number of extra electrons in the silver layer, which is proportional to the intensity of the incident radiation. The current, which is up to 100 μA, can be measured directly by a galvanometer or other sensitive current meter. It is most useful when relatively large amounts of light are present.

The barrier layer cell suffers from several drawbacks. It has low internal resistance due to leakage across the barrier. High resistance in the external circuit causes the current response to be nonlinear, the opposite effect of what happens with most current sources. (Several hundred ohms in the external circuit is its normal operating resistance.) This condition makes the output hard to amplify. Secondly,

the cell has a memory for high radiation levels. Its sensitivity is greatly reduced after exposure to intense light. It also shows fatigue; that is, its output falls gradually with time for the same light level. A shutter is frequently used to control this problem. Finally, the cell responds much better to green light than to red light of the same intensity. This reduces its usefulness in some applications. The barrier layer cell does not respond rapidly and cannot be used with chopper-controlled light paths where the light level changes numerous times per second.

A second detector is the phototube, which is based on the photoelectric effect discovered by Einstein. As the light strikes the cathode in Figure 14-16B, some electrons are knocked off the silvered surface. These electrons immediately find themselves in an electric field of 100 V. They migrate to the anode, thereby causing current to flow. The current flow, which is proportional to the incident radiation, can be measured over a resistor in the power circuit or as we will see later in Figure 14-18.

Phototubes are highly useful for moderate levels of light, but frequently do not have enough sensitivity for measurement of weak radiation. The phototube principle has, therefore, been enhanced to create the photomultiplier tube. Both the schematic and circuit diagram of such a tube are shown in Figure 14-17. As light enters the tube through its window, it strikes a photocathode. As in a phototube, one or more electrons are kicked out per photon. These electrons find themselves in an electric field of 50–100 V between the photocathode and the first of a series of electrodes called dynodes. The electrons are accelerated toward the dynode and strike its sensitive surface with great energy. This causes a larger number of electrons to be emitted. These electrons find themselves in an environment with three electrodes: the very negative photocathode, the dynode they just escaped from, and a second dynode 50–100 V more positive than the first dynode. Naturally, they accelerate toward this second dynode, striking it at high velocity and knocking out even more electrons. This process continues through nine or more stages as the electron pulse continues down the tube, always seeking the most positive of the three electrodes currently in its vicinity. Finally, the electron pulse reaches the anode, which is attached to an amplifier circuit. The final pulse reaching the anode is very large, even though the incident radiation was weak. Such a multiplier approach is very effective in measuring light of low intensity. The electronics of the photomultiplier tube are comparatively simple. A high voltage is applied to the photocathode. This voltage is divided in equal steps to reach ground at the final dynode. The current reaching the anode passes through a large resistor into a differential amplifier and finally to ground. The sensitivity of the photomultiplier tube can be adjusted by varying the voltage across it.

Photomultiplier tubes are several hundred times more sensitive than phototubes and can respond to light pulses only 1 nsec long. This tremendous sensitivity puts significant restrictions on the handling of these tubes. Exposure to strong light can easily

damage such a tube even if such exposure is momentary. As with a phototube, a dark current exists, but such current is much more troublesome. This current gets its name from the fact that it flows through the tube even when no light is incident. It arises from thermal excitation of electrons which then travel through the tube in the same manner as if they had been generated by incident light. Since the presence of such electrons is highly dependent upon the temperature, cooling the photomultiplier compartment is desirable when feasible. Reasonable care must be taken when servicing this compartment due to the presence of high voltage levels.

The choice of detectors is predicated on several factors. These include the intensity of the radiation, its frequency of modulation, its wavelength, and the cost of the detector. Each detector has conditions under which it is quite acceptable, although the photomultiplier tube has the greatest versatility and, therefore, the greatest usefulness.

Section 14-6
THE ELECTRONICS

The electronics that convert the signal from the current produced by the detector to the final output consist of four basic components. The first is an amplifier, which can simply be a variation of the instrumentation amplifier discussed in Chapter 6. It measures the difference between the voltage values on the two sides of the resistor in the external circuit of the detector (between the anode and cathode

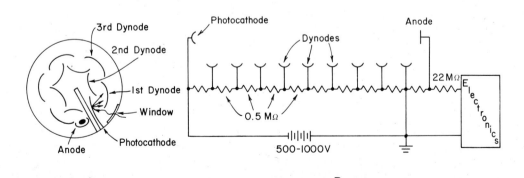

A   **B**

Figure 14-17 Schematic (Part A) and circuit (Part B) diagrams of a photomultiplier tube.

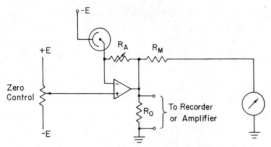

Figure 14-18 A simple circuit for obtaining output from a phototube. The gain can be controlled by adjusting the voltage applied to the cathode or the resistance R_A.

or between the anode and ground). Another approach to amplification is shown in Figure 14-18. The current from the anode of a phototube (or photomultiplier) flows around an amplifier and through a resistor between the inverting input and the output. The current times the negative of the feedback resistance gives the amplifier output voltage which can be displayed, recorded, or further processed. The gain can be adjusted by varying either the voltage over the detector or the resistance in the feedback circuit. An input to the noninverting input allows the dark current to be zeroed.

The output voltage from either of these circuits is then converted to a digital value by an analog-to-digital convertor as described in Chapter 8.

The third electrical component may be as simple as a data latch to hold the data temporarily or as complex as a minicomputer that does sophisticated mathematical procedures on the reading. The most common things this circuitry does is compensate for background, average a number of readings over a period of time to remove the effects of flame fluctuation, and synchronize detector readings with the monochromator output if the same detector is used for several wavelengths. These operations can be done by use of data latches and shift registers without the presence of a full-blown computer.

Finally, the result must be displayed or printed. This involves either a serial or parallel character (digit) transmission to a suitable output device. Printer philosophies were previously discussed in Chapter 9.

Section 14-7
FLAME PHOTOMETRY IN PRACTICE

Now that we have studied all the components of the flame photometer, it is worthwhile to look at some operational considerations. The stability of the flame is paramount. Since flames are easily disturbed, an internal standard is commonly used to compensate for such fluctuations. An internal standard is just another element added to the sample, which has a known concentration. As the flame changes, effects on the internal standard and unknown will be proportional if they are similar in electronic structure. The concentration of the unknown is given by

$$[U] = \left(\frac{R_u}{R_s}\right) [S] \qquad (14\text{-}24)$$

where R_u and R_s are the radiations measured from the unknown and internal standard, respectively, and $[S]$ is the concentration of the internal standard. Most commonly, sodium and potassium are measured in the clinical laboratory by flame photometry, with lithium employed as the internal standard. Because lithium is being increasingly used in medications, its value is more frequently sought. The use of lithium as an internal standard causes lithium salt residue to collect in the burner and affect lithium measurement. Consequently, cesium has been substituted for lithium as the internal standard for some instruments.

The radiation from the flame may be affected by secondary factors (matrix effects) that are not linear in the concentration of the sought-for substances. For example, phosphate will suppress the amount of calcium radiation, presumably by complexing the calcium. EDTA will also lower the apparent concentrations of some metals. A large sodium concentration will enhance the potassium radiation. Excited sodium atoms return to ground by transferring energy to potassium atoms which then radiate the energy. This creates another way to excite potassium atoms and therefore artificially raises the population of the excited state and the radiation seen. Since sodium is 40–50 times as abundant in serum as potassium, a small number of sodium atoms deactivating by this method can have serious effects on potassium measurements. Compensation for these second order effects can be made by use of appropriate standards and calibrations done by either the instrument or the operator.

Physical problems are not totally absent. Orifices and capillaries are subject to blockage by salts, fibrin clots, or dirt and must be checked regularly. The optics and detector are heated by the flame, which can adversely affect their reliability. Components that cannot be physically moved away from the flame may have to be shielded from the heat, particularly if a hotter flame temperature is required. Alignment of the dispersing element, if one is used, is particularly important and can be affected by temperature and handling. Finally, the composition of the optics themselves will be dictated by the wavelength at which the measurement will be made. The requirements for these optics will be discussed in Chapter 15.

This chapter has introduced light emission as a measurement technique and examined its most common usage in the clinical laboratory. The next chapter will discuss the absorption of radiation as a means to measure concentrations. Many of the principles introduced here and much of the equipment will carry over to this methodology.

REVIEW QUESTIONS

1. What is a photon?
2. What are some wave properties of light?
3. What are some particle properties of light?
4. To what is the energy in a beam of light proportional?
5. What is the basic structure of the atom?
6. Why are only certain atomic orbitals stable?
7. What is a quantum?
8. What is the Bohr radius?
9. Define the quantum numbers n, l, m, and s.
10. To what do the suborbitals s, p, d, f, and so on relate?
11. What is the relationship between n and l? Between l and m?
12. How does s differ from the other quantum numbers?
13. Define the quantum number j.
14. Why is the orbital energy of the electron negative?
15. What happens when electrons are excited?
16. How do electrons get excited?
17. Why do atoms radiate only at specific wavelengths?
18. Why are there series of spectral lines?
19. Why don't all possible electron orbital transitions occur?
20. What effect do noncircular electron orbitals have?
21. What produces atomic fine structure?
22. How does one measure a line spectrum?
23. What are the components of a flame photometer?
24. What phenomena contribute to the background radiation from the flame?
25. Explain the terms of the Maxwell-Boltzmann expression.
26. What is the nature of the relationship between the temperature and the population of a given excited state?
27. To what extent is the population of the atomic ground state depleted in a flame?
28. What are the functions of the flame in flame photometry?
29. Why are flame temperatures usually kept low?
30. How is the sample pulled into the flame?
31. Explain how the total consumption burner works.
32. Sketch and label the parts of a total consumption burner.
33. What are the advantages of a total consumption burner? The disadvantages?
34. Explain how the premix burner works.
35. Sketch and label the parts of a premix burner.
36. What are the advantages of a premix burner? The disadvantages?
37. From what are the burners made? What is a disadvantage of each material?
38. How is the gas supply for a flame controlled?
39. What is the purpose of a monochromator?
40. What are the transmission characteristics of a simple filter?
41. What is a cut-off filter?
42. Sketch and label the parts of an interference filter.
43. How does an interference filter work?

44. Why do harmonics of the principal wavelength pass an interference filter?
45. What percentage of the incident radiation passes a simple filter? An interference filter? A multiple interference filter?
46. Why are multiple interference filters so expensive?
47. What limits the narrowness of the bandpass from a prism? List three limitations.
48. How is the nonlinearity of the prism compensated for?
49. Sketch and label the Ebert mounting.
50. Why is a sine bar used with gratings?
51. Diagram two methods of measuring several elements simultaneously with a flame.
52. Explain how the filter wheel instrument works.
53. Why isn't the multislit grating system versatile?
54. Name three types of detector.
55. Sketch and label the parts of a barrier layer cell.
56. Explain how a barrier layer cell works.
57. What are some disadvantages of the barrier layer cell?
58. Sketch and label the parts of a phototube.
59. Sketch and label the parts of a photomultiplier tube.
60. Sketch and label the circuitry of a photomultiplier tube.
61. Explain how a photomultiplier tube works.
62. What problems arise due to the sensitivity of the photomultiplier tube?
63. Discuss two ways to read the output of a phototube.
64. What are some functions of the electronics after the phototube?
65. Why is an internal standard needed in flame photometry?
66. List several matrix effects.
67. Why is cesium sometimes used in place of lithium as the internal standard?
68. What physical problems plague flame photometry?

PROBLEMS

1. If the wavelength of light is 487.6 nm, what is the energy of the light?
2. If the energy of the radiation is $5.000 \cdot 10^{-12}$ ergs, what is the wavelength?
3. What is the momentum of light that has a wavelength of 677.5 nm?
4. What is the Bohr radius for a helium atom?
5. Give the quantum numbers for the electrons of boron.
6. Give the quantum numbers for the electrons of fluorine.
7. Give the quantum numbers for the electrons of silicon.
8. What is the energy for the $n = 2$ orbital of hydrogen?
9. What is the energy for the $n = 3$ orbital of helium?
10. What is the wavelength of light given off as an electron falls from the $n = 2$ to $n = 1$ orbital of helium?
11. What is the wavelength of light given off as an electron falls from the $n = 4$ to $n = 2$ orbital of lithium?
12. At 3000°C what percentage of each atomic concentration of the following elements is in the excited state indicated? Assume that j has the higher of possible values.
    a. Li $2p$ $\lambda = 671$ nm
    b. K $5p$ $\lambda = 404$ nm
    c. Na $3d$ $\lambda = 364$ nm
13. At what temperature does the indicated orbital of the specified atom hold 0.0100% of the total atoms present? Assume j has the higher of possible values.
    a. Li $3d$ $\lambda = 319.5$ nm
    b. Na $4p$ $\lambda = 330$ nm
    c. K $4p$ $\lambda = 768$ nm
14. If 0.027% of an element was in a particular excited state at 3000°C, what would be the wavelength of the atomic transition? Assume that j goes from $\frac{3}{2}$ to $\frac{1}{2}$.

CHAPTER 15
ABSORPTION AND FLUORESCENCE

If all measurements could be made from line spectra that were simple and representative of only the substances being sought, clinical chemical analysis would be a mundane affair. Alas, the substances of interest most frequently are compounds that do not give line spectra. When atoms combine to form compounds, their electron structures change drastically. This makes their emission spectra extremely complex and unusable for analysis. As a consequence, we must adopt a different approach.

Section 15-1
MOLECULAR RADIATION

Let us begin searching for another method of making light measurements of compounds by examining what happens when two atoms of oxygen are bonded together. Each oxygen atom originally had two $1s$ electrons, two $2s$ electrons, and four $2p$ electrons, one p orbital being full and the other two having one electron each (Fig. 15-1). To form the molecule, these orbitals must hybridize to give 3 sp^2 orbitals, two of which have two electrons and one of which has one electron, and a p orbital that has one electron. The half-full sp^2 orbitals from the two oxygens overlap and interact to form two new molecular orbitals, of which the one with the lower energy gets the two electrons. The half-full p orbitals also overlap and interact to form two new orbitals with the electrons again going into the lower energy orbital. This gives the configuration in Figure 15-2, which should be studied carefully. Since the $1s$ electrons are in full shells, they do not take part in the bonding and are, therefore, omitted from the diagram.

The key to forming bonds is a favorable energy change, that is, energy being given off (exother-

mic). Oxygen will not enter the higher energy sp^2–p configuration unless it can form bonds that will lower the overall energy in the molecule. Orbitals are always conserved, so there must be as many orbitals in the final molecule as were in all the component atoms. Since there were four orbitals in the L shell of each oxygen, there must be eight orbitals in the L levels of the final molecule. Electrons are, of course, also conserved. Between the two oxygens there are 12 L electrons to be placed into the molecular orbitals.

The orbitals shown in Figure 15-2 fall into three categories. The molecular sp^2 (σ) and p (π) orbitals are "bonding" orbitals that hold the molecule together. The four sp^2 orbitals are "nonbonding" orbitals, because the electrons are localized to one or the other of the atoms and do not contribute to the bonding. The sp^2 (σ)* and p (π)* orbitals are "antibonding" orbitals because electrons in these orbitals will weaken rather than strengthen the molecular bonds. Note that since the sp^2 orbitals in the molecule have a slightly higher average energy than the component orbitals in the original unhybridized atoms, they are actually slightly antibonding, although not significantly so. When electrons are placed into such an energy level environment, they naturally fall into the lowest levels possible. This means that the bonding and nonbonding orbitals are filled, but the antibonding orbitals are empty. Such a situation yields a stable molecule. If we would try the same thing with two neon atoms, they would have 16 electrons to place in the L levels. This would fill all the available energy levels, including the antibonding levels. Since the antibonding orbitals raise the energy for bonding more than the bonding orbitals reduce it, the molecule falls apart. This explains why neon will not form diatomic molecules.

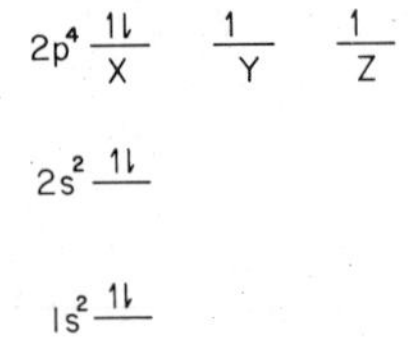

$$2p^4 \quad \frac{1\downarrow}{X} \quad \frac{1}{Y} \quad \frac{1}{Z}$$

$$2s^2 \quad \frac{1\downarrow}{}$$

$$1s^2 \quad \frac{1\downarrow}{}$$

Figure 15-1 The ground state configuration of an oxygen atom.

In order to look at the radiation emitted by molecules, it is advantageous to consider a simpler molecule. We will examine diatomic hydrogen. For a pair of bonded atoms, there is an optimum separation distance between the nuclei. This distance is the compromise reached between the repelling force of the charged nuclei that tries to increase the distance and the contracting force of the electron bond that tries to decrease the distance. For H_2 this distance is 0.746 Å.

The two nuclei of a diatomic molecule are not held fixed at the end of a stick. It is quite possible for the nuclei (and their inner shells of electrons for larger atoms) to move back and forth along the axis of the bond, the classic definition of vibration. Figure 15-3 shows the constraints upon this vibration as a diagram of the potential energy versus the nuclear distance. The horizontal lines tie together points of equal potential energy. If two nuclei started at the distance apart indicated by point A with no kinetic energy, they would move apart until they reached point B and then begin to move together until they reached point A again. This is similar to the harmonic oscillation that a perfect spring or pendulum will give. It is therefore called the harmonic oscillator model of a diatomic bond.

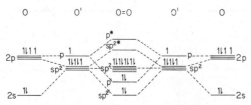

Figure 15-2 Oxygen orbitals must hybridize (O') and can then form molecular orbitals (O=O).

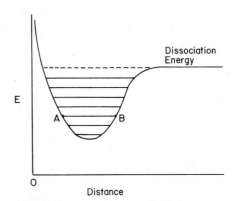

Figure 15-3 The potential energy E is plotted against the internuclear distance. The tie lines indicate the location of stable vibrational levels. This structure is called a potential well.

Because the electrons which form the bonds in which such oscillation occurs must still travel in such a manner as is consistent with their wave properties, only certain oscillation frequencies are permitted. These are related to specific potential energy levels by the equation

$$E_v = (v + \tfrac{1}{2})h\nu_0 \qquad \textbf{(15-1)}$$

where v stands for the vibrational quantum number ($v = 0, 1, 2, \ldots$) and ν_0 is the fundamental vibrational frequency, which is a function of the nuclear masses and effective charges. As can be seen, there can never be a total lack of vibration. Even if $v = 0$, as would be the case at absolute zero, the vibrational energy is positive and vibration occurs.

Before we proceed, it is well to note the horizontal asymptote on the right of Figure 15-3. As the bond stretches beyond a certain point, it ruptures and the atoms fly apart. The energy associated with this occurrence is called the bond dissociation energy. If the vibrational energy exceeds this value, the molecule will dissociate during its first vibrational cycle.

A diatomic molecule permits rotation as well as vibration. Since rotation is much slower than vibration, for modeling the process we can consider the bond length (r) to be the average atomic distance. If one computes the effective moment of inertia I as a function of the nuclear masses and distances

$$I = \frac{m_1 m_2}{m_1 + m_2} r^2 \qquad \textbf{(15-2)}$$

and takes into consideration the restriction imposed by the wave properties of the electron (Schrödinger equation), one finds that the energy associated with rotation is

$$E = \frac{h^2}{8\pi^2 I} j(j + 1) \qquad \textbf{(15-3)}$$

The coefficients are constant for a particular molecule and can be combined into a single entity K. The rotational quantum number j (not the same j as for atoms) can have the values 0, 1, 2, and so on. Therefore

$$E = K j(j + 1) \qquad \textbf{(15-4)}$$

Note that there does not have to be any rotation around the center of mass, since if $j = 0$, $E = 0$. This is referred to as the "rigid rotator" model, because the molecular bond is assumed not to vibrate but to remain of rigid length. Rotational energies are smaller than vibrational energies.

If we combine the two models, we get the rigid rotator-harmonic oscillator model diagrammed in Figure 15-4. Each vibrational level has a series of rotational levels associated with it. Taken together, these yield a large number of energy levels in which a molecule in its ground state can reside. Transitions between these levels occur as the result of collision and are not accompanied by radiation.

When we discussed the hybridizing of molecular orbitals, we dealt with only those electrons in the L shell because this is the valence shell for oxygen. Orbitals in all the other shells also undergo hybridization and incorporation into molecular orbitals. Since there are no electrons to occupy them, however, they are ignored in the discussion of bonding. It is entirely possible, nonetheless, for an electron to be excited into one of these higher molecular orbitals just as it can be excited into a higher atomic orbital in a free atom. In its new electronic level, it can also experience the effects of vibration and rotation in the molecule. Figure 15-5 shows the relationship between a ground and excited potential diagram.

When the electron excitation occurs, there is no relationship that must exist between the molecule's position among the vibrational and rotational states in the ground state potential well versus its position among these states in the excited state potential well. Similarly, when the electron returns from the excited state potential to the ground state potential, there are no rules governing from which state the molecule must start and in which it must end, except that j must be ± 1. Moreover, when an electron is knocked into the excited state, the molecules may undergo several nonradiation transitions within the excited state through further collision

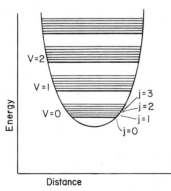

Figure 15-4 The combined potential energy of vibrational and rotational levels versus the internuclear distance.

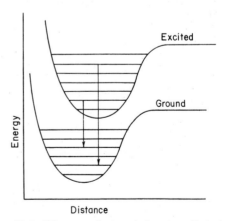

Figure 15-5 When an electron is in an excited state, the energy versus internuclear distance diagram shifts upward and slightly to the right. Radiation is emitted when the electron returns to the ground state, but many separate paths are available for this transition.

before the electron returns to ground. This produces the possibility of a large number of radiation wavelengths relatively close together in the spectrum. Moreover, the Doppler effect, which lengthens or shortens the wavelengths depending on whether the electron is moving away from or toward the observer at the time of emission, causes each of the lines to broaden, so that, in effect, they overlap. Going from hundreds of excited states which differ only slightly in energy to hundreds of ground states which differ only slightly in energy with Doppler broadening of the wavelengths yields a continuum of light rather than a sharp light spectrum as is emitted from unbonded atoms. What is true for diatomic molecules is even more true for polyatomic molecules in which the rotational and vibrational levels are far more complex.

Section **15-2**
MEASURING MOLECULAR CONCENTRATION

We must now apply this theory to make measurements of molecular species. The standard method for measuring the concentration of an atomic species is to heat the specimen to excite the electrons into higher orbitals and then measure the emitted radiation. The same straightforward method will not work with compounds because collision energies sufficient to cause such molecular excitation will also cause bond dissociation and chemical reactions that will make accurate measurements impossible. Consequently, the most common way of measuring compounds using light is to irradiate them and see how much light they will absorb. This is possible because energy transition processes are reversible. If a certain transition x gives off a certain radiation wavelength y when it occurs, then the wavelength of light y will cause an electron to undergo transition x if it strikes an atom or molecule which has an electron in the ground state for the transition. When light of an appropriate wavelength is sent through a compound which can use the energy represented by light of that wavelength, some of the light will be absorbed to excite molecules of the compound present. This will reduce the intensity of the initial beam. Such reduction will be a

function of the amount of the compound present. The compound will reradiate the light, but it will do so randomly in all directions while, under experimental conditions, it will absorb light in only one direction. Therefore, the reradiation of light will have a negligible effect on the measurement of the absorption.

Figure 15-6 shows the light intensity of a beam of radiation that has passed through a specimen versus the wavelength of the light. The amount of light that makes it through the specimen is called the percent transmittance (%T). The areas where the %T is less than 100% are characteristic of the functional groups present in the compound. The depth of the troughs is a function of the amount of the compound present.

All the light incident to the specimen will be seen by the detector except for that absorbed by the specimen. An ideal detector will respond to all wavelengths of light, some perhaps better than others. If a wide spectrum of radiation (Fig. 15-7A) falls on the specimen, the change in the amount of radiation seen with the change in specimen concentration will be very small. While specimen x may contain twice the concentration of the sought for substance as specimen y, the difference in the light measured in the figure is only about 2%. Since we are, in effect, taking the difference between two large numbers to find our answer, much of our significance, and therefore our sensitivity to the change of concentration, is lost. This is bad because the quality of our measurement is its sensitivity to change, which is just the amount of signal we get compared with the noise or background:

$$\text{Sensitivity} = \frac{\text{signal}}{\text{noise}} \qquad \textbf{(15-5)}$$

The problem in Figure 15-7A is that the fraction of the spectrum being used is too great. The range of

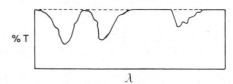

Figure 15-6 A typical absorption spectrum for a compound.

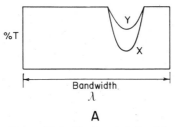 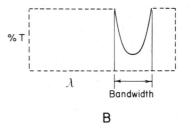

A   B

Figure 15-7 The bandwidth of the incident radiation affects the amount of background that will be transmitted.

wavelengths included in the incident beam is called the bandwidth, as noted in Chapter 14. If we reduce the bandwidth by eliminating much of the radiation in the regions in which no absorption occurs, we decrease the background and, therefore, increase the sensitivity of our measurements (Fig. 15-7B).

We are still using the wrong approach to the problem, however. We are, in effect, trying to find out how much of the cake was taken when only a sliver is gone. This means that we must be able to determine how much cake was there originally and how much now remains. We are still dealing with two large numbers, and our sensitivity is still poor. The correct approach is rather to measure the depth of the well by placing a measured stick down the middle of it. This approach is shown in Figure 15-8. If the bandwidth is small enough, the bottom of the absorption trough is flat relative to the bandwidth, and the amount of radiation absorbed is a direct function of the depth of the trough.

Let us start by defining the fraction of light transmitted (called transmittance, T) as the ratio of the emergent intensity (I) to the incident intensity (I_0).

$$T = \frac{I}{I_0} \qquad (15\text{-}6)$$

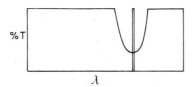

Figure 15-8 A very narrow bandwidth eliminates background radiation and gives a measurable transmittance, which is a function of the concentration.

The percent transmittance then is the transmittance times 100%.

$$\%T = \frac{I}{I_0} \times 100\% \qquad (15\text{-}7)$$

The absorbance (A) is a measure of the amount of light that is not transmitted and is therefore an inverse function of transmittance:

$$A = \log \frac{1}{T} = -\log T = 2 - \log\%T \qquad (15\text{-}8)$$

The absorbance is proportional to a compound-specific constant (a), the length of the path through the sample (b) in meters, and the sample concentration (C) in moles per liter. The general form of this equation is

$$A = -\log T = abC \qquad (15\text{-}9)$$

This is called the Beer-Lambert law, although Lambert is frequently slighted by the omission of his name. The constant a is usually called the "molar absorptivity," and less frequently the "molar extinction coefficient." The units of a are liters mole^{-1} meter^{-1}.

The Beer-Lambert law can only be used if the bandwidth is narrow enough to assume that the bottom of the trough is flat. If this is not the case, then Eq. 15-6 is no longer true. The logarithmic relationship between transmittance and absorption means that the average absorption cannot be calculated from the average transmittance without knowledge of the shape of the curve. The product of Eq. 15-6 and the equation of the curve would have to be integrated over the bandwidth to give an accurate overall relationship. Consequently, the Beer-Lam-

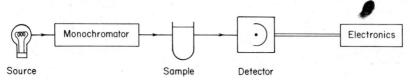

Figure 15-9 Block diagram of the components of a spectrophotometer.

bert law is restricted to light that is effectively 1 wavelength (monochromatic).

The fact that the Beer-Lambert law is a negative logarithmic expression somewhat restricts its usefulness. If the concentration is low, then very little light is absorbed, and we are left with the subtraction of two large numbers to find the small difference. Sensitivity is very poor. If the concentration is high, very little light is transmitted, and these light levels are of the order of the noise inherent in the detection circuitry. This also yields poor sensitivity. The range with the best sensitivity is between $A = 0.7$ to 1.0. Many laboratory methods are designed specifically to take advantage of this part of the absorption range.

Section **15-3**
RADIATION SOURCES

We are now ready to study instruments which use light to make absorption measurements. All such instruments are called photometers, and those that derive the radiation used from separating out a portion of the light given off by a source of wide bandwidth are called spectrophotometers. The parts of a spectrophotometer are shown in block diagram form in Figure 15-9. The monochromator and detectors are the same as for flame-emission measurements and were discussed in Chapter 14. The electronics of the data reduction circuitry are also similar to those used with the flame and will be discussed only briefly later. This leaves the radiation source and the specimen for detailed study. Both entities differ radically from those encountered in flame photometry.

The source is composed of two portions, the power regulator and the emission device. Historically, the power for the radiation source was supplied by batteries, but, except in remote research

stations or for military use, it is now common practice to use wall current. Power supplies of the type discussed in Chapter 7 are used for this purpose. Since the energy radiated is proportional to the square of the current through the radiation source (Eq. 1-9), however, it is frequently desirable to further stabilize the voltage to prevent current fluctuations. This is made more necessary by the fact that photometric measurement procedures sometimes require relatively long periods of time (minutes) to complete. One way that such stabilization can be accomplished is shown in Figure 15-10. If the unregulated voltage attempts to rise, transistor T1 will begin to conduct more strongly, which will cause transistor T2 to conduct more strongly and increase the voltage at point A.

This will have the effect, if unchecked, of increasing the power dissipated by the lamp and adversely affecting the measurement. Since point A is also attached to the inverting input of an operational amplifier, that amplifier will suffer a drastic decrease in output voltage as point A rises. This output is used to control transistor T1. A precipi-

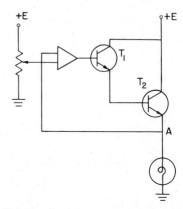

Figure 15-10 This circuit controls voltage drift and permits adjustment of the voltage across the source.

tous drop will reduce the flow of current through T1 and in turn through T2. This will return point A to a lower voltage, virtually identical to the initial voltage existing before the unregulated voltage rose.

The amplifier also has a voltage level present at the noninverting input. This comes from the contact arm of a potentiometer which is attached between ground and a very constant voltage source. Changing the position of the arm will increase or decrease the output of the amplifier and, therefore, the current through the transistors and the energy radiated by the source. This control is used to set 100% T in a classic spectrophotometer and will have to be adjusted as one moves through the spectrum, as will be seen shortly. Increasing the control voltage will increase the radiated power, but such action will also stress the lamp and cause it to deteriorate more quickly.

The radiation source itself consists of a heated filament in an evacuated bulb or of a gas in an envelope with two electrodes that have a high enough potential between them to cause an electrical discharge. To be useful for a variety of measurements, radiation of all wavelengths is needed so that the monochromator can select the appropriate radiation to stimulate the substance of unknown concentration. This broad-band radiation is called "white light." Not all sources are equally effective at producing such radiation. Figure 15-11 is a graph of the relative intensity plotted against the wavelength for some of the more common radiation sources. The Nernst glower is a bar composed of zirconium and yttrium oxides that radiate when heated by current to 2000°K. It and the hotter tungsten filament lamp (3000°K) suffer from the deficiency of having only 10–15% of their radiation in the usable visible part of the spectrum. The rest is in the infrared region. The common tungsten lamp, which resembles a small light bulb in appearance, cannot be used below 350 nm. Shorter wavelengths (i.e., 250 nm), can be obtained by the more complex tungsten–iodide lamp.

Arcs are required for most UV measurements. The high pressure mercury lamp allows 220 nm to be reached, but it suffers from the fact that it has a line spectrum imposed on the emission curve. High-pressure hydrogen and deuterium discharge tubes work well between 180 and 375 nm, with the deuterium source emitting several times as much radiation as the hydrogen, but also being more expensive. These sources emit far too little visible light to be used in that region. The xenon arc is the ideal source. At 6000°K it emits large quantities of radiation from 150 nm well up into the infrared. It

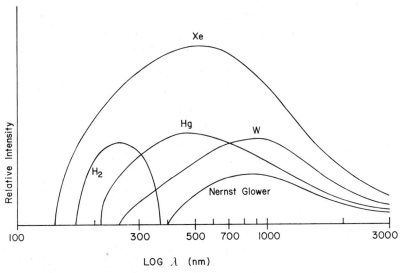

Figure 15-11 Relative radiation intensities of several sources plotted against the wavelength.

has demanding power and heat-shielding require-ments.

The reason all these sources are able to give so broad a band of radiation is that electrons are stripped from the atoms at the high operating tem-peratures, and these electrons are then captured at some later time. As can be seen in Figure 15-12, the energy levels of the outer atomic orbitals are very close together as one approaches the ionization po-tential. Free electrons give up unquantized amounts of energy as they are captured. Outer elec-trons have many available decay paths, further adding to the number of wavelengths emitted. Dop-pler broadening does the rest to form the continu-ous spectrum observed. The most favorable path-ways dictate the output characteristics of the device. These are affected to some extent by oper-ating temperature, but are more significantly af-fected by the electron structure of the atom or mole-cule involved.

Another source of radiation that is becoming common is the laser (*light amplification by stimu-lated emission of radiation*). In a steady-state equi-librium, the number of atoms in each excited orbital is given by Eq. 14-21.

No level contains a large number of atoms rela-tive to the ground state even at flame temperatures, and very few photons of light are emitted relative to the total number of atoms present. The light that is emitted is by a random process of decay, and there is no relationship between the phase of the light waves emitted, although the wavelength is obvi-ously the same if transitions are made between the same orbitals. The light is called incoherent be-cause it does not behave as a unit. The intensity of incoherent light photons is additive.

Coherent light, on the other hand, has all photons traveling together as a cohesive unit. While inco-herent light strikes an object just as waves strike a shore, coherent light strikes an object like a tidal wave. The exact structure of coherent radiation is beyond the scope of this book, but we can look at how, in principle, a laser generates such intense energy.

To gain coherency, all the emissions must be in the same direction at the same wavelength with the same wave phase. This can be accomplished only by "stimulating" the electron transition from a higher to lower energy level. But as we have just noted, relatively few atoms exist normally in ex-cited states to be stimulated to emit. We must, therefore, create an unsteady state by pumping electrons into a higher energy level and creating a population inversion (larger population in excited state). That is to say, we must supply energy through mechanical, optical, or electrical means to cause a large quantity of electrons to leave the ground states of these atoms and to create a supera-bundance of excited atoms at a suitable energy level. If a larger number of atoms are left in the lower state, they will absorb the stimulating radia-tion and quench the laser.

If only two energy levels are involved, it is very difficult to build a population inversion, since sup-plying more energy usually serves only to hasten the equilibrium process by lowering the activation energy barrier. If, however, we use a system with a suitable third energy level, a population inversion can more readily be built (Fig. 15-13A). The energy is pumped into the ground state as close to the exci-tation frequency of λ_1 as possible. Excited state 1 is very unstable, however, and rapidly decays to ex-cited state 2. This state is much more stable, per-haps, 1,000 times or more so, and therefore, it col-lects a large number of atoms relative to the total population. Random emission will occur to allow electrons to return to the ground level from excited state 2. An even better arrangement than Figure 15-13A is where a third state exists above the ground state. If state 3 decays to ground much more readily than state 2 decays to state 3, it is very easy to create a population inversion between states 2 and 3.

Such a situation can be taken advantage of if the element, in the form of a gas or solid, is in a reso-nant cavity. Such a cavity is a relatively long (sev-

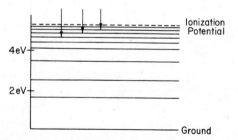

Figure 15-12 Orbital energies become closer to-gether and approach a continuum as one approaches the ionization potential.

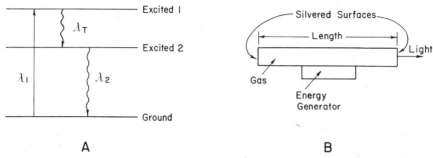

Figure 15-13 The necessary energy levels for building a population inversion (A) and block diagram of a laser (B).

eral centimeters), narrow tube or crystal that has ends which are high-quality mirrors (Fig. 15-13B). The length of the cavity is an exact multiple of the fundamental frequency of interest. When random decay of an excited level (called "relaxation") occurs in the longitudinal direction, it will be reflected back and forth over the length of the cavity and become a standing wave. As this wave encounters other excited atoms, it will stimulate them to emit in phase with this wave. If a large population of excited atoms exists, this wave will become huge as it oscillates between the two mirrors. When it is finally allowed to escape, it represents a tidal wave of energy on a very narrow pathway.

The energy input to the laser can be in the form of an electric and/or magnetic field which forces electrons into a higher energy level or of an intense source of incoherent radiation of a suitable wavelength to cause the first excitation. Sometimes one element is excited and used to excite a second element. The helium–neon laser works this way. Helium is excited to a metastable state that transfers its energy to neon. The excited neon atoms then decay by stimulated emission.

Lasers are becoming more popular. Dye lasers in particular, which are even "tunable" of wavelength to some extent, are coming into use for routine analysis due to their intense light. Lasers are commonly used for turbimetry and nephelometry. The study of lasers is a course in itself, and only the greatest generalizations have been given here.

Several practical considerations narrow the selection of light sources. Obviously the wavelengths needed for the analysis of interest are the predominant consideration. The light source must have adequate intensity at these wavelengths or no measure-

ment can be made. If one source will not cover the range of interest, interchangeable sources will be necessary, such as deuterium and tungsten. In better spectrophotometers this change is made by use of mirrors rather than physical manipulation which could damage the sources. The intensity needed is also a function of the monochromator and detector. Filters can diminish the light to an unusable level, while the dispersing system can be so selective as to leave little light remaining. If a barrier layer cell is used as the detector, more radiation will be required than if a photomultiplier tube is used. Within limits, raising the voltage over the source and photomultiplier tube can improve a low radiation situation. Heat and cost are both limiting factors. If they weren't, everyone would use the xenon arc. Heat can destroy the optics and make the photomultiplier tube noisy. The higher the temperature, the greater is the shielding problem. Water cooling of the source housing and heavy insulation may be necessary, which will make the device both bulky and expensive. Ease of source replacement should also be considered to prevent extensive downtime.

Section **15-4**
SPECIMEN CONSIDERATIONS

Certain factors in the design of a photometer or spectrophotometer are dependent upon the nature of the specimen, and we will explore them under the general heading of specimen considerations. The key to the selection of equipment for an absorption determination of a compound is the spectrum of the compound. Figure 15-14 contains several spectra, each illustrating a consideration

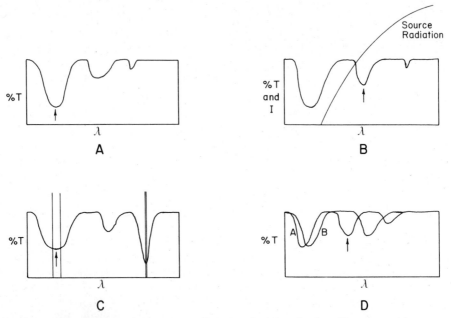

Figure 15-14 Various complications affect wavelength selection. The arrow points to the best choices in each case.

affecting the choice of instrumentation and measurement philosophy. Figure 15-14A shows a specimen with several absorption maxima (transmission minima). If all other factors are equal, one chooses to make the measurements at the strongest maximum (deepest trough). This gives the best signal-to-noise ratio for the measurement. However, one also wants to arrange the experimental conditions to try to make the measurements in the range from 0.7–1.0 absorption units for the reasons previously discussed. Stronger maxima are advantageous because they give greater flexibility in experimental conditions and the ability to measure small quantities accurately.

Figure 15-14B plots the absorption spectrum of the compound of interest and the spectrum of radiation intensity of the source on the same graph (note that the units on the y axis will be different for the two lines). All other factors being equal, the area of the spectrum with the most intense radiation (far right) is the one to select for the measurement. Frequently, the area of highest light emission of the source will not correspond to the area of the great-

est absorption maximum of the sample (left trough), and it will be necessary to select a compromise (middle trough). If very little radiation is present at the absorption maximum, then some less sensitive area must be selected since inadequate radiation makes a measurement impossible.

Figure 15-14C shows another problem. For the measurement to obey the Beer-Lambert law, the bottom of the absorption trough must be flat relative to the bandpass of the radiation. If the absorption maximum is broad (left trough), then a poor monochromator will provide a sufficiently narrow radiation band for the measurement. If the maximum is sharp (right trough), then a narrow band monochromator is needed. The availability or the procurement expense of an instrument with an adequate monochromator may be the determining factor in selecting at which wavelength to make a measurement.

Figure 15-14D shows the most common constraint on wavelength measurement, the ability to measure the sought-for substance without interference from other solution components. Strong absorptions are generally caused by functional groups that may be the same in both the reactants and products. It makes solution measurements extremely difficult when the loss of absorption due to the decrease of a reagent is matched by the increase in absorption of a product. The body fluids analyzed in the clinical laboratory are complex and contribute many absorbing species. Secondary choices for measurement wavelengths are often necessary. Even then, nonreacting species may contribute such significant background interference from overlapping absorption spectra that it is necessary to use a sample blank to set 100% transmittance and thereby to eliminate this constant factor.

It is essential to realize that all the factors in Figure 15-14 come into play at the same time for every measurement. The selection of methodology and instrumentation is therefore critical to accurate measurement. Inconsistencies between different instruments and methods are frequent, and their origins must be understood so that the results which a laboratory reports are a dependable representation of the actual species concentrations within the specimens.

By forcing the choice of a certain wavelength for the measurement procedure, the specimen also dictates the selection of optics. Below 350 nm, ordinary glass will not transmit light. It, therefore, cannot be used for any of the optics within the measurement system. This means not only the specimen cell, but also the lens, prisms, and back-surface mirrors must be made from quartz or fused silica. Such requirements, therefore, add greatly to the expense of the instrument and the care that must be taken in its use. For UV measurements, Corex glass can be used down to 300 nm and quartz down to 210 nm. Fused silica can be used as low as 185 nm, but the whole instrument must be closed so that nitrogen or argon can be used to flush out the oxygen of the atmosphere which absorbs in this region. Such complications in the performance of measurements in the far UV region make them impractical for most common laboratory procedures.

In trying to eliminate all factors other than the concentration of the sought-for substance from the final result, even the geometry of the specimen container cannot be overlooked. Specimen cuvettes should be matched in size and shape. Moreover, the thickness of the glass or quartz should also be

the same, since the container itself will absorb some radiation, and this should be invariant between specimen containers. Many instruments have flow-through cells so that the light path is always identical. Rectangular containers are preferable to circular containers because there is less chance of surface reflection giving scattered radiation.

The reduction of such scattered radiation or stray light is paramount to any successful photometric measurement. Detectors will record light photons regardless of the path they followed to the detector, yet only those which come through the specimen are affected by Beer's law of absorption. Stray radiation therefore means trouble. It usually shows up in terms of high dark current, nonlinearity, or drift in the instrument setting. It greatly increases the uncertainty of the measurement. The problem is attacked by painting all surfaces flat black to minimize reflection. All openings to the light path, especially the sample compartment, are lined with black foam or other compressible sealant. Instruments are frequently designed to use front-surface mirrors made of polished metal rather than back-surface mirrors made of glass or quartz. These latter devices give reflections each time light tries to cross an interface, thereby scattering light, which through devious routes can reach the detector. Minimizing scattered light is also a reason for selecting gratings over prisms since the light need not pass through the former.

Section **15-5**
DATA REDUCTION

The electronics for the first four components of a photometric measuring device have been discussed here and in Chapter 14. The data reduction and representation circuitry is similar to that of the flame emission devices, with one major exception. The result from the absorption process is in the exponential form. The logarithm of the observed light intensity must be taken before other computations can be performed. This can be accomplished by one of two methods. The first is by a logarithmic amplifier, which is a transistor circuit where the current between the collector and emitter is the logarithm of the voltage applied to the base. This current value is changed to a voltage value by passing it through a resistor and is converted to the digital representation by an ADC. The second method is to first convert the detector output to digital and then compute the logarithm by the series expansion or by interpolation from an abbreviated logarithm table. Manipulations then are performed as described in the previous chapter.

More and more laboratory instruments are now featuring various descriptive information attached to the results, such as units and normal ranges, which must be stored internally as ASCII and printed at the appropriate time. Diagnostic information is also handled by the output circuitry and used to flag or suppress the results. Some older spectrophotometers still feature a D'Arsonval meter display in terms of transmittance, with a secondary scale in absorbance units. These are now encountered only in the smallest laboratories and are time consuming to use, but their operating mechanism should be obvious in terms of material previously presented.

Some circumstances render inadequate the general scheme just elaborated. In such cases, the demands of precision are too great for available components and methodology. One such situation is when the reaction occurs over a long period of time (e.g., half an hour). The drift in the circuitry may be a significant contributor to the measured rate of a reaction of a low-concentration catalyst such as an enzyme. Secondly, sometimes it is not possible to find a wavelength which is free from other absorbances. In the presence of such background interference, Beer's law will not be obeyed. Finally, one may want to be able to scan the spectrum to find the absorption maxima by turning the wavelength dial through the spectrum on an instrument. Since the amount of radiation is also a function of wavelength, this will not work as expected. The observed spectrum will be the difference between the source emission and the absorption spectrum of the compound.

A means of handling these situations is with an approach called "dual beam" (Fig. 15-15). The light is split after the monochromator and passes through two separate specimen compartments. It is then either recombined or fed into two separate detectors. In the former case, the electronics must be synchronized so that the circuit knows which beam it is seeing, as in flame photometry. In the latter case, the readings from the two detectors are converted to numeric values and the ratio is taken. The first approach is more desirable because it eliminates detector drift as well as source drift, while the second approach is easier to implement. In either case, the light passing through cell 1 is assumed to be 100% transmitted (I_0 = the blank), and the light (I) through cell 2 is diminished by absorption. Therefore, the operator places water or an appropriate mixture minus the initiating reagent

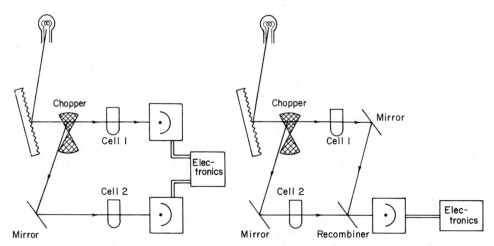

Figure 15-15 Two methods of dual-beam analysis.

in cell 1 and the reaction mixture in cell 2. Source drift and detector drift (in the single detector case) do not affect the result because the ratio I/I_0 will not change.

When significant absorption occurs from other species, this absorption will also occur in cell 1, and its only effect will be to decrease the magnitude of I_0 for both pathways. Equations 15-8 and 15-9 will still hold. Finally, as the spectrum is scanned, any change in the incident light for cell 2 will also be the same change for cell 1 and the ratio I/I_0 will be unaffected. Thus dual-beam spectrophotometry can improve the results which would be obtained from single-beam analysis.

Section **15-6**
ATOMIC ABSORPTION

Now that we have introduced the concept of absorption measurements and have seen its implementation in molecular measurements, we will return to the analysis of atomic species in the flame. The flame is successful at exciting perhaps 1 or 2% of the ground state atoms into the excited states that radiate and are measured. At any given moment most of the atoms are not available to participate in the measurement because they are not in a state that produces radiation. If we could measure these ground state atoms instead of the excited atoms, we should be able to greatly improve our sensitivity since there are so many more atoms to count. This is made an even more appealing approach when one is interested in the elements which are not in the first column of the periodic table. The alkali metals have but a single valence electron to excite with low excitation energies, and this leads to simple spectra with most of the excited population in a few lower orbitals. Other materials have numerous electrons that may be excited independently to give very complex spectra. As a result, no one excited state contains a very high percentage of the total atoms (Eq. 14-21). To increase the population of the states in order to obtain sufficient sensitivity requires the input of tremendous amounts of energy by means of an arc or spark emission device. Such devices are more difficult to use and are not practical for routine clinical laboratory analysis.

The problem is that atoms in the ground state will not radiate. It is therefore necessary to supply them with radiation that they can absorb and then use the Beer-Lambert law to determine their concentration. We could, it would at first seem, design our apparatus like that for the photometric measurement shown in Figure 15-9 by replacing the specimen cell with the flame. Unfortunately, this approach is doomed to failure because the monochromator cannot give an adequately small bandpass. Atoms absorb very precisely at one wavelength with very little Doppler or pressure broadening. Most of the light from even the best monochromator would not be of the correct wavelength to be absorbed by ground-state atoms and would be measured by the detector as background. The signal would vary only a few tenths or hundredths of a percent and would be indistinguishable from noise. The problems discussed in Section 15-2 would strike with a vengeance.

The solution to this difficulty is to find a better source of radiation of the single correct wavelength than a conventional monochromator. Fortunately such a source is available in the form of the element of interest itself. If we excite a separate quantity of the atoms of this element and direct the resulting radiation through the sample vaporized in a flame, some of the radiation will be absorbed, and this loss can be measured. This is the principle of atomic absorption. The block diagram for the apparatus is shown in Figure 15-16.

The source of radiation is called a hollow cathode lamp, sketched in Figure 15-17A. The cathode, from which the name is derived, is a hollowed cylinder that points toward the window of the lamp. The cathode is coated with the metal whose spectrum is sought. Sometimes several metals are combined to give more versatility if their spectra are adequately different. The anode is made of tungsten and is positioned so that a discharge to the cathode will occur at a potential of several hundred volts. The tube contains an inert gas, such as neon or argon, at 1–2 torr. An optical window made of glass or quartz (as necessitated by the wavelength) allows the light to emerge. The other sides of the lamp can be darkened to reduce stray radiation.

When an adequate potential is applied, the gas in the tube becomes positively ionized and collides with the cathode with enough force to dislodge sur-

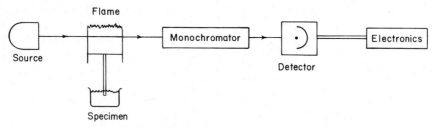

Figure 15-16 A block diagram for atomic absorption.

face atoms. This process is called sputtering. These atoms are excited through collision and radiate their characteristic wavelengths. During nondischarge periods, these atoms settle out onto the sides of the lamp or return to the electrode surface. The operating current is only a few milliamperes. If the current is increased, line broadening results from the increased collisions. This produces light that is less likely to be absorbed and therefore only adds to the background radiation. Increased intensity can be gained by making a lamp with more electrodes, just as the performance of the triode was improved by more electrodes. The equations for the hollow cathode lamp are

$$Ar^+ + M \rightarrow Ar^+ + M^* \qquad \textbf{(15-10)}$$

$$M^* \rightarrow M + h\nu \qquad \textbf{(15-11)}$$

where M is a metal atom, M^* is an excited metal atom, and $h\nu$ is emitted light.

Although essential to atomic absorption, the use of the hollow cathode is not without difficulties. As with any discharge source, control of operating conditions is essential because the amount of radiation varies dramatically with the amount of energy being dissipated. The lamp is very slow to come to steady state, since a constant "atmospheric" concentration of metal atoms must be produced. Continual bombardment of the cathode will cause the lamp to age. Then, too, the spectra of the inert gas atoms and ions will be superimposed on that of the desired element. With proper techniques all these problems can be solved.

In contrast to flame emission photometry, where the intensity of the emitted light is linearly related to the concentration of sought-for species, atomic absorption is governed by the Beer-Lambert relationship. From this law it is clear that the amount of radiation absorbed is directly dependent on the path length of the cell. In atomic absorption the cell is the flame. We can increase the path length, and therefore the sensitivity, by making the flame as long and narrow as possible. As Figure 15-17B shows, we can improve our sensitivity even more by passing the light through the flame several times. This gives more of the large population of atoms in the ground state a chance to absorb passing photons. A flame of constant width is essential.

In Figure 15-16 there is no monochromator before the flame, but instead there is one after it. Clearly, light from the hollow cathode lamp is already more monochromatic than any conventional

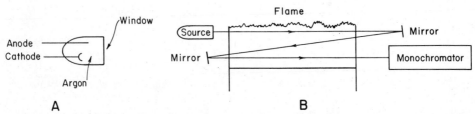

Figure 15-17 The hollow cathode source (A) and the multiple paths through the flame (B).

monochromator can produce, and so one is not needed here. The other wavelengths present in the beam (e.g., from inert gas atoms) will not interfere with the absorption process and can be removed later. A monochromator after the flame, however, is essential. First, of course, there are those other wavelengths from gas atoms and ions in the hollow cathode lamp which must be removed as well as those of perhaps other elements in the cathode and of other orbital transitions from the sought-for element itself. For a good hollow cathode source, these will be significantly different from the desired wavelength and easily disposed of. There is also, however, the radiation from the flame to be eliminated. Since it will emit radiation in a continuum, including wavelengths close to the measurement wavelength, a monochromator or interference filter is necessary to reduce this background radiation. Even so, the monochromator or filter is only a first step in completely removing flame background.

To eliminate the maximum amount of background, it is necessary to again use the dual-beam approach. In this case we place the dual pathways between the source and the monochromator, as shown in Figure 15-18. The beam that passes through the flame (R_1) contains the radiation of the flame (R_F) as well as that of the source (R_S), but it has been reduced by the amount of radiation absorbed in its passage through the flame (R_A) (Eq. 15-12). The beam passing around the flame (R_2) also contains the light of the flame (it gets added in at the recombiner) and the light of the source, but suffers

no absorption (Eq. 15-13). Both are augmented by the dark current of the detector (R_D).

$$R_1 = R_S + R_F - R_A + R_D \qquad \text{(15-12)}$$

$$R_2 = R_S + R_F + R_D \qquad \text{(15-13)}$$

These equations are not sufficient to yield an answer, since it is necessary to know the radiation from the source (R_S) to determine what percentage has been transmitted. R_S can be measured by placing a shutter between the flame and the recombiner at position B. As the beam splitter continues to operate, we get both the source radiation (when the source light passes around the flame) in Eq. 15-14 and the dark current (when the source light enters the flame) in Eq. 15-15.

$$R_3 = R_S + R_D \qquad \text{(15-14)}$$

$$R_4 = R_D \qquad \text{(15-15)}$$

The radiation of the source and the amount absorbed can easily be calculated. The fact that the source drifts for an extended period after being turned on makes the use of a second chopper at point B, one out-of-phase with the beam splitter, desirable. This allows all four values necessary to solve Eqs. 15-12 through 15-15 to be gathered continuously.

The sensitivity and quick response needed for atomic absorption make the photomultiplier the detector of choice. The detector electronics must be synchronized with the choppers to tally the various

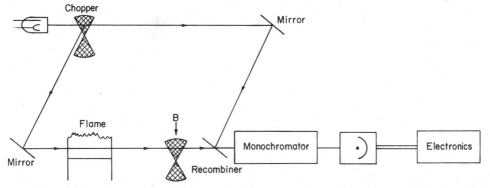

Figure 15-18 A block diagram of the use of optical choppers to interrupt and redirect the light in atomic absorption.

signals at the correct time. This motion can be detected by photodiodes appropriately positioned or by digital timing technology. Background subtraction is done first, followed by logarithmic conversion, digital conversion and division to yield a reportable result. Further enhancements in calculations and representation are being added with the advancement of computer technology.

Calcium is the element most commonly measured by atomic absorption in the clinical laboratory. Heavy metals (e.g., lead, mercury, copper) can also be measured for toxicological purposes. The relative sensitivity versus flame photometry varies with the element being measured and the energy available for excitation. While many more atoms are in the ground state than the excited state, the overall probability of having a measureable transition will favor emission in certain instances. Each method is superior for certain elements.

One of the complicating features of atomic absorption is atomic emission. Atoms excited by the absorption of light can reemit light at the same wavelength. This light is indistinguishable from the source radiation and will cause deviation from Beer's law if detected. Fortunately, the amount of this radiation traveling in the direction of the detec-

tor is small and not significant compared with the other radiation emitted by the flame.

Section 15-7
FLUOROMETRY

This principle of absorption and reemission of radiation can be used to advantage in molecular measurements. (While atomic fluorometry is possible, it is not generally used in the clinical laboratory and will not be discussed further.) The theory is illustrated in Figure 15-19A. Molecules in the ground state absorb radiation and are moved to the excited state because (1) there are many rotational and vibrational levels in each electronic state, (2) numerous transitions are possible, and (3) a broad band of radiation can be absorbed. The excited molecule may then lose some of this energy by collision or by delocalizing it to other bonds (if it is more than a diatomic molecule). While still electronically excited, it has reduced its vibrational and rotational excitement. Even so, it must eventually give off energy and return to a vibrational and rotational level in the electronic ground state. If this can be done through further collisions and delocalizations,

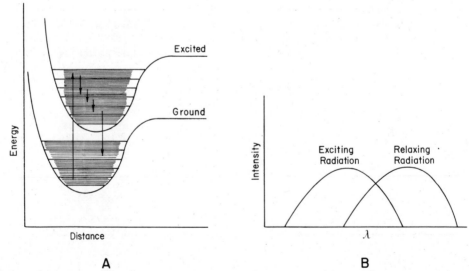

Figure 15-19 Fluorescence depends upon the relaxation radiation being less energetic than the exciting radiation.

as is common, nothing further is seen of the molecule. If, however, the lower excited state gives off radiation as a means of returning to the ground state, then that radiation must be of lower energy than the exciting radiation and consequently be of longer wavelength (Fig. 15-19B). This process of absorbing and reemitting light is called fluorescence and occurs in 10^{-9}–10^{-4} sec. If in the process of excitation the electron spin is inverted, the molecule enters a more stable intermediary state from which it can take much longer to return to the ground state. This process is called phosphorescence and is responsible for the glow-in-the-dark effect some substances exhibit. Because there is so much time for deexcitement (relaxation) through other pathways, phosphorescence is not used too frequently for analytical measurements.

Fluorescence, on the other hand, is quite useful. If we can excite molecules in proportion to their concentration and if they will radiate after a short time, then we have a situation very similar to flame photometry with excited molecules instead of excited atoms. The emitted radiation will be directly proportional to the concentration; moreover, there is no flame radiation to interfere with the measurement.

Figure 15-20 shows the layout of a fluorometer. The source must generate light over a large area of the spectrum, particularly the lower end. The mercury arc is commonly used because it has four strong emission lines in the UV and lower visible region (366, 405, 436, and 546 nm), as well as a continuum over the whole range. The xenon arc is a good source, but it suffers from the previously mentioned heating problems. Tungsten can be used, but it is weak in the lower end of the spectrum at wavelengths needed to excite many compounds.

Two monochromators are needed for fluorometric measurements. The excitation monochromator must limit the light to wavelengths that will cause molecules in the lower vibrational levels of the ground state to move to the higher vibrational levels of the excited state. Other wavelengths will only introduce stray light to the measurement process. After the fluorescence has occurred, the light will enter the fluorescence monochromator. This device must allow the passage of only those wavelengths that result from the relaxation between the lower vibrational level of the excited electronic state and the higher vibrational levels of the ground electronic state. Consequently, it must totally exclude those wavelengths which were able to pass through the excitation monochromator. In short, no light can pass both monochromators. These monochromators can be either filters, gratings, or prisms, depending on the quality of the instrument and the narrowness of the gap between the peak exciting and fluorescing wavelengths.

The need to prevent the exciting radiation from reaching the detector is paramount. The exciting radiation must be intense to give good sensitivity

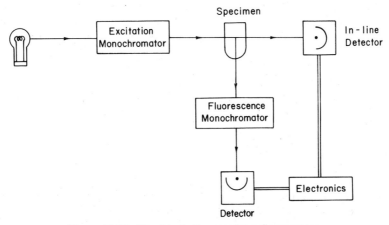

Figure 15-20 The block diagram for a fluorometer.

and will therefore greatly overwhelm the much weaker fluorescent radiation, which is further diminished by being emitted in all directions. The use of monochromators, which together exclude all radiation, is one step to reduce stray light. The second is to place the detector at 90° to the incident beam. Some light will always be reflected off surfaces or scattered by particles in the solution. Such reflection and scattering is at a minimum in the direction perpendicular to the incident beam. Naturally all interior surfaces must be painted flat black and all access doors carefully lined.

The system optics must be, of course, made of the appropriate glass or of quartz to allow light passage. The detector is usually a photomultiplier tube. In fact, it is not uncommon to use two photomultipliers. One is used to measure the fluorescence, and the second is placed in line with the source beam. If the source varies, this in-line detector measurement can be used to correct the fluorescence detector value. The amplification, calculation, and reporting circuitry is similar to that previously seen.

Fluorometry offers important advantages over absorption techniques. First, it is a direct measurement, linearly proportional to the concentration. It is specific for a particular compound or class of compounds. Other substances absorbing at the same wavelength will not interfere unless they also fluoresce at the same observation wavelength. Fluorescence can be made very sensitive by use of a high intensity source and a sensitive photomultiplier. Absorption cannot use this approach because the source radiation would destroy the detector, but the detector in fluorometry will see only the weak fluorescent radiation under similar conditions. The equation for a fluorescence measurement is

$$I = I_0 abC \qquad \text{(15-16)}$$

On the other hand, fluorescence is highly dependent on the solution parameters. Quenching of the fluorescence process can occur from increasing solution temperature, altering the pH, or changing the solvent. Any action that would affect the ability of the fluorescing compound to dissipate the energy of excitation will affect the amount of radiation emit-

ted. The composition of the solution matrix must be kept effectively constant between samples except for the fluorescing compound. Fortunately, electronic sensors now allow us to detect, and in the future should allow us to correct, such physical factors as pH, temperature, and ionic strength to very precise tolerances (± a few tenths of a percent). Spurious protein and bilirubin fluorescence is a problem in biological specimens because it frequently occurs in the same spectral region as the desired radiation.

Fluorescence can also be self-quenching. The radiation given off by fluorescence can be absorbed by another molecule to excite it. This is a net loss of radiation and will affect the linearity of the measurement. It is most prevalent in concentrated solutions and can be avoided by adequate dilution of the specimen.

Having looked at the nature of emission, absorption and fluorescent principles, we will turn our attention to the implementation of such principles, particularly those of absorption, in discrete and continuous flow analyzers. In the process, we will reencounter the ion-selective electrode and the mechanical and electrical control of instrumental processes.

REVIEW QUESTIONS

1. What happens within an atom as it prepares to bond with another atom?
2. How are molecular orbitals formed?
3. How many orbitals exist in the final molecule?
4. How are molecular orbitals populated?
5. What are bonding orbitals?
6. What are nonbonding orbitals?
7. What are antibonding orbitals?
8. Why can't the inert gases form compounds?
9. What two forces determine the bond length in a molecule?
10. What effect does vibration have on a molecule?
11. What is characteristic of the vibrational levels?
12. What is the shape of the bonding potential well?
13. What is bond dissociation energy?
14. Around what does a molecule rotate?

15. What effect does rotation have on the molecular energy level?

16. Why is our model called the "rigid rotator-harmonic oscillator model"?

17. Where do higher molecular orbitals come from?

18. What rules affect radiation transitions between vibrational levels?

19. Why does molecular radiation form a continuum?

20. Why can't molecular concentrations be measured following heat excitation?

21. How are molecular concentrations most commonly measured by radiation techniques?

22. Define percent transmittance.

23. What is sensitivity?

24. Why is broad-band radiation not useful in absorbance measurements?

25. What is bandwidth?

26. What is monochromatic light?

27. State the Beer-Lambert law.

28. Why is monochromatic light needed to use the Beer-Lambert law?

29. What are the practical limitations on the use of absorbance measurements?

30. What are the five components of a spectrophotometer?

31. What parts of a spectrophotometer are similar to those of a flame photometer? What parts are different?

32. What are the two parts of the power supply?

33. Explain how the circuit in Figure 15-10 works.

34. What effects does raising the voltage over the source have?

35. Name the two classes of radiation sources.

36. Define white light.

37. Describe the Nernst glower.

38. What sources are used in the UV range?

39. Why is the xenon arc troublesome to use?

40. How can atomic radiation sources give a continuum?

41. On what principle is a laser based?

42. How does one get coherent light?

43. Describe the construction of a laser.

44. What is peculiar about a helium-neon laser?

45. What are some considerations when selecting a radiation source?

46. Why is the strongest maximum used for radiation measurements?

47. Why does the spectrum of the source radiation play a part in the selection of the wavelength at which a photometric measurement is made?

48. Why does the quality of the monochromator affect the selection of the measurement wavelength?

49. What effect do other absorbing species have on the selection of wavelength for absorbance measurements?

50. Why can't ordinary glass be used for absorbance measurements below 350 nm?

51. What materials can be used to construct measurement cells and optics for UV measurements?

52. List three ways in which the optical elements and/or cuvettes can adversely affect an absorbance measurement.

53. What precautions must be taken to avoid stray light in absorbance measurements?

54. Why is stray light a problem in absorbance measurements?

55. What steps are involved in the electronic manipulation of absorbance data?

56. Give three reasons to use dual-beam spectrophotometry.

57. Describe two dual-beam configurations.

58. Why does the dual-beam approach eliminate drift?

59. Why does the dual-beam approach eliminate background absorption?

60. What is measured in atomic absorption?

61. Why can't an ordinary monochromator produce the radiation for atomic absorption?

62. Describe the operation of a hollow cathode source.

63. Sketch and label the parts of a hollow cathode.

64. What are the important reaction equations in a hollow cathode source?

65. What are some difficulties in using the hollow cathode?

66. Why is the source radiation passed through the flame several times in atomic absorption?

67. Why is a monochromator needed after the flame in atomic absorption?

68. Explain why the complex chopper arrangement

is needed in atomic absorption to compute the answer.

69. Why does atomic emission affect atomic absorption?
70. What is the physical principle behind fluorescence?
71. Why is broad-band radiation suitable to stimulate fluorescence?
72. What is phosphorescence?
73. Sketch and label the parts of a fluorometer.
74. Why is a mercury arc lamp a good source for fluorometry?
75. Why are two monochromators needed for fluorometry?
76. What is the reason for the geometry of the fluorometer?
77. What is the function of the in-line detector?
78. What are some advantages of fluorometry? Disadvantages?
79. What is self-quenching?

PROBLEMS

1. Draw the orbital and electron configuration for N_2.
2. Draw the orbital and electron configuration for F_2.
3. Draw the orbital and electron configuration for CO.
4. What is the absorbance when the $\%T$ is 37.9%?
5. What is the $\%T$ when the absorbance is 1.02 units?
6. If $\%T$ is 42.6%, the molar absorptivity 3.72 · 10^4 liter mole^{-1} meter^{-1}, and the cell thickness 1.72 cm, what is the concentration of the light-absorbing substance?
7. If the concentration of x is 0.0671 M, the cell thickness is 0.98 cm, and the molar absorptivity is 1,284 liter mole^{-1} m^{-1}, what is the $\%T$ of the solution?

CHAPTER 16
DISCRETE ANALYZERS

We have spent most of our time up to this point discussing the methodology and principles of measurement and the supporting electronics. In the next few chapters we will look at the technology that enables the sample or the reaction stream to be manipulated for measurement. Thereafter, for the most part, we will combine the principles and technology of measurement approaches into single units.

All chemical analysis can be divided into two classes: discrete analysis and continuous flow analysis. In the former, reagents and sample are combined in a cell (e.g., test tube, cuvette), and this mixture is then measured. In the latter, the reagents and specimens are mixed as they flow through the system and are measured as they move past a designated point. Discrete analysis is discussed in this chapter, while continuous flow analysis is examined in Chapter 17.

Discrete analyzers can be divided into four classes: test tube, prepackaged, centrifugal, and in situ. The first of these goes back to the early days of chemical analysis, while the rest have arisen in recent years as the result of various technological breakthroughs. All these methods have been enhanced by the growth of computer technology. We will study each of these approaches in the following pages. Due to the large number of discrete analyzers available, we will attempt to discuss them in a generic manner, except where a product is unique enough to merit special description. The analyzers discussed are used primarily for blood serum and urine, although some can also measure blood plasma, whole blood, spinal fluid, or other body fluids.

Section 16-1
TEST TUBE ANALYZERS

The principles of the test tube analyzer are among the earliest learned in experimental science. One mixes chemicals together in a beaker, flask, or test tube and observes what happens. By using this qualitative approach, each of us learned about precipitation and color reactions. As we progressed, we learned that even reactions that we could not see with the unaided eye could be carried out in this fashion and measured by colorimeter, calorimeter, or pH meter. The approach could thus be made quantitative.

The basic implementation of the modern test tube methodology is shown in Figure 16-1. Specimens for analysis are usually placed in a circular tray by the technologist. This tray is advanced one position each time that a sample is aspirated. Such trays or plates are mounted on the instrument with sample cups filled, or cups can be placed in position on the plate while the instrument is operating if it does not process specimens too rapidly. The identity of the specimen in the cups on each plate must be recorded by the technologist, so the results can later be matched to the patients. On some instruments a machine-readable label can be attached to the sample cup so that the instrument can read the patient identification at the time of sampling and pair it with the results when they are measured later.

A measured amount of each sample is aspirated by a pipet. This amount will vary with the type of analysis and the amount of miniaturization realized

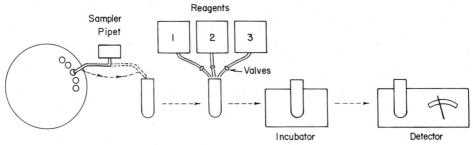

Figure 16-1 Block diagram of a test tube analyzer.

in the instrumentation. This sample is injected into a cup by reversing the pressure within the sampling pipet. The aspiration of the sample is frequently controlled by a stepping motor that drives a syringe, as shown in Figure 8-9. The positioning of a stepping motor is extremely accurate because the motor is wired so that the armature will stop only in specific positions when the current is shut off. The length of time that the motor drives in one direction is linearly proportional to the distance that an attached syringe (or piston) will more. To withdraw a designated amount of sample, power is applied to the motor for the appropriate length of time. To dispense the sample, one of two philosophies can be employed. In the first, the original stepping motor drives in only one direction. A second motor, attached to the sampler pipet by a *T*, expels the sample and usually a measured amount of diluent by driving in the other direction (Fig. 16-2). This approach uses relatively simple motors, and the equipment is washed by the flow of diluent each time a sample is expelled.

In the second approach, one stepping motor is driven in both directions by reversing the polarity of the motor's magnetic coils. If diluent is used in this arrangement, it must be drawn up before the sample either through the pipet or by the use of a valve which switches between the sample and the diluent reservoir. The second approach can also be used in the case when different analyses are done on the same sample at the same time (multichannel). Here measured portions of the original sample drawn up in the pipet are dispensed into adjacent cuvettes. In this usage the addition of diluent with the sample is not possible.

After placing specimen in one or more reaction vessels, the test tube analyzer adds appropriate diluents and reagents to bring the final concentrations and volumes up to specific levels. Such quantities can be added by automated digital pipets (as was the sample), by peristaltic pumping, or from pressurized reagent reservoirs. A pressurized reagent reservoir has a constant pressure applied to the reagent and a tube of specified diameter running to a

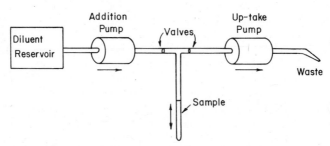

Figure 16-2 The use of two unidirectional pumps to add sample flushed with diluent to reaction tubes.

solenoid valve, which is controlled by a microprocessor or a more elementary relay system. The amount of each reagent added to each reaction tube is determined by the pressure, the size of the connecting line, and the time the reagent is allowed to run into the reaction tube.

Following the addition of all the reagents, the mixture is incubated and measured. Much of the ingenuity of the instrumentation is involved in these steps. From the point the specimen is added, the test tube or cuvette must be moved to where the reagents are added, moved to an incubation station, moved to a reader, and, finally, the specimen must be discarded. In many analyzers the cups are then washed, dried and repositioned to be used again. All these steps add complexity to the instrument, particularly when multiple channels are involved.

One approach to the transport problem is to make the transport path circular and rotate the reaction tubes in a concentric circle with the specimen cups (Fig. 16-3A). At point W the sample is transferred, during interval X the reagents are added, during interval Y incubation occurs, and at point Z the reading is taken. Additional detectors can be added at points Z' and Z'' to make a rate-of-reaction measurement. When all the cuvettes on one plate have been exhausted, the whole plate (specimen and reaction cups) is replaced, and a new group of samples is analyzed. The temperature in such an instrument can be controlled by enclosing the whole instrument in an air bath and by preheating the reagents.

Another approach is to have the original samples placed on a conveyor which moves perpendicularly to the reaction tubes (Fig. 16-3B). As the sample reaches each reaction station, an aliquot is removed and placed in the nearest tube. The tube is transported at a right angle to the sample conveyor. Along the way, reagents are added and the tube goes into a waterbath or is moved between heated metal plates. After several minutes the tube enters a photometer and the appropriate measurement is made. The tube is then washed, dried, and moved back to the sampling station for another specimen. The latter part of the trip will be made in the inverted position to hasten drying. The Parallel made by American Monitor Corporation works basically in this manner.

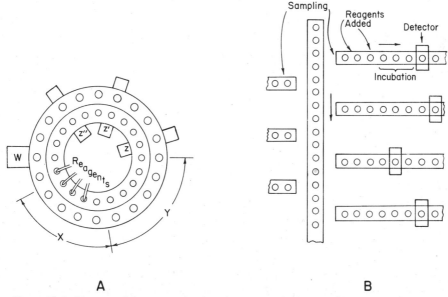

A   B

Figure 16-3   Two possible geometries for a test tube analyzer. Part A shows a concentric arrangement. Part B illustrates perpendicular paths.

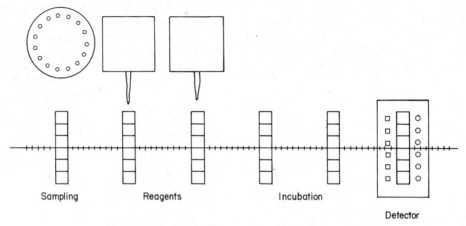

Figure 16-4 Block diagram of lock-step instrument.

A third adaptation is to have the cuvettes used for the various channels move parallel to each other in a block (lock-step approach) (Fig. 16-4). The cuvettes are filled sequentially at the sampler and then move an increment down the conveyor to the next station. Here different reagents are added to each tube so the sample can be tested for several materials simultaneously. The next few steps are used for incubation in a temperature-controlled environment as the reactions proceed to completion. Finally the specimens are moved into parallel detectors where the separate concentrations are read. The Hycel instruments work in this general fashion.

The above description is far from exhaustive, but should give the general idea of the mechanical transport approaches in general use. Each has strengths and weaknesses. The concentric analyzers are basically simple and can be used, with proper programming, to do a wide variety of tests. They are limited to one test at a time, however, and are therefore rather slow. The analyzers where each reaction tube follows its own path give maximum flexibility to the analysis scheme, but also involve a phenomenal amount of mechanical parts, all subject to malfunction. Moreover, sampling time will be spread over a number of minutes and involve numerous probes, adding significantly to the possibility of contamination. The lock-step approach stereotypes the methodology, does not al-low for different temperatures, and makes reagent addition in different time frames more difficult. On the other hand, the lock-step approach requires less manual intervention and has fewer mechanical parts than other approaches. All multichannel analyzers of the test tube variety can be programmed to do only those tests ordered on a patient, thereby saving reagents. This is in marked contrast to the segmented flow analyzers discussed in the next chapter.

Most measurements in test tube analyzers employ light absorbance methods. The use of tungsten light sources is common, and the monochromator is usually some type of glass interference filter. In single-channel instruments, which can run a number of different tests sequentially, the filters are frequently mounted in a wheel that can be rotated into position to give the correct radiation for the different methods (Fig. 16-5). Such positioning must be done manually in the older instruments, but is under microprocessor control in more recent products. The light may be detected by any of the methods previously discussed, ranging from the photodiode to the photomultiplier tube. Because the geometries of the instruments are not always conducive to a linear arrangement of the optical detector, prisms, mirrors, and optical fibers are commonly used to bend the measuring radiation.

Sodium and potassium in several of these instruments are measured by a special flame attachment.

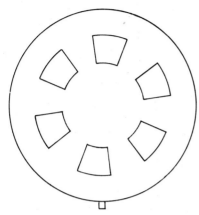

Figure 16-5 A wheel with glass filters for absorbance measurements.

Lithium is added as an internal standard, and the mixture is aspirated into the burner. Ion-selective electrodes can also be used for these measurements after the sample is appropriately buffered.

The container in which the measurements are made is handled in several different ways by the various manufacturers. A common approach is to add the specimen and reagents to this vessel and march it through the whole process. After reading has been made, the cuvette is washed, dried, and reused. Disposable cuvettes are not as good, since they will vary more in wall thickness and diameter than will reusable cuvettes, increasing the error inherent in the methodology. Another approach is to aspirate the reaction mixture and place that sample into a separate measurement cuvette. This allows disposable tubes to be used in the reaction step and can be useful for methods requiring pretreated tubes for successful reaction.

The basic advantage of the test tube instruments is the inherent simplicity of the approach. It mimics traditional manual methods and is therefore easy to troubleshoot. Single-channel instruments are usually not complex in design. Unfortunately, there are also a number of significant limitations. Separation steps, such as dialysis, cannot be readily carried out, limiting the chemical methods that are implementable. A further limitation is the rigid timing of reagent additions and reaction duration. The instruments that feature many channels (10–30) be-

come very complicated mechanically with corresponding operational difficulties. The preparation and preservation of numerous reagents can be a nuisance.

Data reduction and processing is handled by minicomputer or microprocessors in nearly all new instruments, particularly the multichannel varieties. The detector-to-computer electronics are those discussed in the previous chapters. The data correlation and reporting techniques of the larger instruments are similar to those of the Technicon SMAC, which is discussed in Chapter 17.

Section 16-2
PREPACKAGED ANALYZERS

The packet or prepackaged analysis methods have only been developed by a few companies as another approach to containing the reaction mixture. In these methods sample is added to a prepackaged product and the result read. All chemical preparation is eliminated. Different methods can be run interspersed because they depend on the packets chosen, not on how the machine is set up or what reagents are loaded. The prime examples of this approach are the DuPont automatic clinical analyzer (ACA) and the Eastman Kodak Ektachem 400.

A pictorial sketch of the ACA is shown in Figure 16-6. Samples are placed in the top of the sample cup shown in Figure 16-7. The patient identification is placed on the card below the cup. This cup is placed in the sampling area and behind it are placed packets for the analyses desired. These packets (Fig. 16-7) have both a human readable test code and a machine readable test code (binary). Each packet is used to perform exactly one test on one specimen and is then discarded. The packets (or packs) have two special sections. Along the top is an area that can contain a chromatographic or ion-exchange column to do a preanalysis separation. Across the face of the pack are seven dimples containing different reagents in measured amounts (some of the dimples may be empty). These dimples are separated from the outside world by the thick packet wall, but from the interior by only a thin, easily ruptured seal. Twelve to fifteen reagent

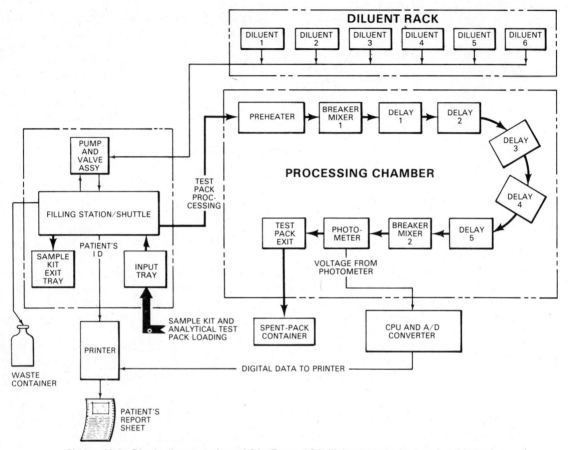

Figure 16-6 Block diagram of an ACA (From ACA III Instrument Instruction Manual. Copyright 1981. Courtesy of E.I. Du Pont de Nemours & Company. Reprinted with permission.)

packs can be placed after the specimen cup before the sample is exhausted.

When a specimen cup reaches the filling station, it is diverted to the left and remains in position until the next specimen cup arrives. The card attached to the specimen cup is photographed and later printed on a film with the results. As a reagent pack arrives, it is identified by an optical reader and sample is pipetted into the top of the pack by a syringe attached to a reversible stepping motor. After the specimen the proper diluent is added from one of the bulk cartons on top of the instrument. If no column is present, these liquids enter the body of

the pack. If a column is present, the sampling needle pipet pierces the end of the column and forces sample and diluent through the column. Most of the diluent and the sought for materials emerge from the other end of the column and enter the pack, while interfering substances remain behind in the column. The pack is then shoved into the thermostated interior of the instrument while the next pack is filled.

Once in the machine, the pack is attached to a chain and moved one step every 37 seconds. The first few steps cause the pack to be warmed to 37°C between two heated metal plates. The pack then

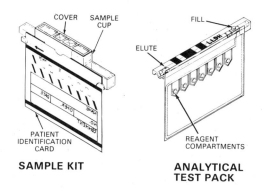

COVER SAMPLE CUP   FILL

ELUTE

PATIENT IDENTIFICATION CARD

REAGENT COMPARTMENTS

SAMPLE KIT   **ANALYTICAL TEST PACK**

Figure 16-7 Specimen cup (left) and reagent pack (right) for the ACA. (From ACA III Instrument Instruction Manual. Copyright 1981. Courtesy of E.I. Du Pont de Nemours & Company. Reprinted with permission.)

enters the first breaker–mixer. Here the first four dimples are broken, and the pack is shaken to ensure complete mixing. Some reagents are already liquids, while the rest are rapidly dissolving solids. Next, the pack waits through several delay steps while any blank or preliminary reaction occurs. The pack then enters the second breaker–mixer, and the remaining three dimples are broken. The pack is shaken, and the final reaction occurs. After another cycle, the pack is moved into the photometer press. The press shapes the malleable, transparent pack into a 1.00-cm cell, as well as creating a strain relief bubble for the extra solution. The filter wheel is rotated to the correct position for the pack being processed, and an absorbance measurement is made. The spent pack is then discarded.

The measured value is reduced to a concentration and printed on the output film with the image of the sample identification. A few methods require two packs, and the readings of the two must be subtracted to give the final result. The older ACAs had elementary computing circuits and could handle only 30 different methods at a time. The latest model has a microprocessor which allows 250 different chemistries. It takes about seven minutes for any one pack to pass through the instrument.

The microprocessor usage in the newer ACAs is characteristic of limited computer application. It is intended solely to aid in the operation of the instrument, not to build a patient data base. As such, it monitors various transducers in the instrument and apprises the operator of any malfunctions. It allows easy calibration, tallies the work activity, and prints units and normal ranges on the results. Its keyboard and information display are relatively simple, and it uses function keys to aid user access to the computer.

The advantages of the ACA for small laboratories are numerous. A wide variety of tests can be performed on a one-at-a-time basis. No time-consuming reagent preparation is needed, and there is no reagent waste. The machine can be operated by laboratory personnel after minimal training. Specimen and result pairing is easy. The disadvantages lie in the speed of the machine (100 results per hour) and the cost of the test packs. The latter can be large compared with a multichannel instrument for a large workload. Moreover, the chemical methods are limited to those which have been implemented with two-stage reagent addition at 37°C and relatively short reaction time.

The Ektachem 400 is a much newer instrument. It is based on the concept of coating slides with several layers of chemicals (Fig. 16-8). The top layer allows the drop of specimen added to spread out and soak through at a controlled rate. Below this is the chemical or enzyme layer where the reaction takes place. Below this is the dye or color layer where dye-coupled and two stage reactions form a measurable compound. Finally, there is the slide itself, which acts as the support for the whole system.

The processing is quite simple. The specimen is aspirated from the specimen cup, and a drop is placed on the slide by the sampler probe. The slide is incubated at 37°C while the reaction occurs, and the result is measured by reflective densitometry or potentiometry (in the case of the electrolytes). The color density is measured at the center of the sample spot. This position gives good precision even

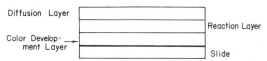

Diffusion Layer

Color Development Layer

Reaction Layer

Slide

Figure 16-8 Chemically coated slide used for the Ektachem 400.

when the sizes of the sample drops are not identical. This is true because the sample tends to spread before it reacts. Reflective densitometry requires the use of a calibration curve or mathematical transform because it is nonlinear. The potentiometric measurements are somewhat more complex and involve a pair of silver–silver chloride electrodes covered with ion selective membranes imprinted on the slide. A potential between the electrodes develops quickly, within several minutes, after one is exposed to sample and the other to reference solution, and this potential is measured and translated into concentration in the same manner as discussed in Chapter 12.

The Ektachem is another step in the process of reducing the amount of bulk chemicals that must be handled in the clinical laboratory. Slides can be stored under refrigeration in compact spaces for long periods and still be ready to use instantly. The widespread use of this methodology depends on tailoring the chemical reactions to stringent measurement conditions, a very difficult task. If it could be accomplished, however, the laboratory could respond immediately to almost any request from its large diversified slide inventory.

Section 16-3
CENTRIFUGAL ANALYZERS

Although the prepackaged analyzers offer diversity and short response time, they suffer from the bane of most single-channel analyzers—they are relatively slow. As such, they are not well suited to the bulk workload that larger laboratories face. If laboratories are to meet such large workloads, then they must either turn to the complexity and high cost of the multichannel test tube or continuous-flow analyzers, or they must use a technology that offers greater speed on a programmable single channel. It would also be desirable if such a faster new approach could do rate as well as the end point measurements which are characteristic of the prepackaged analyzers.

The breakthrough that produced this new instrumental approach was made by Norman Anderson in the late 1960s. He conceived the idea of initiating a reaction with the start of a centrifuge and moni-

toring the various tubes in the centrifuge during the whole reaction process. From these measurements the concentrations can be calculated.

A centrifugal analyzer station actually consists of two major components—the analyzer and a filling station. At the filling station the transfer disk is filled with samples and reagents prior to being placed in the analyzer. The transfer disk is therefore the reaction vessel and the piece of equipment that links the filling station and the analyzer. A diagram of the transfer disk is shown in Figure 16-9. It consists of paired specimen and reagent wells which are cut to facilitate both separate filling and subsequent mixing within the analyzer. The transfer disk is either reusable and made of Teflon or disposable and made of plastic. If the latter is the case, a chamber must be present at point X to act as the reaction vessel. Only the reusable disk will be discussed to avoid confusion. Transfer disks are available in various sizes ranging from 16 to 96 specimen positions. The number is characteristic of each particular instrument and differs among the products of the five companies currently marketing this technology.

At the filling station the transfer disk is placed inside a concentric ring which contains reagent cups. The station is programmed to place the specimen (1–50 μl) and a common reagent into the respective wells by means of a double pipet. If there are inadequate specimens for all the sample positions, a stop is placed on the specimen tray so that when it reaches the sampler, the pipetting of specimens will be terminated. The filling station may fill the rest of the positions with water or reagents if such is needed for balance or if pressure differences are used in the mixing process within the analyzer.

The limitation of the filling station is that it can prepare for only one type of analysis to be run with

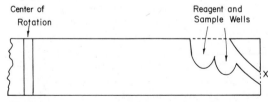

Figure 16-9 Cutaway view of one half of a transfer disk.

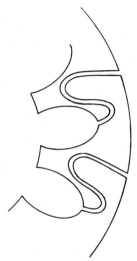

Figure 16-10 Cuvettes and siphons cut into the opaque plate of the rotor (top view).

one transfer disk. The centrifugal analyzer is, therefore, a classical batch analyzer. The filling station is rapidly convertible from one reagent to another, however, and can fill a new transfer disk in less than 10 minutes, depending on the size of the rotor. Since this is of the same time frame that the analyzer takes to process a transfer disk, a large number of different tests can be done in a short time. Moreover, since only those patients who require a certain test need have their cups present on the specimen tray when that test is loaded, this approach allows complete test selectivity.

Once the transfer disk is filled, it is moved to the analyzer. Here it is locked in place in the rotor. An optical sensor can determine which is the first cup from a mark on the rotor. The typical rotor consists of three parts (Fig. 16-10). Tube-shaped notches, one for each sample position, are cut into the middle section, which is both chemically inert and opaque to light. The end of each notch contains a small curved channel which leads to the edge of the rotor and is called the siphon. Above and below this central rotor disk are glass or quartz disks which form the sides of the individual cuvettes.

A cross-sectional view of the transfer disk and rotor is shown in Figure 16-11. As the rotor begins to spin, the reagent and sample are both pulled to-

ward the edge of the rotor. Due to the shape of their wells, they are able to scale the shorter outer walls and quickly move into the cuvette cut into the rotor. The transfer is quantitative since the transfer disks are of nonwetting material. The pressure of centrifugal force contributes to the mixing of the reagents. Unfortunately, such mixing may not be adequate in all cases. Two other approaches are used to facilitate mixing. The first is to rapidly increase and decrease the speed of the rotor within the first few seconds. This causes significant turbulence and effects good mixing. After the initial speed variation, the rotor is brought up to a constant speed that may be as high as 2,000 rpm. Another approach is to use the siphon to induce mixing. The top part of the rotor can be air locked from the rest of the instrument, and its pressure can be changed independently by a tube attached to the center of the assembly. If the pressure is reduced above the rotor, air will be pushed by the high outside pressure through the siphons, which are the only remaining air linkage. These air bubbles help mix the reactants. If some of the cuvettes are completely empty of solution, this approach will fail because the air lock will be broken.

The measurement of the reaction is effected by the optical arrangement shown in Figure 16-12A. Methods based on absorbance or turbidity are the most common. The light source must generate broad band radiation. The monochromators are filters mounted on a filter wheel which can be adjusted mechanically. Quartz must be used for the cuvette walls if UV measurements are made. A photomultiplier tube or photodiode completes the assembly. Wavelengths may range from 200 to 700 nm.

In Figure 16-12B, we see that the position of the

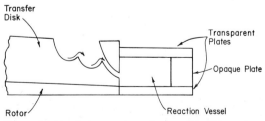

Figure 16-11 Cutaway view of a transfer disk and rotor (side view).

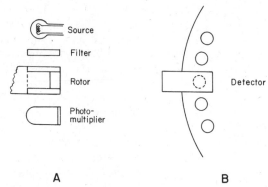

Source

Filter

Rotor

Photo-multiplier

Detector

A

B

Figure 16-12 The optical configuration of the detector (A) and its stationary position relative to the moving rotor (B).

detector is fixed, and that several cuvettes rotate under it continually. As they rotate, the detector sees a rapidly changing scene. Between cuvettes no radiation reaches the detector, giving the dark current or 0% T reading. In the first cuvette a reagent blank is always placed, and this is the 100% T reading. The specimen cuvettes will have readings between these two values. The movement of the rotor is used to trigger the sweep of an oscilloscope, which will record the observation of the photomultiplier tube (Fig. 16-13). This gives the technologist the ability to monitor the progress of the reaction.

The advantages of this type of measurement are tremendous. The analyzer does dual beam monitoring for all channels, as well as taking continual readings of the dark current. All this is accomplished with no moving parts in the optical assembly. This approach gives extremely stable readings that can be enhanced even more by taking multiple readings from each cuvette and averaging them.

In addition to being displayed on the oscilloscope, the readings from each cuvette are converted by an ADC and stored in the memory of the minicomputer controlling the instrument. As mentioned, readings are frequently averaged over successive passes and are corrected on the basis of the dark current. The method by which the data are analyzed is determined by the test being performed and by the parameters selected or specified by the operator. Such choices would include whether to do an endpoint or rate measurement, how many

points to collect per specimen, how many standards to run and their values, and whether to use a nonlinear calibration curve. Once the end-of-reaction conditions are met, the calculations are done, and the results are printed according to cuvette position on a printer.

The centrifugal analyzer finishes each run with a wash cycle. The pressure above the rotor is increased relative to that outside the rotor, which causes the reaction mixtures to exit through the siphon. Wash solution can then be added through the top and siphoned out by air pressure, and the cuvettes can be dried by letting air continue to bleed through the siphons for a short period. Such cleaning is necessary because the cuvettes are not replaceable, but are used again immediately with the next transfer disk.

The temperature is controlled by heating the interior of the instrument and the rotor. The temperature can be monitored by thermostats in the rotor. Slip rings are used to form the contacts on the rotor shaft to permit electrical connections by brushes instead of wires that would be twisted off, just as was done in the case of the generator shown in Figure 3-11.

Computer technology makes the centrifugal analyzer possible. Its operation very closely parallels the hypothetical instrument in Chapter 9. Programs and data are stored on floppy disks or cassette tapes. A keyboard and CRT allow communication with the analyzer, and a separate oscilloscope and printer present the data to the technologist. The data can be edited before transmission to a central computer for filing. The iden-

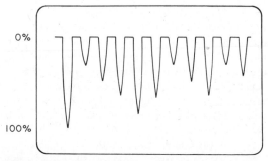

0%

100%

Figure 16-13 The oscilloscope tracing of a typical centrifugal analyzer.

tity of the specimens loaded at the filling station can be entered into the analyzer either before or after the run for pairing with the result. Unlike other modern analyzers, however, there is no way to carry this information in machine-readable form with the specimen through the process, a fact that may eventually prove a major limitation.

Some centrifugal analyzers have been expanded in computer capacity to the point where they are miniature laboratory information systems. Patient demographic information can be entered and stored with the test data, which are measured by the analyzer itself, or which may even be generated by outside sources and be manually entered through the keyboard. Another common capability permits the passing of patient demographic information and test requests to the analyzer from another computer in an operation called "down-loading."

Some effort is now being made to allow the performance of different analyses with one transfer disk. Clearly, the computing power to do this is present, but modifications must be made to the software and in the operation of the filling station to accomplish it. The primary motivation behind this enhancement is to enable the centrifugal analyzer to handle stats. This will reduce the duplication of having one set of instruments for stat and another for batch analyses.

The centrifugal analyzer has some clear advantages over the prepackaged analyzers in throughput and data storage capacity and over the multichannel test tube analyzers in simplicity. There are also disadvantages. Inability to carry along patient identity is one. Very rigid methodology with all reagents added at once is another. The shuffling of samples between sequential loadings of the transfer disks requires care to prevent specimen mix-up. The batch philosophy makes the handling of stats inconvenient on most analyzers.

Section 16-4
IN SITU ANALYZERS

Much of the complexity in discrete analyzers arises from the transport of the reaction vessels through the instrument after the specimen is inserted. In situ analyzers differ from other discrete analyzers in that all measurements for any given test occur in the same cuvette. Sample and reagents are added and allowed to react within the measurement cuvette. The readings are then made, and the cuvette is cleaned in preparation for the next specimen. In many ways the in situ analyzer is a cross between the specimen being isolated by its physical container, which is the measuring mode of the discrete analyzers, and the specimen being isolated by its time of passage through the same space, which is the characteristic of the continuous flow analyzers. The blood gas analyzers, whose measurement technology was discussed in Chapter 12, are in situ analyzers.

Most in situ implementations are basically similar to the Beckman Astra. The Astra aspirates specimen using two probes. This approach has two advantages: (1) the time for sample dispensing is halved, since the probes dispense samples separately, and (2) the conductivity between the metal probes in the sample can be used to detect the presence of sample. If no current flows, the cup is empty or absent from the specimen tray (which is a standard turntable). If three successive cups are empty, the instrument quits trying to sample. Various other approaches are available to detect empty or missing cups, some of which have already been alluded to, and others of which will be covered with continuous flow methods.

The exterior of the sample probe must be cleansed and freed from hanging drops that would alter the specimen volume added. The Astra, using two pistons (syringes) driven by reversible stepping motors, aspirates a slug of air, sample, and more air in each probe. It then moves the probe to a permanent wash cup where the outside of the probe is washed. Then the second air bubble and a small amount of sample are expelled to achieve a reproducible sample-filled probe, which is free of contamination. The wash solution is continually refreshed.

The two probes separate and dispense specimen independently into adjacent reaction cuvettes as the probe holder moves along a track on the front of the instrument. Sample is dispensed only for those tests that have been ordered through the keyboard console. Four or eight test channels are available, depending on the instrument model. After the dispensing step, the probes are emptied and washed at the washing station before another sampling is performed.

The reaction vessels are controlled by a trio of peristaltic pumps (Fig. 16-14), a mechanism that will be discussed further in Chapter 17. These pumps cause liquid to move in one direction only.

After the specimen is in the cuvette, reagents are added. While the Astra adds only one mixed reagent, one could add numerous reagents at the same time or at staggered times if the instrument were so designed. The volume of reagent added may exceed that which is required. The small ex-

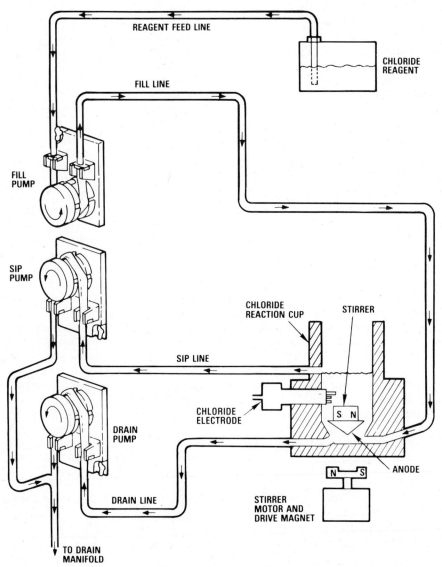

Figure 16-14 Reaction vessel of the chloride channel of an Astra. (Courtesy of Beckman Instruments, Inc., Fullerton, California.)

cess is removed by the second pump, which has an inlet at the correct height above the base of the cup. The contents are then mixed by a magnetic stirrer and the measurement made by electrode or photometrically. Afterward the cup is drained by the third pump, flushed with reagent by the first pump and drained by the third. Periodic flushing and drainage of the reaction vessels occur when the system is idle.

The primary limitation of the in situ analyzers is the speed with which the reaction chamber can be cycled between specimens. It is the bottleneck, and since the various tests are run in parallel, the slowest reaction to reach the measurement point will be the pace setter for the whole instrument. The speed of analysis can be doubled by making the reaction vessel with two chambers. The reaction can be started in the upper chamber and moved to the lower chamber, where the measurement is made. Meanwhile a second reaction can be started in the upper chamber. This method could be expanded to use more chambers, and, in effect, that is what the continuous flow methods discussed in the next chapter do. They use the tubing as a continuous series of chambers.

Instruments like the Astra have benefited from computer control. The selection of tests to be performed is possible by the push of a button and can be programmed into the machine as the run progresses. Stats can be inserted at any time and can be run for any or all of the tests available. Printed results include units and normal ranges.

The primary advantage offered by the in situ analyzers is the constancy of the analysis environment. All the measuring components are permanently fixed. For example, the light path, filter position, and cell walls are identical for each particular type of optical measurement. Using the same components reduces the number of the sources of random error and therefore increases the precision of the measurement. Although it is a time-consuming process, reagents can be added as needed, and each reaction can be carried out in the optimum manner because the lock-step movement from one station to another is not required.

The similarity in the operation of discrete analyzers to that of the manual procedures might suggest that these were the initial methods of laboratory automation. In fact, this is not the case. Test tube, prepackaged, and in situ analyzers are considered to be in the second generation of automated analyzers and centrifugal analyzers in the third. The initial automation in the clinical laboratory was accomplished with the continuous flow analyzer, to which we will turn our attention in Chapter 17.

REVIEW QUESTIONS

1. What are the two basic types of clinical analyzers?
2. What are the four classes of discrete analyzers?
3. What types of samples are used in clinical analyzers?
4. Describe the basic operation of a test tube analyzer.
5. Discuss the operation of a sampler.
6. What two philosophies can be used to power liquid flow in a sampler?
7. What three ways are used to add reagents?
8. Describe the use of pressurized reagent reservoirs.
9. Describe the operation of a circular path analyzer.
10. How are rate measurements done on a circular path analyzer?
11. Explain the operation of the perpendicular transport analyzer.
12. Describe the lock-step parallel analyzer.
13. Compare and contrast the circular, perpendicular, and lock-step transport philosophies.
14. What is the most common means of detection for test tube analyzers?
15. What are the three different cuvette-handling philosophies used in test tube analyzers?
16. Why are reusable cuvettes better than disposables?
17. What are the advantages and disadvantages of a test tube analyzer?
18. Describe the operation of the ACA.
19. How is patient identification attached to the results by an ACA?
20. How does the ACA accomplish protein separation?
21. How does the ACA identify the different test packs?

22. What functions are performed by the ACA microprocessor?
23. Why is two stage addition used by the ACA?
24. What are the advantages and disadvantages of the ACA?
25. Describe the basic principle of the Ektochem 400.
26. Why is sample size less critical on the Ektachem than most analyzers?
27. What two means of detection are used by the Ektachem?
28. What is the limiting factor in the use of the Ektachem?
29. Give the major advantage of the centrifugal analyzer over the prepackaged analyzer.
30. How does the filling station for a centrifugal analyzer work?
31. How would one set up the filling station to run different analyses on the same specimens? The same analyses on different specimens?
32. Describe the transfer disk. What is it made of?
33. Describe the construction of the rotor.
34. What are the three uses of the siphon in a centrifugal analyzer?
35. How do the sample and reagents mix in a centrifugal analyzer?
36. What two methods can be used to facilitate mixing in a centrifugal analyzer?
37. Sketch and label the optics of a centrifugal analyzer.
38. Sketch and label a reagent pack for an ACA.
39. Sketch and label a transfer disk in place on a rotor.
40. Sketch and label the output of a centrifugal analyzer.
41. What are the advantages and disadvantages of a centrifugal analyzer?
42. How are the cuvettes of a centrifugal analyzer cleaned?
43. How is temperature controlled in a centrifugal analyzer?
44. What peripherals does a centrifugal analyzer commonly have?
45. What is down-loading?
46. Why is it important to design centrifugal analyzers which can do more than one test simultaneously?
47. What is the distinguishing characteristic of an in situ analyzer?
48. How are empty specimen cups detected by the Astra?
49. Explain the sampling cycle of the Astra.
50. Describe the mixing and measuring cycles of the Astra.
51. What are the three peristaltic pumps used for on the Astra?
52. What is the principal limitation of an in situ analyzer?
53. What advantages do microprocessors provide to common analyzers?
54. What are the advantages and disadvantages in the in situ analyzer?

CHAPTER 17
CONTINUOUS FLOW ANALYSIS

In Chapter 16 we examined various implementations of discrete analysis. Such analysis is basically just the automation of the test tube methods for performing measurements. A totally different approach is available in the form of continuous flow analysis. This technique, pioneered by Leonard Skeggs in the 1950s and commercially developed by Technicon, has gone through several generations of refinement. It is subclassified into segmented flow analysis and flow injection analysis, depending on the presence or absence of air bubbles in the flowing stream. The former is more common in the clinical laboratory, but both techniques will be examined. Figure 17-1 shows the block diagram of a continuous flow analyzer.

Section 17-1
AUTOANALYZER

The AutoAnalyzer is the initial segmented flow analyzer developed for the clinical laboratory. In its single-channel form it has up to six components: sampler, pump, dialyzer, heated mixing coil, colorimeter, and recorder. We will study each of these in turn.

The sampler is similar to sampling devices encountered previously. The sampler holds a tray consisting of 40 cups that can vary in size from 0.5 to 8.7 ml. A probe is used to aspirate the sample into the apparatus. The timing of the sampler is controlled by a cam (Fig. 17-2). The shape and notching of the cam affect the number of samples aspirated in an hour and the amount of time spent aspirating each one. Between samples, the probe momentarily aspirates air while it is picked up and moved to the wash solution. It aspirates wash solu-

tion until it is again raised to aspirate air on its way to the next sample. The relative size of the cam's teeth to its troughs is the ratio of time that sample is aspirated to the time that the wash solution is aspirated. The cam makes 10 revolutions per hour. The tray is rotated one sample position whenever the probe is moved to the wash solution. A movable metal indicator is used to mark the last cup on the tray. The sampler detects this mechanically and stops sampling when it is reached.

The use of wash solution is essential to the operation of the AutoAnalyzer. While traveling through the small bore of the tubing, the solution is affected by severe velocity gradients. The forward motion of the solution molecules next to the tubing wall is zero, while that in the center is substantial. This velocity gradient causes lateral mixing of the current solution with the previous solution retained near the tubing walls (Fig. 17-3A). This has the same effect as diffusion and causes the sample to spread out into the solution ahead of it and especially behind it. Two adjacent samples will therefore mix to give a phenomenon called "carryover," and the concentration value obtained for the second sample will be inaccurate. The wash segment causes a trough between samples to reduce such distortion of the results and to clearly separate the sample peaks.

The air aspirated between the samples and washes also has an important purpose. Solution will wet the metal probe and, therefore, be carried from sample to wash and vice versa. This will contaminate both samples and wash and, consequently, give inaccurate results. By aspirating air momentarily between samples and washes, the liquid on the probe will be substantially reduced by the suction, and contamination will be much less of

299

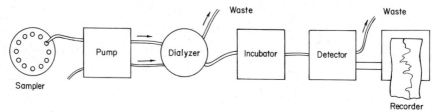

Figure 17-1 Block diagram of a simple continuous flow analyzer.

a problem. Even so, wash solution must be pumped continuously to prevent a gradual build-up of sample concentration.

Unfortunately, the previously mentioned pattern of sample, air, wash, air, sample is still not adequate to prevent substantial mixing from occurring over the long distances involved in AutoAnalyzer tubing. It is necessary to make much more extensive use of air bubbles to segment the solution stream. Figure 17-3C shows how the air bubble works. The air expands to form a seal between the walls of the tubing. Liquid that would otherwise be nearly stationary at the tubing wall is now forced to move at the same speed as that in the center of the channel. Longitudinal transport is therefore consistent throughout the cross section of the tubing, and lateral mixing is diminished. The air bubble greatly increases the integrity of sample segments, but it is not perfect. Solution still leaks around the bubble to some extent because the surface tension of water tries to keep an aqueous film around the bubble. Nonwetting tubing helps to reduce this problem, as do surfactants which reduce the surface tension of water.

To be effective, a dozen or more air bubbles must be inserted into each sample segment. This

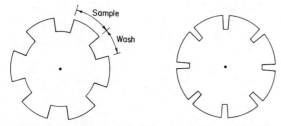

Figure 17-2 Cams control the frequency and length of sampling.

is accomplished by the second component of the AutoAnalyzer, namely the proportioning pump-manifold combination. The principle of the proportioning pump is shown in Figure 17-4. The rollers in the lower part of the figure are driven along by a chain at a constant rate. As they encounter the tubing, they squeeze it against a flat metal plate called a "platen." The pressure is enough to completely close the tubing by forcing the upper and lower walls together. The solution in front of the roller is forced forward by the pressure of the advancing roller, while the solution behind is pulled forward by the partial vacuum created as the roller advances from its previous position. The roller eventually lifts from the platen and allows the motion of the stream to be maintained by the subsequent rollers. Since the pressure on the solution varies cyclically as the rollers move, this mechanism is sometimes called a peristaltic pump. Its use with discrete analyzers was mentioned in the previous chapter.

The key to the success of the pumping action is the thickness of the walls of the tubing (Fig. 17-4B). Regardless of the inner diameter of the tubing, it can be closed completely if its wall thickness is sufficient for two layers of it to take up all the space between the platen and the pump rollers. One can then envision numerous pieces of tubing running through a single peristaltic pumping device and liquid in all of them being pushed along at the same linear velocity (cm/min) if their wall diameters are the same. This is, in fact, precisely what happens in an AutoAnalyzer. The line carrying the sample passes through the pump, but so do lines carrying the reagents and air. While the linear speed of all these fluids must be the same because it is established by the pump, the volume proportions may vary because they are determined by the cross-sec-

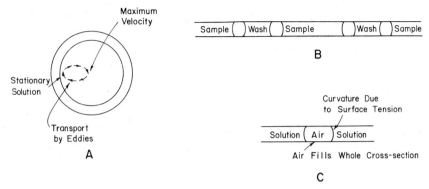

Figure 17-3 Part A shows how liquid diffuses to and from the center of the tubing. Part B illustrates how the fluids are sequenced by the sampler. Part C shows the air bubble as a cleaning agent.

tional area of the inside of the tubing (Fig. 17-4B). Ratios of 2:1, 3:2, 5:3, and so on are easy to obtain simply by selecting the appropriate size of tubing. This gives reasonable flexibility in the establishment of methods. It should be noted that unlike samples, reagents are stored in bottles placed near the analyzer and have tubing coming from them to the pump.

The device on which the tubing is held tightly in place across the platen is called the manifold. The manifold is composed of flat areas before and after the pump and a row of endblocks immediately in front of and behind the pump. Manifolds can be used for any procedure one chooses, but they are diagrammed to be used for specific methods. The diagrams indicate the size of the tubing and what each will carry. In addition, attachments are

present for the necessary coils and Y branches that may be needed for the procedure. These will be discussed shortly. The appropriate pieces of tubing are placed in grooves in the endblocks and tightened when in use (Fig. 17-5). This is possible because plastic tabs are attached near the ends of the pieces of tubing that are placed across the pump. These tabs are hooked over the end blocks. The colors of the tabs indicate the cross-sectional area of the tubing; therefore, the experienced operator can quickly locate the correct sizes of tubing.

The platen of the pump is hinged on the side. When not in use, the platen is raised off the rollers, and the tubing across the pump is loosened. This is done to reduce the stretching and malshaping of the pump tubing. Even so, the pieces of tubing deteriorate from the mechanical action and chemicals, and

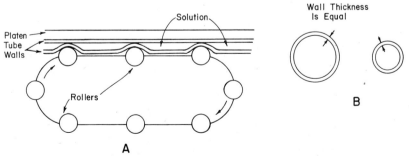

Figure 17-4 The rollers of the proportioning pump squeeze the tubing and force the liquid forward. The wall thickness of all tubing is the same.

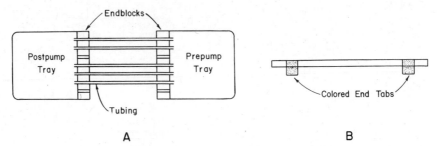

Figure 17-5 The manifold (A) and the pump tubing that fits across it (B).

they must be replaced periodically (i.e., some daily, some weekly, some monthly).

After the reagent, air, and sample streams emerge from the pump, they must be mixed. This is accomplished by Y branches, as shown in Figure 17-6. The air bubbles that will segment the samples are also inserted by a Y branch at this time from a line that is continuously aspirating air. To mix the reagents thoroughly, it is necessary to use a tight glass coil. As the liquids negotiate such a tortuous path, they are folded into each other to make a homogeneous solution, much as the ingredients in a cake batter are blended together with a spoon.

Whether the mixture can be measured at once depends on the nature of the chemical reaction for

the substance to be measured. Some chemical reactions will proceed rapidly to measurable product within a few seconds with no complications even at room temperature. Other reactions suffer from interferences or only proceed at a significant rate at elevated temperatures. For reactions of these latter types, two steps may be necessary before measurement: dialysis and incubation.

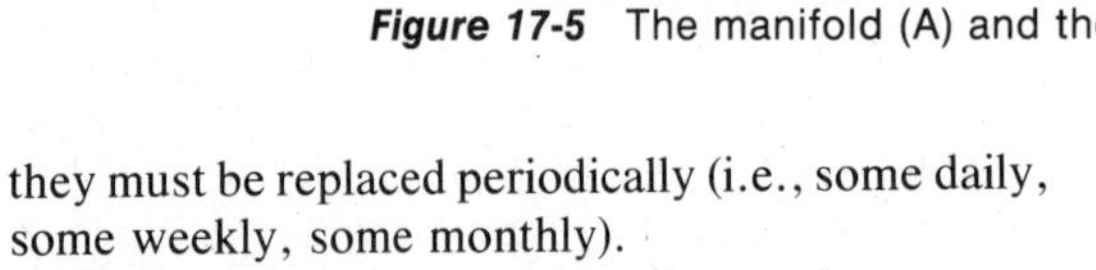

For many years a major hinderance to the development of automation for the clinical laboratory was the presence of protein in the blood serum. This protein interfered with the chemical methods available at the time. To employ the chemical procedures, the protein first had to be precipitated and separated from the samples. This time-consuming procedure was difficult to do through a mechanical means. The introduction of dialysis removed the protein problem.

Dialysis is performed through a semipermeable membrane in a temperature controlled bath. The dialyzer consists of two mirror-image metal plates with spiral channels cut in them (Fig. 17-7). When placed together, the channels form a circular passage through the apparatus. In use, this channel is

Figure 17-6 Y branches (A), metal adapter connecting tubing (B), and mixing coils (C) for AutoAnalyzer.

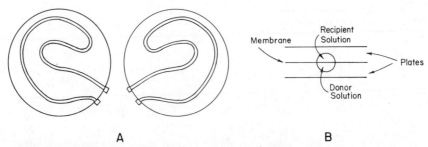

Figure 17-7 View of mirror image plates (A) and cross sections of plates with membrane between them (B).

bisected by a semipermeable membrane, such as cellophane, which is stretched between the plates. Liquid containing the sample moves along one side of this membrane in the channel in one plate, while a second solution is pumped at the same rate along the other side of the membrane. The first solution is called the donor solution, and the second is called the recipient solution.

As the solutions pass along the membrane, some solutes pass through the membrane while others do not. This process allows the separation of these two classes of solutes—the former consists of small ions and molecules and the latter consists of proteins and other large molecules.

The amount of any solute that moves from one solution to the other is 10–20% or less, depending on the nature of the solute, the membrane, and the length of the path within the dialyzer. Diffusion occurs in both directions, but is significant only from the donor solution to the recipient solution because the amount of solute which diffuses from a solution is proportional to the solute concentration within the solution. Normally, the two solutions flow in the same direction through the dialyzer. It is possible to get slightly better results if the solutions flow in the opposite direction (countercurrent) because at one end the spent donor solution is paired with the virgin recipient solution, while at the other end the undepleted donor solution is paired with the already laden recipient solution. In the normal case the best possible transfer of material is 50%, the point where diffusion is equal across the membrane. By use of the counter current approach nearly 100% transfer can occur if the contact pathway is long enough. In an AutoAnalyzer the dialysis does not deplete the donor stream to the extent that the countercurrent method is a substantial improvement. Since the countercurrent approach places more stress on the membrane, causing the upper and lower surfaces to be pulled in opposite directions, it is seldom used in routine clinical analysis. Even so, the periodic replacement of the membrane is essential to successful dialyzer operation.

To get the most reproducible results, it is necessary that the dialysis be carried out isothermally, because the rate of material transport across a membrane is temperature dependent. To accomplish this, the dialyzer is placed in a waterbath held at a constant temperature. To allow the donor and recipient solutions to reach the desired temperature, delay coils are frequently placed before the dialyzer plates within the waterbath.

After emerging from the dialyzer, the donor stream is normally discarded by pumping it to waste. The recipient stream is used for further processing. It is run to the measuring device, an incubator or back to the pump to be combined with an initiating chemical to start the main reaction. In short, dialysis is usually performed to isolate smaller molecules from larger ones that will interfere with the detection reaction. If the undialyzed molecules are of interest and must be separated from smaller molecules before analysis, then countercurrent dialysis in a very long channel is necessary to eliminate the bulk of the dialyzable material from the donor solution.

For those reactions that require a time delay or higher temperature to go to completion, the recipient stream, plus reagents, is run into a delay coil immersed in a heating bath. The coil may be the size of a mixing coil for some reactions and heated in a waterbath. For other reactions, coils 40–80 feet in length may be needed. Such coils are usually heated in mineral oil, which has a higher specific heat than water. This allows the use of temperatures up to 95°C.

By the time the sample reaches the detector, it may have spent 2–15 min within the analyzer. The most common detector is a simple photometer called a colorimeter. The schematic diagram is shown in Figure 17-8A. As the sample enters the colorimeter, the bubbles must be removed since they will cause light scattering within the measuring chamber. This is done by a part of the device called the debubbler. The sample then flows into the light path, where a lamp and dual detectors make the measurement as shown (Fig. 17-8B). The emerging solution is then sent to waste and the results to a recorder. The detector must also be thermostated for good results.

While the colorimeter is the most common detection device, two others are available: the flame photometer and the ion-selective electrode. Both can be used in continuous analysis for the alkali metals but have little application for other materials. These detectors are described in Chapters 14 and 12, respectively.

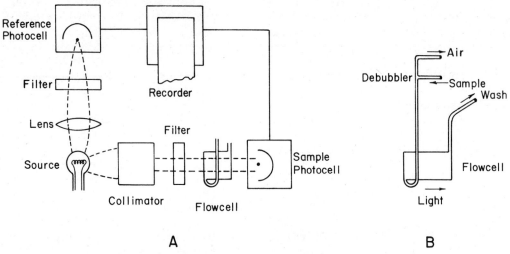

A   B

Figure 17-8 Block diagram of a colorimeter (A) and a debubbler (B).

The signals from the simple AutoAnalyzer are input into a servo-driven recorder (Fig. 17-9). The outputs of two detectors are used to drive the recorder to the position that represents the percentage of light transmitted. These values are then read and interpreted. In normal operation, the AutoAnalyzer runs standards, controls, and samples on each plate. The standards come first and are used to establish the response curve. The controls (known concentration solutions) and the samples (unknown concentration solutions) are then run interspersed. The measured control values are compared against the known values to determine if the instrument is functioning properly before the sample results are reported back to the physicians.

The advantage of a continuous flow device is that all standards, controls, and samples are handled in an identical fashion. As a result, human error in the reagent handling and reaction timing is eliminated. This approach, therefore, gives better reproducibility than manual or most discrete instrumental methods. The system is closed to outside contamination. On the other hand, care must be taken to ensure that all the equipment is in good working order and changeable parts are correctly installed. Standards and controls, which lack the solution matrix of serum samples, may not dialyze to the same degree and can cause erroneous sample readings. Positive sample identification is as much a problem as ever because the identity of the cups placed in the trays must be recorded by the technologist for later correlation with the results.

Section 17-2
MULTICHANNEL ANALYZERS

The simple AutoAnalyzer has proved a very useful tool in the laboratory. However, since many laboratory requests are for numerous tests, this single-test (single-channel) approach to analysis requires a large number of analyzers that soon overflow the available space. Minor modifications to the simple analyzer allow it to handle more than one test at the same time. Laboratories quickly discovered that running glucose and BUN together was cost effec-

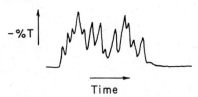

Figure 17-9 Typical recorder output from an AutoAnalyzer.

tive because these tests were frequently ordered at the same time. Similarly, the electrolytes (sodium, potassium, chloride, and carbon dioxide) form a commonly ordered set. By making such combinations, both technologist time and equipment cost could be saved.

The modifications to the single channel instrumentation for dual channel work are not technically difficult. The sample passes through the pump with the necessary reagents for all the tests. The sample is then split into two or more streams, and each stream is mixed with the proper reagents. From this point each sample fraction is processed separately; however, such items as double dialyzers, double coils, and dual-trace recorders are available to reduce the physical space requirements of multichannel analyzers. All these two-channel pieces of equipment are straightforward in design based on the principles previously presented. The dual trace recorder, for example, has two pens with different colors of ink (frequently red and green) driven by different servomotors.

While the above modifications to the basic analyzer meet some needs, it is impractical to expand the number of tests beyond three or four due to the inherent bulk of the apparatus and the volume of specimen needed. A miniaturization of the hardware is needed to accomplish further enhancements. Such enhancements led to the production of the SMA 12/30 and SMA 12/60 as well as the smaller SMA 6/30 and SMA 6/60. (SMA is an abbreviation of *s*equential *m*ultiple *a*nalyzer.) The number before the slash in all cases is the number of tests performed on the sample specimen. The number after the slash is the number of samples that can be analyzed in an hour. Recent models include the SMA II 18/90, SMA II 12/90 and SMA II/C. Rather than discuss each of the analyzers in detail, we will concentrate on the SMA 12/60 as representative of the class and investigate the principles that made the SMA philosophy possible.

Section **17-3**
SMA 12/60

The time savings of the multichannel continuous flow analyzers lies in the fact that there is only one sampler for many reactions. As a result only one sample must be prepared from each patient's specimen to obtain many results. Like the single-channel analyzers, the SMA 12/60s sampler accepts a tray of 40 cups. Unlike the AutoAnalyzer, however, only two standards are used—distilled water and a reference solution—because the operator does a two-point calibration on each channel. The rest of the cups on each plate can be filled with samples and controls. This sampler differs from that of the AutoAnalyzer in that it has a fixed rate (60 cups per hour) and a fixed sample/wash ratio (9:1). The 12/60 aspirates 1.8 ml of sample from each cup. In all other aspects it resembles the sampler of the AutoAnalyzer.

After leaving the sampler, the stream is split into 16 parts and diluted as necessary. There are four proportioning pumps, and each draws reagents for four of the reactions that the instrument performs. The reagents for the reactions are stored under the table, which is the frame of the analyzer, or in an adjacent refrigerator. These and air are drawn through each peristaltic pump and mixed appropriately with the specimen. To get uniform air bubbles into this complex network, an air bar is associated with each pump. This bar crimps the air line for two seconds out of every three, thereby allowing air to enter only one-third of the time. This regular pattern gives more reproducible results. Naturally the tubing through this area is of smaller bore than that which is common in the single-channel analyzer.

The extent of the miniaturization becomes clear when one views the analytical cartridges which rise in the back of the analyzer table. These assemblies contain the plumbing associated with the dialysis and incubation phases of the analyses. The area of the dialyzer plates has been reduced by 90% and the path length along the membrane reduced from several feet to 6 or 12 inches. The heating baths are replaced with heated metal block incubators. Cartridges contain only those instrument components necessary for a specific analysis. These cartridges are replaceable to allow each laboratory to decide which methods it will use for the various tests and in which order they will appear on the report.

After leaving the analytical cartridges, the samples flow into the colorimeters. These devices differ significantly from those of the AutoAnalyzer because they have a blank phototube and four sample

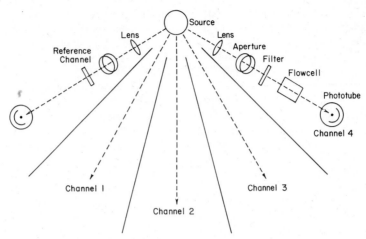

Figure 17-10 A colorimeter for an SMA family instrument.

phototubes to handle the four reaction streams generated by each pump. The block diagram of the assembly is shown in Figure 17-10. Each photocell operates independently of the rest, but receives radiation from the same light source. Each light path has a diaphragm, which allows control of the amount of the radiation reaching the detector. These are adjusted to give optimum detector response. The five resulting signals, one blank and four %T values, are forwarded to the calculating circuitry of the instrument.

The calculating circuitry is called the programmer. The programmer has numerous tasks to perform. It first dispatches the %T signal for each channel to the function monitor. This monitor is a storage oscilloscope that traces the %T of each channel. This continuous monitoring permits problems with the channel to be quickly seen. An example of the trace of one test on a specimen is shown in Figure 17-11. The area raised above the plateau is called the "top hat," and it is during the period when the programmer adds the top hat voltage to the signal that the test is being read for reporting. All 16 channels appear on the same screen and are displayed in two columns of eight each. Usually several cups are shown for each test. When the screen has filled with the tracing, the storage feature of the oscilloscope is cleared; the screen becomes blank and starts tracing again from the left of each test position. The names of the tests appear

along the left and right sides of the screen, and lines are etched on the screen to separate the tests.

The programmer also does a logarithmic conversion on the 16 input signals to change them from %T to absorbance (optical density). The continuous reference to 16 channels when the instrument reports only 12 results may appear erroneous, but it is not. The measurement of four compounds (albumin, total protein, total bilirubin, and LDH) is interfered with by the color and turbidity of the serum. That is, the serum absorbs or scatters too much light in the area of the spectrum used for these measurements. Since the color intensity of the serum is variable, it must be compensated for on a per sample basis. This means that a specimen blank must be used. To measure such a blank accurately, part of the sample must be treated identically to the part of the sample measured for a particular substance except for the presence of the color-developing chemical in the final reagent addition. This blank must be measured just as is the solution with the color reaction and the difference in the absorbance must be found. Each blank therefore requires its own channel. Since there are four tests needing blanks, four extra channels must be present, for a total of 16.

With the blanking done, the results can be reported. If a pen were used for each test, one would need many recorders or would be unable to read the one recording due to the confusion of ink lines.

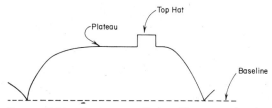

Figure 17-11 The trace on the oscilloscope of a single cup of a single channel on the SMA 12/60.

This problem is circumvented by having one pen record all the data on one chart. This apparently foolhardy enterprise is accomplished by reading each of the 12 test channels for an average of only 5 seconds. The programmer acts as a multiplexer for the tests. To permit such a scheme to work, numerous steps must be taken. First, the response curve must reach the steady-state plateau, as seen in Figure 17-11. This is accomplished by the 9:1 ratio of sample to wash solution used for the 12/60, as well as the miniaturized components of the flow system. Second, some of the values must peak before others. To effect the timing, delay coils called "phasing" coils are placed in the analytical cartridges, with the length of the coil being dependent on where in the sequence the test is to be read. Third, the programmer must correctly sequence through the reading and mark on the function monitor the interval of reading. This interval is nearer the end than the beginning of the plateau to reduce the effects of carryover from the previous sample. Finally, the chart paper must move relatively rapidly to spread the result to a readable degree and must be calibrated in the units of the different tests (Fig. 17-12). Without such calibration it would be impossible to distinguish one test from another or calculate its value. Even the normal range is indicated by a shaded area to aid in interpretation. This output is called the serum chemistry graph.

The most significant point concerning the SMA family is their ability to do many tests on one sample and to report the results in a concise fashion. Many of these analyzers have been interfaced with laboratory computers to correlate the data with other information. The instruments save labor and provide well-controlled results. Their disadvantages lie in the lack of flexibility and the mainte-

nance of the pumping system. All tests are always performed on each sample, even when only one is wanted. This is costly in reagents. The small bore tubing is susceptible to fibrin clots and decays from pumping and strong reagents. Tubing and dialyzer membranes must be replaced frequently. Getting the instrument into proper phasing is necessary whenever tubing is changed. The large number of small components, connections, and reagents means there are many possibilities for malfunction to impede smooth operation. Data handling is elementary compared with newer instruments but can be enhanced with add-on processors.

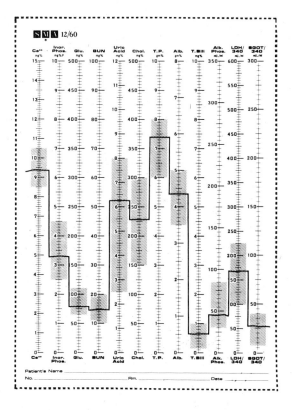

Figure 17-12 The SMA 12/60 recorder gives all the results on a single chart calibrated in units appropriate for each individual result. (Courtesy of Technicon Instruments Corporation, Tarrytown, New York, 10591. Technicon and SMA are registered trademarks of Technicon Instruments Corporation.)

Section 17-4
SMAC

To reduce the sample volume further, increase the speed, and monitor the numerous sources of error more closely, Technicon developed another generation of segmented flow analyzer called the *s*equential *m*ultiple *a*nalyzer with *c*omputer (SMAC). The overall scenario of operation of the SMAC is similar to that of the previously discussed segmented flow analyzers. The major enhancements will be discussed briefly.

The sampler has been redesigned to accommodate 19 racks each holding eight tubes (Fig. 17-13). This large capacity is necessary because the SMAC can sample 150 tubes per hour. A 40-cup tray would only last 16 minutes and would have to be changed hastily between sample aspirations. The eight-cup racks can be added and removed easily during the

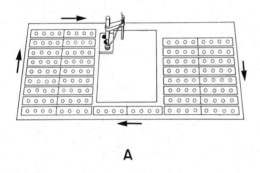

A

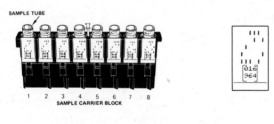

B   **C**

Figure 17-13 The SMAC sampler compartment (A), a sample rack (B), and a sample identification card (C). (Courtesy of Technicon Instruments Corporation, Tarrytown, New York, 10591. Technicon, TECHNICON IDEE and SMAC are registered trademarks of Technicon Instruments Corporation.)

sampling, except for the rack actually being sampled.

The sampler probe control is more complex than on previous analyzers. It is constructed with two refrigerated standard wells and a wash solution well. After finishing each sample the probe is moved from sample to wash while the next specimen is moved into position. The probe is then moved to that sample and raised twice from the sample. This creates four intersample air bubbles. At the same time that the sample is being aspirated, the sample identification is being read by an optical scanner from a card placed in front of the sample. The card has human readable and machine-readable information, the latter being in the 2-out-of-5 code discussed in Chapter 8. The sampler operates at a constant speed and is under the control of the SMAC computer. About 0.5–0.7 ml is sampled to perform 20 separate analyses.

The handling of the air bubbles is more involved on the SMAC compared with the previously discussed instruments. The four initial bubbles are removed by a debubbler and replaced by four larger bubbles. These ensure that some air will be sampled by each of the individual analytical cartridges. After appropriate dilution, the sample passes from the initial table area and proportioning pump up risers to the dual rows of analytical cartridges stacked horizontally up the left side of the instrument. A second set of proportioning pumps samples the specimen streams, draws the reagents, and adds more air bubbles to segment the individual samples. The flow of reagents is controlled by row valves that can be changed under manual or computer control to pump wash solution instead of reagents.

A detailed discussion of the sampling and cartridge plumbing would contribute little to the further understanding of the instrument. All the tubing has been reduced in size, and dialyzers are now as short as 1 inch. Detection is made in the UV and visible regions of the spectrum and by ion selective electrodes for sodium and potassium. The optical technology is radically different from that encountered in previous segmented flow analyzers.

The SMAC has only one visible and one UV radiation source. These are behind the chemical console that houses the analytical cartridges. A block diagram of their operation is shown in Figure 17-14.

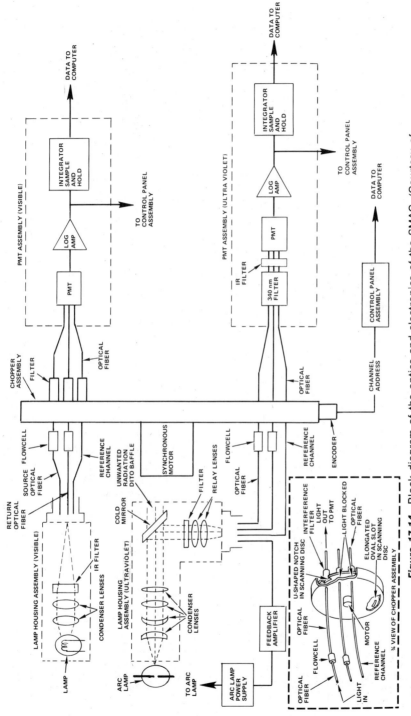

Figure 17-14 Block diagram of the optics and electronics of the SMAC. (Courtesy of Technicon Instruments Corporation, Tarrytown, New York, 10591. Technicon and SMAC are registered trademarks of Technicon Instruments Corporation.)

309

Each source is focused through appropriate filters onto the end of a bundle of optical fibers. The fibers carry the light by means of total internal reflection to the flow cells. The flow cells are frosted glass barrels 0.5–1.0 mm in diameter and 7–12 mm in length. The light beams pass through the flow cells, are picked up by other optical fibers, and are returned to the colorimeter assembly for analysis. Because the data will be acted on by a computer, it is not necessary to debubble the samples before measuring them in the flow cells, a major factor in allowing faster operation.

At the colorimeter the returning light beams are combined by a chopper for a single visible and single UV detector. The radiation is filtered and presented to a photomultiplier tube. Visible filters vary with the reaction, but all UV measurements are done at 340 nm. The channel addresses are encoded on the chopper to permit the computer to credit the measured radiation properly.

The outputs of the P–M tubes enter logarithmic amplifiers and are linearized in absorbance. These values are fed to both the control recorders and the computer, the latter through an integrator sample-and-hold circuit. Two control recorders permit the continuous monitoring of two channels in the manner of the single-channel AutoAnalyzer. These devices are typical stripchart recorders, but they use hot styluses on waxed paper instead of ink. These devices are used only when channels appear to have operational problems. The operator can select which two channels to monitor.

The computer reads each of the channels in a timed sequence. The values are saved and compared to detect drifts, noise, and sample peaks. The drift monitoring is done on the baseline points. If readings on a channel vary outside established tolerances, the operator is notified by a flashing channel light on the console and an audible signal. Noise is continually checked for and is called to the operator's attention if the readings fluctuate beyond a noise threshold. The shape of the response curve is also monitored. The sample curves should resemble the one in Figure 17-15. Each sample should take a specified time to reach its detector after aspiration. If the plateau fails to fall in the prescribed window, a "dwell time" error has occurred and the operator is notified.

The computer in the SMAC is responsible for much of the instrument's operation. It controls the sampler, the pumps, and the row valves. Its prime function, however, is the accumulation and analysis of data. It has a CRT and keyboard attached, which allows the operator to enter requests and demographic data for each specimen that is to be run. The computer will then compare the specimen numbers read by the sampler with the information entered through the keyboard so that it can print only the requested results for each patient. The computer is initially loaded by a cassette tape which permits different SMACs to perform different tests and Technicon to upgrade computer performance by simply issuing a new tape. Other peripherals are the panel lights used to indicate problems, a printer to report the results, and a computer interface to transfer data to another computer.

When reporting the results, the SMAC computer performs many tasks. It must pair the operator request with the identification read by the sampler. It must then time each channel to be certain to report the correct results on each patient. It must convert the absorbance into the correct number for printing based on the automatic standardization it does at the beginning of each run and at fixed intervals thereafter. In the process the interruptions caused by the air bubbles must be eliminated mathematically. It must also calculate the position of the value relative to the normal for range printing (Fig. 17-16) and prepare a separate format for the computer interface. Peculiarities in the results, such as

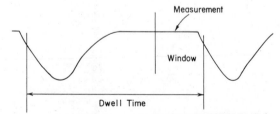

Figure 17-15 Shape of reaction curves on the SMAC. (Courtesy of Technicon Instruments Corporation, Tarrytown, New York, 10591. Technicon and SMAC are registered trademarks of Technicon Instruments Corporation.) Redrawn with permission.

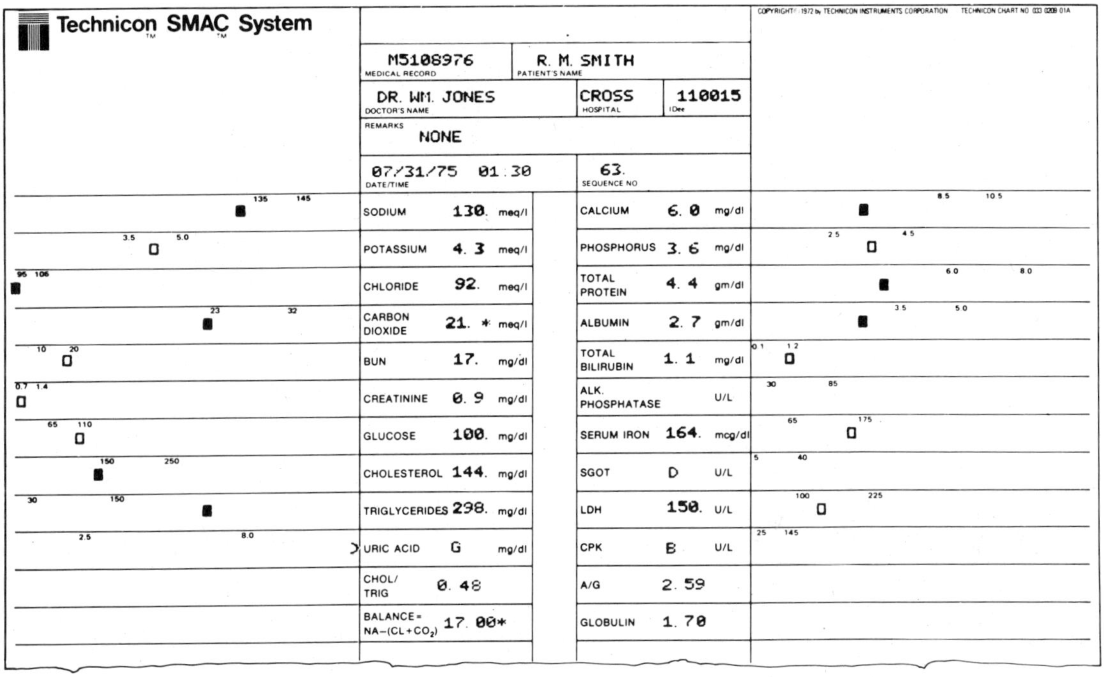

| Technicon SMAC System | | | | COPYRIGHT © 1972 by TECHNICON INSTRUMENTS CORPORATION   TECHNICON CHART NO 003 0208 01A |

| M5108976 | R. M. SMITH |
| MEDICAL RECORD | PATIENT'S NAME |

| DR. WM. JONES | CROSS | 110015 |
| DOCTOR'S NAME | HOSPITAL | IDee |

| REMARKS | NONE |

| 07/31/75   01.30 | 63. |
| DATE/TIME | SEQUENCE NO |

SODIUM	130. meq/l	CALCIUM	6. 0 mg/dl
POTASSIUM	4. 3 meq/l	PHOSPHORUS	3. 6 mg/dl
CHLORIDE	92. meq/l	TOTAL PROTEIN	4. 4 gm/dl
CARBON DIOXIDE	21. * meq/l	ALBUMIN	2. 7 gm/dl
BUN	17. mg/dl	TOTAL BILIRUBIN	1. 1 mg/dl
CREATININE	0. 9 mg/dl	ALK. PHOSPHATASE	U/L
GLUCOSE	100. mg/dl	SERUM IRON	164. mcg/dl
CHOLESTEROL	144. mg/dl	SGOT	D U/L
TRIGLYCERIDES	298. mg/dl	LDH	150. U/L
URIC ACID	G mg/dl	CPK	B U/L
CHOL/TRIG	0. 48	A/G	2. 59
BALANCE= NA−(CL+CO₂)	17. 00*	GLOBULIN	1. 70

Figure 17-16 SMAC output form. (Courtesy of Technicon Instruments Corporation, Tarrytown, New York, 10591. Technicon and SMAC are registered trademarks of Technicon Instruments Corporation.)

turbidity, short-term noise, or a value above the instrument range, must be detected and indicated with the result. Erroneous and nonrequested results must be suppressed from the final report. The memory must then be purged of the patient and specimen information to make room for new specimens.

The SMAC offers clear advantages over previous segmented flow analyzers when large numbers of specimens must be processed. Added speed, smaller sample volume, printed reports, and continuous monitoring for operational errors all contribute to greater capacity and more reliable results. On the other hand, fibrin clots are a more severe problem with the smaller tubing. Any one channel that develops problems will stop the sampler until that channel is disabled. The loss of human review of all the analytical curves bothers some operators. The speed of the instrument requires a well-trained crew to keep it running smoothly.

A later model of the SMAC, called the SMAC II, expands computer capabilities. It allows more methods of data analysis, especially quality control information, and can hold a larger number of patients for longer periods. It features two computers that are loaded from moving-head disk cartridges instead of cassette tape. The sampler has been improved to incorporate controls as well as standards and washes. The general operation of the instrument remains otherwise the same.

Section 17-5
FLOW INJECTION ANALYSIS

Segmented flow analysis (SFA) has proved useful and reliable, but it is susceptible to carryover and has no true baseline region on the graphs when run at high sample rates. Moreover, the volume of sample is significant for some analyses (e.g., in pediatrics) despite continued miniaturization. A means of

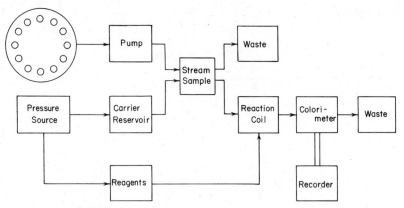

Figure 17-17 Block diagram of a flow injection analyzer.

addressing these problems is by flow injection analysis (FIA). In FIA a small sample, perhaps 10–20 μl, is rapidly inserted into a stream of carrier liquid. Necessary reagents are already present or are added after the sampling. The reaction occurs in the moving stream and is measured by the same techniques as SFA. One possible arrangement of equipment for FIA is shown in Figure 17-17. In the rest of this chapter we will compare the two methods of continuous analysis.

The SFA plumbing is of relatively small bore, but the FIA plumbing is even smaller, 1.0–3.0 mm in internal diameter. The rate of specimen flow is several times faster, but the small bore still allows the overall amount of sample to be smaller. The injection port and the detector must have very small dead volumes (areas where carrier liquid flow is not constricted) to prevent sample mixing. The equipment now being used for FIA comes primarily from high-performance liquid chromatography (HPLC) (see Chapter 22).

To get the process started, a carrier liquid, which may contain the necessary reagents if they are stable, is held under pressure. The liquid is allowed to exit through a filter and flowmeter into a small bore tube. This tube passes through an injection port. The sample may be injected in several ways. Sometimes injection is by hand from a syringe. This technique is discussed in Chapter 22. Another approach is by a slide valve such as the one shown in Figure 17-18. Pneumatics are used to slide the valve rapidly from position A to position B. This causes a precisely measured amount of sample to be transferred from the sample stream to the analysis stream.

The need for reproducibility in sample size is paramount. In FIA the reaction frequently does not reach completion. Therefore, reproducible sampling and mixing are essential to guarantee that each reaction will have gone precisely to the same percentage of completion and therefore, that the measured peaks will be proportional to the sample concentrations. Constant flow rate is similarly critical.

After the sample has been introduced, reagents are added if necessary, and the stream moves into a reaction coil. The slug of sample begins to diffuse into the surrounding reagent-laden stream and re-

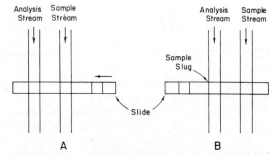

Figure 17-18 A slide valve allows a reproducible slug of sample to be inserted into the analysis stream.

agents enter the sample. The curved path aids the mixing. As the sample reacts, it begins to spread through the tubing longitudinally. Without air bubbles to reduce mixing, this would lead to disaster were it not for the speed of the flow. The sample is swept out of the coil and into the detector before significant carryover can occur. This sweep, however, prevents full reaction from occurring and is the reason that such care must be taken to make conditions identical for the analysis, thereby keeping the percentage of reaction constant. The colorimeter flow cell is 10 mm in length, but only 0.1 ml in volume.

The output peaks shown in Figure 17-19 are sharp and return to the baseline in a properly operating system. They can be output on a stripchart recorder or massaged by a microprocessor. The throughput can be over 100 specimens per hour, putting it in the same league with the SMAC for speed.

Flow injection analysis is a relatively new technique and is not yet in widespread use in the clinical laboratory. This could change rapidly as manufacturers perfect the sampler and develop methods that will be reproducible in a routine work environment. Multichannel capability will also be essential. Since the plumbing technology is well established, kits for build-it-yourself instruments might appear once more chemical methods have been adapted to the technology.

In studying continuous flow analysis, we have seen a contrast to the batch analyzers described in

Chapter 16. There is little doubt that flow analyzers give the capability to handle larger workloads more rapidly. It is also true, however, that flow analyzers are less flexible and must operate on an all-or-nothing basis, because the liquids must be continuously pumped. Each has its place in a diversified clinical laboratory.

We will not drop our flow system investigation with this chapter. Flow need not be continuous to be useful. In Chapter 18 we shall see how interrupted flow analyzers can be used to count cells.

REVIEW QUESTIONS

1. Name the two types of continuous flow analysis.
2. What are the six parts of an AutoAnalyzer?
3. Describe the AutoAnalyzer sampler.
4. What is the sequence in which the sampler functions to aspirate specimen?
5. What controls the sampler?
6. Why does carryover occur in continuous flow analysis?
7. How is carryover reduced on an AutoAnlyzer?
8. How does the air bubble reduce carryover?
9. Sketch and label the parts of a proportioning pump.
10. Describe the operation of a proportioning pump.
11. Why can a single peristaltic pump move different volumes of the reagents at the same time?
12. How are the reagent proportions determined?
13. What is the manifold? Describe its use.
14. What is the purpose of the end blocks?
15. Why does analyzer tubing deteriorate?
16. How are reagents mixed?
17. What is dialysis?
18. Sketch and label the parts of a dialyzer as used in an AutoAnalyzer.
19. Describe how the dialyzer works.
20. What is countercurrent dialysis?
21. What are the advantages of countercurrent dialysis? Disadvantages?
22. Why must dialysis be carried out isothermally?
23. What percent of the material in the donor solution ends up in the recipient solution?

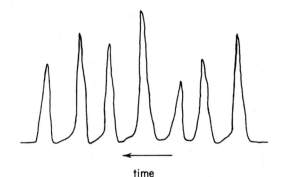

time

Figure 17-19 The shape of the FIA peaks is very sharp and returns to the baseline. Some tailing is observed.

24. How does one proceed if one wants the undialyzable molecules?
25. How is reaction incubation carried out?
26. What is a debubbler? Why is it necessary?
27. What three methods are used for detection in the AutoAnalyzer?
28. Sketch and label the parts of a colorimeter.
29. What are the functions of controls and standards in analytical measurements?
30. What are the advantages of continuous flow analysis? Disadvantages?
31. Describe the basic multichannel flow analyzer.
32. What is a dual-trace recorder?
33. Define the nomenclature of the SMA family.
34. What are the differences between the SMA 12/60 and AutoAnalyzer samples?
35. What is an air bar? Why is it needed?
36. What changes were made to miniaturize the instrumentation for the 12/60?
37. Sketch and label the parts of a colorimeter for a 12/60.
38. What are the functions performed by the programmer?
39. What is the "top hat"?
40. How are the results of the 12/60 returned to the technologist?
41. Why are 16 channels read, but only 12 reported?
42. What channels are blanked?
43. What is a phasing coil? Why are they used?
44. Describe the chart record of a 12/60.
45. Sketch the shape of the curve the colorimetry detector sees for each channel.
46. What are the advantages of the 12/60 class of instruments? The disadvantages?

47. Contrast the specimen trays on the AutoAnalyzer and the SMAC.
48. Describe the operation of the sampler probe on the SMAC.
49. Why is the bubble handling scheme more complex on the SMAC?
50. How does the SMAC measure sodium and potassium?
51. Describe how the SMAC makes optical measurements.
52. At what wavelength are UV measurements made on the SMAC? Visible measurements?
53. Why is debubbling unnecessary on the SMAC?
54. How can the operator of the SMAC monitor problem channels?
55. How does the SMAC respond to error conditions?
56. What are the functions performed by the SMAC computer?
57. How is programming loaded into the SMAC?
58. What are the advantages of the SMAC? The disadvantages?
59. What are some enhancements of the SMAC II?
60. How does flow injection analysis differ from segmented flow analysis?
61. Why must dead volumes be kept to a minimum?
62. From what methodology does most FIA equipment come?
63. List several ways to inject the specimen in FIA.
64. Why is constant flow rate so important in FIA?
65. What are the dimensions of the flowcell in an FIA detector?
66. What is currently limiting the widespread application of FIA in the clinical laboratory?

CHAPTER 18
CELL COUNTING

The measurements that have been made in the previous chapters have dealt with the molecules and ions in the blood. A significant percentage of the blood (approximately 40%) in healthy people is composed of cells rather than chemical-laden liquid. The number and types of these cells, as well as their shape, size, and oxygen-carrying ability, are important to the diagnosis and management of disease. In this chapter we will look at some ways that flow analysis technology has been applied to count these cells and also at the detectors that have been developed for cell counting.

Section 18-1
WHAT CELL COUNTERS COUNT

There are three major particle components in the blood. These are white cells, red cells, and platelets. The white cells are one of the body's major defenses against infection. The body normally contains between 5 and 10 thousand white cells per cubic millimeter of blood. These cells are relatively large (7–20 μm). A count of the total number of white cells present (the white cell count or WBC) is frequently made to determine the existence of infection. Various types of white cells exist, and the classification of white cells by type is called a differential count. Automated ways of doing these will be discussed in the next chapter.

The red cells are the body's oxygen transport system. A healthy person has between 4 and 6 million red cells per cubic millimeter of blood. The red cells are smaller than the white cells (only about $\frac{1}{5}$ their volume on average). The red blood cell count is frequently abbreviated as RBC.

Historically, red and white cells were counted in ruled chambers using a microscope. The chambers had major and minor divisions to facilitate the counting (Fig. 18-1). The cells were sometimes stained to make them easier to see, and a certain number of ruled areas were counted to give an estimation of concentration.

The effectiveness of red cells in transporting oxygen depends not only on their number but also on their size and the amount of hemoglobin they contain. These latter properties are measured by the hematocrit (Hct) and the hemoglobin (Hgb), respectively. The former is the percentage of the blood that is cellular rather than liquid, and the latter is the weight of hemoglobin per volume of blood. Historically, the hematocrit was determined by centrifuging a tube of blood and measuring what fraction of the tube was filled with the red cells that were compacted at the bottom. The hemoglobin was measured by rupturing the cell membrane of the red cells with a lysing agent to release the hemoglobin, reacting the hemoglobin with a cyanide reagent, and then placing the tube into a colorimeter to measure the light absorbed by the resulting cyanmethemoglobin solution.

The information represented in the previous three red cell measurements can also be represented by three other values. These are the mean cell volume (MCV), the mean cell hemoglobin (MCH), and the mean cell hemoglobin concentration (MCHC). The interrelationships between these values (called the red cell indices) and the primary red cell measurements are given by the following equations:

$$MCV = \frac{Hct}{RBC} \qquad (18\text{-}1)$$

$$MCH = \frac{Hgb}{RBC} \qquad (18\text{-}2)$$

$$MCHC = \frac{MCH}{MCV} = \frac{Hgb}{Hct} \qquad (18\text{-}3)$$

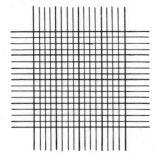

Figure 18-1   Drawing of a ruled slide used for cell counting.

Naturally, the correct units must be used for the equations to work. The pyramid in Figure 18-2 is a useful memory aid for the interrelationships.

Platelets are small cellular fragments that maintain the integrity of blood vessels by aggregating at sites of injury to form hemostatic plugs. Historically, they have been counted like red and white cells. Their normal concentration is 150 to 400 thousand per cubic millimeter.

Section **18-2**
BASIC COULTER COUNTER

The tedium of counting cells on ruled chambers led the Coulter brothers (Joseph and Wallace) to develop an automated approach for cell counting. They devised a reliable counting method and a uniform flow system, both essential to accurate counting. The elementary device is diagrammed in Figure 18-3.

The Coulter counter is based on the principle of conductivity. One electrode is placed inside a glass vessel and another one outside (Fig. 18-3A). There is a small hole or orifice (100 μm in diameter for

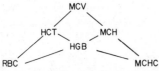

Figure 18-2   The product of two of the functions in a straight line will give the third.

RBC and WBC counts) in the glass vessel. Both the inner and outer vessels are filled with a salt solution, which conducts current between the two electrodes. The circuit obeys Ohm's law, and, therefore, the current is a function of both the voltage and resistance. During the counting the voltage is held constant, so the current is dependent only on the resistance. In Chapter 3 we found the resistance is the inverse of conductivity (σ).

$$I = E\sigma \qquad \textbf{(18-4)}$$

The conductivity is affected by the electrolyte, which remains constant, and the size of the orifice. As long as the orifice remains unblocked, the conductivity and current remain constant. If the orifice is partially blocked, the conductivity and current will decrease. If it is completely blocked, the current will cease. If cells could be moved through the orifice one at a time, the number of current spikes could be tallied and translated into the number of cells present per volume of solution.

There are several steps necessary to accomplish such cell counting. The blood must be diluted with large volumes of the electrolyte. This causes the solution conductivity to be effectively that of the electrolyte (which is constant), rather than that of the blood (which varies with each specimen). It also dilutes the blood so that only one cell will pass through the orifice at any one time. Multiple cells passing the orifice together will be recorded as one pulse, thereby erroneously lowering the total count. A method is needed to force the cells to flow through the orifice in a controlled fashion so the counts are proportional to the number of cells present in the outer vessel. Finally, the observed current spikes must be screened to determine if they are of the appropriate magnitude to be counted.

The initial step in all cell counting is blood collection. The blood for cell counting must be preserved by mixing it with anticoagulant to prevent clotting. EDTA has most commonly been used for this purpose. The second step involves the dilution of blood. In the single-channel Coulter counter, the blood is diluted 1 : 50,000 for red cell counting and 1 : 500 for white cell counting. Due to the large excess of red cells, the presence of white cells usually causes an insignificant error in the red cell count and is not corrected for when counting red cells.

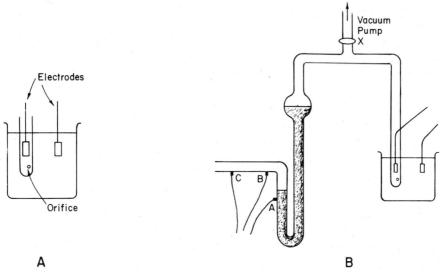

Figure 18-3 Part A shows the main features of the counting chamber, while Part B shows the important portions of the transport system of a Coulter counter.

The red cells are lysed before the white cells are counted and thus are no longer present to interfere with the tally. Platelets can be counted in the presence of white or red cells due to the large size difference between platelets and cells. Automated equipment is available for making the standard dilutions needed for the Coulter counter. Once the specimen is diluted and/or lysed, it is transferred to the outer vessel of the Coulter counter.

The flow of specimen must be uniform, and the volume of sample measured must always be the same. This is accomplished as shown in Fig. 18-3B. A vacuum pump is first applied to draw the mercury back into the reservoir. The specimen that is pulled up during this period while valve X is open is discarded because the flow rate is not uniform enough for accurate measurement. The vacuum pump is then disconnected by closing valve X. When this happens, the mercury begins to fall, and the measurement is made.

The mercury is always in contact with electrode A. As it falls from the reservoir, it contacts electrode B. This makes a circuit through the mercury, which is a conductive metal, and activates the counting procedure. As the mercury proceeds along the glass tube, it reaches electrode C. The current through the circuit between A and C dis-

ables the counting. The volume of mercury required to fill the capillary between electrodes B and C is 0.5 ml. Since the falling of the mercury pulls an equal amount of solution through the orifice, 0.5 ml of solution is counted. The reproducibility of this volume is about 0.1%. Since the viscosity of the sample is always the same, its flow rate through the orifice will be the same, and the counting time will be the same for all samples.

A diagram of the basic electrical elements in the reporting circuit is shown in Figure 18-4. A potential is set across the cell, which acts as a variable resistor. The current through the cell is measured as a voltage over the feedback resistor. This signal is fed into three parallel devices. The first is an oscilloscope, which displays the cells as a series of closely spaced lines of heights proportional to the cell size. The second is a comparator, which is offset from ground. If the voltage change is larger than the offset, the base of the transistor is grounded, causing the voltage at the collector to rise and then to fall as the signal stimulus vanishes. This toggles an UP counter, and the cell is counted. If both upper and lower limits are desired, a second comparator is needed. This approach is discussed more fully in Chapter 20. Finally, the amplifier output can be integrated. This circuitry only exists in more so-

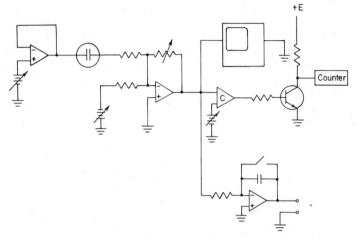

Figure 18-4 Simplified circuit of the detector electronics of a cell counter.

phisticated models and then only for the red cell channel, as will be described shortly.

The actual relationship between the cells counted and the cells present is shown in Figure 18-5. In specimens of higher concentration, the number of cells that pass through the orifice together is increased. This phenomenon is known as "coincidence passage." Since these extra cells are not counted, they must be corrected for by adding an amount to the count either electronically or manually. Because this amount is not a linear function of the concentration, automatic corrections were diffi-

cult before microprocessors were incorporated into the instruments.

The principles of measurement developed by the Coulters were incorporated into a series of single-channel instruments beginning with the Model A and proceeding through the ZBI. In the process the electronics and data representation improved greatly, but the basic sample manipulation plumbing remained essentially unchanged. All models could be used for counting red cells, white cells, and platelets, and some were able also to determine the MCV and Hct by use of a size integrator.

$$MCV = \frac{\Sigma \text{ size}}{RBC} \times \text{volume} \qquad \textbf{(18-5)}$$

$$Hct = MCV \times RBC \qquad \textbf{(18-6)}$$

The volume in Eq. 18-5 is based on a cell size calibration of the instrument.

Section **18-3**
MULTICHANNEL COULTER COUNTERS

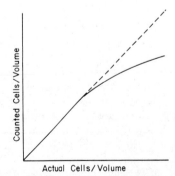

Figure 18-5 Relationship between the number of cells counted and the number of cells actually present.

The number of specimens processed by the Coulter counter would be small if tests for all the blood cell parameters were requested, as is now commonly

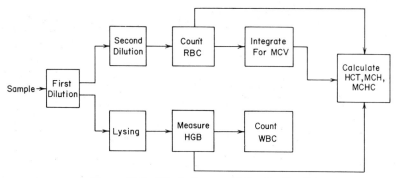

Figure 18-6 Block diagram of the Coulter S.

done. Coulter has incorporated all the common cell measurements into a single instrument. Unlike chemical automation previously discussed, however, each measurement is not made from a separate channel. Only two channels exist—one for red cells (and eventually platelets) and one for white cells and hemoglobin. The family has so far included the Coulter S, S Sr., S Plus, and S Plus II.

The block diagram of the operation of the Coulter S is shown in Figure 18-6. Samples are presented to the instrument one at a time, as there is no specimen rack as part of the sampler. The sample of whole blood is aspirated and diluted 1 : 224 with electrolyte. A separate pipette is available to sample prediluted blood and bypass the first dilution stage. On newer models these pipettes are backflushed with wash solution to prevent carryover. For the counting of red cells the diluted mixture is sampled, and this sample is rediluted to a final dilution of 1 : 50,000. Lysing agent is added to the remaining solution to bring the dilution to 1 : 250. The lysing agent destroys the red cell membranes, releases the hemoglobin, and reacts with it to form a stable colored compound (cyanmethemoglobin) that can be read photometrically. From this point the two samples are processed in a separate, but parallel manner.

The red cell solution passes into a bath (chamber), which contains an electrode and three orifices. The solution is then pulled through each of the orifices into separate aperture tubes, each of which contains an electrode. The potential of all these electrodes in the apertures is the same. As a result, each inner electrode forms a current-carry-

ing electrode pair with the external electrode in the outer bath, which is of a different potential, but not with other inner electrodes, which are of the same potential. The outer electrode creates effective isolation between these circuits. Each circuit is just the simple Coulter circuit, and the number of cells passing through each orifice can be determined by recording the current changes in the corresponding circuit. This gives a triplicate determination of the cell count for each sample. Since nonreproducibility is much more likely to occur in the counting step than the dilution step, this procedure reduces the error in the final measurement. The processing of the output signals will be discussed presently.

The white cell solution is handled identically to the red cell solution to give three replicates of the WBC. In addition, light is passed through the white cell bath to measure photometrically the Hgb released from the lysed red cells. The light originates in a tungsten source, is made monochromatic by a prism, and is measured by a photocell.

The Coulter S family moves solutions by air pressure and partial vacuums generated by a pneumatic power supply unit. The steps are timed by a cam assembly to assure thorough dilutions and complete lysing. The solutions are pumped to waste after measurement. One complete measurement takes 40 seconds.

The data handling differs within the Coulter S family, with the model S Plus using a microprocessor to gain substantially more computing power. In the basic mode S the signals proceed to preamplifier cards, which are large circuit boards. Each amplifier board has one red cell and one white cell channel. These amplifiers measure the voltage difference across the counting orifices (Fig. 18-4). Thresholds eliminate the noise, and the counts are tallied as explained previously. The outputs from the amplifiers are used to drive oscilloscope displays of the cell counting, as was done for the simple Coulter counter. A separate amplifier handles the transmittance data from the hemoglobin measurement. The readings are converted to absorbance and the Hgb is calculated.

The data from the three red cell channels are fed into a voting card, which compares the amplifier values and determines whether the three values are close enough together to be reported. If one count is divergent from the rest, it is regarded as invalid. If one of the values is voted out (invalidated) or absent, the voting card makes its calculation based on the other two. The data from the white cell amplifiers are treated the same way by a second voting card. The RBC and WBC values are then ready to report.

The outputs from two of the red cell cards are fed into an MCV card where they are integrated (Fig. 18-4). This gives the total of the red cell sizes. The two channels are adjusted during calibration so the readings are the same. Using Eq. 18-5, the MCV is calculated from this value, the RBC value, and the effective blood volume before dilution. The MCV value is passed with the Hgb, RBC, and WBC values to the computer card.

The computer card calculates the remaining three values (HCT, MCH, and MCHC) using the equations previously introduced. These values are then converted to three-character BCD representation and sent to the dual printer. No decimal point is transmitted; thus it is necessary to put forms into the printer that already contain the test names, decimal points, and units printed on them, as the printer produces only the three digits sent. The seven test values plus a sequence number and the date, which can be dialed into the machine, are transmitted. The same information can be sent simultaneously through an interface to a laboratory computer by parallel transmission (12 lines—1 per bit). This interface uses binary coding on six other lines to identify the different results (WBC, Hct, etc.) and to indicate when the result lines are to be read.

The Model S Plus does much of the previous calculation using its microprocessor instead of a special purpose circuit board. In addition, it uses a double threshold on the red cell readings to discern the platelets from the red cells. This allows the platelets to be counted and reported with the other cell parameters.

In most ways the Model S Plus is the same as other members of the Model S family. The microprocessor does detect a greater number of distinguishable error conditions and can display the contents of internal registers in hexadecimal. An auxiliary plotter can be attached to the counter for graphic outputs of platelet size distribution. The laboratory computer interface is somewhat more sophisticated.

The most important aspects of the Coulter instrument family are the use of conductivity to count cells, the use of falling mercury to obtain a uniform specimen flow, and the concept of measuring a property other than the one desired to obtain by calculation the value of a property that is more difficult to measure. The Coulter counter, as well as some other cell counters, use interrupted flow analysis. They share with the continuous flow apparatuses the concept that all samples flow through the same plumbing, but they interrupt that flow periodically to allow mixing or to change the driving force of the stream.

Section 18-4
ELT-8

The ELT-8 (Electronic Laser Technology) by Ortho Instruments uses somewhat different methodology than the Coulter counter. Like the Coulter counter, it has no sampler tray. Once aspirated, the blood is split into two streams (Fig. 18-7). The white cell stream is diluted 1 : 19 with Isolac (a diluent) and lysed. The stream is sent through a mixing chamber and held in the plumbing long enough for lysing to be completed before counting. The pumping force is created by a series of pistons that draw up the solution and then expel it. The direction of flow and timing are controlled by a number of valves activated by a set of cams.

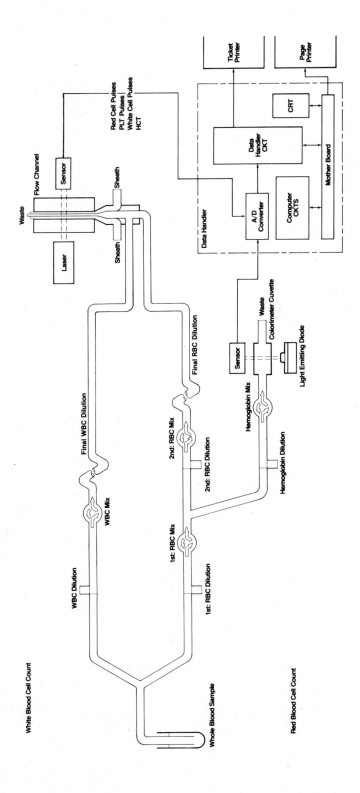

Figure 18-7 Flow diagram of the ELT-8. (All rights are reserved by Ortho Diagnostic Systems, Inc.)

The red cell solution is diluted 1 : 126 by Isolac and split. Part of it is mixed with color reagent (Cyanac), and the hemoglobin is then measured photometrically. The fraction is then pumped to waste. The rest of the sample is diluted further to 1 : 440 in preparation for counting. All additions are accomplished by means of mixing chambers. These chambers use small mechanical stirrers to achieve mixing.

The detector of the ELT-8 is diagrammed in Figure 18-8. The particle-laden stream is forced through a capillary and emerges to find itself surrounded by a fast moving stream of Isolac (Fig. 18-8). Due to the rapid flow and the symmetry of the apparatus, mixing does not initially occur. The sheathing stream is constricted to flow through a tiny neck, which compresses the sample stream within the sheathing stream to only 20 μm. This is known as hydrodynamic focusing. The radiation source is a helium–neon laser, which is focused through the center of the sample and then strikes a blackened shield that protects the photomultiplier from the intense source radiation. As cells pass through this beam, the laser light is scattered in all directions. The light scattered at only a small angle in the forward direction is gathered by the objective lens and transmitted to the light sensor. This forward scattered radiation gives enough information for accurate counting.

The observation of any low-angle forward scattered radiation indicates the presence of a particle in the counting path, since the unreflected laser beam is not seen. The intensity of the scattered light is indicative of the particle volume. The length of time the particle scatters light is proportional to its diameter. Finally, the narrow path size guarantees only one cell-sized particle can be present at any time. Based on this information, the instrument's computer can determine the particle count.

The red cell solution is counted first to give both red cell and platelet counts, based on the relative diameters and refractive indices. The hematocrit is calculated by integrating the volume of the red cells and dividing by the volume of the original sample.

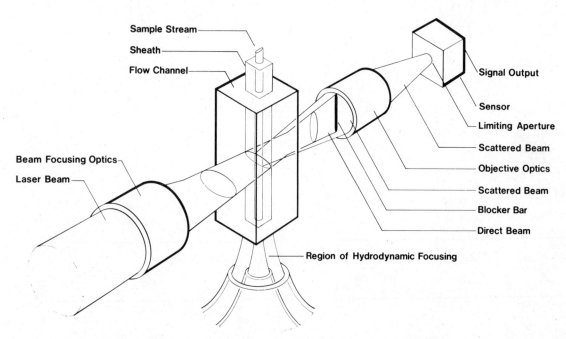

Figure 18-8 Diagram of the ELT-8 counting chamber. (All rights are reserved by Ortho Diagnostic Systems, Inc.)

A valve allows the same detector to then switch to counting the white cell stream. The remaining red cell functions (MCH, MCV, and MCHC) are computed from the red cell measurements and the Hgb using the equations previously introduced. The electronic hardware, including amplifiers, ADCs, CRT, printer, and computer, is similar to that previously discussed in detail.

Section 18-5
HEMALOG AND TECHNICON H6000

The basic principles of the AutoAnalyzer can also be applied to cell counting. The Hemalog and the newer Technicon H6000 are examples of such implementation. The Hemalog uses a circular sample tray containing whole blood samples. Unlike the AutoAnalyzer, however, the sample must be mixed mechanically by a stirrer attached to the sampler arm. Upon aspiration the sample must be strained for debris. These requirements complicate the probe design because stirring and backflush cycles must be added to guarantee representative sampling and to prevent the clogging of the probe.

The sample is moved by means of carefully regulated air pressure rather than peristaltic pumping. Mixing is effected by passing the sample through constricted glass tubing, thereby eliminating the mixing coils of the AutoAnalyzer. Both of these features are used to minimize mechanical damage and changes to the particle-laden stream. The sample is split into separate parts to count red cells, to count white cells and platelets, and to measure hemoglobin and hematocrit. The cell counting is done using forward light scattering, a technique discussed in the previous section, and the hemoglobin is measured photometrically. The hematocrit is measured in the historical way—by centrifuging. The blood is forced into a tube shaped like a J. This is spun at 20,000 rpm, and the height of the cells is read optically. The tube is cleansed by the pressure of an excess of the next sample pushing the current one out. The MCH, MCV, and MCHC are calculated from these measurements.

The Hemalog also performs several other measurements not common to this class of instruments. It measures the conductivity of the whole blood, which is a cell volume measurement and should compare favorably with the hematocrit under normal conditions. It can also measure the prothrombin time (PT) and partial thromboplastin time (PTT) if a tube of citrated whole blood on the same patient is placed next to the blood with EDTA on the sample carousel. A second sample probe aspirates these samples from the inner circle of the tray, and the PT and PTT are done from this separate sample stream.

The Technicon H6000 measures the standard eight blood functions and does the cell differential from the same specimen. The samples are aspirated from a specimen tray which contains machine-readable cards with 2-out-of-5 code in front of the sample for specimen identification. The plumbing is similar to the other Technicon instruments. The specimen is divided into two streams to count red cells and white cells. The counting techniques are relatively similar to the ELT-8 in that the counting is done while sheathing the stream and using forward light scattering. The hematocrit and hemoglobin are measured in a similar fashion to the Coulter counter, and the rest of the functions are calculated. The platelets are measured from the red cell stream by size differentiation. The cell differential technology of this instrument will be discussed in the next chapter.

The interesting aspects of cell counting are the different means that manufacturers devise to process the sample, count the cells, and make the other measurements. Since more results must be reported than will actually be read, it gives the instrument designers some latitude in deciding what to measure as well as how to measure it. Because WBC, RBC, Hct, Hgb, MCV, MCH, MCHC, and platelet are used universally, competing instruments must be able to report all of them. This has led to many similarities, within the bounds of patent law, between all cell counters, including a number not mentioned here.

Up to this point, all instruments discussed in this book have been relatively unintelligent; that is, they have made calculations based on equations that any laboratory worker could easily explain. The exceptions have been the peak detection algorithms used by some chemical analyzers and coincidence counting. In the next chapter we will look at instruments that perform much more complex analysis upon readings which they make.

REVIEW QUESTIONS

1. What percentage of the blood is composed of cells?
2. What are the three major particle components of blood?
3. What is the size of an average red cell? An average white cell?
4. What is the concentration of red cells in human blood? Of white cells?
5. How were cells counted historically?
6. What are the seven major cell functions called? What are their abbreviations?
7. What is the hematocrit?
8. How was the hematocrit measured historically?
9. What is hemoglobin? How is it measured?
10. What are the relationships between the various red cell functions?
11. Upon what principle is the Coulter counter based?
12. Sketch and label the parts of a basic Coulter counter.
13. How large is the orifice for red cell counting?
14. Explain how cells are counted in a Coulter counter.
15. Give two reasons for the large dilution of blood before doing cell counting.
16. Why is blood diluted more for red cell counting than white cell counting?
17. How does one remove the red cells when counting white cells? The white cells when counting red cells?
18. What method does the Coulter counter use to obtain uniform flow?
19. Describe the cell counting process on a Coulter counter.
20. What sample volume does a Coulter counter count?
21. Describe the major parts of the electronics needed for operating a simple Coulter counter.
22. Graph the relationship between the cells present and the cells counted.
23. What is the name of the phenomenon whereby multiple cells pass the orifice at the same time?
24. What cell functions are counted by the Coulter Model S?
25. Describe the sample dilution process on the Coulter S.
26. How are red and white cells physically counted on the Coulter S?
27. How are the other cell functions (aside from RBC and WBC) determined?
28. Trace the handling of the data for each measured cell function in the Coulter S.
29. Describe the ''voting'' process on the Coulter S.
30. How is the MCV computed on the Coulter S?
31. Describe the printed output of the Coulter S.
32. How does the Coulter S Plus measure platelets?
33. What are the major innovations introduced by the Coulter counters?
34. How is the timing controlled on the ELT-8?
35. Describe the solution movement in the ELT-8.
36. How does the ELT-8 mix samples?
37. Describe hydrodynamic focusing.
38. What is forward light scattering?
39. Describe how forward light scattering can be used to measure cell size.
40. Why can all cell counting be done by the same detector in the ELT-8?
41. Describe the sampler on the Hemalog.
42. Contrast the solution movement and mixing of the Hemalog and the AutoAnalyzer.
43. How does the Hemalog measure the hematocrit?
44. Why can the Hemalog measure the PT and PTT as well as the blood cell function?
45. Describe the general operation of the H6000.

CHAPTER 19
INFORMATIONAL TECHNIQUES

In previous chapters the informational content of numbers was alluded to, but the concept was never discussed. The values read from meters, for example, have relative error. Wavelengths on spectrophotometers are selected to get the maximum signal-to-noise ratio. Overlapping peaks cause problems in making accurate measurements. All these are examples of informational problems already encountered, and more will be introduced. The use of informational techniques is the backbone of some laboratory instruments and affects many others in a general way. These informational techniques and concepts will be discussed in this chapter.

Section 19-1
INFORMATIONAL CONTENT

You were introduced to significant figures long ago, and the rules regarding them have been used in this book in the problems we have solved. You know that a number with four significant figures has more "significance" and is known with more "precision" than a number with two significant figures. As you should remember, however, the number of significant figures is not a totally accurate gauge of the precision to which a number is known. For example, 99 has two significant figures and 101 has three significant figures, but the precision to which each is known is approximately the same, 1 part in 100. In the same way, 101 and 999 both have three significant figures, but 999 is known to be an order of magnitude more significant than 101.

The actual precision is always a ratio of the amount of error to the size of the answer. With error represented in this manner, accurate esti-

mates of the precision of the result can be obtained through mathematical manipulations. Unfortunately, these calculations tend to be rather cumbersome. As a consequence, the precision is commonly represented as a number of significant figures, a number that must be modified each time a mathematical manipulation is performed. The resulting estimate of precision as given by the number of significant figures is, therefore, only approximate.

For laboratory measurements the situation is, in reality, much worse than that expressed above. Much of the significance of the number is, in fact, "hollow significance." For example, if one loses 0.1% of one's weekly food budget, one has lost perhaps 3 cents out of 30 dollars. One can afford to write that off without a thought. If the government loses 0.1% of its money on a public works project, that could be one million dollars of a one billion dollar budget. One million dollars should never be lightly written off, because it might be used in this case to corrupt numerous public officials. One expects accounting "down to the penny" no matter how large the number before the decimal point.

In human serum a sodium value of 141 mmol/l is quite normal, but a value of 41 is impossible. In fact, values less than 100 or greater than 180 are virtually incompatible with life. The first 100 positions on the sodium number line are, therefore, meaningless, since they are never used to convey any medically valuable data. One can think of this as the first 100 units of every sodium value being exactly known (0% error) and the total error being in the rest of the value. For example, if the precision is 140 ± 2, the error is not 2 parts in 140, but 2 parts in 40 $(140 - 100)$. This is an error of $\pm 5\%$. This representation is not completely accurate either because errors at the lower end of the range are a much larger percentage of the result than errors of the same magnitude at the upper end of the range. An error of ± 2 is $\pm 20\%$ at 110 but $\pm 4\%$ at 150. Therefore, it is necessary to redraft our previous statements so that we compute the error as the fraction of the range (100–180) represented by the error. In this case, ± 2 is 2.5% of the range (2/80). The functional error of ± 2 in 140 for sodium is almost twice as great as it would seem to be.

The precision of the method or instrument is an important factor in clinical laboratory analysis. Physicians order laboratory tests to differentiate sickness from health and to follow the progress of treatment. In order for these observations to be made, the precision of the instrument must be adequately high. For example, assume patients with sodium values of 137 to 145 mmol/l are normal, while those with sodium values over 150 are significantly abnormal. If the precision of measurement is ± 2, patients will always be correctly classified, even when they fall in the gap. A value of 147 could be 145 or 149, but it could not be 150, so that the patient is borderline abnormal. If, however, the precision of measurement is ± 5, then the same 147 could be 142 or 152. The patient could be normal, borderline abnormal, or significantly abnormal. An instrument with this type of precision is, therefore, worthless for making this determination, although its absolute precision of 5 parts in 147 (3%) is not that bad. Information is only valuable if it allows medically useful decisions to be made. In instrument design or selection, knowing the medically useful precision is essential.

The opposite situation occurs when the measurement is too precise. The human body has many complex equilibria. It is designed to keep a stable internal environment. This environment is constantly being challenged by outside elements such as air temperature, radiated energy, ingested food, physical activity, or even medication. These challenges cause minor alterations in the equilibria and changes in the chemical values of the body. While these changes are usually slight, a very sensitive instrument can measure them. If such measurements were reported, they might cause undue alarm among the medical staff. For example, even if we could measure sodium to ± 0.2 mmol/l instead

of ± 2 mmol/l, reporting it that way would be unacceptable because a body's sodium value can vary 0.2 mmol/l in an hour under normal conditions. Reporting measurements with more precision may, therefore, not always be desirable.

The precision of useful information may vary with its magnitude. Glucose can be almost 0 mg/dl in Reyes's syndrome and reach over 1000 mg/dl in uncontrolled diabetes. Glucose values between 0 and 20 must be very precisely measured (± 2), since recovery will depend on how low on nutrients the brain has been and for how long. Between 800 and 1000, ± 20 will be more than adequate to identify the magnitude of the problem. In cases where there is a fixed bottom to the scale and a very high top, percentage errors based on the result value rather than the range make more sense. In such cases the normals are usually relatively low with abnormals predominantly, perhaps exclusively, above the normal range.

The normal range itself is an arbitrary contrivance to evaluate laboratory data. Presumably 2.5% of the healthy population is above and 2.5% below this range. In other words, 95% of the healthy people are within the normal range. People with values outside this range can be healthy, but one finds few that are. Sick people can be in the normal range and frequently are, depending on the test and the disease. A diabetic might have a normal sodium but an elevated glucose value. The only certain thing is that the further a person is from the normal range, the more likely that the person is ill. The normal range is important to the laboratory as a guide to the standards it must set for its instrumentation. If the precision of the normal results is too low, then the difference between normal and abnormal becomes obscured, as was mentioned before. In fact, without adequate precision, determining a normal range becomes impossible.

Information is not only contained in the value of a number, its relative error compared to the true result, and its relationship to the normal range, but also in the relationship it bears toward other results on the same patient for other tests at the same time or for the same test at other times. For example, a patient with a fasting glucose of 90 may have a glucose of 180 shortly after ingesting a few candy bars. The level may be about 120 after an hour, 95

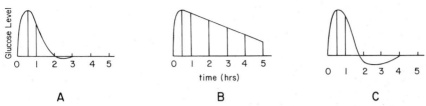

Figure 19-1 Graphs show the reactions of three patients to the ingestion of glucose: healthy (A), diabetic (B), and hypoglycemic (C).

after two hours, and 90 after three hours (Fig. 19-1). A laboratory procedure that measures this is called a glucose tolerance test, and it consists of a number of glucose measurements taken at fixed intervals after carbohydrate is ingested. To be useful, a laboratory instrument must give precise enough results so that the physician can plot the data and determine if the patient is normal, diabetic, or hypoglycemic (Fig. 19-1). The information content of the data in this case is not any one value, but the relationship among them.

A common group of related tests is serum electrolytes, which usually consist of sodium, potassium, chloride, and the CO_2 content. Almost all the extracellular cations are in the form of sodium and potassium, while the principal anions are chloride and bicarbonate. There are also other anions resulting from the ionization of organic acids and negatively charged proteins. Since the body is electrically neutral, an anion gap therefore exists with $[Na^+] + [K^+] > [Cl^-] + [HCO_3^-]$. Various combinations of the results of these tests are possible. Let us look at only two examples. If all values rise except bicarbonate, which decreases ($[Na^+]\uparrow$, $[K^+]\uparrow$, $[Cl^-]\uparrow$, $[HCO_3^-]\downarrow$), a possible diagnosis is uremia (toxic build up in blood due to kidney failure). If, however, the concentration of all the species are depressed ($[Na^+]\downarrow$, $[K^+]\downarrow$, $[Cl^-]\downarrow$, $[HCO_3^-]\downarrow$), then diarrhea would be a more reasonable explanation. The informational content of this data is clearly related not to any one particular value, but to all of them simultaneously. An instrument running electrolytes should, therefore, calculate the anion gap as another result since it is important to diagnosis. Other cases where calculated results are important appear elsewhere in the book.

Section 19-2
SIGNAL DETECTION

Every measurement made by an instrument consists of two parts: signal and noise. The signal results from the analytical process of interest and should bear some relationship to the concentration of a sought-for substance. Noise is signal that arises from other than the process of interest. It is undesirable and must be eliminated or reduced to low levels to permit the measurement.

Noise can be classified into two categories. The first is noise that is repetitive enough to be compensated for to a very high degree. This type of noise is called background. For example, dark current, a current generated by thermal means, will always flow in a photomultiplier tube. This is noise; but if the temperature and voltage are carefully controlled, the dark current can be eliminated from the result by subtracting an amount equal to it somewhere in the calculation circuitry. Similarly, there is always nuclear radiation present in the atmosphere, but by measuring it for a prolonged period, it is possible to get a reliable estimate of this background. The background radiation can then be subtracted from the total counts to give a much more accurate value. While these compensations are not perfect, they reduce noise to the 1% level.

It is not possible to dispose of all noise so conveniently. Noise in the form of short-duration, high-voltage pulses poses real difficulties in measurements. These surges are so infrequent as to be impossible to compensate for by background techniques and are so large as to be a significant portion of the signal. These are called transients. If the signal is of short duration and random, the noise and signal are indistinguishable. In other cases, the noise and signal can only be separated by mathematical techniques. We will review some of these techniques briefly.

The easiest technique to implement is the averaging of values. This can be used when the signal changes slowly but the noise is of high frequency. Figure 19-2 shows an example of this approach. The rate of the reaction is found by computing the slope between x and y. Rather than a line-fitting approach with points taken along the whole line, the two-point method with only points x and y is commonly used. The following equation applies:

$$R = \frac{y - x}{t} \qquad \textbf{(19-1)}$$

If only one reading is taken at x and y, a noise transient can greatly affect the result (Fig. 19-2B). If, on the other hand, five closely spaced readings are taken and averaged to form each point, then the average would show considerably less aberration because of the noise transient.

EXAMPLE 19-1

Point x in Fig. 19-2 is exactly 100 units while point y is 200. If the measurements of point y are 243, 198, 201, 197, 203 and if t is 10.0, what is the relative error of relying only on the first measured point? On the average of the measured points?

Solution:
True value:

$$R = \frac{y - x}{t} = \frac{200 - 100}{10.0} = 10.0 \text{ units/time}$$

Using first point:

$$R' = \frac{243 - 100}{10.0} = 14.3 \text{ units/time}$$

$$\%E = \frac{|R - R'|}{R} \times 100\% = \frac{|10.0 - 14.3|}{10.0} \times 100\%$$

$$\%E = 43\%$$

Using the average:

$$y = \frac{\Sigma P_i}{N} = \frac{243 + 198 + 201 + 197 + 203}{5}$$

$$y = 208.3$$

$$R'' = \frac{208.3 - 100}{10.0} = 10.8 \text{ units/time}$$

$$\%E = \frac{|10.0 - 10.8|}{10.0} \times 100\%$$

$$\%E = 8\% \qquad \blacksquare$$

This result from averaging shows a dramatic improvement over a single measurement of the point, but it is certainly not the best result that can be

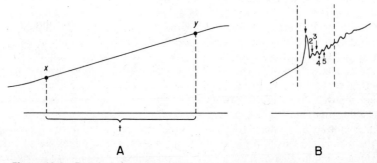

A   B

Figure 19-2 Part A shows a two-point rate measurement. Part B is a blowup of Point y, showing the effect of high frequency transients. If there is a large amount of noise (B), taking several closely spaced readings and averaging them to get the true value of the point are essential to getting good results.

gotten from the data. When several data readings are collected at the same point, any reading that differs more than two standard deviations from the rest by the method of measurement being used is very likely in error due to random noise. Consequently, such points can be dropped from the average. This rule is arbitrary and may be replaced by any convenient rule for removing noise-laden points. This process invariably starts by dropping the point that most differs from the mean.

EXAMPLE 19-2

Drop the first measurement of point y, and calculate the relative error of the remaining values.

Solution: Drop the first point.

$$y = \frac{\Sigma P_i}{N} = \frac{198 + 201 + 197 + 203}{4}$$

$$y = 199.75$$

$$R = \frac{y - x}{t} = \frac{199.75 - 100}{10.0} = 9.975 \text{ units/time}$$

$$\%E = \frac{|R - R'|}{R} \times 100\% = \frac{|10.0 - 9.975|}{10.0} \times 100\%$$

$$\%E = 0.25\% \qquad \blacksquare$$

While the improvement in this case is dramatic and easily justifies the method we have employed, in most cases the improvement is much smaller. Moreover, since the real value under ordinary circumstances will not be known, verifying the improvement will be difficult. As a consequence, the rejection of data points must follow strict guidelines, depending upon the method of measurement, to prevent discarding more accurate points in favor of closely grouped but less accurate points. Nevertheless, the concept of rejecting noise-laden points is extremely important in improving measurements in noisy environments.

As well as securing an accurate measurement of single points, it is possible to enhance the accuracy of a measurement by using numerous points collectively. This technique is commonly called linear regression when used with a straight line and curve

fitting when used with other line shapes. The method employed to accomplish such fitting is to reduce a function of the distance between the theoretical line and the actual points to the minimum value possible. Figure 19-3 shows a curve fitted to some points. The most common method used for such fitting is called least squares. The function being reduced to its minimum is the sum of the squares of the distances (y direction) between the curve and the points. Only one curve of any particular type (straight line, quadratic, cubic, etc.) has such a minimum distance. The general formula is

$$y = f(x), \qquad \textbf{(19-2)}$$

such that $\Sigma[f(x_i) - y_i]^2$ is minimum.

In this equation the x_i's are the values of the independent variable at which the values of the dependent variable (y_i's) were obtained. The quantities x and y are the general variables of the equation.

The derivation of the equation necessary to fit curves to lines is too complex for this book. Moreover, the arithmetic to perform higher order curve fitting is so complicated that it is not worth the time of most students to do it. So that the concepts of curve fitting become clear, however, it is necessary to look at the fitting of a straight line to a series of points.

The equation for a straight line is the familiar

$$y = mx + b \qquad \textbf{(19-3)}$$

Here m is the slope and b is the y intercept. In its more general form, $b = a_0$ and $m = a_1$, where the

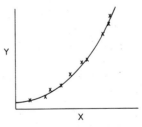

Figure 19-3 A fitted line is the best approximation of the data by some standard, which is called the "norm of fitting."

subscript i of the coefficient matches the power of x.

Therefore,

$$y = a_1 x^1 + a_0 x^0 = a_1 x + a_0 \qquad \textbf{(19-4)}$$

The following equations are needed to find a_0 and a_1 given a group of N (x, y) points.

$$\Sigma y_i = a_0 N + a_1 \Sigma x_i \qquad \textbf{(19-5)}$$

$$\Sigma x_i y_i = a_0 \Sigma x_i + a_1 \Sigma x_i^2 \qquad \textbf{(19-6)}$$

If one realizes that the N in Eq. 19-5 comes from the summing of one N times, $N = \Sigma_{i=1}^{N} 1$, then a pattern should appear obvious that can be carried to higher degree polynomials. For each new coefficient there must be a new term in each of the old equations and a new equation. The general form is as follows:

For $y = f(x^M)$, $M + 1$ equations with $k = 0, 1, \ldots, M$ are needed of the form

$$\sum_{i=0}^{N} x_i^k y_i = \sum_{j=0}^{M} \left(A_j \sum_{i=0}^{N} x_i^{j+k} \right) \qquad \textbf{(19-7)}$$

From this general form all equations necessary to fit any polynomial can be derived.

EXAMPLE 19-3

Find the best straight line through the following five points. (3.0, 14), (5.0, 23), (8.0, 33), (11.0, 47), (15.0, 62). (See Fig. 19-4.)

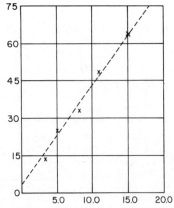

Figure 19-4 Five points and a line fitted to them by least-squares calculations.

Solution: Find the terms necessary for Eqs. 19-5 and 19-6.

$$\Sigma y_i = 14 + 23 + 33 + 47 + 62 = 179$$

$$\Sigma x_i y_i = 3 \times 14 + 5 \times 23 + 8 \times 33$$
$$+ 11 \times 47 + 15 \times 62 = 1868$$

$$\Sigma x_i = 3 + 5 + 8 + 11 + 15 = 42$$

$$\Sigma x_i^2 = 3^2 + 5^2 + 8^2 + 11^2 + 15^2 = 444$$

From Eq. 19-5,

$$179 = 5a_0 + 42a_1$$

From Eq. 19-6,

$$1868 = 42a_0 + 444a_1$$

Solve for a_1:

$$364.4 = 91.2a_1$$

$$a_1 = 4.0$$

And then a_0:

$$a_0 = \frac{179 - 42 \times 4.0}{5} = 2.2 \qquad \blacksquare$$

The ability to fit a curve to a set of data allows us to estimate missing points. This process is called interpolation and is familiar from the use of trigonometric or logarithmic tables. The working curve used in the laboratory is an example of the use of interpolations. The standards form the known points, and the samples are the points for which interpolation must be applied. To construct a working curve, a medical technologist plots the points and draws a straight line with a ruler or a curved line with a French curve. The readings of the samples are then marked on the graph and the corresponding concentrations read.

The computer within an instrument approaches the problem in much the same way. Instead of creating a physical graph, however, it calculates the equation of a curve to fit the standards. From this equation it calculates the concentrations that correspond to the readings for the sample. This information is then printed for the technologist. While interpolation is relatively accurate when a number of standards are run or the procedure is very linear,

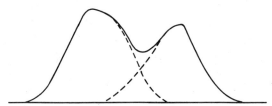

Figure 19-5 Two curves overlap each other, and their areas must be computed by finding the ideal peaks that would give the same results if overlapped appropriately.

extrapolation, the computing of values outside the range of the standards, is considerably less reliable and may suffer from very large errors.

Interpolation can also be used to fill in missing values to make a complete set of data. This method is used in curve smoothing to create a large number of points to display, such as on a CRT. It is also used in pattern matching where part of the pattern may be poorly formed or missing.

Another use of curve fitting is the deconvoluting of overlapping curves. Figure 19-5 shows two incompletely resolved curves. Such curves may result from an incomplete chromatographic separation, for example. To find the area under the curve, which is proportional to the concentration, one can use two curves of the appropriate shape and separation and adjust the parameters until they coincide with the actual curves to a certain quality of fit. The areas under these two curves can then be computed separately with a high degree of accuracy. This process is extremely complex and usually is accomplished by a recursive model starting with initial estimates made by a more elementary formula. Because of this complexity, such resolution without a computer is impractical. Various methods for the manual estimation of such overlapping curves are given in Chapter 22.

Section **19-3**
TIME-AVERAGED SPECTROPHOTOMETRY

Let us look at some applications of information handling techniques. The common spectrophotom-

eters discussed in Chapter 15 have numerous restrictions, such as having to measure the specimen in the dark, being able to measure the specimen at only one wavelength at a time, requiring a reasonably long period to scan a spectrum, and requiring light sources to be changed when going from UV to visible. These restrictions can make working with these instruments slow if one is trying to use the light spectrum to identify compounds or to find relatively low level impurities such as in drug analysis. Information handling techniques allow us to greatly expand the capacities of the UV-visible spectrophotometer.

An example of this new technology is the Hewlett Packard 8450. The optical path of the instrument is shown in Figure 19-6. It uses a tungsten–halogen lamp for the visible light and a deuterium source for the UV radiation. The visible light is shone through the UV source so that both emission spectra are present in the resulting beam. These are reflected through the lamp housing exit slit and routed by an elliptical mirror to the beam director. Note that there is no monochromater present since all the wavelengths of light will be used. Elliptical mirrors are used to better collimate the radiation.

The beam director takes the place of the chopper in a conventional spectrophotometer. This pair of connected mirrors is driven by a torque motor whose position is determined by a shaft encoder. The position is then refined by feedback from a pair of optical detectors on either side of the corresponding slit. The movement from the reference to the sample position requires less than 150 milliseconds.

There are five possible beam positions (Figure 19-7). This allows reference, standards, and sample to be read and compared within seconds. The noteworthy thing about the radiation path through the samples is that it is out in the room light. There is no cover for the sample compartment. This greatly reduces the difficulties surrounding the insertion and removing of the specimens. After passing through the specimen, the light is bent back at a 180° angle so as to pass under the specimen compartment and back to the beam director.

The light, still containing all the wavelengths, is reflected from the lower beam director mirror off

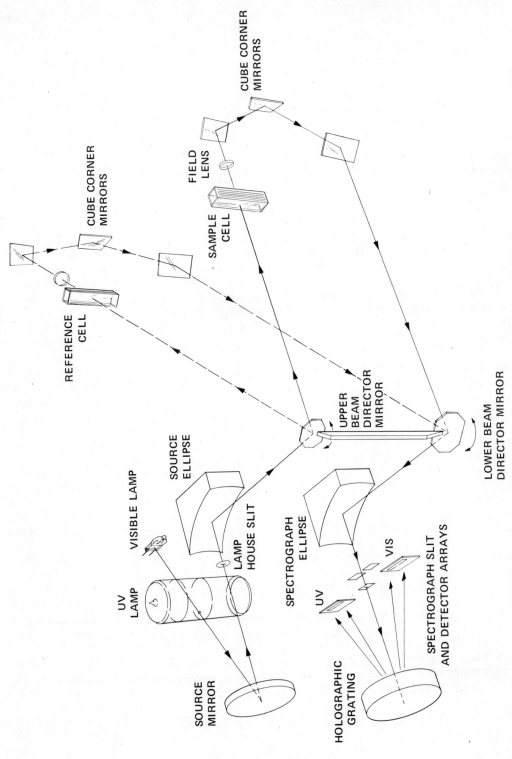

Figure 19-6 Optical layout of the HP 8450 UV-visible spectrophotometer. (Courtesy of Hewlett-Packard. Reprinted with permission.)

CUBE CORNER MIRRORS

CUBE CORNER MIRRORS

FIELD LENS

SAMPLE CELL

REFERENCE CELL

VISIBLE LAMP

SOURCE ELLIPSE

UV LAMP

LAMP HOUSE SLIT

UPPER BEAM DIRECTOR MIRROR

LOWER BEAM DIRECTOR MIRROR

SPECTROGRAPH ELLIPSE

VIS

UV

SPECTROGRAPH SLIT AND DETECTOR ARRAYS

HOLOGRAPHIC GRATING

SOURCE MIRROR

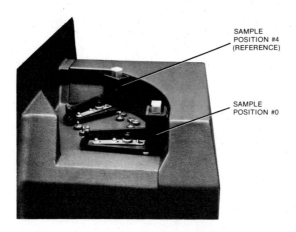

SAMPLE
POSITION #4
(REFERENCE)

SAMPLE
POSITION #0

Figure 19-7 Picture of the sample compartment of the HP 8450, showing five cell positions. (Courtesy of Hewlett-Packard. Reprinted with permission.)

another elliptical mirror and onto a holographic grating. This grating is designed to create a uniform dispersion of radiation so that the distances between wavelengths are the same across the spectrum. Two gratings actually are combined on a common substrate base so that the UV spectrum (200–400 nm) is dispersed in one direction and the visible light (400–800 nm) is dispersed in the other direction.

The spectrum is spread so that 1 nm in the UV covers 60 microns in the detector. The visible light is spread half as much. The mechanism for the detection of the radiation is a matrix of photodiodes. These are 50 microns wide and located every 60 microns. Therefore, each diode matrix must contain a little more than 200 diodes. The circuit for each diode is shown in Figure 19-8.

The capacitor is initially charged at the beginning of a reading cycle. As the light shines on the photodiode, it discharges the capacitor to ground. The amount of charge necessary to restore the capacitor to the original voltage is measured and is proportional to the light energy reaching the photodiode. This is, therefore, proportional to the amount of light transmitted. The fact that a number of milliseconds elapses during the reading cycle eliminates the effects of any high frequency noise.

There are five 100-millisecond measurements of the photodiodes made every second. Two of these measurements occur while the detector is looking at the reference and two while it is looking at the sample. The fifth scan occurs when the radiation sources are blanked out for 100 milliseconds to measure the dark current. The readings from the photodiodes, in turn, are sent through a 14-bit ADC (resolution of 1 part in 16,000) and then stored in the computer memory.

The instrument is controlled by a microprocessor with 28K words of ROM and 16K or 32K words of RAM. Built into the spectrophotometer is a CRT that can be used to display the data collected. The data is initially stored in the unprocessed form. From here it can be displayed or processed with a number of routines. Figure 19-9 shows a typical display. The number on top gives the wavelength of the cursor (pointer). The wavelength range is shown immediately under the plot. In this case the whole spectrum is shown. The Y-axis autoscales to get the highest value found on the screen, and this y scale is given next. Following this is the type of plot, in this case, absorbance. Finally, the type of data transaction appears, in this case, measurement to display.

Another part of the instrument is the keyboard

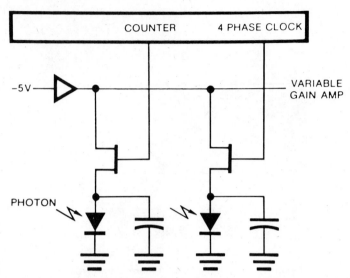

Figure 19-8 The diode circuit for reading information in the HP 8450. (Courtesy of Hewlett-Packard. Reprinted with permission.)

(Figure 19-10), which has a one-piece, touch-sensitive surface to prevent objects or liquids from entering its inner mechanism. This gives the user the option of programming sequences of events and specifying how the data should be handled. Additional hardware can also be attached, such as a plotter to produce a permanent record of the display, a teleprinter to report data tabulation, or a floppy disk drive for long-term storage. These give tremendous versatility to such an instrument.

Let us look at how this type of instrument greatly improves the level of performance one can expect

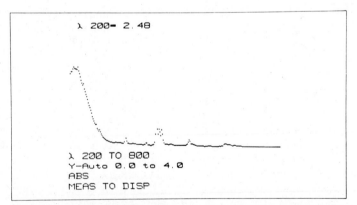

Figure 19-9 Typical wavelength scan, giving the absorbance at 200 nm, the wavelength range, the scale on the *y* axis, the type of measurement, and the type of computer transaction. (Courtesy of Hewlett-Packard. Reprinted with permission.)

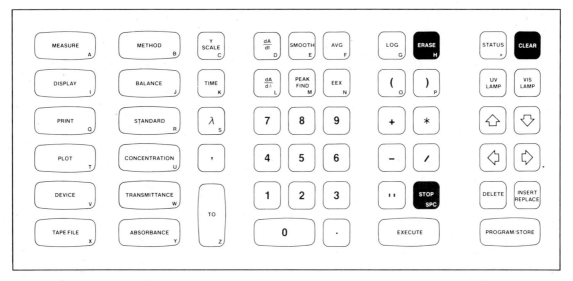

Figure 19-10 Keyboard of the HP 8450. (Courtesy of Hewlett-Packard. Reprinted with permission.)

from a spectrophotometer. First, the manipulation in the source housing is reduced. The need for hardware to switch between the two sources is gone. Such hardware can become misaligned and serve as a source of scattered radiation. Second, the elimination of the monochromator removes one of the most expensive and delicate pieces of apparatus. Misalignment and damage to this critical item are no longer problems, nor is slack in the mechanical linkages used to change wavelengths. The replacement of the chopper with the self-correcting beam director guarantees a uniform amount of radiation reaching each specimen position. In summary, the mechanical portions of the instrument before the specimen cell have been greatly improved by new technical innovation and by the elimination of the need for monochromatic light.

The most astounding feature of the instrument, however, is the ability to make accurate measurements in room light. This is a major advance due totally to the capabilities of the microprocessor and information theory. Stray light has always been a problem in previous designs because of its randomness over the relatively long time (seconds to minutes) that was required to take readings. Several innovations allow this to be circumvented. First,

the readings are taken very rapidly. The process is completed within a second. Second, the reference, dark current, and sample are all read within this period. This means that the zero and full scale values can be determined at effectively the same time as the sample reading is made. Room light is removed as dark current. Third, because each wavelength is read by integration, the effect of any high frequency transient radiation is drastically reduced. Finally, three standards can be measured immediately before or after the sample. Since these too are read relative to the reference and dark current, and since the whole process takes less than 5 seconds, drift is effectively eliminated. Despite this, strong room light or strong radiation entering at a low angle into the specimen is not recommended because it will reduce the sensitivity of the instrument.

The use of a holographic grating eliminates the problem of nonlinear dispersion, which requires a sine-bar in a typical monochromator. Second-order radiation is removed by filters. The use of only half the angle of dispersion in the visible range reduces the cost of the instrument without significantly degrading performance. The advantages of measuring all wavelengths virtually simultaneously are hard to overestimate. It, of course, produces a spectral

Routine #	Calibration Curves (minimum number of stds. needed shown)	Relationship Used in Calculation	Minimum Number of Standards Required
0	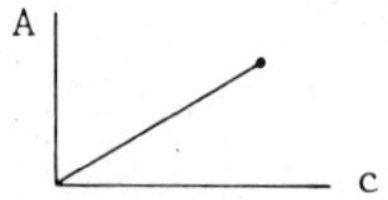	$c = k_1 A$	1
1	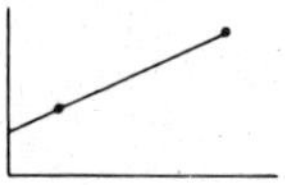	$c = k_0 + k_1 A$	2
2	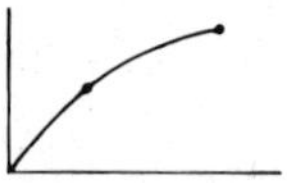	$c = k_1 A + k_2 A^2$	2
3	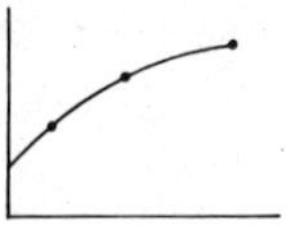	$c = k_0 + k_1 A + k_2 A^2$	3
4	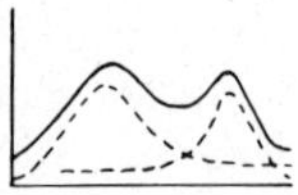	$c = k_1 c_1 + k_2 c_2 + \ldots k_n c_n$ (multicomponents)	12 max @ λ, 7 max @ λ_1 to λ_2

Figure 19-11 Available curve-fitting programs for the HP 8450. (Courtesy of Hewlett-Packard. Reprinted with permission.)

scan of the sample, which is frequently useful. In addition, it permits the measurement of the concentration to be made at numerous wavelengths. This can be important if interferences are present and if it becomes necessary to resort to the use of multiple equations in multiple unknowns. Copies of the complete spectra make excellent documentation of the results and are useful both in later follow-up and in teaching.

Finally, perhaps a brief look should be taken at the calculations that can be performed to find unknown concentrations. Figure 19-11 shows the types of working curves available. These have been alluded to previously in this chapter. Note that they are based primarily on straight line and quadratic fits. The number of standards can be reduced by

one if the curve definitely goes through zero. Since this may not always be the case, a dilution experiment should be performed before making this assumption. One of the options is multivariable analysis. Note that it requires numerous standards. Calculated constants are available from the working curve. In addition, the instrument will report the standard deviation for measurements if requested.

Section 19-4
PATTERN RECOGNITION

While data fitting techniques can give us the ability to drastically improve accuracy in certain measurements, there is another area of informational content technology that is also gaining in importance. This is the field of pattern recognition. Pattern recognition is the science of abstracting information from a series of similar occurrences and finding those keys or facts that are constant among the various occurrences. Moreover, to perform pattern recognition it is also necessary that the facts constituting the pattern in positive occurrences be absent from negative occurrences or nonoccurrences. If this is not the case, the pattern is valid but useless, since it does not distinguish between the two cases that are the subject of the study.

To perform pattern recognition, one can start in the simplest case with the idea that two mutually exclusive sets exist and that all objects fall into one of the two sets. For example, an object is a baseball bat (set 1), or it is not a baseball bat (set 2). One next tries to define attributes that will distinguish items in one set from the other. For example, baseball bats are made of wood or aluminum. Anything that is not made of wood or aluminum is not a baseball bat. On the other hand, everything made of wood or aluminum is not a baseball bat, so this one fact is not adequate to establish a useful pattern. One can improve the discrimination between these sets by looking at more attributes, for example, weight, length, and shape. Each of these will eliminate more and more objects from the set called "baseball bats" and place them in the set "non baseball bats." In fact, the differentiation will go very quickly initially, but trying to eliminate the last items we know clearly are not baseball bats (ax handles, walking sticks, night sticks, etc.) will be much harder. Since all baseball bats are not identical, the pattern, no matter how refined we make it, can never guarantee that the discrimination will be perfect. In most situations this is adequate, because if something fits the description of what is needed closely enough, it can usually be used instead. One can, for example, use a screw driver to open a paint can if one does not have a paint can opener.

A pattern is an abstraction or model of the real world. One abstracts the facts about the set or objects of interest and uses this information for a model of an ideal set member. Because the model should match all set members, it will, of necessity, be somewhat vague. It will appear as if seen through a lens out of focus. The closer the members of a set resemble each other, the sharper the focus will appear to be.

Things become more complex when numerous sets exist and when the differences are slight. Imagine trying to write a description that would distinguish among all the various balls used in playing games throughout the world. There would, in fact, be some overlap, and mistakes in classifying would be common until the patterns were extremely well developed. We will look at this problem in a laboratory context shortly.

Let us first look at some sets and see what the problems with pattern recognition really are. Numeric puzzles are perhaps the classic example of pattern recognition. For example, if the sequence of numbers 0, 1, 1, 2, 3, 5, 8, 13 is given, what is the pattern to the sequence so we can determine if an arbitrary number belongs to it? It does not at first seem obvious, but each number is the sum of the two previous numbers with 0 and 1 given as the first two elements. This is a rather famous sequence called the "Fibonacci numbers," after the thirteenth century Italian mathematician Leonardo Fibonacci who discovered them.

Other sequences may not produce a unique result. For example, the sequence 1, 3, 5, 7 might seem obviously the odd numbers and come from the equation $y = 2x + 1$. However, these could also be the values of equation $y = x^4 - 6x^3 + 11x^2 - 4x + 1$. In the latter case, the next number of the sequence is 33 instead of 9. Hence there are two patterns (equations) that fit the data. It is impossible to decide which pattern is the correct one without more information.

Another example of a pattern is shown in Figure 19-12. Here we have alphabet letters around a circle. Based on what you see, where does the rest of the alphabet go? As it turns out, O P Q R S U go on the inside and N T V W X Y Z go on the outside. The former are all letters with curved-line parts. The pattern here is a bit obscure, but frequently the usable information in pattern matching is not the obvious. For example, topologically a doughnut and a coffee cup are the same, while a sugar bowl is different. The first two each have one hole all the way through the material (handle for the coffee cup), while a sugar bowl has two.

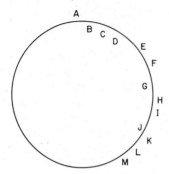

Figure 19-12 A pattern determines which alphabet letters go on the inside and which go on the outside of the circle.

Most of pattern matching research deals with patterns in two and three dimensions. Since laboratory applications also most frequently involve such patterns, we will look at them next. Let us consider the problem of using a computer to read someone's handwriting. This is complex because a computer is essentially a device that thinks in one-dimensional terms and handwriting is a two-dimensional activity. Secondly, not everyone's handwriting is identical. Even one individual's handwriting may vary significantly when he is rushed or writing in an unusual position. Some people, such as the author, have handwriting that is extremely difficult to decipher. Moreover, computers do not understand the context of the materials humans frequently use to resolve conflicts and ambiguities.

Figure 19-13 shows several written letter "a's." Each is clearly an "a," but there are certain differences among them. The first is a nearly perfect "a." It is closed, it is well formed, and it has appropriate connecting strokes. Yet, if one required these of a character to be classified an "a," then the others shown would not be considered "a's." To circumvent these kinds of major difficulties, computer scientists have come up with a variety of

ways of making characters more uniform as they are read by the computer. This is accomplished by using a grid placed over the character as shown in Figure 19-14. This grid must be fine enough so portions of the character are not blurred together, but coarse enough so that matching can occur in a finite time. Once the grid is in place, squares on the grid are marked as 1 (black) if they are predominantly covered with letter and 0 (white) if they are not predominantly covered with letter. This has the effect of sharpening the character as seen in the second part of the figure. It closes slight openings, removes smudges, and makes the edges more distinct. If desirable for a particular application, the representation can be further refined by smoothing techniques to make the thickness of the letter's outline more uniform in width.

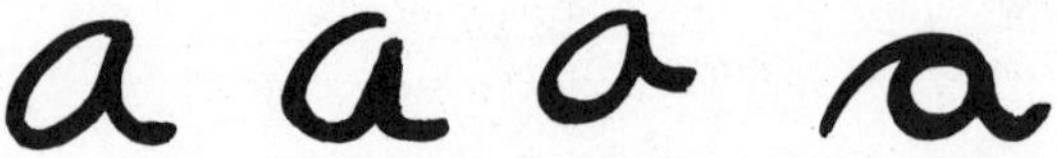

The pattern must now be transferred into a vector, which is just a $1 \times N$ array, where N is the number of squares in the grid. In a simple representation, these entries are the 1's and 0's mentioned in the previous paragraph. In more sophisticated representations these entries might include a weighting factor to indicate how intense the markings were in the grid squares. The logical process that creates this representation is called the sensor.

The above step is relatively simple compared with the second step, the classification of the pattern. There are many approaches available, but we will look at only two rather common ones here, as most are well beyond the scope of this text. The

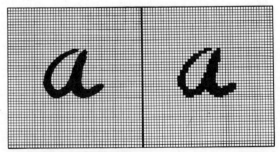

Figure 19-14 The handwritten letter "a" with a grid over it. The second letter "a" is a representation of the first with the blackened area indicating where a 1 would be placed by the sensor because the square was at least half covered with ink.

Figure 19-13 Four handwritten "a's" of varying quality.

first method is that of the decision function. A decision function is an equation that, when applied to the pattern vector, gives a positive result if the pattern is in set 1 and a negative value if the pattern is in set 2. Figure 19-15A shows an example where only two variables are involved. As more variables are involved, as with handwriting, graphic representation of the function becomes impossible, requiring more than three dimensions. The decision function works if the function values for two sets are significantly different from each other. If more sets are involved, additional decision functions will be needed to split up the space into small segments, as we shall see in the next section. Pattern vectors whose values fall near zero, that is, near the decision line, are in danger of being misclassified. The effectiveness of a decision function in classifying pattern vectors depends on the coefficients of the function. Determining these is the most difficult part of this approach. Very frequently known groups of both set 1 and set 2 are used to "train" the function. Training means having the computer adjust the values of the coefficients of the function so that it can distinguish between known members of set 1 and set 2 every time. The function can then be used to evaluate unknown patterns. A second approach is to calculate the distance that a pattern vector is from the ideal pattern vector for a number of sets. This method is shown in Figure 19-15B. The computer obtains an ideal vector to represent each set by averaging the corresponding terms of each pattern known to be in that set. This is like finding the center of gravity of an irregularly cut piece of sheet metal, only in N dimensions, where N is the number of grid squares in the pattern. This vector then points to the center of the pattern group. The distance between an unclassified vector (U) and an ideal vector (K) can be found by taking the square root of the sum of the squares of the differences for each variable.

$$d = \Sigma(U_i - K_i)^2 \qquad \textbf{(19-8)}$$

The vector is classified in that set to whose center of gravity (ideal vector) it is the closest. A difficulty occurs if the members of some sets are less tightly grouped than the members of other sets. This will cause the midpoints between the centers of the sets not to be the midpoints between the edges of the sets and can lead to misclassifications. If this problem arises, a distance weighting factor must be included to compensate for the asymmetry.

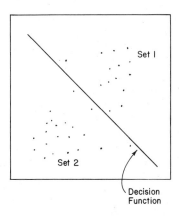

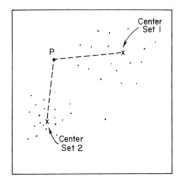

A

B

Figure 19-15 Part A shows the ends of the data vectors (points) separated by a decision function. In two dimensions this is a line. Part B shows the classification of a vector P based on its distance from the ideal vectors, which represent the center of the sets. (*Note:* While vectors originate from the origin, drawing the lines would only confuse the representation.)

Section **19-5**
DIFFERENTIAL COUNTERS

White blood cells come in various types varying in appearance and relative proportions depending on the age of the cells and the disease affecting the person. When counting the various types of white cells, it is necessary to differentiate one from another. This process is called a differential count.

Humans who do such counts have to learn the different patterns of the cells in each category. Because of the way the human brain perceives objects, this is relatively simple. The procedure is much more difficult for a computer. Nevertheless, in the last decade tremendous progress has been made in this area. Automated differential counters have become reliable instruments for counting routine cells, although they experience considerably more difficulty with unusual cells.

There are two automated approaches to differential counting. In the first a slide of the patient's blood must be made and stained with Wright's stain. This slide is then placed, with others, into the differential counter. The slides are moved one by one into the analyzer. The cells to be counted are found by a pattern of slight movements of the slide, which brings different fields of cells into the center of the reading area. The position is then refined to center on a specific cell, using its greater opaqueness to identify its location. The movement of the analyzer is programmed to count a representative sample of the slide without backtracking.

The field is then divided by a grid for pattern recognition. Each square on the grid is measured for light intensity transmitted at two or three wavelengths. This information is stored in an array in the computer memory inside the instrument. Figure 19-16 shows the type of pattern that might result from one of the color scans of the slide. The magnitude of the number represents the relative darkness of the square.

This information is then handled by various processor subroutines. The first one might, for example, try to determine the edge of the cell. This is accomplished by scanning one of the cell matrices and looking for a change of intensity. When this is found, a mark is placed in a corresponding place in another array. After the whole color array has been

```
        2 2
      2 2 2 2
    2 2 2 3 3 2 2 2 2         1
  1 2 2 3 2 3 3 3 2 2 2 1 2
  2 2 3 2 5 6 3 4 2 3 2 1 2 2 2 1 2 2
  2 2 2 6 8 8 7 4 4 3 2 2 2 3 2 2
2 2 2 4 7 9 8 8 8 5 3 2 2 2 3 2 2
2 2 2 5 8 9 9 8 8 5 2 2 2 2 2 2
2 3 2 6 8 8 8 8 4 3 2 2 2 2 2
  2 2 2 7 9 8 8 8 4 2 3 3 2
  1 2 4 8 8 7 3 3 2 3 2 1
    2 2 4 6 7 4 2 3 2
      2 2 3 2 3 2 1
        1 2 3 2 2
          2 2 1
```

Figure 19-16 The density pattern of a cell as indicated by the magnitude of the number at each position.

scanned, the next step is to make sure the outline array is continuous (Figure 19-17). This is done by having a program that fills in edge points if the edge is broken by checking adjacent squares, once an edge square is found, to be certain that at least two of them are also part of the edge. After the edge has been made solid, other cells than the one desired that are wholly or partly in the field are eliminated from all the arrays. The process continues with the isolation of the nucleus. Here again, the finding of the outline is essential. It is done by the same method as before, and the location of the nucleus is then determined. Evaluation of the various points necessary to build the pattern vector can then be started.

There are numerous evaluation parameters, such as cell size and shape. The size can be determined by counting the squares that compose the cell. The shape can be found by measuring the difference between corresponding points on the real cell and idealized cells of the same type. Similar measurements are then made on the nucleus. The ratio of the nucleus to the cytoplasm can be calculated. The average density can be determined by each wavelength at which a measurement was made by adding the value for each square and dividing by the total. Other measurements of texture and granularity can be applied. These are combined to give an ordered set of numbers referred to as the vector of the observed cell.

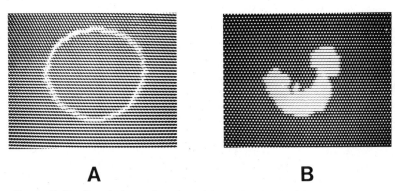

A   **B**

Figure 19-17   Part A shows the edge of the cell as it was detected, and part B shows the nucleus after it was detected and colored in. (Courtesy of Coulter Electronics, Inc.)

To this vector a series of formulae is applied. The goal is to determine which type of cell it most closely resembles. In effect, these equations act as multidimensional planes (hyperplanes) to separate one cell type from another. Because of the complexity of the identification, the equations may not be as simple as those shown with linear coefficients in the previous section. The cell type whose equation gives the optimum value for the result is assigned to the cell, and the total for that type is increased by one in the count. If a cell is not adequately close to any cell model, then it is classified as "other," and its position is saved so it can be reviewed manually. This process is repeated until enough cells have been counted. Usually the total is 100. The tally is then reported via a printer. Frequently characteristics of the red cells and platelets are reported simultaneously, as discussed in Chapter 18.

The differential pattern recognition process in such instruments as the Geometric Data Hematrak or the Coulter diff3 requires dozens of parameters to be evaluated. This gives all the information needed to make a classification. There is so much information that determining how much to weight each piece is a hard decision for the design engineer to make. Presumably, increasing experience with automated differential counters will produce greater reliability in the recognition of more types of cells. This should make them more universally applicable.

A second approach is that used by the Technicon H6000. White cells are diluted and travel in a flowing stream. The stream is split into several portions, each of which is treated with different chemicals. In the peroxidase channel an enzyme–dye reaction occurs which stains the cytoplasm in the eosinophils black and in most other white cells various shades of gray. This stream is then sheathed by diluent and constricted so that cells pass the detection point individually. Light is directed through the sample and measured by two detectors (Fig. 19-18). One of these measures the absorbance of the cell, and the other measures the amount of radiation scattered. The intensity of the scatter is plotted against the absorption, as shown in Figure 19-19. The various types of cells can then be separated by decision planes illustrated in that figure. The differentiation is made due to the cytochemical differences in the various white cells.

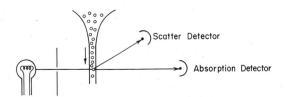

Figure 19-18   The peroxidase channel measures both the light transmitted through the cell and the light scattered by the cell.

Peroxidase X-Y Display

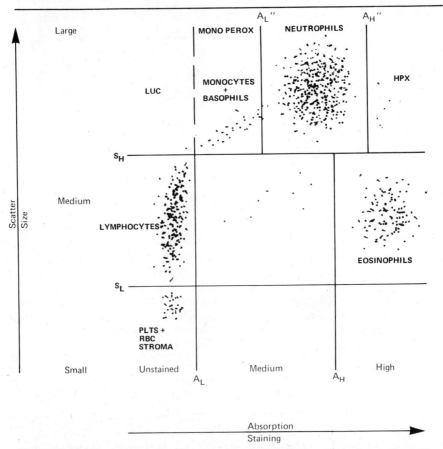

Figure 19-19 The scatter of cells, graphing size against various chemical reactions. (Courtesy of Technicon Instruments Corporation, Tarrytown, New York, 10591. Technicon and Technicon H6000 are registered trademarks of Technicon Instruments Corporation.)

Because of the similarity of the staining of monocytes and basophils in peroxidase, they cannot be distinguished by this method. Therefore a second channel exists; it uses alcian blue to stain the granules of the basophils so that they can be counted separately. The channel is manipulated similar to the peroxidase channel except that it uses two scattering detectors, one in the near infrared and one in the visible spectrum. These are again plotted against each other to separate them from other cells

and platelets. Additional reactions can be used to aid in differentiation, such as myeloperoxidase to detect granulocytes and α-naphthol butyrate esterase to detect monocytes. The H6000 counts 10,000 white cells instead of only 100 to get its percentages to report. This gives a statistically more reliable count of normal cells, but cannot advise the technologist of specific abnormal cells.

Using informational techniques on data to take advantage of the various attributes associated with pieces of data permits measurements that otherwise would not be possible. As computer science perfects more of these techniques, we can expect the "intelligence" of instruments to grow. More and more interpretations of data will be done by the instruments with only very abnormal specimens referred back to humans for evaluation.

REVIEW QUESTIONS

1. How is significance related to significant figures?
2. What is hollow significance?
3. Why must the precision be calculated based on the whole range of viable results?
4. How does the precision of an instrument affect determining whether a patient is "normal"?
5. Why could a result be regarded as too precise?
6. How does one decide what amount of precision is useful?
7. In what cases can a percentage error rather than an absolute error be used?
8. What is the normal range?
9. How does one use the normal range to diagnose disease?
10. What is the purpose of the glucose tolerance test?
11. What informational situation is the glucose tolerance test an example of?
12. What type of information is gained from electrolyte analysis?
13. Define anion gap.
14. Define signal.
15. Define noise.
16. Define background noise. Give some examples.
17. What is a transient?
18. How can one use averaged values to reduce noise?
19. How can one use data exclusion to reduce noise?
20. Why is it difficult to determine the effectiveness of noise rejection?
21. Why can data exclusion sometimes be a dangerous technique?
22. What is linear regression?
23. What is least squares?
24. What does curve fitting accomplish?
25. How is least squares analysis implemented?
26. What are the equations for a least squares solution for a straight line?
27. What is interpolation?
28. How is normal curve fitting accomplished? Contrast this with computer curve fitting.
29. What is extrapolation? Why is it less accurate than interpolation?
30. Define deconvolution. How is it accomplished?
31. What are some of the difficulties with classical spectrophotometry?
32. What are the radiation sources for the HP 8450? How are they combined?
33. Why does the 8450 have no monochromator?
34. How is the light beam on the 8450 positioned?
35. Why can the 8450 measure specimens in room light?
36. What is the holographic grating? What are its advantages?
37. How does the 8450 monitor the whole spectrum at one time?
38. Describe the photodiode matrix of the 8450.
39. How are the photodiodes on the 8450 read?
40. Describe the reading cycle of the 8450.
41. How does the 8450 report the data?
42. What peripherals can be attached to the 8450?
43. How does the 8450 improve spectrophotometric measurements?
44. How does the 8450 compensate for room light in the measuring process?
45. What type of data massaging does the 8450 permit?
46. What is pattern recognition?
47. What is the basic assumption of pattern recognition?
48. What is necessary to be able to separate items into pattern classes?
49. What, in essence, is a pattern?
50. Why is pattern matching frequently difficult?
51. Why is handwriting analysis difficult for a computer?
52. Why are grids used in analyzing handwriting and cells?
53. How is a graphic pattern represented inside a computer?
54. What is a sensor?
55. What is a decision function?

56. What is a pattern vector?

57. Why are training sets used in pattern recognition?

58. How does the vector classification approach differ from the decision function approach?

59. Why are patterns sometimes misclassified?

60. What is a white cell differential count?

61. How does a computer physically carry out a differential count?

62. What information regarding the cells does the computer measure?

63. What steps does the computer follow in cell identification?

64. What are some important factors used in cell classification?

65. Contrast the methods used by the Hematrak and Technicon instruments.

66. What is cytochemistry?

PROBLEMS

For each of the problems 1–4, the rate is determined by a two-point measurement. The value of one point is exactly known, while the value of the other point must be determined by averaging the readings taken. First find the slope of the line using all the data. Second, eliminate the reading farthest from the average and recompute the slope. Finally, estimate the improvement in the measurement assuming that the second computation gives the correct answer exactly.

1. (14.0 sec, 182 units), (23.0 sec, 294, 278, 290, 301, and 287 units)

2. (6.9 sec, 214 units), (41.4 sec, 63, 58, 61, 58, and 57 units)

3. (21.4 sec, 137 units), (39.6 sec, 349, 369, 366, 351, 363, and 346 units)

4. (19.7 sec, 53.3), (33.0 sec, 73.1, 72.8, 73.9, and 71.9 units)

For each of the problems 5–7, the rate is determined by a two-point measurement. The value of each point must be determined by averaging the readings taken. First find the slope of the line using all the data. Second, eliminate the reading farthest from the average for each point and recompute the slope. Finally, estimate the improvement in the measurement assuming that the second computation gives the correct answer exactly.

5. (9.5 sec, 114, 119, 122, 113, and 118 units), (21.4 sec, 208, 211, 206, 210, 213, and 206 units)

6. (21.1 sec, 41.7, 40.9, 42.2, 41.6, 41.5, and 42.0 units), (58.2 sec, 27.3, 26.9, 28.1, 27.8, and 26.2 units)

7. (16.4 sec, 9.8, 10.2, 9.7, 9.4, and 9.9 units), (38.7 sec, 32.2, 32.3, 32.6, 31.7, and 32.6 units)

For each of the problems 8–12, find the best straight line through the points given. Write the equation for the line.

8. (1.30, 26.1), (2.74, 47.1), (3.58, 59.3), (4.21, 67.4)

9. (0.86, 12.2), (1.93, 20.8), (3.01, 28.6), (4.11, 37.8), (4.74, 42.0)

10. (1.11, 2.08), (1.68, 4.61), (2.12, 6.20), (3.41, 11.85), (2.89, 9.29), (1.49, 3.79)

11. (0.67, 0.70), (1.45, 5.91), (2.09, 10.2), (2.88, 15.19), (3.64, 20.0)

12. (0.58, 19.7), (1.16, 14.1), (1.71, 9.8), (2.03, 6.49), (2.50, 2.50)

13. What are the three equations necessary to find the best second order (quadratic) fit to a set of data?

CHAPTER 20
RADIATION MEASUREMENTS

Radioactivity results from the decay of one atom into another. The understanding of the nature of radioactivity constitutes part of the exciting development of atomic physics between the 1840s and the explosion of the first nuclear bomb. In this chapter we will mention the high points in the history of these developments. We start with the discovery of the electron.

Section 20-1
FUNDAMENTAL ATOMIC PARTICLES

Many of the investigations into the nature of matter reached a climax in the 1890s. Zeeman showed that placing a light source in a magnetic field caused certain emitted wavelengths to split into two wavelengths. This indicated that there were magnetic fields in the atom. J. J. Thomson worked with a heated cathode in an evacuated tube. Such a device had long been known to give off particles called "cathode rays." By use of electric and magnetic fields Thomson showed that such cathode rays were negative particles with a charge-to-mass ratio (e/m) of $1.7 \cdot 10^8$ coulombs/g, regardless of what material was used for the cathode. Various people tried to measure the charge of a single charged ion. Millikan finally did it with an oil drop moving under the effects of both gravity and an electric field. His work showed the charge of an ion was always some multiple of $1.602 \cdot 10^{-19}$ coulombs. With the charge known, the mass could be computed.

It was now becoming clear that the atom was composed of more basic particles. The cathode rays, which were clearly the carriers of electricity through an evacuated tube, were called electrons. Their properties are given in Table 20-1. It was also certain that the electron made up very little of the mass of the atom since it was only 1/1800 of the mass of the lightest known element, hydrogen. Moreover, the electron had to be in motion to generate the effects observed when placed in a magnetic field. This naturally led to the Bohr model of the atom with the light electrons orbiting a heavy center or nucleus. The nucleus had to be positively charged to preserve electrical neutrality and provide the attraction necessary to keep the electrons in orbit. The gravitational force generated by these tiny particles was too small to be significant. Further discussion of the electron shells may be found in Chapter 14.

Other physicists turned their attention to the structure of the nucleus. The original periodic tables had been constructed based on the atomic weights of the elements as they were identified. This arrangement of the elements led to some interesting observations. First, if oxygen is set as the standard at exactly 16 daltons (1 dalton = 1 atomic mass unit = $1.66 \cdot 10^{-24}$ g), then most, but not all, elements fall very close to whole numbers of amu's. Second, although the periodic properties of the lighter elements work out appropriately based on their number of electrons, the increase of atomic weight is not uniform among elements. Third, the atomic weight does not always give the right order for the elements. Nickel is slightly lighter than cobalt, but the radiation from transitions of its electrons indicates that cobalt has one less positive charge in the nucleus. Thomson performed another charge-to-mass measurement using perpendicular magnetic and electric fields, but he used the positive ions of neon instead of electrons. He discovered that two distinct weights existed—a strong beam at mass number 20 and a much fainter one at

Table 20-1 Atomic Particles

Particle	Symbol	Rest Mass	Charge	Spin	Magnetic Moment
Electron	e	0.00055	-1	$\frac{1}{2}$	1.00116
Proton	p	1.00728	$+1$	$\frac{1}{2}$	2.7928
Neutron	n	1.00867	0	$\frac{1}{2}$	-1.9130
Neutrino	ν	0	0	$\frac{1}{2}$	
Beta	$\beta^{\pm}$	0.00055	± 1	$\frac{1}{2}$	± 1.00116
Antineutrino	$\bar{\nu}$	0	0	$\frac{1}{2}$	
Alpha	α	4.00249	$+2$	0	
Gamma	γ	0	0	0	0

mass number 22. This demonstrated that an element, although determined by the number of positive charges that it possesses, also has additional but neutral contributions to its mass.

The unit of positive charge was called the proton, and its mass was assigned as that of the hydrogen atom minus an electron (Table 20-1). For every step up the periodic table, one proton and one electron would be added. The number of protons is designated as Z and the atomic mass number as A. To preserve electrical neutrality and account for the extra mass it was originally thought that perhaps the nucleus contained A protons and $A - Z$ electrons. Studies of nuclear spin involving the radiation from larger atoms showed that the proton-electron model of the nucleus was not possible.

Finally in 1932 Chadwick was able to show that a neutral particle with almost the same mass as a proton did exist. This particle was called a neutron, and its vital statistics are given in Table 20-1. The neutron's existence was proven by the discovery that when the beryllium nucleus and helium nucleus collided under controlled conditions, the mass equivalent to a neutron disappeared. For nuclear reactions, atoms of element E are written as

$$^{A}_{Z}E$$

The reaction of interest therefore is

$$^{9}_{4}\text{Be} + ^{4}_{2}\text{He} \rightarrow ^{12}_{6}\text{C} + X \qquad \text{(20-1)}$$

In a cloud chamber (a supersaturated atmosphere between electrical plates), traces can be seen for the charged particles, but not for X becuse it does

not cause ionization of other material. As a consequence, X is a neutral particle called a neutron.

$$X = ^{1}_{0}n \qquad \text{(20-2)}$$

The structure becomes clear. The nucleus is composed of the heavy particles—positive protons and neutral neutrons. A number of electrons equal to the number of protons orbits the nucleus in fixed orbitals. The number of protons determines the element's identity, but the number of neutrons may vary slightly. The relationship between the number of protons and neutrons is the next topic we must investigate.

Figure 20-1 shows a plot of the number of neutrons N versus the number of protons Z in the nucleus. The ratio gradually deviates from unity. This occurs because of the nature of the way the nucleus is held together. The reason that positively charged particles stay in such tremendously close proximity is that they literally cannot leave in one piece. If one could weigh the nucleus, one would find that the mass is smaller than the sum of the component parts!

$$m_A < Zm_p + Nm_n \qquad \text{(20-3)}$$

This missing mass (mass defect Δm) is approximately 0.9% of the nucleus' mass, but it varies among the different types of nuclei. If several nucleons (protons or neutrons) were to leave intact, there would be even less mass, relatively, for the remaining nucleons to share. Since such a further shrinking of mass is not physically possible, nucle-

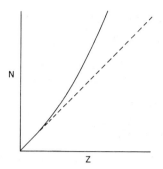

Figure 20-1 The number of neutrons N gradually increases relative to the number of protons Z.

cleus together, because if it were provided, the nucleus would fly apart. This energy equivalent is, therefore, called the binding energy.

If we compute the binding energy based on the mass defect for all the isotopes known, we get the graph shown in Figure 20-2A. This graph is a relatively obvious result of multiplying the mass by 0.9% and by the speed of light squared. If we divide the total binding energy by the number of nucleons, however, we get the graph in Figure 20-2B. This graph is extremely important because, while it shows that the binding energy averages a little more than 8 MeV (million electron volts) per nucleon, it also shows that in light and heavy elements the average is somewhat less than that value. If one would split a very heavy nucleus ($A > 200$ daltons) into two lighter nuclei, for the same number of nucleons, there would be more binding energy. More binding energy implies a greater mass defect. The lost mass cannot leave as a particle; consequently, it must leave as energy since mass and energy together must be conserved. Splitting a heavy nucleus, therefore, releases energy. The binding energy of orbital electrons is only several to a few hundred electron volts, while the binding energy of a nucleon is a few million electron volts. Splitting heavy nuclei produces large quantities of energy, as

ons are prevented from leaving the ground states of nuclei. The mass defect is given by the equation

$$\Delta m = Zm_p + Nm_n - m_A \qquad (20\text{-}4)$$

By Albert Einstein's famous equation for the interconversion of mass to energy, we can discover the energy equivalent to the missing mass.

$$\Delta E = \Delta mc^2 \qquad (20\text{-}5)$$

The quantity c is the speed of light. The energy equivalent to the mass defect is what holds the nu-

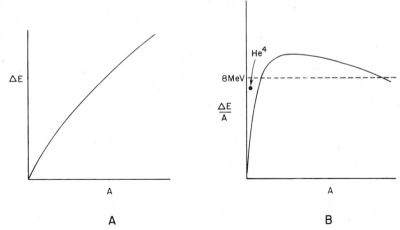

Figure 20-2 The total binding energy (ΔE) and the binding energy per nucleon ($\Delta E/A$) are plotted versus the atomic mass number (A).

atomic bombs clearly demonstrate. This process is called nuclear fission.

If we look at the lower end of Figure 20-2B, we see that if we could combine lighter nuclei ($A < 10$ daltons), we could also produce more binding energy per nucleon and, therefore, release energy. In fact, per nucleon we could release more energy that way than by splitting heavier atoms. This process is called nuclear fusion and is the basis of the hydrogen bomb. The nuclear binding force is indeed powerful.

There are two primary factors affecting nuclear binding energy. The most obvious is electrostatic repulsion. The more protons added to the nucleus, the stronger the repulsive interaction. Since the radius of the nucleus increases only at the rate of the cube root of the rate of the increase of the number of nucleons, it is small wonder that the average binding energy decreases in heavier nuclei as electrostatic repulsion intensifies. On the other hand, attractive forces are a result of complex inter-nucleon exchange reactions. These are called nuclear forces and are very strong, but of extremely short range. As a consequence, the nuclear forces are only effective between near neighbors. With more than 60 nucleons, very few are lacking the maximum number of neighbors, so any additional binding energy per nucleon is offset by charge repulsion.

The action of the attractive forces and the repelling forces is further modified by the magnetic forces resulting from the spinning and movement of the nucleons. Together these force the nucleons into orbitals of a sort around the center of the nucleus. These are not totally similar to electron orbitals since nucleons cannot be treated as point charges, nor do they orbit around an almost fixed object. Nevertheless, shells exist that add to the stability of the nucleus when they are full. Proton and neutron shells fill separately, with full shells occurring at 2, 8, 28, 50, 82, and 126. Let us look at some examples of stability. In Figure 20-2B, we see a point off the line which is $^4_2$He. Both protons and neutrons have full shells (2 nucleons) in $^4_2$He. The configuration is so stable that no five nucleon configuration exists and eight nucleon nuclei fall apart almost instantly into two helium nuclei. Oxygen ($Z = 8$) has three stable isotopes, which is unusual in an element with such a low atomic number, and nitrogen with 8 neutrons is stable. Carbon with 8 neutrons has the longest half-life of any isotope with a low atomic number. Tin ($Z = 50$) has ten stable isotopes. The full shell configuration is indeed very stable. Review of the other full shell configurations shows similar phenomena. These then are the factors that contribute to the structure of the nucleus.

Section 20-2
NUCLEAR RADIATION

The line in Figure 20-1 shows the N/Z ratio that stable or relatively stable nuclei exhibit. But what happens if a nucleus with a higher N/Z ratio comes into being? In effect, such a nucleus would have too many neutrons for the available protons. It is not possible to expel the excess neutrons under normal conditions because of the adverse affect on the binding energy. What then must be done?

One approach, we could imagine, would be to wave a magic wand and convert some of the neutrons into protons. This would restore the N/Z ratio to the appropriate level. In reality, a magic wand is not necessary because the available energy from such a change would be positive, and therefore, the process is spontaneous. In terms of our model, the neutrons are in higher orbitals, which means that their binding energy is less than that of extra protons in lower proton orbitals. Therefore, an increase in binding energy would occur if a neutron were converted to a proton. If that energy is greater than the rest mass of an electron, then the nucleus can afford to create and emit an electron and thereby reach a state of higher binding energy and higher stability.

There are two problems with our model, however. A proton, neutron, and electron each have a spin of $\frac{1}{2}$. Since angular momentum is conserved in nature, a particle with a spin of $\frac{1}{2}$ cannot split to give two other particles which also have a spin of $\frac{1}{2}$. Second, the kinetic energy of the electron and recoiling nucleus is frequently observed to be less than the energy equivalent to the mass difference between the parent and daughter nuclei. Figure 20-3 shows the typical energy distribution for such

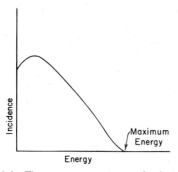

Figure 20-3 The energy spectrum of a beta particle from a typical beta emitter. The maximum energy is equivalent to the total mass lost.

electron emission. To save the basic physical tenets of conservation of energy and angular momentum, it is necessary to postulate that a third particle emanates from the conversion of a neutron to a proton and an electron. This particle has a spin of $\frac{1}{2}$ and is capable of absconding with various amounts of energy, but it has no rest mass, and, therefore, must travel at the speed of light. (Note: $\frac{1}{2} + \frac{1}{2} + \frac{1}{2}$ can equal $\frac{1}{2}$ because spins add as vectors and can have different orientations.)

The net equation for a neutron conversion to a proton is:

$$\,_0^1n \rightarrow \,_1^1p + \,_{-1}^0e + \,_0^0v \qquad (20\text{-}6)$$

The superscripts and subscripts are usually omitted on fundamental particles.

$$n \rightarrow p + e + v \qquad (20\text{-}7)$$

The particle that was postulated, and later discovered, to account for the energy difference and to provide for conservation of angular momentum is called the neutrino and is described in Table 20-1. The type of radiation process here presented was discovered just before the turn of the century and was given the name β radiation because it was the second type of nuclear radiation observed. The electron, the only particle then detectable in the decay, was initially called a "β particle." The identification of the β particle as an electron came shortly thereafter. Since the rest mass of the neutron is greater than that of a proton and electron combined, it would seem reasonable for a neutron

outside the nucleus to also spontaneously decay into a proton and electron. This, in fact, happens. The half-life (the time for half the original amount to decay) is about 12 minutes, with the decay curve being exponential.

Let us look at an example of β radiation. A most useful one is the decay of carbon-14.

$$\,_6^{14}C \rightarrow \,_7^{14}N + \beta^- + v \qquad (20\text{-}8)$$

The half-life of ^{14}C is 5700 years. Because of the low mass defect between the parent and daughter nuclei, the maximum available energy is only 150 keV (thousand electron volts). While ^{14}C has a relatively short half-life compared to some of the heavier elements, its concentration in the atmosphere remains relatively constant due to the nuclear collisions between cosmic rays and atmospheric nitrogen, which creates new ^{14}C and compensates for the material that decays.

This process of reducing the N/Z ratio seems straightforward and reasonable. What happens, on the other hand, if the N/Z ratio is too small? The most logical occurrence would be for the nucleus to expel a positive charge to create another neutron. This would be symmetrical to the previous process. In fact, this does happen in many cases, but it is accompanied by some *prima facie* difficulties. Since the proton is lighter than the neutron, proton to neutron decay outside the nucleus is impossible. Inside the nucleus the instability must be large to permit the loss of an electron mass, the smallest that can carry a charge. The positive particle with an electron mass was first called an antielectron, but the names "positive electron" and then "positron" have become more popular. The same problem with angular momentum and energy occurs as with β^- decay, so another particle had to be formulated to accommodate these properties. This particle is called the antineutrino and has the opposite spin of a neutrino. A typical β^+ decay is

$$\,_7^{13}N \rightarrow \,_6^{13}C + \beta^+ + \bar{v} \qquad (20\text{-}9)$$

Unfortunately, not all parent–daughter pairs that would benefit from β^+ decay have enough excess mass to produce a positron and the energy to expel it. For these another mechanism is available, which requires no mass loss whatsoever. The nucleus merely captures an electron to neutralize one of the positive charges. This is, at best, a tricky procedure because electrons do not readily enter the nucleus to combine with nucleons. Head-on collisions between stray electrons and nuclei are incredibly rare due to an electron shell repulsion, the slingshot effect, and quantum mechanical wave requirements. It is possible under extremely favorable conditions, on the other hand, for a nucleus to capture one of its own electrons to cause the neutralization. The easiest electron to capture is one from the K shell, leading to the name of the process: K capture.

$$e + p \rightarrow n + \bar{\nu} \qquad \text{(20-10)}$$

An example of K capture is

$$^7_4\text{Be} \xrightarrow{K} {}^7_3\text{Li} \qquad \text{(20-11)}$$

Because they accomplish the same thing, K capture and β^+ decay can be competing processes. Some nuclei, such as $^{18}_9\text{F}$, undergo both. The situation is even further complicated by the fact that all nuclei with an odd number of both protons and neutrons, except in the lower part of the periodic table, are unstable, but frequently the isotopes of both adjacent even elements with the same mass number (isobars) are stable. Competing processes also exist here. For example,

$$^{122}_{51}\text{Sb} \rightarrow {}^{122}_{50}\text{Sn} + \beta^+ \qquad \text{(20-12)}$$

$$^{122}_{51}\text{Sb} \rightarrow {}^{122}_{52}\text{Te} + \beta^- \qquad \text{(20-13)}$$

Note that the neutrinos are usually omitted when writing elemental decay equations.

The half-life of most β emitters is so short that their concentration is rapidly depleted. Their existence might have remained undiscovered for many more years had it not been for the α emitters. The heaviest naturally occurring elements (uranium and thorium) are not stable. The intranuclear forces are weakened by the concentrated positive charge to the point where, if given their choice, nuclei of these elements would spontaneously split into two or more stable nuclei. The difficulty with such splitting is that half of a heavier nucleus is not stable either. Take, for example, $^{238}_{92}\text{U}$, the heaviest naturally occurring nucleus. Half of this would be $^{119}_{46}\text{Pd}$, but this isotope cannot even form because it is so highly unstable. Only tin ($Z = 50$) has a stable iso-

tope at 119, but it is four units higher on the atomic number scale. Heavier nuclei, such as uranium, are just too neutron rich to be able to decay by spontaneous fission, at least from their ground states.

Heavier nuclei are not helped by β decay, either. Negative β decay creates more protons, which further strains the binding force. Positive β decay creates more neutrons, which are forced into very high nuclear neutron shells where bonding forces are weak. Neither of these transformations improves the situation. The most logical solution would be to expel a proton or neutron to reduce the mass. Unfortunately, the rest mass of a neutron plus that of the daughter element ^{237}U is greater than that of ^{238}U. Since such a process is endothermic, it cannot happen spontaneously. The situation with a proton and ^{237}Pa is just as bad. In fact, the expulsion of a nucleon from the ground state is not energetically favorable for any of the heavy naturally occurring elements.

Yet uranium is radioactive; in fact, it undergoes the first type of radiation discovered: alpha (α) radiation. This type of disintegration is possible due to the abnormally high binding energy and, therefore, abnormally low mass, of the helium nucleus ^4He. The four particles (two protons and two neutrons) fill the inner nuclear shell for each type of particle. The ability of each of the nucleons to interact with each other further enhances bonding. As a result, if the masses of the helium nucleus and of ^{234}Th are added together, they are less than the mass of the ^{238}U nucleus. Consequently, ^{238}U can spontaneously split into ^{234}Th and ^4He. The bare helium—four nucleons without any electrons—is called an alpha particle (α).

$$^{238}\text{U} \rightarrow {}^{234}\text{Th} + \alpha \qquad \text{(20-14)}$$

EXAMPLE 20-1

If the mass of a proton is 1.00728, of a neutron is 1.00867, and of an α particle is 4.00249, and if 1 dalton is $1.661 \cdot 10^{-24}$ g, 1 eV is $1.603 \cdot 10^{-12}$ erg, the speed of light is $2.998 \cdot 10^{10}$ cm/sec, and the units of the erg are gram centimeters squared per second squared, calculate the binding energy (B.E.) per nucleon of an alpha particle.

Solution: $\Delta m = Z m_p + N m_n - m_A$

$$= 2 \times 1.00728 + 2 \times 1.00867$$

$$- 4.00249$$

$\Delta m = 0.02941 \text{ dalton}$

$\Delta m = 0.02941 \times 1.661 \cdot 10^{-24} \text{ g}$

$$= 4.885 \cdot 10^{-26} \text{ g}$$

$E_e = \Delta m c^2$

$$= 4.885 \cdot 10^{-26} (2.998 \cdot 10^{10})^2$$

$E_e = 4.391 \cdot 10^{-5} \text{ g cm}^2/\text{sec}^2$

$E_e = 4.391 \cdot 10^{-5}/1.603 \cdot 10^{-12}$

$$= 27.39 \text{ MeV/nucleon}$$

$\text{B.E.} = \dfrac{E}{A} = \dfrac{27.43}{4} = 6.85 \text{ MeV/nucleon}$ ∎

The fact that the ^{238}U and other heavy elements can emit α particles does not mean that they do so with great facility. To escape from the nucleus, the α particle must first form and then escape from the local nuclear forces. An elementary sketch of the potential well the α particle faces is shown in Figure 20-4. The mass defect between the parent and

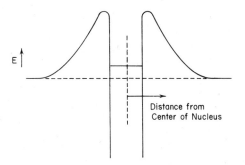

Figure 20-4 The energy level of the nucleus with the mass of the alpha particle as part of it is greater than the total energy after the loss of the alpha particle. A significant energy barrier, however, exists to the decay in the form of nuclear forces, which must be either overcome or tunnelled through.

the daughter components greatly affects the rate of the decay. A 10% increase in the available energy from the mass defect will decrease the half-life by a factor of 100 or more. The half-life of many heavy elements is measured in millions or billions of years.

There are four possible radioactive series among the heavy elements because the mass of the α particle means a leap-frogging of four mass units will occur every time one is emitted. One of these series does not exist because none of the isotopes has a long half-life. The three series that do exist start with ^{235}U, ^{236}U, and ^{238}U, respectively. All of them end in isotopes of lead. The "uranium series," named after the long-lived isotope ^{238}U in the series, is shown in Figure 20-5. Note that the series has some branches resulting from competitive decay routes. In all cases the end product is the same. The tremendous loss of mass (32 amu) and the number of radioactive decays (14) indicate the great instability that exists in the heavier elements. The fact that a closed shell of protons exists at 82 and of neutrons at 126 (for series ending in ^{208}Pb and ^{209}Bi) is probably responsible for the sudden stop to the radioactive decay.

The final type of radiation we must examine is gamma (γ) radiation. Whereas α and β radiation are classical particles, γ radiation is electronmagnetic radiation, as is visible light. The amount of energy in a typical γ ray can vary from several thousand to several million electron volts. Because of the large amount of energy involved, the wavelengths of γ rays are very short. The longer wavelengths are on the order of x-rays.

Since the photon, which is the particle of the γ radiation, has neither rest mass nor charge, it has no net effect on the composition of the nucleus. It arises from the efforts of a nucleus to reach its ground state. Nuclei become excited by nuclear collision or by nuclear decay. When a nucleus finds itself in an excited state, it can use the extra energy to undergo nuclear fission (as ^{235}U does when hit by a neutron), it can expel a nucleon (as ^{18}F does after being formed by a collision of ^{4}He and ^{14}N), or it can eject light radiation (a γ ray) to move to the ground state (as ^{204}Pb does after formation). Energy levels exist in the nucleus much as in the electron

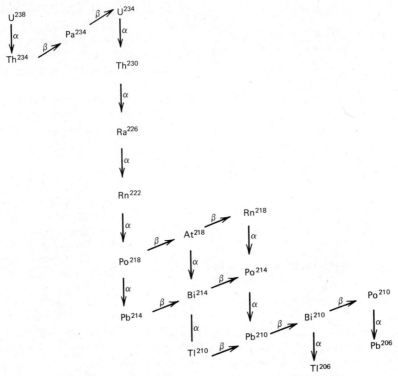

Figure 20-5 The decay series of ^{238}U, the uranium series.

shell, so the wavelengths of γ radiation emitted will reflect the energy differences between levels. The interactions of nuclear radiation with matter, which are necessary to permit detection, lead, however, to significant spectral broadening and not a clean line spectrum. The study of nuclear energy levels is difficult due to the large amount of energy needed to excite nuclei (particle accelerators with millions of electron volts are needed) and the relatively short half-lives of many of the excited states ($\sim 10^{-20}$ seconds).

The mathematics of nuclear decay are relatively simple because such decay is a first-order kinetic process. This means the rate of decay is proportional to the amount of material present at any specified time. This is identical to what we saw when we studied the capacitor. The decay constant, which is the inverse of the time constant as seen with capacitors and inductors, is designated by the symbol λ. The radioactive decay equation is

$$N = N_0 \exp(-\lambda t) \qquad \text{(20-15)}$$

In this equation N_0 is the amount (in moles or grams) of material present originally, and N is the amount of material present after time t.

The decay constant is seldom used to characterize the radioactive process. In its place the time for half the original amount to decay, called the half-life ($t_{\frac{1}{2}}$), is used. We can find it in terms of the decay constant by setting N/N_0 equal to $\frac{1}{2}$.

$$\frac{N}{N_0} = \frac{1}{2} = \exp(-\lambda t_{\frac{1}{2}})$$

$$\ln \frac{1}{2} = -\ln 2 = -\lambda t_{\frac{1}{2}}$$

$$t_{\frac{1}{2}} = \frac{\ln 2}{\lambda} = \frac{0.693}{\lambda} \qquad \text{(20-16)}$$

If both the parent and the daughter are radioactive, as in the uranium series, then the change in the amount of daughter present is equal to the amount being created through the decay of the parent minus that being lost through the decay of the daughter. This yields a complicated equation and will not be considered further.

EXAMPLE 20-2

What amount of ^{90}Sr is left after 18.7 years if its half-life is 28.1 years and 71.4 μmoles were originally present?

Solution:

$$\lambda = \frac{0.693}{28.1} = 0.0247 \ y^{-1}$$

$$N = N_o \exp(-\lambda t)$$

$$= 71.4 \cdot 10^{-6} \exp(-0.0247 \times 18.7)$$

$$N = 45.0 \ \mu\text{moles} \qquad \blacksquare$$

Section **20-3**
RADIATION AND MATTER

For radiation to be measured, it must interact with matter. Such interaction was first observed by Marie Curie when her photographic plates were exposed by contact with pitchblende, an ore containing uranium and its daughter elements. Since then, the ways that radiation affects matter and vice-versa have been extensively studied.

Alpha particles are frequently emitted from nuclei at high energy (several MeV). Due to their relatively large mass and energy, but small size, they will travel in straight lines through the electron cloud of the surrounding atoms. The positive charge will rip electrons out of their orbitals and cause them to scatter. These electrons are referred to as delta radiation, and the particle that causes them is sometimes called ionizing radiation. The effect of dislodging these electrons is to rapidly reduce the energy of the α particle. Eventually that energy is reduced so much that the α particle will actually capture two of the electrons it has freed and will become a helium atom. When it reaches this point, it is no longer distinguishable from other helium atoms. The atoms ionized by the α particle will undergo reactions with their neighbors that they might not otherwise undergo. This is why radiation can cause burns, cancer, and genetic defects. Fortunately, despite their initial energy, α particles interact so strongly with matter that they can be stopped by a piece of paper or the skin of the body. They, therefore, pose a serious problem only in cases of very large exposure or ingestion. This same inability to penetrate, however, makes α particles difficult to measure routinely. The coatings of most probes will completely block this type of radiation.

Beta radiation interacts with matter somewhat differently. Again the electrons are affected, but unlike α particles, which scatter electrons like a bowling ball scatters pins, β^- particles interact with other electrons more like billiard balls colliding. The electrons do not physically collide, but their electric fields do interact at short range, which gives the same effect as an elastic particle collision. The initial energy of the β^- particle is split between itself and the electron with which it collided. The results of such a collision can be calculated by simple vector algebra. After a few collisions in which electrons are kicked out of their orbitals or excited, the β^- particle has slowed enough to be captured by an atom and to disappear as a spent force. Positive β radiation will interact with electrons more like very low energy α particles, but it will physically collide with an electron as it loses energy and be annihilated to form two γ rays. The penetrating power of β radiation is much greater than that of α radiation. It requires 1 or 2 cm of dense material such as a book, a piece of wood, or a human hand to stop a β particle. As such, it poses a more substantial threat to vital body organs. It is also considerably easier to measure because it can penetrate a thin cover to enter a counting chamber.

Of the fundamental types of radiation, γ rays have the weakest interaction with matter. Moreover, there are several distinct ways in which γ rays act upon electrons and vice-versa. The first of these is the photoelectric effect, which garnered its discoverer, Albert Einstein, the Nobel Prize. In it a γ ray strikes an electron and knocks it out of orbit, giving all its energy to the electron and thereby

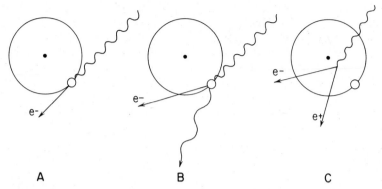

Figure 20-6 Gamma radiation interacts with matter by the photoelectric effect (A), Compton effect (B), or pair production (C).

disappearing (Fig. 20-6A). This event is most likely to occur if the energy of the γ ray is less than 0.5 MeV.

The second way that γ rays interact with electrons is by the Compton effect. A γ ray with energy between 0.50 and 1.02 MeV strikes an electron and knocks it out of orbit (Fig. 20-6B). In the collision a second γ ray with lower energy is created. The direction and momentum of each particle after collision is dependent on the direction and momentum before collision. The variability of energy available to the second γ ray will, therefore, result in a wavelength spectrum for this radiation.

Finally, a γ ray can be split by the electric field near the nucleus to give an electron and a positron

(Fig. 20-6C). This is a classical conversion of energy to mass and must obey Eq. 20-5. To occur, the energy of the γ ray must be greater than 1.02 MeV, which is the rest mass of two electrons. The remainder of the energy is split between the two particles. The electron and positron behave as β^- and β^+ radiation.

The penetrating power of γ radiation is very great. It takes two meters of concrete or many centimeters of lead to stop a γ ray. Due to the weak interaction with matter, γ rays are not as easy to count as β radiation. A dense material is needed to guarantee that the chances of an individual γ ray being seen are large enough to get an accurate count.

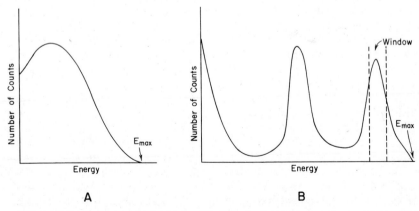

Figure 20-7 Alpha and beta spectra (A) differ from those of gamma emitters (B).

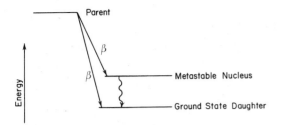

Figure 20-8 Beta decay can leave nuclei in unstable states that lead to subsequent gamma radiation.

The amount of interaction that one can expect between radiation and matter is a function of the energy of the radiation. Figure 20-7 shows the different energy spectra of radiation. Alpha and beta particles have a specific mass, as do the ground state parent and daughter nuclei whose metamorphosis they facilitate. The mass difference, as previously mentioned, must appear as kinetic energy. E_{max} is the maximum energy that an α or β particle can receive if it receives all of this energy. Most particles receive less than the maximum amount of energy. The remaining energy is absorbed by nuclear recoil, neutrino emission, or an excited energy state in the daughter nucleus.

Gamma radiation results from a transition between nuclear energy levels (Fig. 20-8). As a result, it will peak at those numbers that represent the energy differences between two nuclear energy states. Energy spectra of gamma emitters are indicative of the isotopes involved, much as line spectra are indicative of specific elements.

Section 20-4
METHODS OF COUNTING

The original method of nuclear detection was the photographic plate. These plates showed the tracks of particles in the plane of the plate. Such tracks were used to determine the mass and charge of radiation particles. To determine three-dimensional activity, the plates were stacked many layers thick. Electric and magnetic fields were supplied to cause particles with different m/e ratios to curve to different extents or in different directions if they possessed different charges.

These clumsy photographic emulsion stacks have been replaced with cloud chambers (Fig. 20-9A). The atmosphere of the chamber is supersaturated with moisture. An electric field is applied across the chamber, which will cause charged particles to be deflected. As radiation occurs, the ions created along the radiation track will act as the seed to form droplets. This will make the track visible. Because we are only interested in the number of disintegrations per unit time and in the amount of energy they generate (in some cases), we need not use such a complex and delicate detector in the clinical laboratory.

Another type of detector is the Geiger–Mueller (G–M) counter, the device used by prospectors. The detector portion of the instrument is shown in Fig. 20-9B. The tube is made of glass with an extremely thin mica end that acts as a window to let in the radiation. The anode is a tungsten wire in the center of the tube, while the cathode is a copper cylinder. A potential of 1000–2500 V is maintained between the electrodes. The gas in the tube is composed of 80 torr of argon and 20 torr of chlorine or volatile organic molecule.

When ionizing radiation enters the tube, it knocks electrons out of the argon atoms. These electrons are rapidly accelerated in the strong electrical field. Thus energized, they knock additional electrons from argon atoms on their way to the anode. When they strike the anode, they release photons that ionize more argon. As a consequence, within a microsecond a large avalanche of electrons is racing toward the anode and a cloud of argon ions is headed for the cathode. This causes a 1 to 10 volt pulse to occur and the tube to conduct current. Within a short time the argon ions will interact with the chlorine or organic molecules and steal their electrons. These bulkier molecules will then proceed to the cathode. While progressing, however, their positive charge will shield the area around the anode from the negative cathode and greatly reduce the field strength. This will interrupt the cycle of electrons creating photons creating ions which release electrons, the cycle initially causing the tube to discharge. After 200 μsec, the molecular ions will reach the cathode and be neutralized without generating more photons, as might happen with smaller ions. As a result, the discharge is

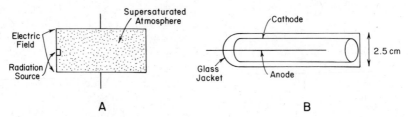

Figure 20-9 Diagram of a cloud chamber (A) and a Geiger–Mueller tube (B).

quenched, and the tube returns to a quiescent state. Due to this large dead time during which additional radiation cannot cause a discharge, the Geiger–Mueller tube has a maximum counting rate of 15 thousand counts per minute. The reactions in the tube are

$$\beta + Ar \rightarrow Ar^+ + 2e \qquad \textbf{(20-17)}$$

$$e + Ar \rightarrow Ar^+ + 2e \qquad \textbf{(20-18)}$$

$$h\nu + Ar \rightarrow Ar^+ + e \qquad \textbf{(20-19)}$$

$$e + W^+ \rightarrow W + h\nu \qquad \textbf{(20-20)}$$

$$Ar^+ + Q \rightarrow Ar + Q^+ \qquad \textbf{(20-21)}$$

The G–M tube is a good counter for moderate and high energy β radiation. Alpha radiation and low energy β radiation, such as that from radioactive elements commonly used in the clinical laboratory, cannot penetrate the mica window. Gamma radiation interacts poorly with the argon atoms, and therefore the G–M tube is not as sensitive to γ rays. The G–M counter suffers from other liabilities regarding its usefulness in the clinical laboratory. With organic quenching agents, molecular dissociation causes the tube to age. The energy level of the radiation cannot be determined because all radiation causes a complete discharge of the tube. For accurate counting the tube must be well shielded from stray radiation. On the positive side, the counting circuitry is simple because the pulses from the tube are large enough not to require amplification.

Beta counting is routinely done in the clinical laboratory by means of a liquid scintillation (LS) counter. Scintillation counters record light pulses occurring when radiation excites light-emitting materials. The light emitted when such scintillators again relax is measured by a photomultiplier tube.

Liquid scintillation counting takes advantage of β particles' relatively strong interaction with matter. After the β particle emerges from the nucleus, it encounters numerous solvent molecules, which it excites by dislodging their electrons. This energy is translated into physical motion. Within the solvent are molecules of a compound called a "fluor," which, when excited by electrons or ions, emits radiation in the UV or visible region of the spectrum and which can, therefore, be readily detected by a photomultiplier tube. Each disintegration will produce a pulse of radiation from the fluors along its trace, and these are counted to give the final result. Liquid scintillation counting is especially useful for weak β emitters, such as ^{14}C ($E_{max} = 150$ keV) and ^{3}H ($E_{max} = 18$ keV). Such radiation has trouble penetrating the cover on other counters and is not detectable by them. These isotopes are useful because they can easily be incorporated in body molecules.

To carry out liquid scintillation counting, it is necessary to get the sample and the fluor both within a suitable solvent, such as toluene or dioxane. Such mixtures are called cocktails. If both sample and fluor are not readily soluble, a stable emulsion may be adequate. The fluor is normally a heterocyclic organic compound whose mole fraction is 0.1 to 1 percent of the cocktail.

The geometry of an LS counter is shown in Figure 20-10. Two photomultiplier tubes monitor the cocktail from opposite sides. The light produced by particles from radioactive decay will be adequate to trigger both photomultiplier tubes. The presence of

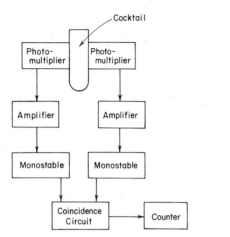

Figure 20-10 Block diagram of a liquid scintillation counter.

two pulses, therefore, indicates a disintegration and is counted. If only one pulse is detected, it is probably the result of a thermal electron in one of the detectors and not of radioactive decay. It is not counted. Thermal noise can be reduced by cooling the counting chamber.

An example of coincidence circuitry is given in Figure 20-11. After amplification, the pulses are extended by monostable circuits to allow for slight time discrepancies (10–20 nsec) and then ANDed.

A pulse will appear at the output and be counted only if the two pulses overlap.

The greatest drawback to LS is quenching, which reduces the count artificially by limiting the number of photons that reach the detector. Quenching can be caused by several factors. Chemical quenching is caused by impurities in the sample or the solvent. The foreign chemicals absorb energy from the excited solvent molecules, but do not transmit it to the fluor, thereby reducing light intensity. Optical quenching occurs in emulsions when suspended material absorbs radiated energy. Dilution quenching results from an insufficient amount of fluor to be excited. Color quenching happens when colored biological material of the sample is present in solution and absorbs the radiation given off by common fluors. Such foreign material can often be detected visually because counting cocktails are normally light blue.

Quenching increases the amount of radiation seen at lower energy and decreases the amount seen at higher energy (Fig. 20-12). The low energy β particles may not produce enough light to be detected. Such an occurrence will lower the overall counting frequency and cause inaccurate results. The counts measured are always lower than the actual counts even under the best circumstances because low energy β particles are not detected. The ratio of the counted disintegrations to the ac-

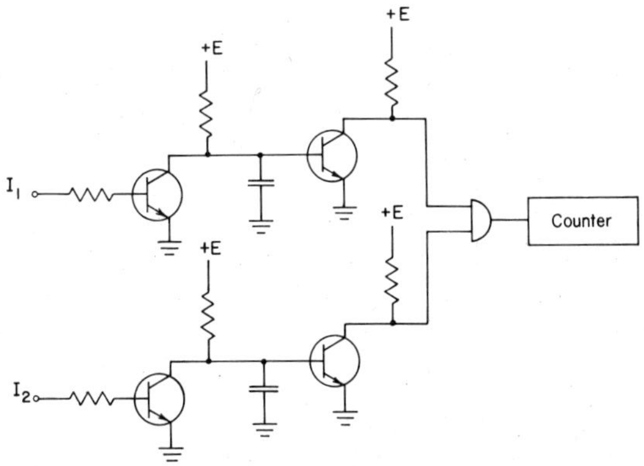

Figure 20-11 Simplified circuit diagram of two monostables and a coincidence counter.

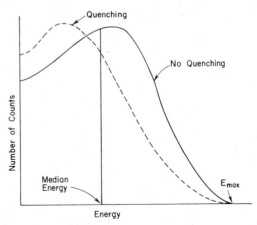

Figure 20-12 Quenching distorts the energy spectrum of beta radiation.

tual disintegrations is called the counting efficiency.

$$\% \text{ Efficiency} = \frac{\text{counted disintegrations}}{\text{actual disintegrations}} \times 100 \quad \textbf{(20-22)}$$

This efficiency will range from nearly 100% for a strong β emitter to less than 50% for ^3H when severe quenching is present. An instrument must normally be calibrated versus standards, and the results must be corrected for counting efficiency even without quenching.

When quenching is present, more complex corrections are needed. The two most common approaches are the standard addition method and channel ratio method. With standard addition the specimen is counted once in the ordinary fashion. Radiation is then added to the specimen in the form of a known amount of sought-for substance (internal standard) or a known number of Compton electrons created by γ radiation from outside the specimen (external standard). It is assumed that these new electrons are quenched to the same extent as the old and, therefore, that the ratio of the added counts (SC) to the added disintegrations (SD) will be the same as the unknown counts (UC) to the unknown disintegrations (UD).

$$UD = \frac{(UC)(SD)}{(SC)} \quad \textbf{(20-23)}$$

The channel ratio method requires that the signal from the detectors be split. One part of the signal is treated normally. The other part is screened with a voltage threshold (Chapter 18), which is set at a voltage level to reject half the pulses detected when counting an unquenched standard (Fig. 20-12). When quenching occurs, the lower half of the energy pulses will grow relative to the upper half. The ratio of the two channels gives the fraction of the counts in the lower half. This number is used with a table that relates the counting efficiency to the channel ratio for a particular instrument, and the table value is used to correct the count for quenching.

Quenching corrections are not always perfect. They suffer from pipetting error, changes of solution matrix, dissimilarities between Compton elec-

trons and β radiation, and the shape of the quenching curve. Quenching and the complexity of sample preparation are two reasons for the declining populatiry of LS versus γ counting.

Gamma counting is another name frequently used for crystal scintillation counting, although crystal scintillation can be used for β counting also. Unlike LS, in crystal scintillation counting, the crystal holds the fluor, but not the sample. Gamma radiation from the sample enters the crystal, excites the fluor by the photoelectric and Compton effects, and causes light to be given off. This is measured by a photomultiplier tube and tabulated to give the result. (Fig. 20-13 shows a diagram of a crystal scintillation counter.) The crystal is very pure NaI with 1% of thallium added as the fluor for counting γ radiation. (Anthracene or stilbene are used as both crystal and fluor for high energy β counting.) Because the crystal is hydroscopic, it must be enclosed in an aluminum case, which also protects it from sample contamination. The crystals are 5–8 cm in diameter, which is long enough for the energy of the scattered electrons to be dissipated and, therefore, to generate the maximum amount of radiation. The sample is placed into a well in the center top of the crystal, and a light-tight cover is placed over the compartment. The crystal is bonded to the window of a photomultiplier tube so that all the radiation will be detected.

The dead time of the P-M tube between counts is roughly 0.2 μsec for sodium iodide crystals and 0.02 μsec for organic crystals. The counting rate can, therefore, be extremely high. The size of the

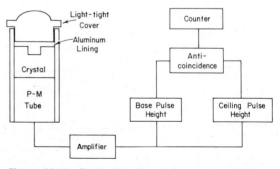

Figure 20-13 Block diagram of a crystal scintillation counter.

pulse from the P-M tube is proportional to the amount of light given off by the fluor, which is proportional to the energy of the radiation. This fact can be used to count one γ emitter in the presence of another.

The output from the photomultiplier tube is amplified and then supplied to two comparators (Fig. 20-14). A different voltage offset is applied to each comparator. As a consequence, pulses that pass the comparator with the lower threshold will not always pass the comparator with the higher threshold, but the converse is always true. The output of these two comparators is fed into an anticoincidence device, which will allow a pulse to pass if one and only one of the comparators produces a voltage spike. From Chapter 8 it should be clear that this device is just an EXCLUSIVE OR gate. The voltage of the lower comparator is frequently called the base discriminator (E_B in Fig. 20-14), and the voltage difference between the two comparators is called the window (E_W).

Gamma radiation occurs at energy levels equal to the difference in energy levels between two nuclear states (Fig. 20-8). The window is set so that only disintegrations with energy levels near a specific transition will be counted (Fig. 20-7). This allows for some energy level broadening through the interactions of the γ radiation with matter, but limits the amount of noise from background radiation and permits the counting of one γ emitter in the presence of another. The windows used are of the order of 0.1 MeV or less. Some instruments attach several pairs of comparators to the output of the P-M tube. This allows one isotope to be counted at several energy levels or several isotopes to be counted simultaneously.

Crystal scintillation counting has a distinct advantage over liquid scintillation counting in ease of use and lack of quenching. The major disadvantage is that the half-lives of the useful γ emitters are short ($^{131}I = 8$ days, $^{125}I = 57$ days). This results from the greater instability of the nucleus, which is necessary to produce the energy needed to give off this type of radiation. Unfortunately, it means that one's measuring tool has a short shelf life and must be reprocured frequently. By contrast, the half-life of ^3H is 12 years and ^{14}C is 5700 years. Gamma emitters also pose a greater health hazard to the technologist, but are generally used in such low quantities as to be extremely safe. Radioactive material is measured in curies, 1 curie being $2.22 \cdot 10^{12}$ disintegrations per minute. Only a small fraction of a curie is used in any laboratory measurement.

Radiation is most commonly used for measurements in immunology and endocrinology. A common technique is radioimmunoassay (RIA). Radiation can also be used to measure the growth of bacteria. Such measurements, as well as those based on other principles, will be covered in the next chapter, which is on microbiological instrumentation.

REVIEW QUESTIONS

1. How did the work of Thomson and Millikan allow the mass of the electron to be determined?
2. What is the relative mass of the electron?
3. What phenomenon concerning atomic mass led to the nuclear theory?
4. How did Thomson discover that neon had isotopes?
5. How is the atomic number of an atom defined?
6. How was the neutron discovered?
7. How does the number of nucleons relate to the atomic number?
8. What is the mass defect?
9. Why does the mass defect hold the nucleus together?
10. What is the nuclear binding energy?

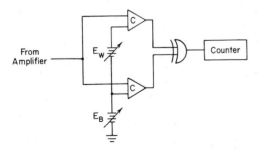

Figure 20-14 Circuit diagram of a pair of pulse height discriminators and an anticoincidence counter.

11. What is the shape of the binding energy-per-nucleon curve?
12. What is the relative binding energy of nucleons and electrons?
13. Why do nuclear fission and fusion work?
14. What two forces affect the nuclear binding energy?
15. What is the nature of nuclear shells?
16. Why are five-nucleon combinations so unstable?
17. What happens when the N/Z ratio causes deviation from the line in Figure 20-1?
18. What is β radiation?
19. How do the two types of β radiation differ?
20. Why must the neutrino exist?
21. What are the properties of a neutrino?
22. Why can a free neutron decay into a free proton, but not vice-versa?
23. What are the decay equations for ^{14}C, n, and ^{13}N?
24. What is K capture?
25. Why does K capture occur?
26. What competitive nuclear decay procedures occur in most nuclei with odd numbers of both protons and neutrons? Give an example.
27. What is α decay?
28. In what elements is α decay most common?
29. Why does α decay occur in preference to other possible forms of radiation?
30. What is a radioactive decay series?
31. What is the relationship between members of a radioactive series?
32. Why do some radioactive nuclei decay so slowly?
33. What are γ rays? Why do they occur?
34. Why is γ radiation so powerful?
35. What equation governs radioactive decay?
36. Define half-life.
37. What type of process is nuclear decay?
38. Describe the interaction of α particles with matter.
39. What is the penetrating power of α particles? β particles? γ radiation?
40. What is delta radiation?
41. How do β particles interact with matter?
42. What happens when a β^+ particle encounters an electron?

43. In what three ways does γ radiation interact with matter?
44. What is the photoelectric effect?
45. Describe the Comptom effect.
46. What is necessary for pair production?
47. At what energy levels do the various γ ray interactions with matter occur?
48. Contrast the β and γ ray spectra.
49. Describe the photographic emulsion stack. Why was it used?
50. Sketch and label the parts of the Geiger–Mueller (G–M) tube.
51. Describe the operation of the G–M tube.
52. What is the maximum counting rate of the G–M tube?
53. What are the principal reactions of the G–M tube?
54. What is scintillation?
55. What are the principles involved in liquid scintillation?
56. Describe the LS cocktail.
57. Describe the counting circuitry of an LS counter.
58. What is quenching?
59. Name and describe several types of quenching.
60. Define counting efficiency.
61. What is standard addition?
62. Describe the use of the channel ratio correction.
63. What are some limits to the effectiveness of quenching corrections?
64. Describe γ counting.
65. Why must the counting crystal have a metal case?
66. Sketch and label the electronic components of a γ counter.
67. Why are energy windows used in γ counting?
68. What are the advantages of γ counting over LS? Disadvantages?

PROBLEMS

1. What are the products of the following β^- decays?
   a. ^{43}K **b.** ^{73}Ga **c.** ^{88}Rb **d.** ^{110}Ag

2. What are the products of the following β^+ decays?
   a. ^{21}Na   **b.** ^{54}Co   **c.** ^{82}Rb   **d.** ^{127}Cs

3. What are the products of the following α decays?
   a. ^{147}Sm   **b.** ^{163}Ho   **c.** ^{192}Pt   **d.** ^{205}Rn

4. What are the products of the following nuclear reactions?
   a. $^2_1$H $+ \, ^2_1$H $\rightarrow \, ^3_2$He $+$?
   b. $n + \, ^{11}_5$B $\rightarrow$ 3? $+ \, ^0_{-1}e$
   c. $\alpha + \, ^{13}_6$C $\rightarrow \, ^{16}_7$N $+$?
   d. $^3_1$H $+ \, ^3_2$He $\rightarrow \, ^4_2$He $+$?

5. ^{235}U decays into ^{207}Pb. Give a reasonable decay series for this change.

6. ^{233}U decays into ^{209}Bi. Give a reasonable decay series for this change.

7. The nuclear mass of ^{72}Ge is 71.9042. What is its binding energy per nucleon?

8. The nuclear mass of ^{11}B is 11.00659. What is its binding energy per nucleon?

9. The nuclear mass of ^{235}U is 234.9938. What is its binding energy per nucleon?

10. If the binding energies per nucleon are the values given below, what are the masses? Make reasonable assumptions about the N/Z ratios.
    a. 7.41 at mass 20
    b. 8.41 at mass 65
    c. 7.91 at mass 194

11. If 14.72% of an element is left after 253 years, what is its half-life?

12. If one starts out with 217.5 g and has 14.57 μg left after 360.2 days, what is the half-life of the substance?

13. If there are initially 0.04377 moles, how much is left after 1.40 days if the half-life is 80.0 minutes?

14. If one starts with 98.1 mg of a substance with a half-life of 64.7 days, how much does one have left after exactly one fortnight?

15. If there are 72.5 μg left after 36.2 minutes, what was the original amount present if the half-life is 20.5 minutes?

16. How much material was present 4.00 hours ago if currently there are 322.6 mg and the half-life is 72.6 minutes?

CHAPTER 21
MICROBIOLOGICAL INSTRUMENTS

The development of instrumentation for microbiology has been slow. In part, this is due to the difference in measuring techniques used in microbiology compared to those used in the rest of the clinical laboratory. In chemistry and hematology what is of interest is already present in large enough quantities to detect by light or electrode measurements. In microbiological analysis, the bacteria or fungi of interest are present in such small quantities that they cannot be readily observed. To grow, identify, and enumerate these microorganisms take time. While instrumentation can reduce this time, it cannot produce the same throughput observed in the other parts of the laboratory.

The development of instrumentation is further complicated by the large number of possible outcomes from a microbiological investigation and the greatly divergent paths that can be followed based on what is found. For example, the only sample-related complication to a glucose analysis is its falling outside the range of accuracy of the instrument. A microbiological analysis may dictate the use of several media and turn up three or four organisms requiring different sets of biochemicals to identify and different antibiotics at different concentration levels to destroy. To be completely automatic, an instrument would have to perform this whole analysis without human intervention. Such a complex instrument does not exist now and may never be built. Instrumentation in microbiology has instead been aimed at assisting the microbiologist in specific phases of the analysis and is, therefore, only semiautomatic. We will examine a number of these instruments to see how previously introduced principles can be applied to the identification and enumeration of bacteria.

Section 21-1
MEASUREMENT BY RADIATION

Johnston Laboratories has created a group of instruments to analyze bacterial growth based on the metabolism of radioactive media. Their instruments are sold under the name Bactec. The analysis is carried out in bottles filled with measured amounts of media containing ^{14}C. These bottles are safe to handle because the weak β^- radiation cannot penetrate the glass bottles. A rubber septum acts as the stopper and entry port for specimen and reagents. The bottle is inoculated by a syringe filled with blood, urine, or spinal fluid, as appropriate, and agitated in an incubator for several hours. During this time any bacteria present and capable of metabolizing the media will release waste CO_2 into the atmosphere of the bottle. Some of this gas will be radioactive.

After the incubation period the bottles are placed in a four-bottle rack inside the Bactec. These bottles are moved sequentially into the sampling mechanism. A two-needle probe pierces the septum of the bottle (Fig. 21-1). A sterile gas of known composition (culture gas) is used to flush the atmosphere of the bottle into an ion chamber. Within the chamber the radioactive decay creates ions. An electrical field is applied within the chamber, and the current is proportional to the amount of radioactive decay occurring. Since the amount of radiation detected is proportional to the amount of bacterial growth in the bottle, a determination of the bacterial concentration is obtained from this measurement. The process can be repeated several times to detect various rates of growth.

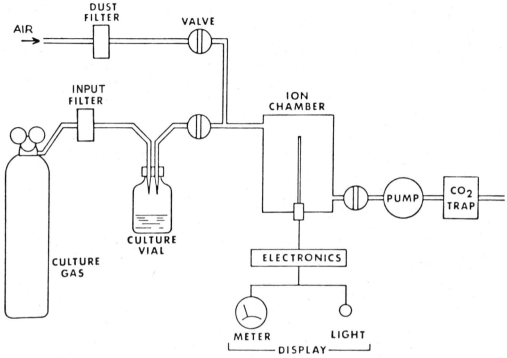

Figure 21-1 Block diagram of the Bactec. (Courtesy of Johnston Laboratories.)

After being counted, the radioactive CO_2 is trapped to prevent it from contaminating the laboratory. The ion chamber is flushed with filtered room air. This air is counted and provides a background correction for the next sample. This correction is applied automatically by the electronics. The sample probes are sterilized at 160° between bottles to prevent cross-contamination.

The reporting electronics of the Bactec are relatively simple. The current measured in the ion chamber is converted to a digital value and corrected for background. The value is then displayed on a meter, printed on a paper strip, and used to activate a panel indicator light if growth has occurred. An attachment is available to record the information on a card for easier filing.

The advantages of the Bactec are its relative ease of use and the speed at which it can detect organism growth. It will detect growth at $5 \cdot 10^5$ to 10^6 bacteria per milliliter. On the other hand, it can only do a limited number of identifications based on different media and cannot determine minimum inhibitory concentrations (MICs) of drugs. Its primary function is the detection of growth. The use of the Bactec also means the presence of radioactive material in the laboratory which, while not dangerous, brings with it numerous new rules of operation and requires additional training.

Section 21-2
OPTICAL METHODS

By far the most popular method of detecting bacterial growth is optical. Numerous manufacturers have adopted this approach, and we will review a few of the principles commonly used. All methods must consist of an inoculation step, some form of incubation, and reading. The reading step may be repeated numerous times, specimens may be reinoculated along the way, and manual transport is almost always necessary somewhere in the process. Some steps may be totally manual.

The simplest form of microbiological instrument is one in which the only automated step is the data analysis. A broth is prepared and placed in a shallow tray. A plastic plate with multiple prongs is placed into the tray to pick up the broth as liquid adhering to the prongs. These prongs are arranged so as to fit into the wells of a prepackaged reagent plate. These wells contain various biochemicals and drugs so that both the identification and MICs can be determined. After overnight incubation, the plate is placed on the reader. The technologist visually inspects each well and pushes the corresponding button if growth has occurred. The instrument codes the responses in terms of an index number, which it looks up in an organism table to find the organism identification. Alternately, it may output the number for the technologist to look up manually. These index numbers consist of one binary digit for each biochemical present. These lists are grouped by 3's to create octal numbers, which are then displayed or printed as the organism identification (Fig. 21-2). Sometimes several organisms are possible, based on these readings, and the result is expressed as a probability for each possibility. The MIC for each relevant drug is also printed based on the dilution that inhibited growth. The Micro-Media Systems, Inc. Micro-Coder I (Fig. 21-3) is an example of such an instrument.

Some manufacturers have enhanced this approach to increase the level of automation. One common method is to automate the sampling step so that a broth tube can be inserted and the well inoculated by the instrument. This can be done either by inoculating a plate containing many wells of different reagents with one specimen or by using many specimens to simultaneously inoculate a plate containing the same reagent in all the wells on the plate. In the latter case, multiple plates are needed for each specimen. A second innovation is the use of optical transducers to measure the presence or absence of growth after incubation. All instruments of this class use microprocessors to do the data analysis, and some permit entry of specimen identification or analytical information gained from other sources.

An optical instrument of the next level of complexity is the Autobac by General Diagnostics. The measurement cuvette used by this instrument is shown in Figure 21-4. The cuvette has 13 chambers and is made of clear plastic. One of the chambers is used as the blank, while the other 12 can have disks containing antimicrobial chemicals loaded by a disk dispenser. After loading the disks, the chambers are capped with a rubberized plug strip. A bottle of culture broth is screwed into the cuvette and the broth distributed among the chambers through a series of channels.

The cuvettes are then placed in an incubator-shaker that causes uniform agitation of the samples for 3–5 hours at 36 ±0.5°C. During this period the antibiotic from the disk mixes with the broth. If the bacteria are susceptible to the drug at the level added, no growth will occur. Otherwise the growth will continue.

After incubation, the cuvettes are transferred manually to the reader. White light from a tungsten halide source is shone through each cuvette chamber. The detector is placed 35° out of line with the incident radiation so that only scattered light reaches the detector (Fig. 21-5). Such scattering is a function of the opaqueness of the broth, which is a function of the bacterial growth. The angle of measurement is chosen to gain the greatest sensitivity while at the same time using the simplest possible optics. This requires small angles that are far

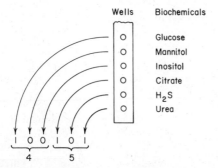

Figure 21-2 Example of the encoding of the index numbers based on growth in chemicals observed visually.

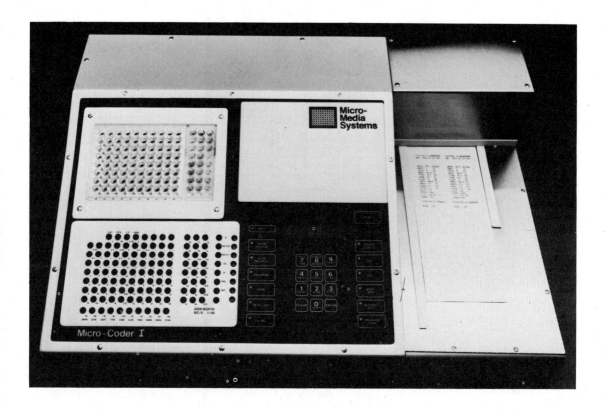

Figure 21-3 Picture of the face of the Micro-Coder I. (Courtesy of Micro-Media Systems. Reprinted with permission).

enough from the incident beam to be easily isolated from the direct source radiation. A 4° arc is subtended by the detector. The light through the untreated broth is used as the no-inhibition value and is assigned a light scattering index (LSI) value of 0.00. Other chambers are measured relative to this value on a log scale. LSI values of 0.00–0.50 are regarded as resistant, 0.51–0.59 as intermediate,

and 0.60–1.00 as susceptible. The readings are converted to numerical form and printed with the interpretation for each cuvette.

The data from the Autobac is most commonly used to determine either sensitivities or MICs of an organism by using the LSIs of multiple drugs or various dilutions of the same drug, respectively. It is also possible to use the instrument to determine

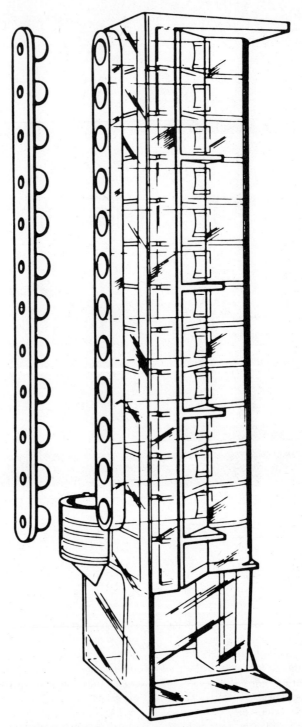

Figure 21-4 Multichannel cuvette for the Autobac. (Reprinted with permission of General Diagnostics, Division of Warner-Lambert Company, Morris Plains, NJ.)

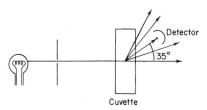

Figure 21-5 Optical diagram of the Autobac.

the identity of the bacteria based on their response to different biochemicals and antibiotics. Patterns of growth can then be matched against known organisms. The advantages of the instrument are its simple operation and rapid analysis. The disadvan-

tages are the amount of manual intervention needed for operation and the alteration of work flow.

An instrument with significantly more automation is the Automicrobic System (AMS) by Vitek Systems. Sample cards for the AMS are shown in Figure 21-6. The specimen is diluted appropriately and placed in a tube in the filling stand as shown. A straw is placed in the specimen and connected to the sample card. A group of filling stands are placed into the filling station where a pressure difference between the inside and outside of the card forces specimen through the capillary channels into the internal chambers (wells) containing media. Some of these wells contain pathogen-specific media, and growth occurs in such wells only if the correct bac-

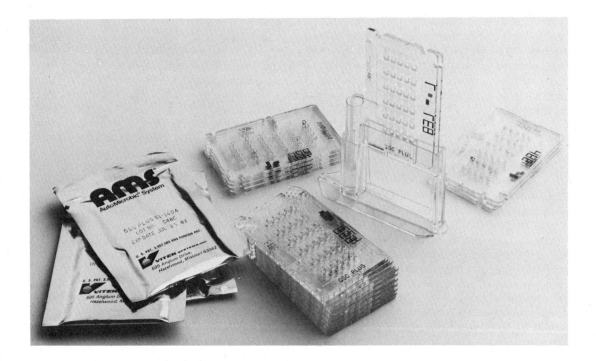

Figure 21-6 Sample cards and filling stand for the AMS. (Courtesy of Vitek Systems, Inc. Reprinted with permission.)

terium is in the specimen. Other wells contain nonspecific media, and growth in these chambers is used for enumeration purposes. The procedure is similar for inoculation of the various types of specimens, although each type of specimen has its own card.

Once a specimen card is loaded, it is placed in a tray in an incubator/reader module. Each tray contains up to 30 cards stacked vertically with four trays per incubator/reader. Here the cards are incubated at 35°C for 13 hours. Once every hour each tray is moved to the reading position for six minutes and the wells on the cards are read by an LED–detector pair. An identification number, which is colored in a special field on the card, is also read at the same time to prevent specimen mixup. A computer then analyzes the data and determines which bacteria are present and in what concentration. The susceptibility of the organism to various antibiotics can be determined by sampling the well that is producing growth and inoculating an appropriate susceptibility card. This card is marked with an identification number and placed in the incubator/reader. After 13 hours, the computer will determine to which drugs the organism is sensitive or resistant.

The versatility of this instrument seems to be quite great, although it is still somewhat restricted in the types of specimens that it can handle (e.g., specimens with multiple organisms) and in its ability to calculate MICs. Its advantages are its high degree of automation and its ability to differentiate between different organisms.

Another instrument featuring substantial automation is the MS-2 by Abbott Laboratories. The cuvette is plastic and disposable (Fig. 21-7). It is composed of an upper chamber into which the broth is poured and eleven lower chambers separated from the upper chamber by a hydrophobic membrane. The lower chambers are loaded with antibiotic disks prior to the addition of broth by a disk loader/sealer module.

Once the broth is added, the cuvette is placed in an analysis module, which functions as an incubator (35°C), an agitator, and a detector. An LED and detector are used to monitor the upper broth until growth is detected. A partial vacuum is then created in the lower level to transfer the broth down-

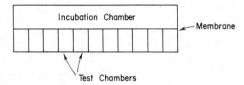

Figure 21-7   Diagram of a cuvette for the MS-2.

ward. Ten chambers contain reagent disks while the eleventh acts as a control. Each of these chambers is monitored periodically (every five minutes) for the duration of the run by separate LEDs and detectors.

The results are measured and tabulated by a microprocessor for each chamber of each cuvette. Growth rate and MICs can be calculated based on the growth activity observed. Biochemicals can be used in place of drugs to determine patterns of growth for identification purposes. The advantages of the MS-2 are that it requires no manual intervention once the broth is introduced into the upper chamber and that it will print the MIC values and sensitivities automatically.

Our discussion of microbiological instruments has been brief. Most of the physical principles of measurement have been encountered before, and the automation is still relatively primitive compared to other laboratory areas. The cost/benefit ratio has still not reached the point for any instrument where its presence in the laboratory is almost mandatory. This may well happen in the coming years, however. We will next turn our attention to instrumentation which is much better established, namely that involved in doing separations.

REVIEW QUESTIONS

1. Why can't bacteria be analyzed in the same way as chemicals or blood cells?
2. In what role do most microbiological instruments function?
3. What is the principle behind the Bactec?
4. How does the Bactec perform its measurements?

5. Sketch and label the parts of the Bactec sampling system.
6. How does the Bactec prevent cross-contamination?
7. Why must all gases from the Bactec be filtered?
8. What are the primary uses of the Bactec?
9. What is the most popular method of growth detection?
10. Give the basic steps in an automated optical method for a microbiological measurement.
11. Explain the operation of the simplest optical detector.
12. Describe the coding of the index numbers.
13. What is the newest innovation for simple optical instruments?

14. What are the two ways to evaluate multiple specimens against the same battery of biochemicals?
15. Describe the operation of the Autobac.
16. How does the Autobac detect growth?
17. Describe the Autobac cuvette design.
18. What is the light scattering index?
19. How is the MIC determined by the Autobac?
20. Sketch and label the sample card of the AMS.
21. Describe the processing of the AMS sample card.
22. How does one do sensitivities on the AMS?
23. Describe the operation of the MS-2.
24. How are the results measured on the MS-2?
25. Give a major advantage of the MS-2.

CHAPTER 22
CHROMATOGRAPHY

Many times it is necessary to separate a species from the rest of the sample in order to identify and quantify it. This is particularly true when the sought-for substance is present in low concentrations or can only be measured by methods with which other specimen components interfere. In the case of drug levels, the identity of the sought-for substance may be unknown, and a general method of separation must be applied to obtain an isolated species whose identity can then be deduced and whose concentration can then be measured.

Chromatography represents a family of methods that can be used to perform separation. In the family are column chromatography, thin layer chromatography, high-performance liquid chromatography (HPLC), paper chromatography, and gas chromatography. We will first look at the general principles of all chromatographic separations and then study gas chromatography and HPLC in particular.

Section 22-1
THEORY OF SEPARATION

Figure 22-1A shows a basic distillation apparatus used for the simple separation of two liquids. It will give nearly pure liquid X if the boiling point of X is much lower than that of Y, the other component. If the boiling point of liquid X is only slightly lower than that of liquid Y, then the resulting distillate will be more concentrated in X than the original solution, but it will also contain a significant amount of Y.

The phenomenon described above is illustrated by Figure 22-2. This is a boiling point–composition diagram for any mixture of X and Y from pure X to pure Y. It represents any two liquids, except those which form azeotropes. The upper curve represents the vapor composition at the boiling point of the liquid mixture, while the lower curve represents the liquid composition. The horizontal line CB, tying the curves together, represents the boiling temperature (isotherm).

The diagram is used by starting with a known mixture A (liquid composition) in the lower container of Figure 22-1. As this is heated, the vapor pressures of the two components increase independently until their sum equals the atmospheric or room air pressure. At this point (B) the solution boils, and the vapor concentration (C) can be found by following the constant temperature line to the vapor composition curve. If this vapor is then removed from the boiling environment (as in simple distillation) and recondensed, the new liquid composition will be D, which is the same as the vapor composition.

As can be seen from the above discussion, the separation that results from a single-step distillation process is not very effective unless liquid Y has a relatively high boiling point. However, one can take the distillate of the first simple distillation and redistill it. This gives us the isothermic boiling line DE and the isoconcentration line EF. As can be seen, the concentration of X at point F is greater than that at points A and D because it has been doubly enriched. If we repeat this process numerous times, we will continue to move toward distillate of higher X concentration. After enough redistillation, the final solution will be effectively pure X.

The problems with this approach are that it takes a large amount of time and equipment and that most of the original solution is lost in the numerous pot mixtures left behind as distillations are completed.

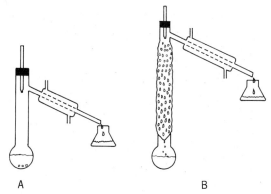

A   B

Figure 22-1 Part A shows a simple distillation apparatus, while part B includes a fractional distillation column.

These problems can be overcome if all the distillations are carried out at the same time from one pot mixture using a fractional distillation column as shown in Fig. 22-1B. As the vapor from the first distillation rises it meets the cooler column and recondenses. Since this condensation produces heat, the temperature at the bottom of the column gradually rises to the point where some of the condensed liquid reevaporates and moves farther up the column. Again the vapor recondenses and the process is repeated. Each time the process occurs, a simple distillation is, in effect, carried out. The pro-

cess is continuous with no clearly defined boundary where one distillation stops and the next starts. Eventually the distillate, now almost pure X, evaporates into the tube at the top of the column and is condensed into a separate container. To compare the effectiveness of fractional distillation columns, the term "theoretical plate" is used to indicate the equivalent of one simple distillation, and a column is rated on the number of theoretical plates to which it is equivalent. More theoretical plates imply the equivalence of more simple distillations and therefore better separation. Since all separation processes are basically similar to a series of simple distillations, the concept of theoretical plates is routinely used to measure the effectiveness of all separation techniques.

Distillation is an example of a two-phase process. Part of the sample is in the liquid phase and part in the gas phase. Each compound has a different concentration or mole fraction in the two phases. In the case of distillation, the two phases themselves are completely composed of the sample to be resolved. This, however, need not be the case to have a two-phase system. Solvent extraction is an example of a sample that is split between two independent phases (usually organic and aqueous) and can be used for separating substances of different relative solubilities. Solvent extraction, as done by a separatory funnel, produces results similar to simple distillation. To separate pure X from a sample com-

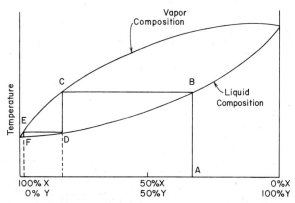

Figure 22-2 A boiling point–composition diagram shows the relationship between vapor composition, liquid composition, and boiling point.

posed of both X and Y may require numerous extractions. Consequently, this method too has been made a nearly continuous process in a procedure called counter-current extraction.

To have a continuous separation process, the two phases used to cause the separation must be in contact with each other over a long narrow area. One of the phases has to move through this separation area (device), propelling the sample with it and causing the sample to undergo numerous transitions between the two phases. If several substances are present in the sample, each will spend a different amount of time in the two phases depending on its affinity for the materials making up the phases. Those substances that have relatively more affinity for the moving phase will reach the end of the device sooner than those that have relatively more affinity for the nonmoving phase.

Let us formalize the previous description in the traditional terms. The moving phase is called the mobile phase while the nonmoving phase is called the stationary phase. The relative affinity of a substance for the two phases is expressed as a partition coefficient K, which is the ratio of the concentration of the substance in the stationary phase to that in the mobile phase.

$$K = \frac{C_s}{C_m} \qquad \text{(22-1)}$$

At each point in the separation device (hereafter called a column, although the device could be a strip or plate, etc.) an equilibrium is assumed to exist between the substances in the mobile phase and the stationary phase. As the mobile phase moves the sample along the length of the column, its components equilibrate with the stationary phase. As the sample is carried further along the column, more and more is lost until the mobile phase is effectively depleted of sample. After the sample has been applied to an area of the column, more mobile phase containing no sample arrives. The material in the stationary phase now reequilibrates with the mobile phase, causing a loss of sample from the stationary phase to the mobile phase. As more sample-free mobile phase passes, the supply of sample in the stationary phase at a point is gradually depleted by constantly being lost in the equilibrium process. This sample that has come out

of the stationary phase is swept along the column by the mobile phase until it reaches a point where its concentration in the mobile phase is excessive compared to the concentration in the stationary phase. At that point the sample will move back into the stationary phase. The result of this process is that the initial slug of sample is carried along the column, spending some of its time in the mobile phase and some in the stationary phase. The more time it spends in the mobile phase, the faster it moves. When the K values for various substances in a sample differ, it is possible to achieve separation of the components as they move down the column. Fig. 22-3 shows how separation occurs in a column over time and column distance. The rate (R) at which a sample component travels is the velocity of the mobile phase (v) times the fraction of time ($\%t$) the component spends in the mobile phase.

$$R = v \cdot \%t \qquad \text{(22-2)}$$

The fraction of time spent in the mobile phase is the ratio of the concentration in the mobile phase to the total concentration.

$$\%t = \frac{C_m}{C_m + C_s} \qquad \text{(22-3)}$$

If we solve Eq. 22-1 for C_s and substitute, we get

$$\%t = \frac{1}{1 + K} \qquad \text{(22-4)}$$

and the rate of movement becomes

$$R = \frac{v}{1 + K} \qquad \text{(22-5)}$$

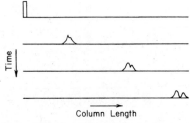

Figure 22-3 The separation of two compounds occurs and the peaks broaden as time passes and the materials move farther down the column.

If this method worked perfectly, then the tracing of a recorder attached to a detector measuring the material coming from the end of the column would be as shown in Figure 22-4. Such sharp separation, where each output component is the width of the specimen slug and its height is proportional to the concentration, never occurs in practice for four reasons common to all forms of separation. These are noninstant equilibrium, diffusion, nonuniform surface contact, and nonlinear detector response.

The equilibrium process is never instantaneous. Even in nuclear chain reactions, an interval exists between the initial critical situation and the final expended reaction mixture. Similarly, physical processes involving electrical attraction and the crossing of interfaces do not happen instantly because it takes time for all the species involved to reach the appropriate position. The equilibrium state in a continuously changing system will, therefore, not normally be reached. The faster the rate that the mobile phase moves, the greater the deviation from the equilibrium condition. Deviations from equilibrium decrease the effective K and make the separation less clean.

A drop of dye placed in the middle of a beaker of water will gradually spread out, even if there is no motion in the liquid. This phenomenon is called diffusion, because the dye molecules move from an area of high dye concentration to one of low dye concentration. In a column the same thing occurs, only the effects are limited to one dimension, the axis of transport. The fact that one phase is moving has no bearing on the process, since the diffusion process is affected only by a concentration gradient and not by translational movement. Diffusion occurs in both the mobile and stationary phases. As a result of this diffusion, the initial well-defined slug

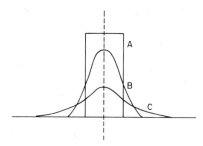

Figure 22-5 As time passes, a slug of specimen with concentration profile A will diffuse to profile B and then to profile C.

of sample begins to spread out over a larger area, with a tail forming in each direction (Fig. 22-5). This distribution will approximate a normal distribution if the equilibrium is rapid compared with the transport rate.

In a race all runners have the same distance to cover. In a chromatographic separation the distance any particular part of the moving phase travels is affected by the obstacles it encounters. If some pathways are more twisted than others, some portions of the mobile phase will have to move farther. This means that some portions of the carrier stream will bring their sample to the detector later than other portions, causing a spreading of the sample over a larger area. In the case of gas chromatography, the uniformity of pathlength is affected by the uniformity of the column packing. A column with gas pockets or packing of nonuniform size will lead to significant broadening of the sample peaks and, therefore, poor separation.

Nonlinear detector response will be discussed when detectors are reviewed later in this chapter.

It is possible to combine the effects of equilibrium, diffusion, and pathlength variation to give an indication of how well a column is performing a separation. First, however, we must define a new quantity. When we examined fractional distillation, we rated columns by the number of theoretical plates they had. If we double the height of a column, we should logically expect to double the number of theoretical plates. This is, in fact, what happens, which gives rise to the concept that in a particular column of uniform construction each theoretical plate has a specific height. We call this the

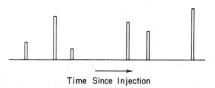

Time Since Injection

Figure 22-4 The ideal output from a separation process. The peak width is the same as the sample slug width (length), and the peak height is proportional to the concentration.

*h*eight *e*quivalent to a *t*heoretical *p*late (HETP), and it is given by

$$\text{HETP} = \frac{\text{height of column}}{\text{number of theoretical plates}} = \frac{L}{N} \quad \textbf{(22-6)}$$

The smaller the value of the HETP, the more theoretical plates are present in a fixed length of column. Conversely, if the number of theoretical plates necessary for a specific separation and the HETP for the column type are known, then the length of the column needed to perform the separation can be found.

It is possible to relate HETP to the factors previously discussed. This is called the Van Deemter equation, the abbreviated version of which is

$$\text{HETP} = A + \frac{B}{v} + C \cdot v \quad \textbf{(22-7)}$$

The *A* term is the eddy diffusion term. It is caused by uneven pathways and mixing due to mobile phase turbulence. This value is effectively independent of the velocity of the mobile phase and, therefore, constant for any particular column. The *B* term is caused by longitudinal diffusion. Since *v* is the velocity of the mobile phase, it is clear that as the rate increases, this term, for which *B* is a constant coefficient, decreases. This occurs because at a higher carrier rate, the sample has less time to diffuse. Consequently, it appears at the detector as a tall narrow peak. The final term is a constant *C*, which is related to the speed of the equilibrium, times the velocity. As the velocity increases, the time for equilibrium to be achieved at any point

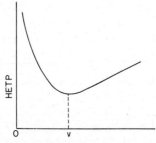

Figure 22-6 The Van Deemter plot. As the velocity decreases, diffusion reduces the effective resolving power; as the velocity increases, lack of equilibrium has the same effect.

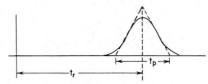

Figure 22-7 The retention time is a property of the compound, and the peak width shows the effect of diffusion while the compound is in the column.

decreases. This means a higher proportion of the sample remains in the mobile phase at any point, and the effective separation power of the column is decreased.

As can be seen from the equation, the velocity of the mobile phase has two opposite effects on the HETP. At slow rates the diffusion increases the HETP while at fast rates the lack of equilibrium increases the HETP. It seems that there must somewhere be an optimum velocity for the mobile phase that will give a minimum for the HETP and, as a result, a maximum number of theoretical plates in a given length of column. The graph of Eq. 22-7 in Figure 22-6 shows this to indeed be true. The minimum can be determined, using calculus, by differentiating HETP with respect to the velocity. This gives the optimum velocity for separation as

$$v = \sqrt{\frac{B}{C}} \quad \textbf{(22-8)}$$

The HETP can seldom be calculated from the Van Deemter equation because *A*, *B*, and *C* are usually unknown for a particular column. To find the HETP, it is more useful to use Eq. 22-6 after getting an estimate of the number of theoretical plates (*N*) in a column. This can be done by using Eq. 22-9 on the output as seen by the detector (Fig. 22-7).

$$N = 16\left(\frac{t_r}{t_p}\right)^2 \quad \textbf{(22-9)}$$

In this equation t_r is the retention time, that is, the average time the sample component is retained by the column. The zero point for this measurement is the time when the mobile phase present at the point of sample injection reaches the detector. In other words, the time it takes the mobile phase to reach the detector after injection is subtracted from the time it takes the sample component to reach the detector after injection. The quantity t_p is the peak width at the base expressed in units of time.

Section 22-2
SEPARATION AND MEASUREMENT

The separation of compounds by any form of chromatography depends on some molecules being more strongly attracted than others to the stationary phase. There are various mechanisms in which this attraction can occur. In the final analysis all of these attractions are based on electrostatic charge. The easiest attraction to understand is the dipole–dipole interaction. The positive end of one molecule is attracted to the negative end of another. Depending on the strength of the dipole, these attractions between polar molecules can be quite strong. Polar compounds are, therefore, generally relatively easy to separate from nonpolar molecules and from each other.

If one molecule has a dipole and another does not, inductive forces can still cause electrostatic attraction to occur. The positive end of one molecule will cause the electrons in a neighboring molecule to be shifted toward it. This will induce a temporary dipole and tend to hold the molecules together, although less strongly than if both molecules had permanent dipoles.

For those molecules too nonpolar to have permanent dipoles, temporary dipoles can still exist from bond vibrations within the molecule. Electronic shifts as the molecules vibrate and rotate can cause oscillating dipoles that will align with similar oscillations in other molecules.

Positional forces can also cause molecular attraction. The most common of these is hydrogen bonding, where the hydrogen orbitals overlap those of several other atoms. This creates hybrid molecular orbitals, which can link molecules together. This is particularly important if oxygen or nitrogen is present in the compounds.

Another form of positional force is the formation of complexes and cages. In these cases molecules wrap around each other or imprison each other to fill coordinate sites left by empty orbitals. This is particularly common with metal-containing compounds.

All forms of molecular attraction are adversely affected by temperature. As the temperature rises, the energy contained as molecular vibration, rotation, and translational velocity increases, and collisions between neighboring molecules disrupt the orderly arrangement of the molecules drawn together by the various attractive forces. This results in lower retention times on the column and provides one way to get a higher molecular weight material through the separation column.

When the sample components finally reach the detector, it will give an appropriate response. If the separation process is nearly ideal, each resulting detector response will resemble Figure 22-7. The retention time of a particular compound will be the same each time it is run on the same column under the same conditions. This time can, therefore, be used to identify a specific compound in a sample with several compounds. This is useful in drug analysis if the ingested drug is unknown, but it is also important in establishing which peak belongs to which compound even if all the compounds present are known. The area under the peak will be proportional to the amount of substance present. This statement is true for the peak of each substance provided the linear response region of the detector is not exceeded. It is not necessarily true between compounds because most detectors do not respond equally well to all compounds. The reason for such variation will be discussed later. If the response does vary between compounds of interest, calibration factors may be necessary to correct the measured values. Sometimes an internal standard of known retention time and concentration is added to compensate for variations in column operation and detector response.

The area under the curve may be approximated in a number of ways. One of the oldest is to do the recording on a paper of uniform weight. After the analysis is done, the peaks are cut out and weighed, and then the weight is multiplied by the appropriate calibration factor to give the concentration. This method suffers from the problem of humidity affecting the weight of the paper. The area can also be found by use of a planimeter, a mechanical device to calculate the area based on traversing the perimeter. A method requiring more skill, but which can be accomplished with pencil and ruler, is triangulation. If the peaks are completely resolved,

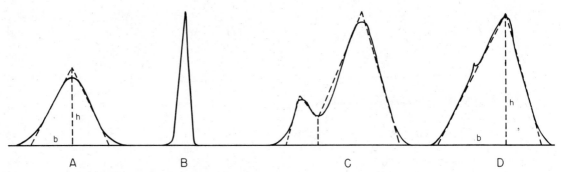

Figure 22-8 Various peak shapes challenge the measuring skill of the experimenter.

as in Figure 22-8A, a triangle is constructed from the base and tangents through the midpoint of the two sides. The height and base are measured and the area calculated. If the peak is extremely sharp, its height can be used instead of the area to calculate the concentration (Fig. 22-8B). If two peaks overlap (Fig. 22-8C), then a perpendicular is dropped from the center of the trough, and the areas of the trapezia are measured. If one peak appears as a shoulder of another, the area of the larger peak can be found by smoothly cutting off the smaller one (Fig. 22-8D). The area of the smaller one can also be calculated, but it is likely to be significantly in error. In recent years the use of electronic integration (Chapter 6) to compute peak area has become very common. The drifting of the baseline used to be a significant problem with this approach, but the use of the microprocessor to calculate and compensate has permitted accurate baseline extrapolation and removal. Curve fitting techniques also improve the resolution of overlapping curves and give a better estimate of shoulder peaks (Chapter 19). Compensation for detector response can also be programmed in, and the final results are reported as digital numbers.

Section 22-3
CARRIER GASES

A gas chromatograph is composed of a number of components, each of which is important to its operation. These will be discussed in the following sections. Gas chromatography is actually gas–liquid

chromatography. The mobile phase is an inert gas, while the stationary phase is a substance that is liquid at the column operating temperature, but that may be solid at room temperature. As a support for this stationary phase, the column is packed with inert material. Transfer of sample back and forth between the gas and liquid phases constitutes the method of separation. Figure 22-9 is a pictorial diagram of a gas chromatograph.

The selection of the carrier gas is important to gas chromatography. Unlike other forms of chromatography, solubility of the sample in the mobile phase is not a consideration because the sample is vaporized before the separation process. The nature of the gas does affect the process for two reasons, however. First, certain types of detectors require specific carrier gases. This will be explained when detectors are discussed. The second reason is that the density of the carrier gas affects the quality of separation. High-density gas will enhance the separation efficiency by reducing diffusion, while low-density gas will maximize the speed of column operation. The most commonly used gases are hydrogen, helium, nitrogen, argon, and carbon dioxide.

The quality of the gas is highly important. Since the detector will be set to treat the pure carrier gas as the baseline, any impurities will appear as noise. Purity is essential; any materials in the gas storage tank or picked up on the way will cause problems. For most separations the presence of water vapor is unacceptable, and traces of water vapor and hydrocarbons that are in the system are removed with a cold trap or a molecular sieve.

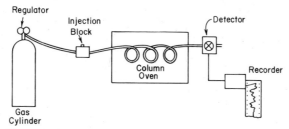

Figure 22-9 Pictorial drawing of a gas chromatograph.

The rate of gas flow through the column is controlled by the gas pressure at the start of the column. Since the bulk storage tank may contain several thousand pounds of pressure per square inch, this must be reduced in stages to the several pounds per square inch necessary to maintain a reasonable flow rate through the column. Frequently, a needle valve is then employed to further control the pressure. The actual flow rate is usually measured by a soap film flowmeter, which can be attached to the end of the chromatograph. The flow rate is computed from the length of the time that it takes a soap bubble to move between two marks. New instruments also have meters giving estimated flow rate. Fluctuations in flow rate appear as baseline drift on the output.

Section 22-4
COLUMNS

The stationary phase of gas chromatography is built on an inert material used to pack the column, called the support. The support is a material capable of holding a condensed liquid phase; consequently, it must have a large surface area. It must be composed of granular particles that pack well, but not too tightly, and are nearly uniform in size and shape. It must be stable under large temperature changes and not deteriorate under packing conditions.

There are a number of commercially available supports prepared especially for gas chromatography. The most elementary is powdered firebrick sold under the name Chromosorb-P. It is a silicon–oxygen polymer with the outer edges terminated by hydroxy groups, as shown below.

$$-O-\underset{|}{\overset{OH}{Si}}-O-\underset{|}{\overset{OH}{Si}}-O-\underset{|}{\overset{OH}{Si}}-O- \qquad \text{(22-10)}$$

Because of the strength of the oxygen–silicon bond and the electronegativity of oxygen, it is the O—H bond that can most easily be ruptured. This makes Chromosorb-P relatively acidic.

A second very common support is Chromosorb-W, which is made from diatomaceous earth. (Diatoms are single-celled algae with silicified skeletons.) This is treated by the manufacturer with an alkaline flux to reduce the acidity. It has somewhat less surface area per unit than Chromosorb-P.

Other materials can be used, but they generally suffer from lower surface area (glass microbeads), difficulty of coating (powdered Teflon), or plain messiness (graphitized carbon). One can even change the nature of the chemical surface to improve conditions if one chooses. For example, the hydrogen in Chromosorb-P can be replaced by a trimethylsilo group ($-Si(CH_3)_3$) to give the trimethylsilo ether. This places a very inert group on the surface, making the surface nonpolar and unreactive.

The choice of the column (physical container) will depend on the nature of the separation, the purpose of the separation, and the amount of material available. On the low end are the tubular columns that are 0.25–1.5 mm in diameter and 15–35 m long. In these the tubular wall acts as the support, and the columns are made of glass. The most common column size is 0.30–1.00 cm in diameter and 1–15 m long. These are composed either of glass bent in the shape of a "U" or of metals, such as aluminum, copper, or steel, bent into a coil. These arrangements allow different-sized columns to fit into the same-sized column oven. Columns used for compound separation after synthesis may have column diameters greater than 2.5 cm. These are used as a substitute for conventional distillation for difficult-to-separate compounds. In all cases the number of theoretical plates that the column contains must be adequate to accomplish the desired separation for the column to have any merit.

The most important material in the separation is the stationary or liquid phase. There is a wide choice of materials, but certain requirements apply to all of them. The first and foremost property a good liquid phase must have is that it must permit the compounds in the sample to be resolved. This means that the partition coefficients of the various components of the sample must be sufficiently different to permit each compound to form a separate peak. Generally, polar compounds will be better liquid phases for separating polar compounds, and nonpolar compounds will be better liquid phases for separating nonpolar compounds. In some cases the latter separation may be little more than a classical distillation under gas chromatographic conditions.

There are other requirements for a good stationary phase. The material must be thermally stable. Decomposition of the liquid phase will alter the partition coefficients as time goes on, making the column nonreproducible, and will give an increasing baseline drift as the temperature rises. The liquid phase must be nonvolatile, having a vapor pressure of less than 0.1 torr at column operating temperature. This generally implies a boiling point 200–300°C above the column operating temperature. The liquid coating must also be chemically inert to the components in the sample, because if reaction occurs, some components will be lost and/or replaced by others that are products of the chemical reaction. There is a distinct difference between chemical attraction needed to cause the separation and a chemical reaction leading to different products. The liquid phase-support matrix must be porous to gas movement so that it does not form a plug, causing the gas to stop flowing. Finally, the liquid phase must coat the support uniformly and reproducibly. It should be a single compound, or a family of closely related compounds, which will form a predictable configuration with the support so the column appears the same to the sample over its entire length. The liquid phase must have enough adhesion to the support to prevent being dislodged by the pressure of the carrier gas. Some common liquid phases are SE-30 (silicone rubber gum), Carbowax 20M (polyethylene glycol), DC-550 (silicone oil), and squalene (hexamethyl tetracosane).

Preparing the column is in itself frequently a challenge. While commercially prepared columns are available, many people prefer making their own. The liquid phase (coating material) must be dissolved or uniformly suspended in a low boiling liquid (sometimes warming is necessary). The support is then blended in, much as flour is when making a cake. After thorough mixing, the packing material (as it is now called) is slowly dried with heat and usually under reduced pressure. Once the product is no longer sticky, it is sized by using an appropriate sieve and poured into the column. To ensure adequate mixing, a mechanical vibrator is commonly used to shake down the packing material. Extreme care must be taken to prevent the development of cracks or air pockets in the final column. The ends are then stuffed with glass wool, and the column bent, if necessary, into the correct shape to fit into the column oven. The bending of a metal column must be done with great care to prevent distorting the packing material or kinking the column, thereby causing an eddy. Once in place in the chromatograph, the column must be "cured" by operating at an elevated temperature for several hours to several days. It is advisable to disconnect the detector during this initial conditioning process to prevent it from becoming fouled from the material that bleeds out of the column. The carrier gas is turned on to perhaps twice its normal pressure, and the temperature is gradually elevated until it is significantly (50–100°C) above the operating temperature. This allows excess liquid phase to be blown out of the column, a process called column bleeding. After the column has reached a stable state with no more bleeding occurring, it is ready for use.

A tubular column is made by passing a dilution of the liquid phase through the column so that it will adhere to the walls. The column is then dried by the passage of carrier gas and conditioned as are the packed columns.

Section 22-5
COLUMN OPERATION

To study column operation we must look at three elements of the gas chromatograph. These are the injection block, the column oven, and the detector oven. The purpose of the injection block is to get the sample into the gas phase. The sample may be injected directly or dissolved in a low boiling liquid and injected into the injection block (Fig. 22-10) with a syringe through a rubber septum. The contents of the needle are ejected as quickly as possible at the bottom of the block, which is heated by an electrical circuit to 50–100°C above the operating temperature of the column. This causes flash evaporation to occur. All the solvent and solute are placed into the vapor phase and are immediately swept into the column by the carrier gas stream.

There are several items that need noting. While it is imperative that the sample be rapidly vaporized, it is equally as important that the sample not be pyrolyzed. Such heat decomposition of the specimen will prevent separation since the original compounds are no longer intact. Second, the width of the specimen slug on the column will be reflected in the width of the final peaks. It is desirable to get as compact a slug of sample as possible into the column. This is the reason the specimen is injected as quickly as possible and is flash heated. It is also desirable to have as little volume in the injection

block and column head as possible, since this is dead volume where diffusion and eddies can increase the width of the sample slug. Care should be taken not to introduce so much sample as to overload the column's separation capacity.

The column oven can be operated in one of two modes. The first is the constant temperature mode. Here the temperature is held very constant (less than 0.1°C variation) in a highly insulated box. This is the most efficient mode of operation when compounds of similar boiling points are being separated since it allows for new samples to be injected as soon as the old ones emerge. Unfortunately, it is sometimes necessary to separate compounds whose boiling points vary drastically. If one runs these separations at high temperatures, low boiling compounds come out so quickly that they are not completely resolved or will sometimes even be lost under the large solvent peak. If one runs the separation at low temperatures, the first peaks are well resolved, but the high boiling components may not come out for hours (days) and may produce such diffuse and broad peaks as to be unmeasurable. The solution to this dilemma is to program the temperature so that initial compounds emerge while the temperature is low, but raise the temperature quickly to force out the rest of the material. Common programs call for the column oven temperature to rise at 1–20°C per minute. The obvious disadvantage to this approach is that the column oven must be opened after each analysis to cool the column prior to the next separation. This can be time-consuming, but not nearly so much as waiting for high boiling peaks to emerge at low temperatures.

The detector is also kept in an oven. The temperature here is usually 25–50°C above the column temperature to keep the gas from the column from being retained in the detector and to prevent compounds from condensing and fouling the detector.

Section 22-6
DETECTORS

In order to know when and how much material emerges from the gas chromatographic column, some type of device must be available to monitor

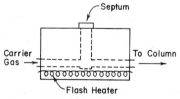

Figure 22-10 Schematic drawing of an injection block.

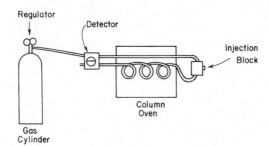

Figure 22-11 The thermal conductivity detector must measure both the input and output streams.

the stream and detect the presence of other than the carrier gas. A number of detectors are in common use, and we will examine four of them. Detectors may pose additional constraints on column operation to those discussed above.

An extremely common type is the thermal conductivity detector. It detects the presence of material based on its ability to remove heat from a metal filament. It is implemented by taking a platinum or tungsten wire and holding it at a fixed length so it will not change length with temperature changes. The wire is then heated to a specific temperature by passing a current through the wire. As the carrier gas moves past the wire, it removes some of the heat from the wire. The change in the resistance of the wire is proportional over a small range to the change in temperature. The pure carrier gas reading is used as baseline. If the carrier gas has other compounds in it, these will be less efficient at removing the heat from the wire, and the wire's tem-

perature, and therefore its resistance, will rise. At constant voltage, this will cause a measurable current change.

Things are not as straightforward as they would seem. The temperature in the environment of the detector will affect the temperature of the wire. The rate of carrier gas flow is also important because changes in flow rate will also produce changes in cooling. At best this will mean baseline drift, but it can also affect area measurement if a rapid change occurs as a peak is emerging. To solve these problems, several steps must be taken. The first is to eliminate the flow rate variation by measuring the pure carrier gas stream as a reference as it enters the chromatograph. Flow rate changes will thus affect both the sample and the reference detector in the same way. A diagram of such an arrangement is shown in Figure 22-11. Second, the reference and sample detectors must be balanced against each other when pure carrier gas is flowing through the gas chromatograph. Since these are both resistance measuring devices, a Wheatstone bridge is the appropriate means to balance the circuit. Therefore, each detector is made one leg of such a bridge. In fact, a greater advantage can be gained by placing sample detectors in the opposite branches of the bridge and reference detectors in the other two branches, as shown in Figure 22-12. As the resistances in the sample detectors rise, the bridge gets twice as far out of balance as if only one pair of detectors were used. This enhances sensitivity. The null point detector in the bridge can be replaced by an instrumentation amplifier that drives

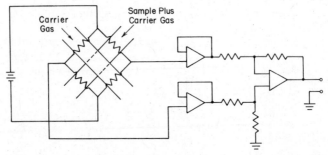

Figure 22-12 A Wheatstone bridge is used in a thermal conductivity detector to measure the difference in the cooling ability of the two gas streams.

a servorecorder or a digital convertor attached to a microprocessor to store the data.

Because of its high thermal conductivity, the best gas to use with a thermal conductivity detector is hydrogen. Because of other considerations (reactiveness), hydrogen is frequently replaced by helium, where available. Nitrogen can be used, but is much less efficient due to the small difference in thermal conductivity between it and organic compounds. The detector's sensitivity is of the order of 10^{-8} moles of solute. Because the thermal conductivity of all measured compounds is not the same, correction for this nonuniformity of response may be necessary.

A second type of detector is called the flame ionization detector and is diagrammed in Figure 22-13. This detector makes use of the fact that a flame acts as a solution, permitting the free movement of ions that are, therefore, able to carry current between two electrodes. The background flame will be created by the combustion of hydrogen by air or oxygen. As a consequence, the operator has the option of using hydrogen as the carrier gas or introducing it at the time of combustion. Gas mixing must be carefully controlled to keep the response of the detector proportional to the sample present.

The detector is sensitive to the amount of ionic material generated by the combustion. Ideally this should be proportional to the number of organic molecules that undergo partial combustion, which should, in turn, be proportional to the number of organic molecules present. Unfortunately, as organic molecules become more complex, they tend to give off more ions during controlled combustion. This causes the flame ionization detector to be more sensitive as the carbon content rises. On the

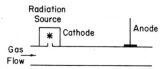

Figure 22-14 The basic design of the radioactive source detectors.

plus side, the detector is not sensitive to water since that is the major product of the combustion. This detector is sensitive down to 10^{-10} to 10^{-15} moles of solute, depending on its construction.

The electronics of the detector are similar to those used for the polarography of oxygen. The voltage difference is fixed by the output of an operational amplifier holding the voltage constant. The current (of the order of 10^{-12} A) is then measured by the changes it induces in the circuit of a difference amplifier. Due to the high voltage and low current, the actual circuits are extremely complex to guarantee stability and suppress transients from the flame.

Figure 22-14 contains the working sketch for the last two types of detectors to be discussed. The first is called the argon ionization detector and the second the electron capture detector. Both use radioactive elements to cause a background current. A change in the current is caused by the presence of a sample, and this change is proportional to the amount of sample present.

In the argon ionization detector a radioactive source, such as ^{63}Ni, is positioned upstream from the anode. The source and the surrounding environment are 1000 V more negative than the anode. The β particles coming from the radioactive decay cause argon atoms to ionize. These ionized atoms are then accelerated by the strong electric field and collide with other argon atoms, forcing some of them in an excited state. If nothing is present but argon, the excited atoms are constantly swept out by the bulk gas movement, and only a low baseline current occurs. If organic molecules are present, the argon, in its high excited and fairly stable (called metastable) state (11.6 eV above ground), will return to ground by giving its energy to the organic molecules. The organic molecules cannot dissipate this much energy without ionizing. The bulky organic ions will be swept out of the chamber

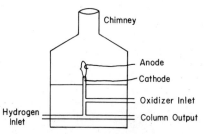

Figure 22-13 Schematic drawing of flame ionization detector.

by the carrier gas, but the electrons will migrate to the anode to give a current proportional to the number of ionizable organic molecules present. This current will be converted to a voltage, amplified and reported to a recorder or microprocessor. The relevant reactions are

$$\beta + Ar \rightarrow Ar^+ + 2e \qquad \textbf{(22-11)}$$

$$Ar^+ + Ar \rightarrow Ar^+ + Ar^* \qquad \textbf{(22-12)}$$

$$Ar^* + Org \rightarrow Ar + Org^+ + e \qquad \textbf{(22-13)}$$

A few things about the argon ionization detector are worth noting. Argon, of course, must be used as the carrier gas. The detector will not respond to very small molecules or fluorocarbons. The detector can be made reasonably sensitive and is linear over five orders of magnitude.

The electron capture detector has the same general electronics as the argon ionization detector, but the voltage difference between anode and source is only 10–100 volts. It is the reverse of the argon detector, however, in that it measures the decrease, rather than the increase, in current flow. The electrons emitted by the tritium source are slow (low energy), but are able to ionize the nitrogen that is used as the carrier gas, creating more slow electrons. These electrons would normally migrate to the anode while the positive ions are swept from the chamber. If a compound containing electronegative elements or groups, such as halogens, oxygen, or nitrate, is present, it will soak up the free electrons and be swept past the weak anode without yielding the electron. Therefore, the current is reduced. The relevant reactions are

$$N_2 + \beta \rightarrow N_2^+ + 2e \text{ (slow)} \qquad \textbf{(22-14)}$$

$$Org\text{-}X + e \rightarrow Org\text{-}X^- \qquad \textbf{(22-15)}$$

The detection limits are around 10^{-12} moles of solute.

Section 22-7
LIQUID CHROMATOGRAPHY

In recent years another form of chromatography, high performance liquid chromatography (HPLC), has come into greater use. Like gas chromatography (GC), HPLC can be used to separate drugs and other complex compounds for analysis and identification. Unlike GC, however, this separation can be done at lower temperatures and without the danger of pyrolysis, which exists when samples must be made gaseous. The components necessary to carry out HPLC are shown in the block diagram in Figure 22-15.

HPLC is based on the use of a liquid mobile phase and a liquid or solid stationary phase, which is bonded onto the column packing. The mobile phase is stored in a reservoir (~500 ml) made of stainless steel or glass. The liquid is kept at a constant temperature using a heater controlled by a temperature sensor, and it is sometimes stirred by a magnetic stirrer. It is frequently desirable to degas the mobile phase to remove oxygen or other dissolved gaseous species. One method of degassing is to apply a vacuum to the reservoir while heating and vigorously stirring the contents. The liquid phase is frequently filtered upon exit from the reservoir to remove micron-sized particle contaminants.

The driving force in HPLC is the mobile phase pump. This pump must be able to perform at 500–5000 psi to force the mobile phase through the densely packed column. Pumps are usually made with working parts of Teflon or stainless steel. (The former is usable only at lower pressures.) Various factors are important to good pump performance. The pump should deliver solution at as constant a flow rate as possible. Since most pumps are piston-driven (reciprocating) and generate a pressure gradient similar to the voltage of a half-wave rectifier, it is necessary to use a multiple piston pump or have an effective damping system to keep the pressure uniform. The pump should be resettable to the same flow rates so that the results of different runs can be compared. The pump must have good short-term precision of flow rate and have only small flow rate drift over several hours. A pump should deliver a flow rate of up to a minimum of 3 ml/min with a reproducibility of substantially less than 1%.

Between the pump and the column are several auxiliary components used to enhance the quality of the measurements. A pressure gauge is useful to diagnose system problems, such as plugged columns or leaky connectors, before more serious damage is done. It also facilitates adjusting conditions for optimum separation. A line filter with 2

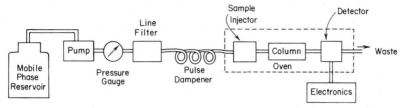

Figure 22-15 Block diagram of a high performance liquid chromatograph.

μm pores is useful to prevent particles from clogging the column inlet. Pulse dampeners composed of several meters of capillary tubing (0.25 mm) will reduce the magnitude of the pressure gradients produced by a reciprocating pump. This is important to prevent column deterioration and to permit the use of some types of detectors. If various mobile phases are used interchangeably, it is important that the internal volume of these auxiliary components be minimized to reduce the amount of solvent washout time required to change mobile phases.

Unlike GC, high temperatures are seldom needed for HPLC. Nevertheless, maintaining the temperature at a constant level is important for many liquid chromatographic applications. This is especially true in those applications where one is relying on a partition coefficient between two phases to effect separation. Such coefficients are temperature dependent and require temperature precision of $\pm 0.2°C$. Other forms of separation, such as size-

exclusion or ion-exchange chromatography, may need to be carried out above room temperature. The temperature control is accomplished by placing the sample injector, the column, and the detector into an oven. As in GC, such ovens are generally air baths.

There are several techniques available for the introduction of samples into the flowing stream. The simple slide valve was introduced in Chapter 17 in connection with continuous flow analysis. The use of this principle of placing a sample into a short cylindrical plug or a longer tube (Figure 22-16) and then rapidly making this sample-filled vessel part of the liquid flow path has become the preferred way of sample addition. It causes only a minimal disruption of the flow while allowing a precise volume of sample to be inserted. The leading alternative to such sampling valves is needle injection through a septum, just as in GC. The approach has an inherent uncertainty of several percent and cannot be

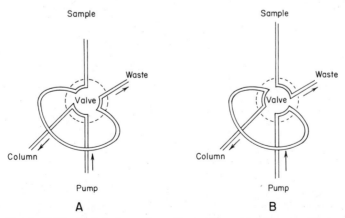

Figure 22-16 Part A shows the valve positioned to allow sample to be inserted into the sampling loop, and Part B shows the valve positioned to make the sampling loop part of the mobile phase path.

used directly above 1500 psi due to sample leakage around the plunger. At higher pressures special techniques must be employed, such as septumless injection, which permits a quantity of sample to be measured and injected by a special attached syringe, or stopflow, where the mobile phase pump is temporarily turned off while the injection is made. Automated samplers, which pierce sample vials, extract a measured amount of sample, and insert it as a slug into the mobile phase, are available for unattended batch analysis.

The key to the separation is the packed column. The column is made of stainless steel or, sometimes, reinforced glass. The column is straight and 10–150 cm in length. The inner diameter is between 0.2 and 1.0 cm, and the internal wall must be polished to reduce surface effects for maximum performance. The column ends are fitted with porous frits or screens to retain the column's packing. Particle packings are divided into two basic categories. Some are called pellicular because they are built around a silicone core to which appropriate functional groups are attached. Such pellicular particles are frequently spherical, and columns packed with them are relatively permeable to mobile phase flow. Other packing material is completely porous and irregular in shape. Such particles tend to give more tightly packed columns with less permeability. Hard gels based on polystyrene are used in some applications such as ion exchange. Particle size ranges from 2–75 μm, depending on the application, but should vary no more than ±50% within one column. The choice of packing material for a particular separation is based on the same type of consideration used for GC. Several column packing methods are employed depending on the nature and size of the packing material, but the goal of all of them is to prepare uniform columns with no pockets that foster mobile phase eddies.

Good detectors for HPLC are sensitive, not affected by changes in temperature and pressure, and able to measure over a wide range of solute concentrations. As for GC, numerous detectors exist, and a detailed analysis would be repetitive of material previously covered. Photometric and spectrophotometric measurements, particularly in the UV, are the most commonly used techniques. Another frequently used approach is differential refractometry, which compares the refractive indices of the column effluent to the pure mobile phase stream. Various methods of comparison are available. Other detectors are more specialized. A flow-through scintillation counter can be used to measure radio-labeled compounds. Fluorescence and infrared detectors will work with compounds that have appropriate absorption characteristics. Amperometric detectors can be used for reducible and oxidizable species (see Chapter 12), and conductivity detectors are applicable for some ions. The latter detectors require conducting mobile phases that will not foul the electrodes.

As with GC, HPLC instruments now contain microprocessors for instrumental control as well as for data acquisition, reduction, analysis, and representation. Such microprocessor use has been de-

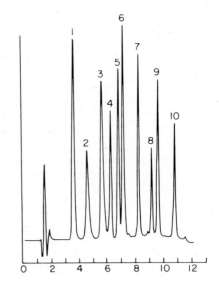

Key

1. Demoxepam
2. Oxazepam
3. N-Desmethylchlordiazepoxide
4. N-Desalkylflurazepam
5. N-Desmethyldiazepam
6. Chlordiazepoxide
7. Diazepam
8. Internal Standard
   (Benzophenone of Lorazepam)
9. Prazepam
10. Endogenous Serum Peak

Figure 22-17 Typical drug panel with numerous drugs present.

scribed extensively in connection with other instruments.

Chromatography is an excellent method for separating and quantitating a group of unknowns. It lacks good ability at identification, however, because numerous compounds will have nearly the same retention time. The example of drug analysis shown in Figure 22-17 will bear this out. Other devices, such as the mass spectrometer discussed in the next chapter, are needed to simplify identification. Fortunately, advancing technology has allowed us to attach separation and identification devices together so both can be brought to bear simultaneously on a sample.

REVIEW QUESTIONS

1. What is simple distillation?
2. Under what two conditions will simple distillation fail?
3. Draw a boiling point-composition diagram and label the parts.
4. What is an isotherm?
5. Explain the distillation process using the boiling point-composition diagram.
6. Explain how fractional distillation works.
7. What is a theoretical plate?
8. Why is batch extraction similar to simple distillation?
9. How is continuous separation effected?
10. Define the partition coefficient.
11. Describe the separation process inside a chromatographic column.
12. How is the rate of sample transport in a column calculated?
13. Give four reasons why separation is not as clean as in Figure 22-4.
14. Why is equilibrium never obtained in a flowing system?
15. Define diffusion.
16. Why are the pathlengths in a chromatographic column nonuniform?
17. Define HETP.
18. Write the Van Deemter equation. Define the constants.
19. What effect does the mobile phase velocity have on the separation of the sample?
20. What is the optimum mobile phase velocity?
21. Define retention time.
22. How does the number of theoretical plates depend on the retention time and the peak width?
23. What is the basis of all mechanisms of attraction in chromatographic separation?
24. Give five means of sample–stationary phase interaction.
25. How is a dipole induced?
26. How does hydrogen bonding work?
27. What effect does temperature have on chromatographic separation?
28. For what is retention time used?
29. What is the area under the peak proportional to?
30. What are internal standards? Why are they sometimes used in chromatographic separation?
31. Describe several manual ways to calculate the peak area.
32. Describe the apparatus used for gas chromatography.
33. Give several reasons why the selection of carrier gas is important to gas chromatography.
34. How are impurities removed from the carrier gas?
35. How is the carrier gas flow rate controlled?
36. How is the carrier gas flow rate measured?
37. What is a support? List several.
38. List the requirement for a good support.
39. Describe the chemical properties of powdered firebrick.
40. What is Chromosorb-W?
41. Describe several different column types.
42. What factors influence the choice of column type?
43. What is the stationary phase?
44. What are the properties of a good liquid (stationary) phase?
45. What effect does the thermal decomposition of the liquid phase have on gas chromatography?
46. What are the volatility constraints on the liquid phase?
47. List some common liquid phases.
48. Describe the steps in the packing of a column.
49. Why is a column cured or conditioned? How is this done?
50. Why is the detector disconnected during conditioning?
51. Why is the specimen flash heated?

52. What is pyrolysis? How does it affect gas chromatography?
53. At what temperature should the injection block be kept?
54. What is the effect of dead volume? Why?
55. What two modes of column operation are commonly used?
56. Describe isothermal operation.
57. Describe the use of programmed temperature.
58. When are programmed temperatures used?
59. At what rate is temperature commonly programmed?
60. What is the major disadvantage of temperature programming?
61. Why is the detector oven kept warmer than the column oven?
62. List four types of detectors for gas chromatography.
63. How do thermal conductivity detectors work? Sketch one.
64. What gases are most effective with thermal conductivity detectors?
65. What problems must be overcome with thermal conductivity detectors?
66. Explain how the Wheatstone bridge is used in a thermal conductivity detector. Sketch it.
67. How does a flame ionization detector work?
68. Sketch and label the parts of a flame ionization detector.
69. Why is a flame ionization detector more sensitive to more complex organic molecules?
70. How is the signal from a flame ionization detector measured?
71. Sketch and label the parts of a radiation-based detector.
72. How does an argon ionization detector work? Give the reaction equations.
73. What are the limitations of an argon ionization detector?
74. How does an electron capture detector work? Give the reaction equation.
75. How does electron capture differ from argon ionization as a means of detection?
76. What are the detection limits of the various detectors?
77. What is the major limitation of using gas chromatography for compound identification?

PROBLEMS

1. If the velocity of the carrier gas is 3.04 m/sec and the peak takes 82 sec to emerge from a 10.0 m column, what is the partition coefficient?
2. The rate of travel of a sample component is 0.269 of the carrier gas. What will the rate be if the partition coefficient is increased by 58%?

3. If 71% of a substance is in the mobile phase and its concentration in the stationary phase is 3.65 mg/l, what is the concentration in the mobile phase?
4. If the HETP is 1.88 cm, the eddy diffusion contributes 2.6 mm, the longitudinal diffusion coefficient is $1.53 \cdot 10^{-2}$ m²/sec, and the equilibrium speed factor is $3.72 \cdot 10^{-3}$ sec, what is the carrier gas velocity?
5. The eddy diffusion is 3.7 mm, the longitudinal diffusion coefficient is $8.0 \cdot 10^{-3}$ m²/sec, and the carrier gas velocity 2.43 m/sec. If the HETP is at a minimum under these conditions, what is its value?
6. There are 361 theoretical plates in a column 7.0 m long. If the eddy diffusion is 4.3 mm, the longitudinal diffusion coefficient is $1.39 \cdot 10^{-2}$ m²/sec, and the carrier gas speed 1.75 m/sec, what is the equilibrium speed factor?
7. What would be the number of theoretical plates in the column in Problem 5 if the carrier gas velocity were increased by 31% and the column were 6.29 m long?
8. If there are 346 theoretical plates in a column and a compound has a retention time of 114 sec, what is the width of the peak if the chart drive runs at 20.0 cm/min?
9. A column has a longitudinal diffusion coefficient of $1.03 \cdot 10^{-2}$ m²/sec. When the column is operating at minimum HETP, substance X, which has a concentration of 1.21 mg/l in the gas phase and 18.7 mg/l in the liquid phase, has a rate of travel of 4.2 cm/sec. What is the equilibrium speed factor?
10. Derive an equation to express the partition coefficient in terms of the column length, HETP, carrier gas velocity, and peak width.

CHAPTER 23
MASS SPECTROMETRY

The gas chromatograph gives an excellent means of separating compounds, but it gives only marginal information about their identity. Since many compounds have similar retention times under a given set of conditions, positive identification is possible only if the number of candidates is very restricted. In the clinical laboratory, particularly when doing drug analysis, this is not the case. Therefore, in the past it has been necessary to do complex separations before a gas chromatograph could be used. Such separations were time-consuming, were difficult due to the small amount of sample present, and were frequently inconclusive.

Mass spectrometry gives the ability to identify compounds after they have been separated by gas chromatography. The information in a mass spectrum gives clues to the identity of the various pieces of a molecule and how they were put together. By applying rules related to atomic masses and valences, and by matching known spectra, compounds can be readily identified. Mass spectrometry resulted from the work of J. J. Thomson and F. W. Aston in England in the early twentieth century (Thomson's work was previously mentioned in Chapter 20).

Section 23-1
THEORY OF MASS SPECTROMETRY

If a molecule is impacted by an electron of sufficient energy, it will be ionized by the loss of an electron from one of its orbitals. In addition, the molecule will be left with some extra energy from the collision. If there is enough energy available, weaker bonds in the molecule will be ruptured, and parts of the molecule will break off. This disintegra-

tion will produce uncharged simple molecules (H_2O, NO_2, HCN), neutral radicals ($\cdot CH_3$, $\cdot C_2H_5$, $\cdot OH$), and charged ions of smaller size than the original molecule. The first two categories of species are called "leaving groups" or fragments and cannot be measured directly. The charged fragments can be collected after separation and measured by their mass-to-charge ratio (m/z) at the detector.

To identify the various charged fragments, it is necessary to measure their mass-to-charge ratios. The first step in this process is to accelerate the charged particles in an electric field. While most ions will have the same charge ($+1$), the mass will depend upon how much of the molecular ion has been lost in the form of leaving groups. This, in turn, will be a function of the structure and composition (functional groups) of the original molecule. Through techniques discussed later the accelerated ions are sorted by their acquired energies so that ions of different mass-to-charge ratios can be measured separately.

The detector response is plotted against the mass-to-charge ratio (expressed in atomic mass units), as in Figure 23-1, to give mass peaks. If present, the parent peak (that is, the original molecular ion) is located to establish the overall molecular mass. The mass difference between the parent peak and other peaks is computed to identify leaving groups ($\cdot OH = -17$, $\cdot CH_3 = -15$). The effects of naturally occurring isotopes (^2H, ^{13}C, ^{37}Cl) are used to identify the elemental content of major peaks. Finally, the clues are fitted together to give a tentative identification. Confirmation is obtained by running a sample of the pure compound under identical conditions and getting an exact spectral match.

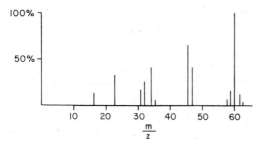

Figure 23-1 A typical mass spectrum.

Section 23-2
SAMPLE IONIZATION

The sample for mass spectrometry may come from a gas chromatograph, or it may simply be injected into the device. In the former case, it will already be in gaseous form ready for ionization. In the latter case, it must be vaporized so that it will be a gas at the operating temperature and pressure of the ionization chamber. For liquids and solids this can be accomplished by placing them in large reservoirs (1–5 liters) and allowing them to evaporate at a suitable temperature in an oven that encloses the reservoir. The temperature must be low enough to prevent decomposition. Another method of injecting a solid is by a direct insertion probe. The solid is dissolved and evaporated on the end of a gold-tipped probe (or placed there as a solid crystal), and the probe is inserted into the ionization chamber. The solid is vaporized by controlled heating.

The sample enters the ionization chamber through a pinhole leak or other device to maintain the source pressure in the 10^{-5}–10^{-7} torr range. In a gas chromatograph this leak is placed after the detector, while in other applications it is controlled by a valve to the sample reservoir. The carrier gas does not cause problems provided the evacuation system can keep the overall pressure low enough inside the mass spectrometer. Sometimes tubing permeable to hydrogen and helium is used to remove some of the excess gas and concentrate the sample before admission to the ionization chamber. The sample leaks into the ionization chamber from the source chamber because the source pressure is 1000 times greater than that in the ionization chamber.

Inside the ionization chamber the pressure is kept around 10^{-5} torr by the vacuum pump. Of the original sample in the source chamber, which may be only a fraction of a micromole, only 2–3% will enter the ionization chamber. Of that, only 0.1% will be ionized. A schematic drawing of the ionization chamber appears in Figure 23-2. As the gas molecules enter from the pinhole leak, they are drawn into the chamber by the reduced pressure. When molecules wander into the electron beam moving between the heated filament cathode and the counter electrode, they may collide with electrons accelerated between these two plates and be ionized.

$$M + e^- \rightarrow M^+ + 2e^- \qquad (23\text{-}1)$$

At potentials from 6–14 volts, simple ionization occurs for most samples, and the molecular mass can be determined. If the potential difference is raised to 50–70 volts, then the molecules fragment, giving the mass spectrum of the compound. Other methods of ionization, such as chemical ionization, are beginning to be used more extensively for some applications, because less fragmentation and greater intensity of ions related to the molecular ion are observed.

Once formed, it is imperative to get the ion fragments out of the ionization chamber and into the analyzer (flight tube), where the actual separation will occur. This is accomplished by the use of charge. Repeller plates on the walls away from the flight tube are given a positive charge so that the positive ions will tend to avoid them. Negative accelerator plates are placed on the analyzer end of the chamber. The first accelerator plate has a small

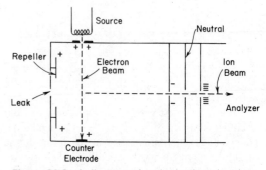

Figure 23-2 A diagram of an ionization chamber.

negative potential, and many of the ions are lost by collision and neutralization with the first accelerator plate. The second plate has no charge at all and serves to collimate the beam of ions. The final accelerator plate is several hundred to several thousand volts more negative than the first. As a consequence of the strong electric field, the ions experience a dramatic acceleration similar to that of electrons in a CRT. The ions are at this point in a narrow beam travelling at high speed. (It should be noted that, for safety reasons, it is desirable to have the flight tube and detector at ground potential. Therefore, in practice, the whole ionization chamber is biased to a high positive potential so that the final acceleration plate is at ground relative to the outside world.)

The exact speed of each molecular fragment will depend on its mass. The amount of kinetic energy (E_k) available from an electric field is the voltage of the field times the charge on the particle (z) being accelerated.

$$E_k = zE \qquad (23\text{-}2)$$

On the other hand, the kinetic energy can also be expressed in terms of the mass and velocity.

$$E_k = \frac{mv^2}{2} \qquad (23\text{-}3)$$

If we solve these equations for v, we get

$$\frac{mv^2}{2} = zE$$

$$v = \sqrt{\frac{2zE}{m}} \qquad (23\text{-}4)$$

By carefully setting the voltage and measuring the velocity in some manner, we can compute m/z, the mass-to-charge ratio.

$$\frac{m}{z} = \frac{2E}{v^2} \qquad (23\text{-}5)$$

Section **23-3**
METHODS OF ION SEPARATION

To accomplish the separation we must use some sort of flight tube. The shape and length of the tube will depend on the nature of the method of separation. Under any methodology the tube must be clear of molecules that might collide or otherwise interact with the ion beam and thereby interfere with the measurement. To accomplish this the pressure of the flight tube is reduced to 10^{-8}–10^{-7} torr. Such low pressure is difficult to maintain because molecules from otherwise innocuous material become significant, such as grease from the seals, oil from the vacuum pump, or residue of previous specimens remaining on surfaces. Removing these contaminants by heating and pumping can be very time-consuming.

There are numerous methods of separation available. One of the most common involves the use of a magnetic field to bend the ion beam. As you will recall from Chapter 3, the force (F) applied to a charge moving in a magnetic field was proportional to field strength (B) and the charge. The final factor in this equation is the velocity.

$$F = Bzv \qquad (23\text{-}6)$$

This force causes the particle to bend its path perpendicular to both its original path and the direction of the magnetic field. If the magnetic field is large enough, the particle will move in a circle and return to its original position and direction. A counter force, called centrifugal force, will oppose this action.

$$F = \frac{mv^2}{r} \qquad (23\text{-}7)$$

At balance, we will have

$$Bzv = \frac{mv^2}{r}$$

or

$$v = \frac{Bzr}{m} \qquad (23\text{-}8)$$

If we now combine this with Eq. 23-4, we can eliminate the velocity:

$$\sqrt{\frac{2zE}{m}} = \frac{Bzr}{m}$$

$$\frac{2zE}{m} = \frac{B^2z^2r^2}{m^2}$$

$$\frac{m}{z} = \frac{B^2r^2}{2E} \qquad (23\text{-}9)$$

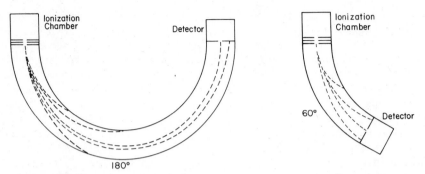

Figure 23-3 Two types of single-focus mass spectrometers, each employing a magnetic sector. The magnetic fields are perpendicular to the plane of the paper.

Using the above equation, it is very easy to separate any mass-to-charge ratio from the rest. A device with a magnetic sector of some standard size, such as 60° or 180° (Fig. 23-3), is used to provide the fixed magnetic field B. Similarly, the radius of the flight tube path to the detector is also fixed. If the electric field E is changed, the m/z ratio necessary to impact the detector will change. By scanning the voltage through the relevant m/z ratios, all the ion peaks can be focused on the detector in succession. A clear disadvantage is the nonlinearity of the m/z ratio with the potential, which means that as one moves to higher mass-to-charge ratios, their separation becomes progressively smaller until they are indistinguishable. It is also difficult to extrapolate the positioning of the peaks from nonlinear spectra. The need to have carefully mounted large permanent magnets is an additional drawback. Nevertheless, this approach has proven highly practical in many applications. Useful information can be gathered for m/z ratios up to a thousand dalton/electron charge unit.

Single-focus mass spectrometry, as the above is frequently called, is limited in resolution, however, because all the ions do not have the identical initial velocity or trajectory. The randomness of the velocity with which the ions enter the accelerating electric field causes a spectrum of energy levels in the ion beam as it enters the analyzer and a broadening of the mass peak. If one wishes to accurately determine atomic masses or separate two peaks with the same mass number (CH_2 from N, for example), then this energy distribution of ions is unsatisfactory. To eliminate it, an electrostatic separator is used (Fig. 23-4). As the ion beam leaves the ionization chamber, it passes curved plates that create an electric field. Only those ions with the ideal velocity will travel the arc of the circle and pass through the slit into the magnetic focusing area. The rest of the ions, which cannot be focused

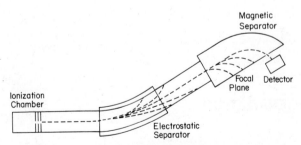

Figure 23-4 A dual-focus spectrometer uses both electrostatic and magnetic fields to separate the ionic masses.

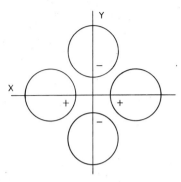

Figure 23-5 A cross-sectional view of a quadrupole analyzer. The ion beam enters this separator along the Z axis.

by the electric field, will collide with the charged plates or miss the slit. The remaining ions will be of highly uniform velocity and will give very sharp peaks. Resolution of 1 part in over 40,000 to 150,000 is instrumentally possible. Because many of the ions are rejected by the separation, the ion currents measured at the detectors are relatively small. This approach is called double-focus mass spectrometry and was developed by Mattauch and Herzog.

One can perform separation of ions without a magnet by use of a four electrode system called a "quadrupole." As shown in Figure 23-5, this device has the opposite electrodes of the same polarity. A high frequency ac (radio frequency) voltage, in addition to their dc voltage, is applied to the electrode pairs. This causes ions travelling in the z direction (which is down the center of the rod structure) to oscillate around that axis. Only those of a specific m/z ratio will make it through without impacting an electrode or the chamber walls. The mass spectrum can be scanned by varying the ac frequency. By appropriate design, quadrupole spectrometers can be made relatively compact.

There are also other means of separation available. The cycloidal-focus mass spectrometer uses crossed electric and magnetic fields to generate a cycloidal, rather than circular, path. A radio-frequency spectrometer uses a pulsating electric field to sort out the masses. The omegatron accelerates the ions in a spiral in a crossed radio frequency

electric field and a magnetic field. The time-of-flight spectrometer has no active separation element, but relies on the length of time it takes for particles of the same energy but different mass to cover a fixed distance. Each of these methods has specific uses and is the preferred method under certain conditions and within certain price constraints.

Section 23-4
METHODS OF DETECTION

The ion current that reaches the detector is of the order of 10^{-15}–10^{-10} A. At one time the whole spectrum was measured simultaneously, at least on the single-focus instruments, by use of photographic plates. These have been replaced by devices that monitor one mass number at a time. One such device is the Faraday cage (cylinder). It collects charge, as a capacitor, which is then amplified by an electrometer tube. Another popular method is the electron multiplier tube. The basic multiplier principle is similar to that of the photomultiplier, but more care must be taken in accepting incoming particles because of the varying amounts of energy they possess.

For recording the results, the use of recording galvanometers with multiple pens or light beams was popular for some years. Each recording channel was 3 to 10 times more sensitive than the previous one so that peaks of varying magnitude could be seen on the same recording. With the advent of digital data reduction methods, most instruments now use digital printouts and normalized spectral displays to present the data to the operator.

Section 23-5
METHODS FOR DETERMINING EMPIRICAL FORMULAE

In the common kind of low-resolution mass spectrometry the purpose is to identify the compound. The key to this identification is finding the "parent peak," since this gives us the mass of the compound. At low voltages of the electron beam in the ionization chamber, this peak, which is just the singly ionized molecule, will predominate. It is not, however, the only peak even if no molecular degradation occurred. Let us assume the compound is pure atomic carbon. The peak at mass-to-charge ratio 12 would be large, but a definite peak 1.12% as tall would be at m/z ratio 13. This peak cannot be eliminated by instrumental means because it represents the portion of carbon that naturally occurs as carbon-13. This peak at the principal mass plus one ($M + 1$) is, in fact, extremely useful because it gives us a clue as to the composition of the peak at M. If we have a peak with N carbons, the next mass number will have a peak of 1.12% N times the height of the first due solely to the natural abundance of heavier carbon-13. This is known as the "isotope effect."

Carbon is not the only element to have a natural isotope distribution. Hydrogen, nitrogen, oxygen, sulfur, chlorine, and bromine are other commonly occurring elements that have such heavier isotopes. The situation is made more complex by the fact that not only are peaks at $M + 1$ significant, but those at $M + 2$ may also be significant. For example, oxygen, sulfur, chlorine, and bromine all have their principal heavy isotope at two mass units above their most common isotopes. Moreover, if more than one atom is present, the usual case, then it is possible that each will be present as a heavier isotope, and the result must be calculated from the binomial expansion.

$$y = (a + b)^N \qquad \text{(23-10)}$$

In this equation y is the total amount under the peaks, while a is the relative size of the peak of the light isotope, b is the relative size of the peak of the heavier isotope, and N is the number of atoms of a given element. For two carbons we would have

$$y = (1.0000 + 0.0112)^2$$

$$y = 1.0000 + 2(0.0112) + (0.0112)^2$$

The value 1.0000 represents the peak at 24 (100%). The next value is the relative size of the peak at 25 ($2 \times 0.0112 \times 100\% = 2.24\%$), and the last value is the relative size of the peak at 26 [$(0.0112)^2 \times 100\% = 0.012\%$].

When more elements are present, the amount that will fall at each mass location must be calculated from more complex formulae. The relative

Table 23-1   The Relative Size of Secondary Peaks due to the Isotope Effect of One Atom

	$M + 1$	$M + 2$
H	0.015%	—
C	1.12%	—
N	0.37%	—
O	0.037%	0.20%
S	0.80%	4.44%
Cl	—	32.4%
Br	—	97.9%

abundances of the isotopes for common elements are given in Table 23-1.

EXAMPLE 23-1

What would be the mass spectrum for a bromine molecule, assuming the parent peak is 50.0 units tall and no splitting of the molecule occurs?

Solution: We must use the binomial expansion with $N = 2$. The parent peak for Br_2 is caused when two isotopes of mass 79 are present. This is mass 2×79 or 158.

$$P_{158} = 50.0$$

The $M + 2$ peak will be twice the Br_{81} percentage (since two bromine are present) times the abundance of the parent peak.

$$P_{160} = 2 \times 0.979 \times 50 = 97.9$$

The $M + 4$ peak will be the square of the Br_{81} percentage, since it will only occur when both atoms are Br_{81}, times the abundance of the parent peak.

$$P_{162} = (0.979)^2 \times 50 = 47.9$$

These are the only peaks present. ∎

To use the values in Table 23-1 to calculate the values of peaks at $M + 1$, $M + 2$, etc., one must add together the contributions of each species. For a compound of the form $C_w H_x N_y O_z$, the % ratio of the $M + 1$ peak to the parent peak is

$$\% \frac{P_{M+1}}{P_M} = 1.12w + 0.015x + 0.37y + 0.037z$$

(23-11)

It should be clear that the hydrogen and oxygen contribution will be insignificant in small molecules, but will be discernible in larger molecules with more of these atoms present. For the $M + 2$ peak,

$$\% \frac{P_{M+2}}{P_M} = 0.006w(w - 1) + 0.004wy$$

$$+ 0.002wz + 0.20z \quad \textbf{(23-12)}$$

The hydrogen contribution is insignificant, the carbon is significant only at large numbers, but the oxygen will be readily discernible. The $M + 2$ peak becomes prominent only if sulfur, chlorine, or bromine are present. The above formula is a simplification of a complex expansion formula, and its derivation need not concern the reader.

EXAMPLE 23-2

A compound $C_wH_xN_yO_z$ has a parent peak of 100 (exactly, by definition) at 62 and peaks of 2.50 at 63 and 0.42 at 64. What is the empirical formula for the compound?

Solution: First let us determine the maximum number of carbons present.

$$\max w = \frac{62}{12} = 5$$

If this were the case, we would have C_5H_2 and the peak at $P + 1$ would be

$$\% \frac{P_{M+1}}{P_M} = 5 \times 1.12 + 2 \times 2 \times 0.015 = 5.66\%$$

This number is much bigger than 2.5, so C_5H_2 is not our compound. Since carbon is the greatest contributor to $M + 1$, one can get an estimate of the carbon content by dividing $\%P_{M+1}/P_M$ by 1.12% (the relative abundance of ^{13}C). This gives 2, a reasonable guess, and it leaves us with 38 ($62 - 24$) mass units to account for. If we subtract the contribution of two carbons from P_{M+1} and P_{M+2}, we have $P_{M+1} = 0.26$ and $P_{M+2} = 0.41$. Since everything in the compound contributes a little to P_{M+1}, very little more can be learned from it. The only thing contributing significantly to P_{M+2}, on the other hand, is oxygen. If we divide $\%P_{M+2}/P_M$ by 0.20% (the relative abundance of ^{18}O), this also gives 2. If the compound has 2 carbon and 2 oxygen, it must have 6 hydrogen to make up the rest of the mass ($24 + 32 + 6 = 62$) and the formula is $C_2H_6O_2$. Obviously, this means that there is no nitrogen present and $y = 0$. The most reasonable structure is ethylene glycol (HO—CH_2—CH_2—OH). ∎

The method of identification is relatively straightforward. Estimate the number of carbons from the size of the $M + 1$ peak and the molecular weight. Estimate the presence of oxygen and heavier elements from the size of the $M + 2$ peak. Make up the mass difference with hydrogen and nitrogen.

Because other debris may end up at the $M + 2$ peak, determination of the number of oxygens versus nitrogens as NH_2 can sometimes be difficult. Nature fortunately gives a hint by what is called the nitrogen rule. Except for nitrogen, all common isotopes have either even mass and even valence (C, O, S, Si) or odd mass and odd valence (H, F, P, Cl, As, Br). As a result, if a stable compound has an odd mass, it must have an odd number of nitrogens; if it has an even mass, it must have an even number of nitrogens. This rule is applicable to any parent peak.

EXAMPLE 23-3

What is the empirical formula of a compound $C_wH_xN_yO_z$ with a parent peak of 100 at 59 and peaks of 2.75 at 60 and 0.25 at 61?

Solution:

$$\text{Estimated carbon} = \frac{2.75}{1.12} = 2$$

$$\text{Remaining weight} = 59 - 24 = 35$$

$$\text{Odd weight} = \text{odd nitrogen, only 1 possible}$$

$$\text{Remaining weight} = 35 - 14 = 21$$

$$\text{Estimated oxygen} = \frac{0.25}{0.20} = 1$$

Remaining weight = 21 − 16 = 5 hydrogen

The formula is C_2H_5NO. ∎

Section 23-6
STRUCTURAL DETERMINATION

Finding the empirical formula, however, is seldom enough. It has been possible to do this for years by degrading the compound chemically to get the ratio of the coefficients and then finding the molecular weight by freezing point depression. While the mass spectrometer can determine such information more quickly, its real contribution is in the area of structural identification. Compounds with the same formula can have vastly different chemical properties. Ethanol (C_2H_6O) and dimethyl ether (C_2H_6O) have considerably different effects on the human body. Structural determination is therefore essential.

One chemical relationship that aids in identification is called, for short, the ring rule. This rule tells how many degrees of unsaturation exist in a molecule. A ring or a double bond will contribute one degree, while a triple bond will contribute two degrees. The relationship starts with 1 and subtracts $\frac{1}{2}$ for each monovalent atom. It adds $\frac{1}{2}$ for each trivalent atom, 1 for each tetravalent atom, $\frac{3}{2}$ for each pentavalent atom, and 2 for each hexavalent atom. Divalent atoms cause no change in the saturation status. For the simple compound $C_wH_xN_yO_z$, the rule is

$$R = 1 + w + \frac{y - x}{2} \qquad \text{(23-13)}$$

Table 23-2 shows how other atoms fit the formula.

Table 23-2 The Effect of Atoms in the Ring Rule

Factor	Atom (oxidation state)
$-\frac{1}{2}$	H, F, Cl, Br
0	O, S (−2)
$+\frac{1}{2}$	N, P, As (−3)
$+1$	C, Si
$+\frac{3}{2}$	N, P, As (+5)
$+2$	S (+6)

EXAMPLE 23-4

Find the number of degrees of unsaturation in the molecule in Example 23-3. Suggest possible structures.

Solution: Formula C_2H_5NO:

$$R = 1 + 2 + \frac{1 - 5}{2} = 1$$

Numerous structures are possible. Here are six:

1. $CH_3 - \overset{\overset{\displaystyle O}{\|}}{C} - NH_2$ 4. $CH_3 - CH_2 - N = O$

2. $H\overset{\overset{\displaystyle O}{\|}}{C} - CH_2 - NH_2$ 5. $CH_3 - O - CH = NH$

3. $\overset{\displaystyle O}{H_2C - CH} - NH_2$ 6. $\overset{\overset{\displaystyle OH}{|}}{CH_2 = CH - NH_2}$

∎

To fragment the molecule in the ionization chamber, excess energy must be imparted to the molecule. This energy will cause bonds to stretch and then rupture. Since there are many bonds in even a moderate-sized molecule, it is necessary to determine which ones will be most likely to break. This has been studied extensively, and certain definite statements can be made. The following rules, while not exhaustive, can be helpful in interpreting splitting patterns.

1. Aromatic rings are very stable. Splitting will occur preferentially beyond the first side chain (α) carbon.
2. Conjugated bonds are relatively stable, and splitting will tend to occur between the first and second carbon outside the conjugated system.
3. Alicyclics are more stable than unbranched chains, which are more stable than branched chains. Tertiary carbonium ions are most easily formed.
4. Small molecules and radicals make the best leaving groups. The charge tends to remain behind on the larger fraction of the molecule.
5. Aliphatic chains will tend to come apart at each

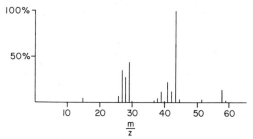

Figure 23-6 A mass spectrum of the unknown discussed in Example 23-5.

bond, leaving a whole family of peaks 14 units apart on the mass spectrum.

If the rules are applied, simple compounds can be easily identified. More complex molecules may still present problems because they disassemble into large fragments, which are of unknown structure. If such is the case, chemical means may be necessary to separate molecules into suitable pieces for examination by mass spectrometry.

In the next few pages we will examine some mass spectra and identify the molecules. This will give you a feel for this type of analysis, which is very much like detective work. To make spectra more comparable, they are normalized. The largest peak is set to exactly 100, and the rest of the peaks are given in proportion to this peak. Sometimes this is the parent peak. If it is not, it is called the base peak. Finding the parent peak is essential to identification. There may not always be a parent peak, however. In such cases, if a molecular weight is not also given, it may be impossible to determine the original structure. At times the parent ion will be determined by a separate low voltage run and be

given as separate information along the $P + 1$ and $P + 2$ peaks.

EXAMPLE 23-5

Find the compound whose spectrum is given in Figure 23-6 and Table 23-3.

Solution: The parent peak appears to be at 58. The peak at 59 is 4.5% as large and the one at 60 is insignificant. This eliminates most of the heavy elements and makes 4 carbons probable.

Remainder: $58 - 4 \times 12 = 10$ hydrogen

Possible formula: C_4H_{10}

This is the alkane butane. To confirm this formula we look at 43, which would indicate one methyl group lost, and find it is large, in fact, the base peak. Peaks at 41 and 42 support the concept of a lost methyl group and one or two more hydrogens. The peak at 15 also supports a lost methyl group. The size of the peak at 44 supports the isotope effect of three carbons in the ion at 43. Since the mass peaks congregate around four m/z ratios, the presence of four carbon-sized atoms (C, N, O, and F) is strongly suggested. Oxygen is eliminated by the lack of peaks at key $M + 2$ positions (45 and 60), and fluorine is eliminated because the mass gaps are too small. Since the molecular weight is even, if any nitrogen were present, there must be two present. This, however, would not account for key $M + 1$ peaks (44 and 59). Butane is clearly the compound, but which isomer is it—*n*-butane or methylpropane? While the easy loss of a methyl group might seem to indicate the latter, the strong peak at 29 indicates an ethyl group (C_2H_5) intact.

Table 23-3 Data for Example 23-5

m/z	Relative %	m/z	Relative %	m/z	Relative %
15	5.3	37	1.0	44	3.3
16	0.1	38	1.8	45	0.05
26	6.1	39	12	51	2.4
27	37	40	1.6	58	12
28	32	41	27	59	0.54
29	44	42	12	60	0.01
30	1.0	43	100		

Table 23-4 Data for Example 23-6

m/z	Relative %	m/z	Relative %	m/z	Relative %
14	8.3	31	1.4	48	0.2
15	51	32	.5	60	4.0
16	5.6	43	3.1	61	53
27	7.0	44	4.7	62	0.9
28	6.3	45	6.2	63	0.2
29	8.0	46	35		
30	100	47	0.2		

This is only possible in *n*-butane, so this is our compound. ∎

EXAMPLE 23-6

Find the compound whose spectrum is given in Table 23-4.

Solution: The parent peak is at 61. It is a good idea to divide the molecular mass by 15, a mass characteristic of the carbon class elements, to get an idea of how many of these atoms might be present. This number is chosen because fragments common to the class (CH_3, CH_2, CH, C, NH_2, NH, N, O, OH) have an average mass of about 15. If heavier elements are present, this will not work until the heavier elements are subtracted from the mass. In this case,

$$\text{Atoms} = \frac{61}{15} = 4$$

By the nitrogen rule we know that one or three of them must be nitrogen. If we look at peak 62, we see that it is less than 2% of peak 61. Since some of this is caused by ^{15}N, it is likely only one carbon is present. If we look 15 units down the mass scale at 46, we find another large peak. The peak at 47 is less than 0.5% of peak 46, so no carbon is in it. Taken together, these facts suggest that a methyl group can easily be lost. So far we have identified CH_3 and N. If we subtract these,

$$\text{Remainder} = 61 - 15 - 14 = 32$$

The most likely candidates are one sulfur or two oxygens. Sulfur is ruled out because the peak at 63 is too small and because there is no way to explain the peak at 30. The existence of a measurable peak at $P + 2$, however, does tend to rule out three nitrogens. The $M + 2$ peaks at 48 and 63 are consistent with two oxygens, and the $M + 2$ peak at 32 with at least one oxygen. Therefore, CH_3NO_2 is consistent with the spectrum. The structure of nitromethane is further confirmed by the lack of a major peak at 31, which would arise if a CH_3O were present. ∎

EXAMPLE 23-7

Find the compound whose spectrum is given in Table 23-5.

Solution: The parent peak appears to be at 178. Dividing by 15 tells us there are roughly 12 carbon class atoms possible. The peak at 179 indicates that they could all be carbon, but the peak at 180 suggests that some may be oxygen. The lack of a really large peak at 180 rules out chlorine and bromine. An even number of nitrogens is present. A large peak occurs at 77, which is indicative of a phenyl group (C_6H_5) because of the great stability of the benzene ring. The $M + 1$ peak at 78 is consistent with this assignment. The base peak at 105 suggests a very stable ion. Since $105 + 77 > 178$, this ion must include the benzene ring. The mass of the side chain is $105 - 77 = 28$. From the $M + 1$ peak 106 we see that we are limited to seven carbons. This leaves a remainder of 16 ($105 - 77 - 12$), which is undoubtedly made by oxygen since it is both consistent with the peak at 107 and with the valence of carbon. A ketone group adjacent to a benzene ring is stabilized by inclusion in the ring resonance,

while a $-\overset{|}{\underset{|}{C}}-NH_2$ group would not be (NH_2 is the only other combination that yields 16).

Table 23-5   Data for Example 23-7

m/z	Relative %	m/z	Relative %	m/z	Relative %
27	3.5	76	2.0	123	68
28	2.5	77	37	124	5.0
29	5.0	78	3.0	125	0.5
41	6	79	5.0	135	1.3
42	0.3	105	100	136	0.5
43	0.9	106	8	178	2.0
55	2.7	107	0.5	179	.25
56	19	121	0.3	180	.02
57	1.5	122	17		

We now have $\phi-\overset{\overset{\text{O}}{\|}}{\text{C}}-$ as a structure. The remaining mass is $178 - 105 = 73$.

The larger peaks at 122 and 123 deserve attention, but are not easy to interpret. The peak at 123 can contain only seven carbons because of the size of the $M + 1$ peak at 124. The mass difference (17 and 18 from the peak at 105) can therefore only be made up by a nitrogen or an oxygen. However, neither oxygen and two protons nor nitrogen and three protons are easy to add to the previous structure in a logical way. Therefore, we will drop this approach for awhile.

If we subtract 123 from 178, we get 55 as the remaining mass. No significant peak exists here, but there is one present at 56, which means that there must be some sort of proton exchange when the two pieces separate. The lack of an $M + 2$ peak at 58 rules out oxygen and most of the heavier elements. The peak at 41 is 15 units from 56 and indicates a methyl group. Fragments in the area of 27–29 suggest the presence of an ethyl (C_2H_5) or vinyl ($CH_2=CH$) group, perhaps both. The fact that the ion readily fragments into 1, 2, and 3 member carbon units indicates the n-butane structure that was seen before. Mass 56 is consistent with C_4H_8, which is butane. This determination and the nitrogen rule force us to assign oxygen as the mystery atom since we cannot have only one nitrogen. We can now compute the final formula based on the carbon-class atoms present. Six carbons from the ring, one from the ketone, and four from the butane chain gives 11 carbons for a mass of 132. There were two oxygens for a mass of 32. This plus 132 gives 164 mass units, or 14 left over for hydrogen in

the final structure. Five of these are on the benzene ring, so the other nine must be on the side chain. This means its formula is really C_4H_9, and it must have suffered some rearrangement before splitting. The structure, therefore, is

$$C_6H_5\overset{\overset{\text{O}}{\|}}{\text{C}}-O-C_4H_9 \text{ (n-butyl benzoate)} \quad \blacksquare$$

While it is hard to give precise rules for spectral interpretation, some things are always worth looking for. These include the following:

1. Finding the parent peak, if present, and estimating the number of carbon-class atoms possible and the number that could be carbon.
2. Identifying the tell-tale patterns of chloride and bromide.
3. Finding evidence of aromatic or substituted aromatic rings.
4. Looking for the loss of methyl groups and other carbon chain units.
5. Using the nitrogen rule.
6. Being aware of the number of atoms possible due to isotope effect in each major peak.
7. Using the ring rule to give clues to common structures.
8. Not forcing unusual structures upon the data, as some rearrangement may occur on ionization.
9. Confirming your analysis against the spectrum of the pure compound if possible.

A few complicating factors should be mentioned. Occasionally an ion will become doubly charged. This is most likely to happen in a molecule which has two separate areas that can withstand electron loss. The m/z ratio is cut in half for such ions since the charge has doubled, and they will fall on the mass spectrum at half their actual mass, since it is the ratio, not the mass, that affects separation. Second, all ions do not disassemble instantly. Some do not undergo disintegration until in the flight tube. This means that the initial velocity imparted to them is not proportional to their final m/z ratio. This causes such ion fragments to end up at unusual places in the spectrum and frequently to have a significant peak width because they do not all disassemble at one time. These are called metastable peaks. Third, the possibility of molecular rearrangement exists in ions with excess energy. We have already seen this happen in the last example. These rearrangements are difficult to predict and create peaks that are hard to explain. Occasionally they put the person trying to interpret the spectrum completely on the wrong track. Finally, impurities either in the sample or the spectrometer may add spurious peaks to complicate interpretation. The presence of multiple compounds makes spectra difficult and challenging.

One hardly expects the average medical technologist to be an expert at mass spectra interpretation. Those who work in toxicology laboratories have the aid of computer calculations and library matching to reduce the number of possibilities. Nevertheless, the final decision on what is reasonable must rest with the technologist.

REVIEW QUESTIONS

1. Why are gas chromatography and mass spectrometry complementary?
2. Why is gas chromatography frequently ineffective at compound identification?
3. What happens when an energetic electron strikes a compound?
4. What is a leaving group?
5. What types of substances are common leaving groups? Give some examples.
6. Why are the ionized fragments accelerated in an electric field?
7. What is the parent peak?
8. How are mass spectral identifications confirmed?
9. What are several sources for the gaseous molecules needed for mass spectrometry?
10. How and why does the specimen enter the ionization chamber?
11. How are some carrier gases removed prior to sample insertion?
12. What is the pressure in the ionization chamber? In the flight tube?
13. What fraction of the specimen is actually ionized?
14. What potential is needed to create a molecular ion? To fragment a molecular ion?
15. Sketch and label the components of the ionization chamber.
16. Describe the operation of the accelerator plates.
17. What is the relationship between the molecular mass and speed? Why?
18. Why is low pressure so difficult to maintain?
19. What effect does the magnetic field have on the ion beam? Why?
20. Why does a magnetic field cause different mass-to-charge ratios to separate?
21. How does one "scan" the mass spectrum?
22. Why is the mass spectrum nonlinear?
23. What are the disadvantages of single-focus mass spectrometry?
24. What is the function of the electrostatic separator in dual-focus mass spectrometry?
25. What is the resolution of the various forms of mass spectrometry?
26. Explain how a quadrupole mass spectrometer works.
27. What is the magnitude of the ion current?
28. Describe several detectors for mass spectrometry.
29. What is the physical evidence of the isotope effect in a mass spectrum?
30. What is the binomial expansion? Write out the expansion for $a = 1.0000$, $b = 0.11$, and $N = 4$.
31. Which elements give significant $M + 1$ peaks?
32. Which elements give significant $M + 2$ peaks?
33. What is the nitrogen rule? Why does it occur?
34. What is the general form of the ring rule?
35. What does the ring rule tell us?
36. Give the relative order of stability of carbon structures.
37. Where does a side chain tend to cleave from an aromatic ring?

38. What is the base peak?

39. How is the spectrum normalized?

40. What are the rules for configuration identification?

41. How does one estimate the number of carbon-class atoms present?

42. What effect do doubly charged ions have on the spectrum?

43. What causes metastable peaks?

44. What is the effect of multiple compounds in the mass spectrometer at the same time?

PROBLEMS

Identify the following compounds based on their simplified mass spectra.

1. m/z	%	2. m/z	%	3. m/z	%
12	1.5	12	3	12	1
13	2.5	13	4	13	1.5
14	3	14	4	14	3
15	2	16	1	15	4
24	2	28	29	16	2
25	6	29	100	24	1
26	50	30	89	25	3
27	54	31	1.5	26	23
28	100	32	.2	27	34
29	2.5			28	100
				29	20
				30	26
				31	.6

4. m/z	%	5. m/z	%	6. m/z	%
12	2	14	6	14	13
13	1.5	15	31	15	1.5
14	8	16	2	16	4
15	1	26	4	28	10
24	1	27	7	29	2
25	2	28	1	30	33
26	3	29	3	31	2
27	1.5	39	3	44	100
28	3	40	2	45	.5
38	6	42	6	46	.5
39	13	43	100		
40	48	44	2.5		
41	100	45	.2		
42	3	57	1		
		58	34		
		59	1.2		
		60	.1		

7. m/z	%	8. m/z	%	9. m/z	%
15	6	14	8	37	6
27	25	15	23	38	8
28	2	16	23	39	9
29	10	26	5	45	7
30	1	27	5	49	3
39	15	28	13	50	30
40	2	29	3.5	51	46
41	31	38	3	52	5
42	87	39	2	74	9
43	100	40	7	75	4
44	4	41	4	76	5
55	5	42	7	77	64
71	16	43	100	78	6
72	1	44	2.5	94	4
86	3	45	.5	105	100
		54	34	106	8
		55	1	107	.3
		56	.1	121	1
		69	32	122	77
		70	1.5	123	6
		71	.1	124	.4

10. m/z	%	11. m/z	%
26	1	19	6
27	1	25	2
37	3	31	4
38	3	50	12
39	2	69	100
50	11	70	1
51	3	88	1
55	6		
73	9		
74	11		
75	22		
76	1.5		
84	3		
85	3		
110	39		
111	3		
112	13		
113	1		
146	100		
147	8		
148	65		
149	6		
150	11		
151	1		

	m/z	%		m/z	%		m/z	%		m/z	%
12.	16	14	**13.**	18	13	**14.**	25	1	**15.**	26	3
	17	71		26	21		26	1		27	49
	42	6		27	62		37	1		28	3
	43	26		28	100		38	2		29	1
	44	72		29	85		39	9		33	4
	45	1.5		30	16		50	11		34	2
	46	.2		31	4		51	13		35	12
	60	100		39	3		52	15		38	4
	61	2		41	4		74	3		39	26
	62	.3		42	5		75	1		40	4
				43	8		76	3		41	5
				44	6		77	18		42	13
				45	55		78	100		43	100
				46	5		79	7		44	3
				47	3					45	9
				55	16					47	4
				56	16					58	5
				57	30					59	2
				73	48					60	2
				74	79					61	37
				75	3					62	1.5
				76	.4					63	2
										76	70
										77	3
										78	4

APPENDIX A
GENERAL MATHEMATICS AIDS

The ability to perform algebra and trigonometry is essential to the understanding of scientific principles. This appendix reviews commonly applied techniques.

Quadratic Formula

With a linear equation $ax + b = 0$, we can quickly find x by dividing minus b by a ($x = -b/a$). This is a first-order or first-degree equation. Less common, but nevertheless sometimes encountered, is the quadratic equation $ax^2 + bx + c = 0$. Many years ago a means of solving this general equation was derived and is given by the formula

$$x = \frac{-b \pm \sqrt{b^2 - 4ac}}{2a}$$

There is nothing magical about this equation, but it is extremely useful. It is derived in the following way:

$$ax^2 + bx + c = 0$$

Multiply by a:

$$a^2x^2 + abx + ac = 0$$

Subtract ac:

$$a^2x^2 + abx = -ac$$

Add $b^2/4$:

$$a^2x^2 + abx + \frac{b^2}{4} = \frac{b^2}{4} - ac$$

The left side has been made a square and can be factored.

$$\left(\frac{ax + b}{2}\right)^2 = \frac{b^2}{4} - ac$$

Place both components of the right side over the same denominator:

$$\left(\frac{ax + b}{2}\right)^2 = \frac{b^2 - 4ac}{4}$$

Take the square root:

$$\frac{ax + b}{2} = \frac{\pm\sqrt{b^2 - 4ac}}{2}$$

Subtract $b/2$:

$$ax = \frac{-b \pm\sqrt{b^2 - 4ac}}{2}$$

Divide by a:

$$x = \frac{-b \pm\sqrt{b^2 - 4ac}}{2a}$$

To use this equation, x can be any unknown quantity. For example, in the equation $7.3 \log^2 x - 14.2 \log x - 3.1 = 0$, the term "$\log x$" can be replaced by z to give $7.3z^2 - 14.2z - 3.1 = 0$. When z is found, it can then be set equal to $\log x$ and the final value for x computed. In reality, what we have is

$$z = \log x$$

$$= \frac{+14.2 \pm\sqrt{(14.2)^2 + 4 \times 7.3 \times 3.1}}{2 \times 7.3}$$

Simultaneous Equations

Simultaneous equations are sets of equations that are true at the same time. These sets of equations come in three types: independent, dependent, and inconsistent. Independent equations are equations that can all be true independently of each other.

For example,

$$5x + 3y = 11$$

$$4x - y = 2$$

These equations represent two lines in a plane that intersect at $x = 1$, $y = 2$.

Dependent equations are combinations of each other. For example,

$$x + 2y + 3z = 12$$

$$2x + y - z = 8$$

$$3x + 3y + 2z = 20$$

The third equation is just the sum of the previous two and therefore dependent on them. It contributes no new information.

Inconsistent equations are equations that cannot be true at the same time. For example,

$$2x + 3y = 11$$

$$2x + 3y = 13$$

These equations form parallel lines in a plane and therefore cannot both be satisfied at once. To solve a set of simultaneous equations in order to find n unknowns, we must have n independent equations. Several methods to effect the solution are available, but one of the easiest is the elimination of variables one at a time. The method works as illustrated for the following equations:

$$5x + 4y - 2z + w = 11 \qquad (1)$$

$$2x - y + 3z - 2w = 1 \qquad (2)$$

$$-x + y + z + 3w = 16 \qquad (3)$$

$$3x + 2y - z - w = 0 \qquad (4)$$

We first pick a variable to eliminate (such as x) and pick an equation that is easy to work with (such as Eq. 3). We then multiply the equation by a factor such that when the chosen equation is added to another equation, the chosen variable disappears. If we multiply Eq. 3 by 5 and add it to Eq. 1, we get

$$9y + 3z + 16w = 91 \qquad (5)$$

If we multiply Eq. 3 by 2 and add it to Eq. 2, we get

$$y + 5z + 4w = 33 \qquad (6)$$

If we multiply Eq. 3 by 3 and add it to Eq. 4, we get

$$5y + 2z + 8w = 48 \qquad (7)$$

We must now choose a new variable (such as y) and a new equation (such as Eq. 6) to reduce this set of equations from 3 to 2 variables. By multiplying Eq. 6 by -9 and adding it to Eq. 5, and by 5 and adding it to Eq. 7, we get

$$-42z - 20w = -206 \qquad (8)$$

$$-23z - 12w = -117 \qquad (9)$$

If we now multiply Eq. 8 by 6 and Eq. 9 by -10 and add them, we get

$$-22z = -66$$

From this it is clear that $z = 3$. We can now back substitute into any equation because all of them are true.

From Eq. 9,

$$-12w = -117 + 23z = -117 + 23 \times 3 = -48$$

$$w = 4$$

From Eq. 5,

$$y + 33 - 5z - 4w = 33 - 5 \times 3 - 4 \times 4$$

$$y = 2$$

From Eq. 3,

$$x = -16 + y + z + 3w = -16 + 2 + 3 + 3 \times 4$$

$$x = 1$$

This completes the solution.

Successive Approximation

Equations with transcendental functions, such as $y = x \log x$, are common. If the value of x is known, it is simple to determine y. If, on the other hand, y is known, x cannot be solved for directly. No closed-form solution for x as a function of y exists.

To determine x, we must resort to successive approximation. No one method of successive approximation will work for all cases, so no set of operational rules can guarantee finding an answer. Nevertheless, the approaches discussed below will probably work in all problems encountered in the clinical laboratory.

METHOD 1

First rearrange the equation to isolate an x on the left side.

$$x = \frac{y}{\log x}$$

Substitute for the knowns (assume y is 5 in this case).

$$x = \frac{5}{\log x}$$

Next make an educated guess of the value of x (guess $x = 3$ in this case) and substitute it into the right side of the equation.

$$x = \frac{5}{\log 3}$$

Calculate x.

$$x = 10.480$$

Now assume this is the new approximation (guess) of x and substitute it into right side of the equation and calculate a third approximation of x.

$$x = \frac{5}{\log 10.480} = 4.900$$

Since 4.900 is closer to 10.480 than was 3.000, it looks like our approximations are getting closer (converging). In fact, the next few iterations of the process give

$$x = \frac{5}{\log 4.900} = 7.244$$

$$x = \frac{5}{\log 7.244} = 5.814$$

$$x = \frac{5}{\log 5.814} = 6.540$$

If the process is repeated 17 times, the value 6.271 will be the value of x to 3 decimal places, and it will not change upon further repetitions. Therefore, $x = 6.271$, as can be seen by substituting into the initial equation.

If we try to apply the same process to the equation $y = x^3$, we will not have much luck. Method 1 gives the following results for $y = 27$.

$$x = \frac{y}{x^2}$$

$$x = \frac{27}{x^2}$$

Guess $x = 2$ and do repeated calculations for x.

$$x = \frac{27}{2^2} = 6.75$$

$$x = \frac{27}{6.75^2} = 0.5926$$

$$x = \frac{27}{0.5926^2} = 76.89$$

Instead of converging, our estimates of x are getting farther apart. Further iterations will not produce a useful result.

METHOD 2

After isolating x on the left side, add Nx to each side and divide the equation by $N + 1$.

$$x = \frac{y}{x^2}$$

$$x + Nx = \frac{Nx + y}{x^2}$$

$$(N + 1)x = \frac{Nx + y}{x^2}$$

$$x = \frac{Nx + y/x^2}{N + 1}$$

Select a value for N and estimate x as in Method 1 (for this case, let $N = 1$ and $x = 2$ as before) and calculate x.

$$x = \frac{1 \cdot x + 27/x^2}{1 + 1}$$

$$x = \frac{x + 27/x^2}{2}$$

$$x = \frac{2 + 27/2^2}{2} = 4.375$$

Repeat the process with N remaining unchanged, but substituting the new x on the right side of the equation.

$$x = \frac{2 + 27/(4.375)^2}{2} = 2.893$$

$$x = \frac{2 + 27/(2.893)^2}{2} = 3.056$$

$$x = \frac{2 + 27/(3.056)^2}{2} = 2.970$$

Six more iterations are necessary to reduce the error to <0.001 and give a close approximation of 3. If we had chosen $N = 2$, only 2 iterations of the method would have been necessary for adequate conversion. If N were greater than 2, however, convergence would have been slower again. Choosing the appropriate N and making a good initial guess take some practice, but any values that cause conversion will get the job done. A good choice for N is frequently the largest power of x in the denominator of the right side of the equation if such a power term exists. N need not even be an integer, but it must be positive.

It should be noted that Method 1 is really a special case of Method 2 with $N = 0$. Method 1 nevertheless should not be disdained, for it is both simpler to use and is far superior to Method 2 in those instances where the convergent series of numbers are approaching the answer from only one side (all values less than the convergent value, for example). Problems involving inverse trigonometric functions frequently fall into this category.

Significant Figures

When working with numbers, it is essential that we have an estimate of the precision with which the numbers are known. For precise theoretical work, there are numerous statistical methods available to estimate very accurately the uncertainty in the numbers being manipulated. These methods are too laborious for common usage.

In most analyses in the clinical laboratory, not enough information is available to apply precise statistical methods, yet it is imperative that we have some measure of our precision before reporting a result. We communicate our estimate of our precision by the number of significant figures we report. The number of significant figures, however, is only an approximation of our measuring precision. A far better estimate is what is called the sig-

nificance. The significance is the ratio of the amount of error to the amount of signal. If we know a result is the number 243 ± 3, then the measurement is good to (significant to) 3 parts in 243. Usually this is reduced to the lowest terms and called 1 part in 81. Significance is our gauge in selecting the number of significant figures.

A few examples will show what happens when arithmetic operations are performed on measured values. Let us start by multiplying 20 ± 1 times 20 ± 1. The product is 400, but what are the error limits? At worst both numbers could be either 19 or 21. These would yield 361 and 441, respectively. Therefore the result of the multiplication is 400 ± 40. The original significance was 1 part in 20 for each of the numbers, yet the significance for the answer is 1 part in 10. Therefore the product may be less precisely known than the original terms. Division can have a similar effect. Fortunately, the probability of both errors being maximum is very small, and the actual statistical decrease in significance is considerably less than the maximum possible. *Nevertheless, the result should never be regarded as having more significance than the least significant of the operands from which it was obtained.* We will use this as our basic rule for multiplying and dividing in this book.

Addition yields a closely related situation. For example, if we add 3285 ± 1 to 9 ± 1, we get 3294 ± 2. Our significance has dropped from 1 part in 3285 to 1 part in 1647. Here again, the chances of the errors being maximum are small. We will use the rule that the significance of the sum cannot exceed *the significance of the most significant addend.* If the sum is used in further computation, the final result should be referenced back to this original most-significant addend.

Subtraction poses even sterner constraints. If we subtract 9862 ± 1 from 9879 ± 1, we get 17 ± 2. From a significance of one part in nearly 10,000, we have a significance of less than 1 part in 10 after the subtraction. Subtracting two large and nearly equal numbers devastates significance. Therefore, *after subtraction the significance can be no greater than the average error of the operands over their difference.* Further computation must reference this difference to determine the limits of significance.

If we could always do our computation using significance reduced to its lowest terms, it would be relatively easy to keep a good estimate of the true significance. Unfortunately, we are constrained by our number system, base ten, to deal with numbers in terms of a specific number of decimal places. These are what we call the significant figures of a number. We must therefore formulate rules to use significant figures to estimate the significance to which we know the number. The following rules should be used:

1. Assume that the significance of each number, except exact numbers, is to 1 part in the mantissa of the number (e.g., 12.3 is known to 1 part in 123).
2. Never round a number during computation so that the significance is less than the original number, which limits the significance by the rules given previously.
3. Identify the number that governs the final significance by the rules previously given.
4. If that number is x, round the result y so that in significance

$$2.5x \geq y \geq \frac{x}{4}$$

Let us look at a few examples. If we start with 18.7 and get for a result 397.2, we could report 397.2, 397, or $4.0 \cdot 10^2$. Our comparison values are $18.7 \times 2.5 = 47.8$ and $18.7/4 = 4.7$. This yields

$$3972 > 478 > 397 > 47 > 40$$

Note well that the position of the decimal point is ignored when calculating the number of significant figures. Clearly 397 is the number that fits between the limits, and therefore 397 has the correct number of significant figures.

Let us assume that we started with 47 and now have 129.5. We could report $1.3 \cdot 10^2$, $1.30 \cdot 10^2$, or 129.5. Our references in this case are 118 (47×2.5) and 12 (47/4). This yields

$$1295 > 130 > 118 > 13 > 12$$

The correct answer here is 1.3×10^2. Note that one limit is always 10 times the other, which is necessitated to cover all cases in base 10. In case of a close decision, it is better to err on the side of keeping an extra digit.

Rules Governing Transcendental Functions

EXPONENTS

$$x^a \pm x^b = x^a(1 \pm x^{b-a})$$

$$x^a x^b = x^{a+b}$$

$$\frac{x^a}{x^b} = x^{a-b}$$

$$x^a \cdot y^a = (xy)^a$$

$$\frac{x^a}{y^a} = \left(\frac{x}{y}\right)^a$$

$x^a \pm y^a$ cannot be simplified

$$x^a y^b = (xy)^a y^{b-a}$$

$$x^{a^b} = x^{ab}$$

LOGARITHMS

$\log (x \pm y)$ cannot be simplified

$$\log xy = \log x + \log y$$

$$\log \frac{x}{y} = \log x - \log y$$

$$\log x^a = a \log x$$

If $y = x^a$, then $a = \log_x y$

TRIGONOMETRIC FUNCTIONS

$$\text{sine (sin) } \theta = \frac{\text{opposite side}}{\text{hypotenuse}}$$

$$\text{cosine (cos) } \theta = \frac{\text{adjacent side}}{\text{hypotenuse}}$$

$$\text{tangent (tan) } \theta = \frac{\text{opposite side}}{\text{adjacent side}}$$

$$\text{cotangent (cot) } \theta = \frac{\text{adjacent side}}{\text{opposite side}}$$

$$\text{secant (sec) } \theta = \frac{\text{hypotenuse}}{\text{adjacent side}}$$

$$\text{cosecant (csc) } \theta = \frac{\text{hypotenuse}}{\text{opposite side}}$$

$$\sin \theta \csc \theta = 1$$

$$\cos \theta \sec \theta = 1$$

$$\tan \theta \cot \theta = 1$$

$$\tan \theta = \frac{\sin \theta}{\cos \theta}$$

$$\sin^2 \theta + \cos^2 \theta = 1$$

$$\sin (\theta + \phi) = \sin \theta \cos \phi + \sin \phi \cos \theta$$

$$\cos (\theta + \phi) = \cos \theta \cos \phi - \sin \theta \sin \phi$$

$$\sin \tfrac{1}{2}\theta = \pm \sqrt{\frac{1 - \cos \theta}{2}}$$

$$\cos \tfrac{1}{2}\theta = \pm \sqrt{\frac{1 + \cos \theta}{2}}$$

$$\sin (-\theta) = -\sin \theta$$

$$\cos (-\theta) = \cos \theta$$

APPENDIX B
SYMBOLS

Symbol	Meaning	Units or Value
A	atomic mass number	integer
A	absorbance	unitless
A	ampere	1 coulomb/second
A	amplification	unitless
A	amplifier gain	unitless
A	area	in meters^2
A	eddy constant	in meters
$\mathring{A}$	Angstron	10^{-10} meters
ADC	analog-to-digital convertor	
a	activity	in moles/liter
a	molar absorptivity	in reciprocal meter moles
a_o	Bohr radius	in Angstroms
a_H	Bohr radius of hydrogen	0.5292 $\mathring{A}$
a_i	general coefficient	
ac	alternating current	
amu	atomic mass unit	$1.6598 \cdot 10^{-24}$ grams
B	longitudinal diffusion coefficient	in meters^2/second
B	magnetic flux intensity	in gauss
BJT	bipolar junction transistor	
b	base of transistor	
b	cell length	in meters
C	capacitance	in farads
C	concentration	in moles/liter
C	coulomb	$6.24 \cdot 10^{18}$ electron charges
C	equilibrium coefficient	in seconds

Symbol	Meaning	Units or Value
C	flip-flop clear	
°C	degrees Celsius	
CRT	cathode ray tube	
c	collector of transistor	
c	speed of light	$2.998 \cdot 10^8$ meters/second
cm	centimeter	10^{-2} meters
D	data input of flip-flop	
D	image distance from eye	in meters
DAC	digital-to-analog convertor	
d	a change in	
d	distance	in meters
d	drain of FET	
d	electronic subshell	third
d	resolving distance	in meters
d	thickness	
dc	direct current	
d_f	depth of field	in meters
E	Electromotive force potential	in volts
E	energy	in ergs or joules
E	optimum viewing distance of eye	in meters
$\bar{E}$	average voltage	in volts
E^o	standard potential	in volts
E_-	voltage of inverting input	in volts
E_+	voltage of noninverting input	in volts
$\%E$	percent error	
$E\%$	relative error	%

407

Symbol	Meaning	Units or Value	Symbol	Meaning	Units or Value
E_B	potential over battery	in volts	h	height	in meters
			h	Planck's constant	$6.6262 \cdot 10^{-27}$ erg seconds
E_k	kinetic energy	in ergs or joules			
E_o	output voltage	in volts	$\hbar$	energy quantum	$h/2\pi$ $(1.0546 \cdot 10^{-27}$ erg seconds)
E_p	peak voltage	in volts			
E_p	primary voltage	in volts			
E_{p-p}	peak-to-peak voltage	in volts	I	current	in amperes
			I	ionic strength	in moles/liter
E_{rms}	root-mean-square voltage	in volts	I	light intensity	
			I	moment of inertia	
E_s	secondary voltage	in volts	I_f	feedback current	in amperes
E_T	potential over tube or transistor	in volts	IR	infrared	
e	charge of an electron	$4.8029 \cdot 10^{-10}$ esu	J	joule	1 newton meter (1 kg m^2/sec^2)
e	electron		j	quantum number	rotational
e	emitter		j	quantum number	spin-orbital coupling
e	natural constant	2.71828			
erg	erg	10^{-7} joules (1 g cm^2/sec^2)	K	dielectric constant	unitless
			K	electronic shell	$n = 1$
esu	electrostatic unit	$3.336 \cdot 10^{-10}$ coulomb	K	equilibrium constant	
eV	electron-volt	$1.6021 \cdot 10^{-12}$ erg	K	partition coefficient	unitless
F	farad	1 coulomb/volt	K	1024	in bytes or words
F	faraday	96,522 coulombs	°K	degrees Kelvin	
FET	field effect transistor		k	kilo	10^3 times
f	electronic subshell	fourth	k	Boltzmann constant	$1.3804 \cdot 10^{-23}$ J/°K
f	focal length	in meters			
f	frequency	in hertz	k	indefinite constant	
f_e	focal length of eyepiece	in meters	L	electronic shell	$n = 2$
			L	inductance	in henries
f_o	focal length of objective	in meters	L	length of microscope or column	in meters
G	giga	10^9 times	LED	light emitting diode	
g	electronic subshell	fifth			
g	gate of transistor		l	quantum number	angular momentum
g	gram				
g	force of gravity	9.8 meters/second^2	ln	natural logarithm (base e)	$2.303 \cdot \log$
g_i	statistical factor	unitless			
			log	logarithm to base 10	
H	henry	1 joule/ampere			
HETP	height equivalent to a theoretical plate	in meters	M	electronic shell	$n = 3$
			M	magnification factor	unitless
Hz	hertz	1 cycle/second			

Symbol	Meaning	Units or Value
M	mega	10^6 times
M	metal atom	in reaction
M	molar	1 mole/liter
M_e	magnification of eyepiece	unitless
M_o	magnification of objective	unitless
m	mass	in kilograms or grams
m	mass of electron	$9.1094 \cdot 10^{-28}$ grams
m	meter	
m	milli	10^{-3} times
m	order of refraction	unitless
m	quantum number	angular momentum in z direction
mm	millimeter	10^{-3} meter
m_A	mass of nucleus	
m_e	mass of electron	$9.1094 \cdot 10^{-28}$ grams (0.00055 amu)
m_n	mass of neutron	1.00867 dalton
m_p	mass of proton	1.00728 dalton
N	electronic shell	$n = 4$
N	newton	1 kilogram meter/second^2
N	number present	(frequently atoms)
N.A.	numerical aperature	unitless
N.C.	normally closed	
N.O.	normally open	
n	electron-abundant semiconductor	
n	nano	10^{-9} times
n	neutron	
n	quantum number	principal
nm	nanometer	10^{-9} meter
O	electronic shell	$n = 5$
OA	operational amplifier	
P	partial pressure	in atmospheres
P	power	in watts (joules/second)
P_M	height of peak at mass M	normalized %

Symbol	Meaning	Units or Value
P_{M+1}	height of peak at mass $M + 1$	normalized %
p	electronic subshell	second
p	hole-abundant semiconductor	
p	momentum	in kilogram meters/second
p	object distance	in meters
p	pico	10^{-12} times
p	proton	
pH	$-\log[\text{H}^+]$	unitless
$p_\angle$	angular momentum	in kilogram meters^2/second
p_z	angular momentum	in z direction
Q	flip-flop output	
Q	organic molecule	in reaction
$\bar{Q}$	negation flip-flop output	
q	charge	in coulombs
q	image distance	in meters
R	amount of radiation	
R	gas constant	8.314 J/mole · °K
R	rate (slope)	in units/second
R	resistance	in ohms
R_f	feedback resistor	in ohms
R_g	ground resistor	in ohms
R_i	input resistor	in ohms
r	radius of circle	in meters
r	radius of curvature	in meters
r	ripple factor	unitless
rf	radio frequency	
S	flip-flop set	
SCE	saturated calomel electrode	
SCR	silicon-controlled rectifier	
SHE	standard hydrogen electrode	
S_o	object distance	in meters
S_i	image distance	in meters
s	electronic subshell	first
s	second (unit of time)	
s	quantum number	spin

Symbol	Meaning	Units or Value	Symbol	Meaning	Units or Value
s	source of FET		α	radiation	helium nucleus (4.00249 amu)
sec	second				
T	flip-flop trigger		β	angle of resultant ray	in degrees
T	temperature	in degrees (Kelvin or Celsius)			
T	transmittance	unitless	β	radiation	electron (positron)
t	time	in seconds	γ	radiation	high energy light
t_r	retention time	in seconds	Δ	the difference between	
t_p	peak width	in seconds			
$t_{\frac{1}{2}}$	half-life	in seconds, days, or years	δ	radiation	secondary electrons
$\%t$	time fraction	unitless	ε_o	permittivity of free space	$8.85 \cdot 10^{-12}$ farad/meter
UART	universal asynchronous receiver-transmitter		θ	angle	in degrees
			λ	decay constant	in reciprocal seconds
UV	ultraviolet light	<400 nm	λ	wavelength	in meters
V	volt	1 joule/coulomb	μ	index of refraction	unitless
VOM	Volt-Ohm meter		μ	micro	10^{-6} times
v	quantum number	vibrational	μ	micron	10^{-6} meters
v	velocity	in meters/second	ν	frequency	in reciprocal seconds
W	watt	1 joule/second			
W	work (energy)	in joules	ν	neutrino	
w	general variable		$\bar{\nu}$	antineutrino	
			Π	product notation	
x	horizontal axis		π	natural constant	3.14159
x	general variable		σ	conduction	in mho (reciprocal ohms)
X	reactance	in ohms			
X_C	capacitive reactance	in ohms	ρ	density	in kilograms/meters^3
X_L	inductive reactance	in ohms	Σ	summation notation	
y	vertical axis				
y	general variable		T	torque	
Z	impedance	in ohms	τ	time constant	in seconds
z	3-space axis		Φ	magnetic flux	in webers
z	charge of nucleus	in electron charges	ϕ	angle	in degrees
z	charge of ion	in electron charges	Ω	ohms	1 volt/ampere
z	general variable		∞	infinity	
α	activity coefficient	unitless	$+$	OR	
α	angle of aperature	in degrees	$\cdot$	AND	
α	angle of incident ray	in degrees	$\oplus$	EXCLUSIVE OR	
			$-$	NOT	

APPENDIX C

ANSWERS TO SELECTED PROBLEMS

1-2 $3.6 \cdot 10^6$ J

1-3 2.0 mA

1-5 85 Ω

1-7 25 Ω

1-9 $E_{R_1} = 0.50$ V, $E_{R_2} = 2.5$ V, $E_{R_3} = 1.0$ V

1-11 17.3 mA

1-14 $1.5 \cdot 10^2$ V

1-17 $E_A = 20.0$ V, $E_B = 12.5$ V, $E_C = 10.0$ V, $E_D = 20.0$ V, $E_E = 15.0$ V

1-20 150 Ω

1-21 3.8 mA

1-23 $\%I_1 = 43\%$, $\%I_2 = 35\%$, $\%I_3 = 22\%$

1-25 30 Ω

1-27 67 W

1-29 $I_1 = 0.78$ mA, $I_2 = 0.47$ mA, $I_3 = 0.31$ mA, $I_4 = 0.31$ mA, $I_5 = 0.31$ mA, $I_6 = 0.47$ mA, $I_7 = 0.78$ mA

1-31 $I_1 = 16.6$ mA, $I_2 = 8.7$ mA, $I_3 = 8.7$ mA, $I_4 = 7.9$ mA, $I_5 = 7.9$ mA, $I_6 = 16.6$ mA, $E_G = 0$, $E_A = 21.6$ V, $E_B = 9.3$ V, $E_C = 19.0$ V, $E_D = 7.4$ V, $E_E = 3.0$ V, $E_F = 1.5$ V

1-33 $I_T = 0.77$ A, $I_1 = 0.30$ A, $I_2 = 0.027$ A, $I_3 = 0.33$ A, $I_4 = 0.44$ A, $I_5 = 0.47$ A, $I_6 = 0.47$ A

1-35 (A) $R_A = 70.$ Ω, $R_B = 87$ Ω, $R_C = 100.$ Ω

1-36 (A) $R_{AB} = 99$ kΩ, $R_{AC} = 111$ kΩ, $R_{BC} = 290$ kΩ

1-38 7.1 V

1-40 $I_1 = 17.3$ mA, $I_2 = 44.2$ mA, $I_3 = 26.9$ mA

2-1 1.45 Ω

2-3 710 Ω

2-5 1700 Ω

2-9 41%

2-11 561.8 Ω

4-1 3.98 V

4-4 28 μF

4-6 $C_1 = 12$ μF, $C_2 = 16$ μF, $C_3 = 22$ μF

4-9 6 μF

4-11 $\tau = 0.183$ sec, $E_r = 0.25$ V

4-13 2.78 μF or 11.0 μF

4-15 0.203 Hz

4-19 268 H

4-21 $\Delta Z = 29.0$ kΩ, $\Delta \phi = 26.5°$

4-23 1.64 nF

4-25 22 Hz

5-1 Current will flow through R_L unless both A and B are high (+).

5-3 If A is low (0), nothing happens. If A is high (+) and B is low (0), current will flow through T_3. If A is high (+) and B is high (+), current will flow through R_L, but not through T_3.

5-9 -50 V

5-11 $\Delta E_R = -3.8$ V, $A = 3.8$

6-2 0.15 mA

6-4 9.0 V

6-6 2.54 kΩ

6-9 182 kΩ

6-13 0.251 V

6-16 -0.85 V

6-18 -0.279 V

6-20 69.6 kΩ

6-22 0.067 V

7-2 $E_P = 142$ V, $\bar{E} = 90.$ V, $E_{rms} = 100.$ V

7-4 $I_P = 23.1$ mA, $I_s = 57.3$ mA

7-6 22.8 Hz

7-9 45.6 V

8-6 a. 101001   d. 10101001000

8-7 a. 38   d. 1132

8-8 a. 65   d. 2323

8-9 a. 44   d. 1482

8-10 a. 10111   d. 1011111101

8-11 a. 33   d. 1422

8-12 a. $A + \bar{B}$ d. $A + C$

8-13 Reduce to simplest terms first.

    a. $\overline{A \cdot B \cdot C}$ c. $\bar{B} \cdot \bar{C}$

8-14 Reduced expression: a. $\overline{\overline{A \cdot \overline{A} \cdot C} \cdot \overline{B}}$

8-15 Reduced expression:

    c. $\overline{\overline{A + B} + \overline{\overline{A + C} + \overline{B + C}}}$

8-20 2.01 V

9-1 a. 7642

9-2 a. -1406

9-3 a. 4624

9-4 a. -141

9-5 a. 0563

9-6 a. 3760

9-7 a. $M = 2402,\ E = 12$

9-8 a. 59.78

9-9 b. $42 - 17 - 17 - 20 - 23 - 41 - 42$

9-10 b. THE DOOR IS RED.

9-11 a. $122 - 145 - 155 - 145 - 155 - 142 - 145$
    $- 162 - 040 - 164 - 150 - 145 - 040 - 115$
    $- 141 - 151 - 156 - 145 - 041$

9-12 a. New York City

9-13 a. DF4

9-14 a. 2623

10-1 $q = 15.9$ cm, $S_i = 3.1$ cm, in front of mirror

10-3 19.8 cm

10-5 $q = 25.6$ cm, $S_o = 3.71$ cm, behind the mirror

10-8 10.2 cm convex

10-10 1.71

10-12 4.02 cm

10-15 38.7 cm

10-17 $p = 60.5$ cm, $S_i = 21.9$ cm

10-20 69.1 cm

10-23 $q_2 = 255$ cm, $S_i = 94$ cm, beyond L2

10-25 $p_i = 53.6$ cm, $S_o = 24.0$ cm, left of L1

10-28 $\lambda_2 = 143$ nm

10-30 25.0°

11-2 21.1 cm

11-4 53.5 cm

11-6 6.1%

11-8 209 nm

11-10 1310

12-2 b. $2.52 \cdot 10^{-3}\ M$ e. $0.065\ M$

12-3 b. $\alpha_{\text{Na}} = 0.944,\ \alpha_{\text{SO}_4} = 0.796$
    e. $\alpha_{\text{NO}_3} = 0.746,\ \alpha_{\text{Ba}} = 0.310$

12-4 -1.369 V

12-7 $2.34 \cdot 10^{-2}\ M$

12-9 -0.549 V

12-12 $4.6 \cdot 10^{-2}$ g

13-1 1.602

13-3 31.54°

13-5 1.738

14-1 $4.074 \cdot 10^{-12}$ erg

14-3 $9.780 \cdot 10^{-21}$ g cm/sec

14-5 $n = 1$ $l = 0$ $m = 0$ $s = +\frac{1}{2}$
    $n = 1$ $l = 0$ $m = 0$ $s = -\frac{1}{2}$
    $n = 2$ $l = 0$ $m = 0$ $s = +\frac{1}{2}$
    $n = 2$ $l = 0$ $m = 0$ $s = -\frac{1}{2}$
    $n = 2$ $l = 1$ $m = 0$ $s = +\frac{1}{2}$

14-8 $-5.4 \cdot 10^{-12}$ erg

14-10 30.4 nm

14-12 a. 0.286%

14-13 a. 4096°C

14-14 490 nm

15-5 9.5%

15-6 $5.8 \cdot 10^{-4}\ M$

19-1 3%

19-5 0%

19-8 $a_0 = 7.8,\ a_1 = 14.3$

20-1 a. ^{43}Ca

20-2 a. ^{21}Ne

20-3 a. ^{143}Nd

20-4 a. n

20-7 8.74 MeV

20-10 a. assume ^{20}Ne, 20.0003 amu

20-11 92 years

20-14 84.4 μg

22-1 24

22-3 8.9 mg/l

22-5 1.03 cm

22-7 $6.0 \cdot 10^{2}$ plates

23-2 Formaldehyde (CH_2O)

23-6 $N_2O(N^- = N^+ = O)$

23-9 Benzoic acid (ϕ—C(=O)—O—H)

23-12 Urea ($(NH_2)_2C = O$)

23-15 2-propanethiol ($(CH_3)_2$ CH SH)

GLOSSARY

Absorbance   The optical density of a substance, which is equal to the negative logarithm (base 10) of the transmittance.

Accumulator   A register in a computer used to temporarily hold operands and results during the computation process.

Accuracy   The closeness of the measured value to the actual value.

ADC (analog-to-digital convertor)   A circuit that changes an analog voltage into the appropriate digital representation.

Alphanumeric   A character set that includes alphabetic and numeric symbols and frequently also punctuation and printer control characters.

Alpha radiation   The spontaneous emission of a helium-4 nucleus from a heavier nucleus.

Alternating current   A current that periodically changes direction within the circuit.

ALU (arithmetic logical unit)   The computational portion of a computer.

Amplifier   A circuit that outputs a signal of larger magnitude than the input signal.

Analog   A representation that has a continuum of values.

Anode   A positively charged electrode; the plate of a vacuum tube.

Armature   The rotary part of a motor or generator.

Array   A serial arrangement of data in rows and columns.

ASCII (American Standard Code for Instrument Intercommunication)   A standard way of coding alphanumeric information in binary form.

Background   A random, but relatively constant level of signal indigenous to the local environment and independent of the occurrence being measured.

Bandpass (bandwidth)   The part of the light spectrum able to pass through a monochromator, usually defined as the width of a peak at half its maximum.

Bar code   A method of coding numbers by the position and/or thickness of parallel lines.

Baseline   The level of signal indigenous to an apparatus when none of the sought-for substance is present.

Battery   A chemical device that creates a relatively constant potential difference between external connections and supplies electrons for an external circuit between them.

BCD (binary coded decimal)   A method of representing the digits 0–9 in binary form.

Beta radiation   The spontaneous emission of a positive or negative electron from the nucleus of an atom.

Bias   In electronics, voltage applied to a circuit element to control current flow through that element. Analytically, the difference between two values.

Binary   A system having two parts or stable states; a number system based on two digits.

Bit   A binary digit, one binary position.

Blaze angle   The angle between the cut of the lines of a grating and the face of the grating.

Broadening   A phenomenon causing radiation lines and chromatographic peaks to spread in width and become more difficult to measure.

Bus   In electronics, a wire or group of wires carrying signals common to numerous parts of an instrument.

Byte   A group of bits, frequently equivalent to one alphanumeric character in length.

Calibration curve   A line showing the relationship

between the measurement response and the concentration of a sought-for substance. This relationship, after being identified by standards, is used to determine the concentration of unknowns.

Capacitance A physical property permitting electrical potential difference to be stored as charge on two conductors separated by a nonconductor.

Card reader A device capable of converting the marks and holes in a card into corresponding electrical signals.

Carousel A circular tray that holds specimens and is rotated to present the specimens sequentially to a sampler probe.

Cathode A negatively charged electrode.

Chopper A component that, through periodic motion, changes one or more constant signals into alternating signals for the purpose of comparison.

Chromatography A method of separation using a mobile phase to carry specimen at a uniform rate over a stationary phase, which retards the movement of the various specimen components to different degrees.

Circuit A closed path through which electrons or ions can flow.

Cocktail A mixture of organic solvent, radioactive compound, and fluor used for liquid scintillation counting.

Coincidence Events occurring at effectively the same time and therefore being masked, as to number, from the detector.

Colligative properties Vapor pressure, osmotic pressure, boiling point elevation, and freezing point depression.

Collimate To direct scattering radiation into a beam of parallel rays.

Colorimeter A device for measuring radiation of a particular bandpass (color) passing through a specimen.

Common mode A signal present in all inputs to a circuit element.

Compton effect The phenomenon of a gamma ray ejecting an electron from an atom and simultaneously producing a lower energy gamma ray.

Computer A device capable of producing results from the input of variable data and whose output is based on a changeable set of instructions.

Computer language A group of legal instructions that a computer can convert to an internally executable format.

Conductance The ability of a substance to transmit electrical current.

Continuous flow An analytical technique in which samples are introduced sequentially into a continuously flowing stream of reagents to facilitate the sequential measurement of a given analyte for each sample.

Control A sample of known or expected value that is analyzed repeatedly to monitor the precision and accuracy of a method or instrument.

Coulometry A titration where the titrant is electrochemically generated in the reaction vessel.

CPU (central processing unit) The heart of the computer, which contains the logical control unit (LCU), the arithmetic unit (ALU), and high-speed memory.

Critical angle The incident angle to the normal of an interface at which light is bent along the interface of two media when it approaches that interface in the medium of higher refractive index.

Curie A measure of radioactivity ($3.7 \cdot 10^{10}$ disintegrations per second)

Current The flow of charge (either electrons or ions) through a circuit element, wire, or solution.

DAC (digital-to-analog converter) A circuit that creates an analog voltage proportional to a digital input.

Dark current A background current generated in a photodetector when no light is falling on the detector.

Decimal A number system having 10 digits.

Dialysis The process whereby small molecules move through a semipermeable membrane from a solution of higher concentration to one of lower concentration while larger molecules do not.

Diffraction grating A polished surface with precisely cut parallel lines used to disperse light into its component wavelengths.

Diffusion The movement of ions or molecules from areas of higher to lower concentration.

Digital A numeric representation in which the magnitude of a quantity is represented in discrete steps (i.e., by digits).

Diode A device that allows current passage in one direction but not the other.

Direct current A current that flows in one direction only.

Discrete analyzer An instrument that measures each specimen in a separate container or in some other mechanically separated manner.

Disk A rotating storage medium with concentric magnetic tracks to hold data in computers. A rotating device containing samples and reagents in centrifugal analyzers.

Dispersion The separation of light into its component wavelengths.

Dissociation constant A value that is equal to the product of the product concentrations divided by the product of the reactant concentrations.

Drift Unidirectional fluctuations in the baseline with time.

Electric field A potential difference between points within a localized area.

Electrochemical The descriptive word for processes in which electrons and chemicals react to give other chemicals.

EMF (*electromotive force*) The potential difference that drives current.

Emission spectrum The wavelengths of light (lines or bands) given off when a substance is excited by thermal, electrical, or some other type of energy.

Emitter A heated cathode or a doped semiconductor that acts as the source of electrons or holes in a circuit element.

Encoder An electrical or mechanical device that reorganizes information into a different data representation.

Endpoint method A method of analysis in which the reaction must reach equilibrium before the measurement is made.

Equilibrium The state at which the probability of the reactants interacting to form the products is equal to the probability of the products interacting to form the reactants. No macroscopic reaction is observed.

Excitation The process of raising an electron or nucleus from a stable ground state to a less stable state of greater potential energy.

Excited state A quasistable configuration, position, or orbital that has more energy than the ground state of the excited entity.

Exponential decay A process of deterioration or change in which the rate of change of a substance is governed solely by the amount of material initially present and a decay constant.

Feedback The process in which the output signal of a device is used to modify the input signal to the device to reduce drift.

Filter A device to remove unwanted signal, such as electrical noise or unusable wavelengths.

Fixed-head A disk configuration in which each concentric information track has its own reading head.

Flame A combusting mixture of gases that acts as a plasma or solution for ions and free atoms.

Flip-flop A bistable device that can readily be moved between states and used to store information.

Floating point A mathematical representation in which the decimal (binary) point is always located at the same place in the bit patterns and a separate exponent tells how far to shift the decimal point to retrieve the actual value.

Floppy A type of flexible disk used with laboratory instruments.

Flow cell A cuvette positioned in the light path of an instrument through which all the reaction mixtures are pumped sequentially to be measured.

Fluor A compound that can readily be induced to absorb energy and fluoresce, and which can be used for nuclear decay measurements.

Fluorescence The act of absorbing radiation at one wavelength and subsequently emitting light at a longer wavelength.

Frequency The rate at which repetitions of the same event occur.

Gain The amount of amplification in terms of the ratio of the magnitude of the output to that of the input.

Galvanometer A wire-wrapped core that will rotate a distance proportional to the current flowing through it.

Gamma radiation The spontaneous emission of a high-energy photon from the nucleus of an atom.

Grating A polished surface with precisely cut parallel lines used to disperse light into its component wavelengths.

Ground The electrical lead designated as having zero potential, frequently attached in some manner to the earth.

Ground state The electronic or nuclear state with the lowest potential energy consistent with all equilibrium forces.

Half-life The period of time required for half the initial quantity of material to decay or change by exponential decay or first-order kinetic reaction.

Hard copy Material printed on paper by an instrument.

Hardware The electronics and mechanical components of an instrument.

Head The electromechanical device used to read and write information from a disk or tape.

Heat of fusion The energy needed to break the crystal structure of a solid and permit to to melt.

Heat sink A large piece of metal used to absorb and radiate the heat generated by electrical components.

Impedance The total opposition to the flow of current in an ac circuit.

Index of refraction The ratio of the velocity of light in vacuum to the velocity of light in another substance.

Inductance The electrical potential generated by the change in current flowing through a wire coil.

Induction The generation of a magnetic field around a current-carrying wire or coil.

Infrared The radiation wavelengths above the visible light (800 nm) and below the radio wavelengths.

Input A signal that enters a circuit element or instrument.

Instruction set The group of legal operations that a computer can perform.

Integrated circuit A group of electrical components that performs a complex task and is sealed inside an epoxied envelope.

Interface The physical boundary between two objects or the electrical connection between two instruments.

Intrinsic carriers Current-carrying electrons and holes in semiconductors that exist even when no external electric field is applied.

I/O (*input output*) Some aspect of entering or retrieving information.

Ion current The stream of ionized molecular fragments generated in the ionization chamber of a mass spectrometer.

Ionization The process of removing an electron from an atom or splitting up ionic substances.

Ionization potential The energy necessary to remove an electron from an atom.

Ion-selective electrode An electrode that responds only or primarily to the activity of one ionic species.

Isotope A specific combination of protons and neutrons forming the nucleus of an atom.

Iterative The repetitive application of a specified set of steps or rules.

Junction potential The voltage difference that develops over an interface of two dissimilar materials due to electron migration.

Kinetic energy The energy represented by the motion of atomic particles or bulk objects.

LCU (*logical control unit*) The operational sequencing unit of a computer that decodes instructions and fetches and stores data.

Least squares A technique to find an equation that best represents a set of data.

Line printer A device that prints all the characters on a line virtually simultaneously before advancing the paper.

Logarithmic amplifier A circuit with an element that responds with an output which is proportional to the logarithm of the input signal.

Lyse To destroy the cell membrane and allow the cell contents to mix with the exterior solution.

Machine-readable A property of data representation permitting it to be directly deciphered by computer peripherals without manual interpretation.

Magnetic field A structured area of space created by the flow of current through a wire or coil or by a permanent magnet that will affect magnetizable objects.

Mainframe A main portion of a computer, usually

synonymous with the CPU, generally used to describe large computers and minicomputers, but not microcomputers.

Mantissa The value of a data representation without regard to the position of the decimal point.

Mark-sense The use of pencil marks on a computer card to transmit information to the computer via a card reader.

Memory A group of bistable devices used to store instructions and data needed by the computer as it operates.

Memory effect The loss of sensitivity of a transducer due to its exposure to a previous signal stimulus.

Meter A transducer for converting electrical signals into mechanical motion proportional to the stimulus.

Microprocessor The basic ALU and LCU of a computer with a short word length and very limited instruction set.

Mnemonic A shorthand representation of instructions or data using a few alphanumeric characters.

Mobile phase The moving fluid (liquid or gas) used to propel a sample through a chromatographic analysis.

Molar absorptivity A constant that represents the ability of a substance to absorb light at specific wavelengths.

Monochromatic light Light containing only one wavelength.

Monochromator A filtering or dispersion device that tries to remove all but one wavelength of light, but in reality allows a group of closely related wavelengths to pass (bandpass).

Moving-head A disk configuration in which each concentric information track does not have its own reading head, and the heads must move over numerous tracks to find the correct one.

Nephelometry The measurement of light, usually at 90° to the incident beam, which is reflected or scattered by the particles within a solution.

Node The branch points in an electrical circuit or data tree.

Noise Fluctuation in the input signal that is not caused by the specimen being measured.

Nomogram A plot of data on a complex chart that relates various chemical species or properties, for example, blood gas data.

Normal range A reference interval of numbers containing the measured results of 95% of the people tested who are deemed to be free of disease that would alter the amount of the species being analyzed for.

Nucleon An atomic particle residing in the nucleus of an atom, usually the generic name for protons and neutrons.

Octal A number system having 8 digits.

On-line A state in which data generated by an instrument is automatically transferred to a computer without human intervention.

Optical density The amount of light absorbance of a substance.

Osmotic pressure A colligative property describing the pressure that would have to be placed on a solution to prevent pure solvent from passing through a semipermeable membrane from the other side to further dilute the solution.

Osmolality The number of moles of particles (molecules and ions) in 1000 grams of solution.

Output The signal produced by a circuit element or instrument.

Pair production The splitting of a high-energy gamma ray into a positron–electron pair by the electronic field near a nucleus.

Parameter A variable or an adjustable constant.

Partial pressure The pressure of a component of a gaseous mixture.

Percent transmittance The percentage of incident light passing through a sample.

Periodic Subject to recurrence at regular intervals.

Peripherals Devices attached to a computer to facilitate storage and communication.

Phase A physical state of some material that does not mix with other physical states of the same or different materials (e.g., gas phase, organic phase).

Phase angle The relative position of the voltage maximum to the current maximum in an ac circuit in terms of polar coordinates.

Photodetector An object that produces a current when exposed to electromagnetic radiation.

Photoelectric effect   The process in which high-energy radiation knocks an electron out of orbit and gives it all of the available energy.

Photometer   A device to measure the quantity (intensity) of light.

Photomultiplier tube   A multielectrode tube that causes a large current pulse for every photon that enters it.

Photon   A particle of light of zero rest mass whose movement generates electromagnetic waves.

Polarography   A method in which the cathode is made progressively more negative in a uniform fashion to cause a reduction of reducible species diffusing to the cathode. The rate of diffusion of the reducible species to the cathode limits the observed current for a given concentration.

Positron   A particle with the mass of an electron but with a positive charge.

Potential   The driving force that causes events to occur (e.g., electrical potential causes current to flow, gravitation potential causes things to fall).

Potentiometer   A device used to accurately set or measure the potential in part of a circuit.

Power   Energy expended per unit time.

Power supply   A circuit, usually involving a transformer, rectifier, filter, and regulator, that produces dc voltage of the proper level.

Precision   The reproducibility of repetitive measurements of the same entity.

Printer   A device that, by impact, ink spitting, or hot stylus, places characters on paper.

Prism   A glass or quartz solid with nonparallel sides that causes light to split into its component wavelengths.

Program   A coordinated set of instructions that causes a computer to perform some desired task. These instructions are stored within the computer when in use.

PROM (*programmable read only memory*)   A ROM that can be programmed using special equipment by the PROM user.

Quantum number   An integer describing some facet of orbiting electrons in an atom or molecule.

Radioactivity   The amount of spontaneous emission of particles and energy by an atomic nucleus.

RAM (*random access memory*)   High-speed memory in which all words can be accessed equally rapidly.

Rate method   A method of analysis in which numerous measurements are taken over time and the slope of the measured values versus time is the desired information.

Reactance   The effective resistance to current flow in an ac circuit caused by the presence of capacitance and/or inductance.

Real time   The measurement, recording, and interpretation of events as they occur.

Record   A grouping of information on a storage medium.

Recorder   A device that makes a continuous record of analog information.

Reference electrode   An electrode of a known potential that is not affected by the solution into which it is inserted.

Register   A group of bits within a computer that is treated as a single unit.

Relay   An electrically operated switch that mechanically switches one or more other electrical circuits.

Resistance   The opposition to the flow of current through a substance due to imperfect pathways and inadequate charge carriers.

Resolution   The ability to discern the difference between two closely spaced objects.

Resonance   The periodic vibration of current magnitude and direction in a circuit containing both capacitance and inductance.

Retention time   The length of time that a substance is held within a chromatographic column due to interaction with the stationary phase.

Rheostat   A variable resistor for adjusting current within a circuit.

ROM (*read only memory*)   A RAM that has specific data or instructions permanently set in its registers.

Root-mean-square   The power effective voltage equal to the peak ac voltage divided by the square root of 2.

Salt bridge   A tube with an immobilized salt solution used to create a path for ionic movement between solutions.

Scale factor The factor an instrumental result must be multiplied by to give the actual result in the correct units.

Scintillation The emission of light after a fluor has been excited by radioactive decay.

Self-absorption The reabsorption by a solution of radiation given off by another part of the same solution.

Semiconductor A substance that does not conduct electricity as well as a metal but considerably better than an insulator. Such materials have complex electrical properties.

Sensitivity The number of discernible increments of response that can be reliably determined for the substance of interest or the lower limit of detectability for a measurement.

Servo-driven recorder A recorder that self-corrects its position using feedback to prevent overshooting the true value.

Shunt A pathway to permit most of the current to bypass a circuit element.

Signal The component of the input information that is a result of the substance of interest.

Signal/noise ratio A measurement of the sensitivity of an observation (the ratio of the magnitude of the signal to the magnitude of the noise or background).

Slit A narrow opening in an optical device to control the size of the light beam or bandpass.

Software The computer programming.

Solenoid A relay (valve) that controls the flow of liquid current rather than the flow of electrical current.

Specific gravity The density of a substance relative to the density of water at 4°C.

Spectrophotometer A device that measures the amount of radiation that is absorbed from a slice of the spectrum made by a dispersing element (prism or grating).

Spectrum A plot depicting the variation in the magnitude of the primary component of a system as a function of some other component; for example, light intensity as a function of wavelength, or ion intensity as a function of the mass-to-charge ratio in mass spectrometry.

Stack A data structure in which only the top element is directly accessible by a stack pointer, which keeps track of the top of the stack.

Standard A specimen of known value used to calibrate an instrument before unknowns are measured.

Stationary phase The nonmoving phase in chromatography that interacts with the sample in the mobile phase.

Steady state A state where conditions (e.g., concentrations, temperature), although not necessarily at equilibrium, are so constrained that they can be accurately known relative to the initial conditions.

Stray light Radiation that reaches the detector without having traversed the specimen on the proper path.

String A data structure consisting of sequential characters that can be matched, replaced, or added to similar structures.

Substrate A reactant in an enzyme reaction or the coating material placed on the support to create the stationary phase of a chromatographic column.

Supercooled A liquid cooled below its normal freezing point due to the absence of nucleation sites necessary to seed crystallization.

Support The inert material used to fill the column volume in chromatography and hold the substrate that interacts with the specimen in the mobile phase.

Tailing The shifting of a chromatographic peak to produce a long tail due to uneven retention of specimen by some parts of the column.

Tape A long, narrow storage medium with longitudinal magnetic tracks that must be searched sequentially from the beginning to find information.

Teleprinter A device that, by impact, ink spitting, or hot stylus, places characters sequentially on paper.

Terminal A teleprinter or CRT with an associated keyboard for two-way communication with computers.

Thermal conductivity The temperature-dependence of the conductivity of a metal or semiconductor.

Thermister A device whose resistance is temperature-dependent.

Thermocouple A device producing a junction potential across itself that is a function of its temperature.

Transducer A device that maps the value of an entity in one domain (e.g., physical) into the value of a different entity in another domain (e.g., electrical).

Transformer A device that, through inductance, changes the relationship of ac voltage and current in a secondary winding to that which exists in the primary winding.

Transistor A three-electrode semiconductor device in which the current or potential at one electrode controls the current flow between the other two electrodes.

Transmittance The ratio of the amount (intensity) of light passing through a specimen to the amount of light entering the specimen.

Tree A data structure in which each piece of information (record) can have pointers to several other records.

Triode A vacuum tube that has three electrodes, with the potential of the grid controlling the amount of current flowing between the other two.

Turbidity The measurement of the amount of light transmitted by a cloudy solution.

Ultraviolet The radiation wavelengths below the visible light (<400 nm) but above X-rays.

Vapor pressure The partial pressure of gas above its liquid or solid phase.

Venturi principle The law that fluids moving past the end of a small tube cause a suction on the contents of that tube.

Wavelengths The distance between successive peaks of a light wave.

Word length The number of bits in a word.

Working electrode The electrode whose potential is established by the sought-for species in a solution.

Worksheet A list of specimens and the tests to be performed on them.

Zener breakdown The enormous increase in current that occurs when the potential in the reverse direction over a diode exceeds its ability to resist current flow.

BIBLIOGRAPHY

ABL Customer Training Manual, Radiometer/Copenhagen, Copenhagen, Denmark, 1979.

ACA II Instrument Instruction Manual, DuPont Company, Wilmington, Delaware, 1980.

Ackerman, P. G., *Electronic Instrumentation in the Clinical Laboratory,* Little, Brown, Boston, 1972.

Alpert, N. L., *Clinical Instrument Systems,* **1,** 3, (1980).

Autobac MTS Operator's Manual, Pfizer Inc., New York, 1979.

Bauer, H. H., G. D. Christian, and J. E. O'Reilly, *Instrumental Analysis,* Allyn & Bacon, Boston, 1978.

Benford, J. R., *The Theory of the Microscope,* Bausch & Lomb, Rochester, New York, 1965.

Blaedel, W. J. and V. W. Meloche, *Elementary Quantitative Analysis,* 2nd ed., Harper & Row, New York, 1963.

Bueche, F. *Principles of Physics,* 3rd ed., McGraw-Hill, New York, 1977.

Chloride Chemistry Module Operating and Service Instructions, Beckman Instruments, Brea, California, 1979.

Coulter Counter Model S-Plus Operator's Reference Manual, Coulter Electronics, Hialeah, Florida, 1981.

French, A. P., *Principles of Modern Physics,* Wiley, New York, 1958.

Gall, L. S. and W. A. Curby, *Instrumented Systems for Microbiological Analysis of Body Fluids,* CRC Press, Boca Raton, Florida, 1980.

Garber, C. C. and R. N. Carey, "Automation in the Clinical Chemistry Laboratory—Classification and Examples," in Manka, D. P. (editor), *Automated Stream Analysis for Process Control,* Academic Press, New York, 1982.

Grab, R. L., *Modern Practice of Gas Chromatography,* Wiley, New York, 1977.

Greene, E. S., *Principles of Physics,* Prentice-Hall, Englewood Cliffs, New Jersey, 1962.

Handbook of Chemistry and Physics, 60th ed., CRC Press, Cleveland, Ohio, 1980.

Hayt, W. H. Jr. and J. E. Kemmerly, *Engineering Circuit Analysis,* 3rd ed., McGraw-Hill, New York, 1978.

Hicks, R., J. Schenken, and M. A. Steinrauf, *Laboratory Instrumentation,* 2nd ed., Harper & Row, Hagerstown, Maryland, 1980.

Lee, L. W., *Elementary Principles of Laboratory Instruments,* Mosby, St. Louis, 1978.

Lewin, D., *Theory and Design of Digital Computer Systems,* Wiley, New York, 1972.

Lurch, E. N., *Fundamentals of Electronics,* 3rd ed., Wiley, New York, 1981.

Malmstadt, H. V., C. G. Enke, and S. R. Crouch, *Control of Electrical Quantities in Instrumentation,* Benjamin, Reading, Massachusetts, 1973.

Malmstadt, H. V., C. G. Enke, and S. R. Crouch, *Digital and Analog Data Conversion,* Benjamin, Reading, Massachusetts, 1973.

Malmstadt, H. V., C. G. Enke, and S. R. Crouch, *Electronic Analog Measurements and Transducers,* Benjamin, Reading, Massachusetts, 1973.

Malmstadt, H. V., C. G. Enke, and E. C. Toren, Jr., *Electronics for Scientists,* Benjamin, New York, 1962.

McLafferty, F. W., *Interpretation of Mass Spectra,* Benjamin, New York, 1967.

Microcomputer Processor Handbook, Digital Equipment Corporation, Maynard, Massachusetts, 1979.

Operation and Maintenance Manual for the Bactec 460, Serial MF 1187 and Up, Johnston Laboratories, Cockeysville, Maryland, 1979.

OS Osmometer, Fiske Associates, Uxbridge, Massachusetts, 1975.

Page, L. B. and P. J. Culver, *A Syllabus of Laboratory Examinations in Clinical Diagnosis,* Harvard University Press, Cambridge, 1961.

Pecsok, R. L. and L. D. Shields, *Modern Methods of Chemical Analysis,* Wiley, New York, 1968.

Product Labeling Technicon SMAC System, Technicon Corporation, Tarrytown, New York, 1979.

Programmed Instruction for the Basic AutoAnalyzer, Technicon Corporation, Tarrytown, New York, 1969.

Programmed Instruction for the Technicon SMA 12/60 System, Technicon Corporation, Tarrytown, New York, 1970.

Rotochem IIa Centrifugal Fast Analyzer Operator's Manual, American Instrument Company, Silver Spring, Maryland, 1978.

Shortley, G. and D. Williams, *Elements of Physics,* 5th edition, Prentice-Hall, Englewood Cliffs, New Jersey, 1975.

Skoog, D. A. and D. M. West, *Analytical Chemistry,* 3rd ed., Saunders, Philadelphia, 1979.

Snyder, L. R. and J. J. Kirkland, *Introduction to Modern Liquid Chromatography,* Wiley, New York, 1979.

Strobel, H. A., *Chemical Instrumentation,* Addison-Wesley, Reading, Massachusetts, 1960.

Tietz, N. B. (editor), *Fundamentals of Clinical Chemistry,* Saunders, Philadelphia, 1976.

Toren, E. C., Jr. and A. A. Eggert, *Computers in the Clinical Laboratory,* Dekker, New York, 1978.

Tou, J. T. and R. C. Gonzalez, *Pattern Recognition Principles,* Addison-Wesley, Reading, Massachusetts, 1974.

Triebel, W. A., *Integrated Digital Electronics,* Prentice-Hall, Englewood Cliffs, New Jersey, 1979.

8450 UV/VIS Spectrophotometer Operator's Manual, Hewlett Packard, San Diego, California, 1981.

Williard, H. H., L. L. Merritt, Jr., and J. S. Dean, *Instrumental Methods of Analysis,* 4th ed., Van Nostrand, Princeton, New Jersey, 1965.

INDEX

423